高等学校教材

Fundamentals, Approaches and Breakthroughs in R & D Genetically Engineered Biotherapeutics

基因工程药物研发的原理、途径与突破
（中英文双语版）

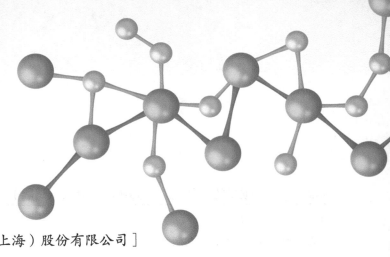

主　编　王春晓

副主编　吴文惠　李晓晖

编　委　（按姓名汉语拼音排序）

郭锐华（上海海洋大学）

金　亮（中国药科大学）

李晓晖（上海海洋大学）

李新宇［益方生物科技（上海）股份有限公司］

吕正兵（浙江理工大学）

钦传光（西北工业大学）

王春晓（上海海洋大学）

王　峰（暨南大学）

吴文惠（上海海洋大学）

U0332252

北京大学医学出版社

JIYIN GONGCHENG YAOWU YANFA DE YUANLI、TUJING YU TUPO（ZHONGYINGWEN SHUANG YU BAN）

图书在版编目（CIP）数据

基因工程药物研发的原理、途径与突破：汉、英 / 王春晓主编 . — 北京：北京大学医学出版社，2023.8

ISBN 978-7-5659-2859-8

Ⅰ . ①基… Ⅱ . ①王… Ⅲ . ①基因工程 - 药物学 - 高等学校 - 教材 - 汉、英 Ⅳ . ①R977 ②Q78

中国国家版本馆 CIP 数据核字（2023）第 034784 号

基因工程药物研发的原理、途径与突破（中英文双语版）

主　　编：王春晓

出版发行：北京大学医学出版社

地　　址：（100191）北京市海淀区学院路 38 号　北京大学医学部院内

电　　话：发行部 010-82802230；图书邮购 010-82802495

网　　址：http://www.pumpress.com.cn

E－mail：booksale@bjmu.edu.cn

印　　刷：北京信彩瑞禾印刷厂

经　　销：新华书店

责任编辑：法振鹏　　责任校对：靳新强　　责任印制：李　啸

开　　本：850 mm×1168 mm　1/16　印张：33　字数：952 千字

版　　次：2023 年 8 月第 1 版　2023 年 8 月第 1 次印刷

书　　号：ISBN 978-7-5659-2859-8

定　　价：138.00 元

云深逐序

文 / 王春晓

砺翅寒暑兮草稿枕，字痕香发兮黑白换。

银丝闪耀兮极思泽，灵犀汇集兮后辈传。

灵均问天兮孰斡旋，而今天问兮访星船。

基因组序兮有时尽，生命探索兮无穷绵。

基因突变兮致疾患，生物工程兮调核酸。

基因功能兮深发掘，蛋白从新兮待殊观。

基因重组兮巧制药，止民疾患兮生命灿。

* 云深，取自"寻隐者不遇：松下问童子，言师采药去。只在此山中，云深不知处。"

Fundamentals, Approaches and Breakthroughs in R & D Genetically Engineered Biotherapeutics《基因工程药物研发的原理、途径与突破（中英文双语版）》是经过精心梳理和编写而成的英汉双语教材。本书主要介绍了基因工程药物的发展沿革及进展趋势、基因工程技术的原理以及基因工程药物的制备过程，重点阐述了基因工程和下游技术应用于药物开发和制备过程中的关键技术。在阐述上述原理、技术方法的同时，还插入纵观生物药物开发历史上的妙招、灵巧构思，使读者们不仅能一览生物药物研发如何从种子长成幼苗，再发育成枝繁叶茂的大树，还能逐步靠近这棵树，一点点看清主干、侧枝；优选了某些小细枝、开或未开的花朵、熟或未熟的果实，甚至对来到树上欢唱的小鸟，做了一系列的特写、细观。使读者不仅对生物制药的大致过程有一定的了解，还可以了解、欣赏、学习前人的成就与思路，启迪他们未来在生命科学领域的科研之路。

本书以英文为书写语言，对个别单词、术语辅以中文注释。此举是为了方便读者阅读，特别适合作为本科生或研究生开设本课程的双语课教材，可以使他们在学习专业课的同时，提高专业英语水平；也可以作为本科生或研究生开设本课程的全英文课的教材，供师生使用（中国学生或外国留学生皆可）；也可以作为相应专业的专业英语教材，选取部分章节使用。另外，对于一些对专业英语有提升要求的人群，或对生物药物的研发有兴趣的人群，仔细研读本书也一定开卷有益。

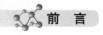

　　由于时间、精力及各种其他限制，我们搜集到的资料可能并不全面。另外，科学技术永远在向前推进。科学家及工程师们彼时的最佳路线极可能会被更新，被更好的办法所更替。笔者在细致又细致、更新再更新的资料搜集、整理中，难免还会有一些瑕疵或遗漏。因此，本教材中的不足之处，希望得到大家的谅解！同时，非常欢迎读者们为本书提出宝贵意见。

　　感谢上海海洋大学王永杰教授与编者关于病毒的讨论；感谢百奥泰集团梅晓丹博士组织的2021生物医药产业大会以及会议茶歇与三优生物的谭永聪博士关于噬菌体展示制备全人源抗体的讨论；感谢药渡网韩雪松给予相关数据支持；感谢许广文老师朋友圈分享公众号"知识分子"文章"两只小鼠的江湖"以及该文章作者"金淘沙拣"；感谢《中国药物化学杂志》和《沈阳药科大学学报》原执行主编兼编辑部主任王玉珠教授生前对本教材编写的指导；感谢全国各地图书馆文献传递部门工作人员为我们提供了近千篇相关文献，同时特别感谢所有这些论文、书籍的作者（因篇幅所限，不能列出所有参考文献）；感谢金银哲博士、武万强博士参与个别专业词汇的探讨；感谢研究生祝宝华及留学生 Md Moktadirul Alam 在本教材编写过程中给予的帮助；感谢编者团队成员的携手共进、彼此照耀；感谢暨南大学国际学院和药学院同行专家以及北京大学医学出版社的认可，在此一并致谢。

编　　者

Contents

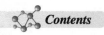

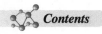

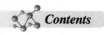 *Contents*

Chapter 1
Overview and Prospects of Biopharmaceutics

Modern biotechnology

The rapid development of modern biotechnology has been successfully promoting scientific progress and economic development, changing people's way of life and way of thinking as well as the development of human society. The fruits of modern biotechnology are being applied more broadly in medicine, food, energy, chemicals, light industry and environmental protection and other areas. Biotechnology is the core of the revolution in the 21st century, with huge economic benefits and potential productivity. In the past decade, biotechnology industry has gradually become one of the pillar industries in the world economic system as predicted. Bio-technology is a comprehensive science and technology, which utilizes living organisms to create new species in biological systems, and to process and produce biological products on the basis of life sciences and engineering principles. Broadly speaking, modern biotechnology includes **genetic engineering, protein engineering, cell engineering, enzyme engineering,** and **fermentation engineering.** The most vigorous of the core technology is **genetic engineering.**

Genetically engineered pharmaceuticals（基因工程药物）refer to those therapeutics developed and produced using genetic engineering techniques, which mainly include:

1. Recombinant peptide and protein drugs（重组蛋白多肽药物）

2. Antisense therapeutics（反义核酸药物）

3. DNA drugs（DNA 药物）

4. Genetically engineered antibodies（基因工程抗体）

New peptide and protein drugs（新型多肽及蛋白质类药物）

Peptide and protein drugs comprise among others proteins isolated from human sources. With the advent of biotechnology, peptides and protein drugs have generated much medico-pharmaceutical interest. Peptides and proteins made by biotechnology include **monoclonal antibodies, recombinant human hormones, cytokines** and **growth factors.** In the field of **vaccine,** development and innovation are taking place as well.

There have been two leading developments in the field of peptide and protein drugs: hybridoma technology for the preparation of drugs and vaccines, as well as receptors. Hybridoma technology provided the opportunity to produce highly specific monoclonal antigen binding proteins with potentialities for site-specific delivery to organs. The objectives for applying recombinant DNA-technology may be various: to produce existing products in purer form and more efficiently and cheaply (*e.g.,* insulin), or to produce proteins in commercially interesting amounts that would be otherwise very scarce (*e.g.,* interferons, plasminogen activators, blood clotting factor Ⅷ). Another option is to produce viral protein subunit vaccines as (safer) substitutes for viral vaccines and, particularly, to produce vaccines against viruses that cannot be cultured (*e.g.*, hepatitis B). Recombinant DNA technology has created possibilities to produce receptors as well as protein structures, which are extremely useful for pharmacological investigations and also possibly in pharmacotherapy as drugs because of their ability to bind pathogens.

It should be realized, however, that peptide and protein drugs have already constituted part of the pharmacotherapeutics regimen (养生法) for many years [example: insulin, plasma protein fractions (蛋白分段), polymyxins (多黏菌素)]. Moreover, a number of drugs exist, some of them already for a long period, with strong structural resemblance to peptides (*e.g.*, angiotensin-converting enzyme (ACE) inhibitors) and endorphins (内啡肽).

Up to 1996, more than 143 biotechnology drugs and vaccines were under way or awaiting approval. The number is greatly increased these days, 10 times greater up to 2021, while peptide and protein drugs composed the most prominent (重要的) biotechnology drugs. On the other hand, it is not to be expected that all protein drugs will be prepared by biotechnology in the near future. A number of peptides [*e.g.*, the gonadotrophin (GnRH) analogues] is synthesized by chemical synthesis. The biotechnological and chemical synthesis of these products has addressed the issue of scarcity for a number of these drugs (*e.g.*, growth hormone), although they still remain expensive. Meanwhile a substantial number of protein drugs are still isolated from human material despite the advances in biotechnology. The underlying conditions are either a lack of knowledge, or the complexity and/or cost to synthesize these drugs biotechnologically.

Optimal application schemes of these drugs may not have been reached and (clinical) pharmacists should contribute to the optimization. Since recombinant technology has abolished scarcity for a number of these drugs — especially 'physiological' substances — special ethical problems regarding an unlimited application or expansion of the indications may arise.

Peptides and proteins made by biotechnology
Monoclonal antibodies

Through the development of the hybridoma technology by Köhler and Milstein it became possible to produce identical, monospecific antibodies in almost unlimited quantities. These monoclonal antibodies are, in contrast to polyclonal antisera, directed against a single antigentic determinant and are constructed by the fusion of B-lymphocytes, stimulated with a specific antigen, with immortal myeloma (骨髓瘤) cells. The resultant hybridomas can be maintained in culture and are capable of producing large amounts of antibodies. From these hybrid cells, a specific cell line or clone producing monospecific immunoglobulins can be selected.

In clinical trials, antigenic modulation (调控) on tumor cell surface and anti-murine antibody responses are frequently reported as complicating factors. The success of antibody therapy is dependent on a). the binding capacity *i.e.*, specificity and affinity and b). the accessibility of the antibody to the target antigen. Many monoclonal antibodies directed against tumor are not entirely 'tumor-specific' but cross react with normal tissue. Clinical applications created for unconjugated monoclonal antibodies are rather diverse, *e.g.*, antithrombotic agents, immunosuppressive agents used in organ transplantation, agents used to modulate TNF-α, and agents used to reduce mortality rates in Gram-negative sepsis (败血症).

Several monoclonal antibodies coupled with radionuclides (放射性核素) have been found in routine clinical application in diagnostic nuclear medicine, whereas radioimmunotherapy and immunotherapy with targeted cytotoxins are mainly confined to clinical trials. One of the first monoclonal antibodies approved in Europe was Myoscint, an antimyosin （抗肌球蛋白抗体） used for the assessment of myocardial infarction. Diagnostic imaging with monoclonal antibodies appears to have certain advantages in the staging and early detection of recurrences of colorectal and ovarian cancers. On the other hand, many studies have failed to demonstrate radioimmunoscintigraphy （放射免疫闪烁扫描术） to be superior to other diagnostic modalities.

Experience over the past decades has helped scientists to understand the advantages and limitations of monoclonal antibodies, which has led to a variety of 'designer' antibodies, such as chimeric and humanized antibodies, immunoadhesins （免疫黏附素）, single-chain antigen binding proteins and hypervariable region peptide molecules (molecular recognition units) thus optimizing specificity and affinity, increasing target accessibility, and decreasing immunogenicity.

Recombinant human hormones
Somatropin (recombinant human growth hormone)

Recombinant human growth hormone has been a registered drug since about 1986. Roughly, its action may be characterized as affecting the metabolism of protein, carbohydrate and fat. The formally registered indications （适应证） for the use in children are limited, but in practice an increasing number of applications is proposed, making a good case for eventually administering growth hormone to every child of short stature. The growth response of a child, however, depends on a number of factors, like pretreatment growth velocity, the dose of growth hormone used, the frequency of administration and the condition during the treatment. To date, no hard predictive parameters are known. Generally, administering growth hormone to children other than those with growth hormone insufficiency rarely results in a consistent increase in growth velocity over the years and may even shorten the growth period.

Cytokines and growth factors

The cytokines comprise a rather diverse class of signal polypeptides which represent a major communication network in living organisms. They act as autocrine, paracrine and endocrine hormones and are involved in the regulation of a variety of physiological and pathological conditions, such as normal and malignant cell growth, recognition and elimination of pathogens by immune cells and inflammation.

Growth factors produced by recombinant DNA technology are now being used clinically and include GM-CSF, G-CSF, interleukin-3, M-CSF, SCF (stem cell factor) and epoetin （重组人肾红细胞生成素）.

Vaccine

The classic concept of a vaccine derives from the field of viral vaccines. Two types of "classical" viral vaccines may be distinguished: either virulent （致命的） virus particles that have been inactivated or live particles of virus strains that have been alternated or weakened. These vaccines are supposed to no longer cause disease but still be able to immunize against virulent strains. Accidents may occur, however, especially when one or more virus particles have escaped inactivation. Moreover, contamination deriving from the animal cells where the vaccine has been grown may elicit adverse reactions in some recipients. Since the surface proteins of the virus particles are the major antigens that induce immunity, it was realized that it should be possible to use these surface proteins instead of the virus particles. A novel approach to immunization is presented by **DNA vaccines**. DNA vaccines provide protective immunity through expression of a foreign protein within the host. Host cells appear to take up the DNA after direct DNA inoculation, express the encoded antigen, and present it to the cells of the immune system. Thus, the immunogen is synthesized within the host by cells which have taken up the antigen-encoding DNA. The *in vivo* protein synthesis allows the processing, modification and presentation of the antigen to the host's immune system in a manner that would be similar to that which would occur during a natural infection.

For viral vaccines, individuals are immunized against viral agents before encountering the pathogenic virus. Such a strategy is feasible with viruses because viral genomes are relatively simple, with a limited number of defined antigens. This does not apply to tumor vaccines as most tumor cells are weakly antigenic. Immunodeficient and immunosuppressed patients develop more tumors of certain tissues. In contrast to viruses, for most tumors the potential universe of antigens can be virtually unlimited. Therefore, in the case of tumor vaccines, the most common clinical setting is one in which induction of a systemic immune response by the vaccine must occur subsequent to, rather than before, the antigenic result. The (experimental) use of cancer vaccines is still at its infancy. In up to 90% of cases of carcinoma of the uterine cervix the human papilloma-virus (HPV) is found in the tumor. Recent developments in molecular virology and immunology have allowed the detection of HPV peptides that can be used to elicit an immune response. In an animal model system a vaccination protocol utilizing HPV peptides has been developed which effectively prevents the outgrowth of HPV-16-induced tumors. Based on these findings, clinical trials in humans have been conducted investigating the feasibility of an ultimate goal — the development of antigen specific vaccines for cancer chemotherapy. And from 2016 to 2019, 2-valent, 4-valent and 9-valent HPV vaccines have been marketed successively in China.

Antisense technology and antisense therapeutics （反义 RNA 与反义药物）

Antisense oligonucleotide (ASO) is a short (12~24 nucleotide) oligonucleotide that can base-pair with complementary RNA and trigger different post-hybridization mechanisms to modulate gene expression. It can be either single-stranded or double-stranded. Small interfering RNAs (siRNA，小干扰RNA) is a short (~21 base pairs) RNA duplex that can trigger the degradation of RNAs containing homologous sequences through endonucleolytic cleavage by Argonaute (AGO) proteins.

Antisense RNA plays an important role in inhibiting the expression of deleterious genes and overexpression of uncontrollable gene, or upregulating the production of desirable mRNA and the encoded proteins. Antisense RNA may be introduced into a cell to inhibit translation of a complementary mRNA by base pairing to it and physically obstructing the translation machinery, or alter splicing (*e.g.*, promote exon skipping). In the case the target region for base pairing is within an ORF, this effect is therefore stoichiometric （化学计量的）. Antisense RNA has long been thought of as a promising technique for disease therapy.

How antisense works compared with conventional drugs

The approximately 20 000~25 000 genes in our human genome can be transcribed into about 85 000 different mRNA, each used in the cell as a template to synthesize a different protein. Conventional pharmaceutical drugs (small chemicals), peptides, or proteins (for example, hormones), and antibodies (which are very large proteins) typically bind to the target protein directly to treat a disease.

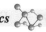

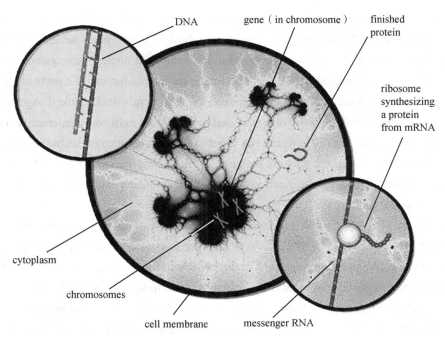

Fig. 1-1   Genes, proteins and the drug discovery process.

Antisense drugs are designed to bind to the mRNA of a target protein, or other kinds of RNA required for the translation of proteins, pre-mRNA splicing, pre-rRNA processing, RNA modification, mRNA stability, inhibiting or promoting the protein production process and participating in various biological processes (Fig. 1-1, Fig. 1-2). The completion of the sequencing and initial analysis of the human genome through the HGP provides a resource for the design of antisense drugs without requiring the complex and time-consuming analysis of the structure of the target protein which is required for conventional (small molecule) drugs.

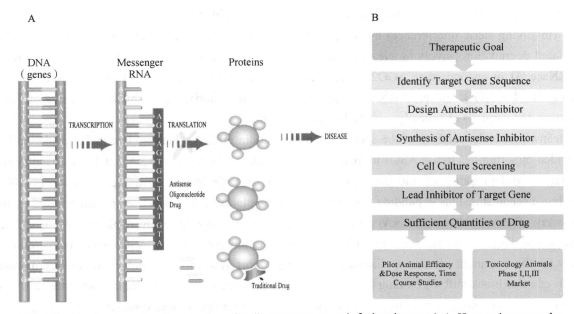

Fig. 1-2   Mechanism of antisense drug, its discovery, research & development. A. How antisense works; B. Antisense drug discovery and research and development.

The antisense concept originates from a study reported in 1978, while efforts to convert the concept into a drug discovery platform did not begin in earnest until the late 1980s, when several 'antisense' companies were formed. Antisense compounds were designed to have the right nucleotide sequence to bind specifically to and interfere with its associated mRNA, the instructions for the production of a particular protein. To create antisense drugs, special chemically stabilized nucleotides were synthetically linked together in short chains (called oligonucleotides). Each antisense drug was designed with the right complementary genetic code to bind to a specific sequence of nucleotides in its mRNA target to form a short area of double strands.

Antisense RNA has undergone various technical refinements. Based on an understanding of nucleic acid structure and biochemistry, modifications of the phosphodiester backbone and the 2′ position in the sugar have been major foci.

Phosphorothioate (PS, 硫代磷酸) linkages and the modifications in phosphorodiamidate morpholino oligomers (PMOs, 磷酰二胺吗啉代寡核苷酸) are two such modifications that have been widely applied in ASOs as backbone modification. The first ASOs to reach clinical trials in the 1990s were either PMOs or PS ASOs without 2′ modifications. Although the unmodified PS ASO fomiversen (administered intravitreally) gained FDA approval for treating retinitis (视网膜炎) caused by cytomegalovirus (巨细胞病毒) in patients with HIV infection in 1998, unmodified PS ASOs have since been largely abandoned because of their limited potency and their pro-inflammatory effects following systemic administration. Among the many 2′ modifications that have been investigated, a 2′-O-methoxyethyl (2′-MOE) group has proved particularly useful, resulting in increased potency, longer tissue elimination half-lives, and reduced pro-inflammatory effects. Another more recent area of development has been the conjugation of ligands to ASOs to promote delivery to specific organs and cells and thereby enhance their potency in these organs and cells. Overall, the advances in medicinal chemistry have broadened the potential therapeutic applications of the technology.

Mechanisms of action. The formed double stranded region can inhibit the production of protein by a number of mechanisms. Advances in RNA biology have supported the development of ASOs that work via various post-RNA-binding mechanisms, which can be divided into two broad groups: occupancy only (involving steric interference) by stopping the ribosome from reading the message; or occupancy-mediated degradation (involving cleavage of target RNAs) by leading to the destruction of the mRNA by RNase H1 or endonuclease AGO2, which destroys such double-stranded nucleotides. Either RNase-H1-mediated or AGOs-mediated RNA degradation represents an antisense mechanism focusing on RNA targeting and employs chemically modified oligonucleotides.

Meanwhile, understanding of the specific elements within mRNAs that regulate their translation has provided opportunities to use ASOs to increase the translation of specific mRNAs, and new insights into the regulated degradation of mRNAs support the design of ASOs to take advantage of new post-RNA-binding-mechanisms, thus expanding the versatility of the platform. This has been complemented by the discovery of the microRNA (miRNA) pathway and the numerous roles this pathway plays. ASOs have been designed to directly bind and inhibit specific miRNAs, and miRNA-targeting ASOs have entered clinical trials for the treatment of various diseases, including Alport syndrome and polycystic kidney disease. ASOs can also block miRNA binding to target mRNA by masking the miRNA-binding site in the mRNAs.

Antisense technology is now beginning to deliver on its promise to treat diseases by targeting RNA. Nine single-stranded antisense oligonucleotide (ASO) drugs representing four chemical classes, two mechanisms of action and four routes of administration have been approved for commercial use, including the first RNA-targeted drug to be a major commercial success, Nusinersen. Although all the approved drugs are for use in patients with rare diseases, many of the ASOs in late- and middle-stage clinical development are intended to treat patients with very common diseases. ASOs in development are showing substantial improvements in potency and performance based on advances in medicinal chemistry, an understanding of molecular mechanisms and targeted delivery. Moreover, the ASOs in development includes additional mechanisms of action and routes of administration, such as aerosols and oral formulations.

By 2021, 13 RNA-targeted oligonucleotide drugs have received regulatory approval: nine single-stranded ASOs — Fomivisen（福米韦生）(1998), Mipomersen（米泊美生）(2013), Eteplirsen (2016), Nusinersen (2016), Inotersen (2018), Golodirsen (2019), Volanesorsen (2019), Viltolarsen (2010) and Casimersen (2021) — and four siRNAs — patisiran, givosiran, lumasiran and inclisiran. The ASO Nusinersen has revolutionized care for patients with spinal muscular atrophy (SMA，脊髓性肌萎缩) since its approval in 2016 and is the first antisense drug to be sizeable commercial success, a 'blockbuster'(Fig.1-3).

A key advantage of PS ASOs is that they can be administered by essentially any route for both local — intrathecal（鞘内注射），aerosol, rectal, intravitreal, intradermal — and systemic applications — *i.v.* infusion, oral administration. Moreover, as the medicinal chemistry of oligonucleotides advanced and created more potent PS ASO chemical classes, these advances were incorporated into many of the delivery approaches.

Like all drugs, antisense drugs can have side effects. The side effects are generally predictable, occur at high doses and are well understood.

Prospect

Antisense technology represents an important breakthrough in the way we treat disease. The explosion in genomic information led to the discovery of many new disease-causing proteins and created new opportunities accessible only to antisense technology. Once we have identified a therapeutic application and corresponding gene target, an antisense lead inhibitor compound can be rationally designed within hours suitable for use in research and clinical trials. This compares with traditional drug discovery approaches, which can take years to produce such a lead compound.

With over 30 years of technology refinement, antisense is a mature drug discovery and therapeutic platform. Antisense is an innovative platform for drug discovery. Platform technologies combine all the elements necessary to rapidly and efficiently create a stream of new products. Substantial progress in understanding the molecular mechanisms of activity, distribution, cell uptake, subcellular distribution, and toxicity provides an exciting framework from which additional advances in the technology should arise.

The rapid development of antisense technology offers almost unlimited scope for the development of new and highly specific therapeutics. Antisense Therapeutics therefore is well positioned to play a significant role in the progression of antisense technology for drug development in human diseases.

DNA Drugs

Turning DNA into a therapeutic treatment usually means delivering the genetic material directly into cells, where it can act as native DNA does, coding for needed proteins. Now researchers are using DNA in a new class of drugs that rev up（加快转速，使更活跃）the immune system, potentially helping to

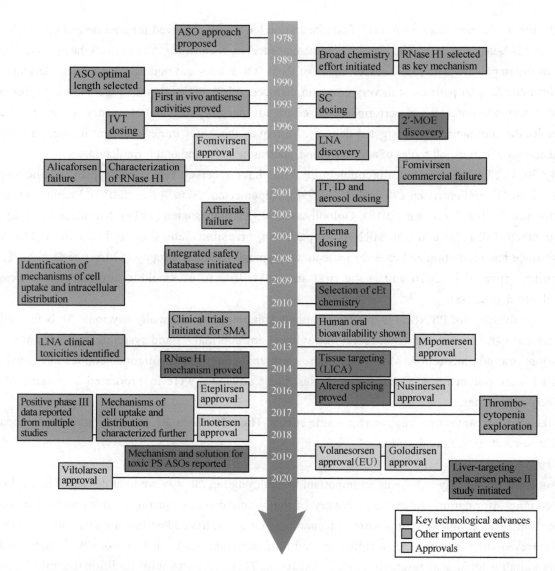

Fig. 1-3 An overview of progress in antisense technology. Key technological advances, drug approvals and other important events and setbacks (挫折) are highlighted. Some dates are approximations of the timing of events, and recent advances are too frequent to fit easily on the schematic. As the performance of antisense oligonucleotides (ASOs) has improved, the breadth of therapeutic opportunities has increased to encompass both rare and common diseases as well as essentially any delivery route. 2′-MOE, 2′-O-methoxyethyl; cEt, constrained ethyl; ID, intradermal; IT, intrathecal; IVT, intravitreal; LICA, ligand-conjugated antisense; LNA, locked nucleic acid; PS, phosphorothioate; SC, subcutaneous; SMA, spinal muscular atrophy.

boost vaccines′ power and even to fight cancer — all without even entering a cell.

The new drugs consist of short synthetic DNA segments that mimic gene sequences found only in bacteria. The segments bind to receptors on the surface of immune cells; the cells interpret the molecules as signs of a bacterial infection and respond by ramping up (增加, 使增加) the body′s defenses. The first use of the technology in humans is likely to be with vaccines, in order to boost the immune system′s response to inoculation, says Ethan Shevach, an immunologist at the National Institute of Allergy and Infectious Diseases. In tests on animals, the DNA segments are "unbelievably good", Shevach says.

Dynavax in Emeryville, CA, has completed early human-safety trials of an immune-stimulating DNA sequence, which when combined with a standard hepatitis B vaccine, seems to help the vaccine take effect faster and with fewer injections. Because slightly different DNA sequences may preferentially trigger specific elements of the immune system, the drugs can be tailored for particular uses such as activating natural killer cells, which attack cancerous cells. Shevach believes that the DNA fragment technology "will have a stand-alone（独立的）drug", but even that would be greatly welcomed by researchers.

Antibodies and genetically engineered related molecules

Genetically engineered antibodies

The mammalian immune system has a vast repertoire of antibodies, and the technology for exploiting it is well-advanced. B lymphocytes, however, have been constrained by evolutionary pressures so that they produce whole antibodies that differ from each other only in the fine sequences of their variable regions and their class type. Predetermined changes in amino acid sequences can quite easily be brought about by the use of recombinant DNA techniques. Furthermore, by genetic manipulation, molecules could be generated in which, for example, the cloned variable region from a mouse antibody could be joined to a cloned constant region from a human antibody. Such molecules could overcome the problems associated with the administration of heterologous antibodies for therapeutic purposes. Indeed, this approach is not limited to whole antibodies. Fab or other fragments could be produced directly, perhaps fused to useful effector molecules such as toxins that could have value in cancer therapy. The cloning and expression of immunoglobulin genes, therefore, provides new opportunities for investigating the structure and function of antibodies and creates the starting point for the generation of novel immunoglobulin-related molecules.

Despite early failures of murine products, chimeric, humanized and fully human monoclonal antibodies are now viable therapeutics. A number of genetically engineered antibody constructions have emerged, including molecular hybrids or chimeras that can deliver a powerful toxin to a target such as a tumor cell.

1.1 Development of genetically engineered pharmaceutials （基因工程药物发展概况）

1.1.1 A brief history of the development of the world biopharmaceutical industry and current situation（世界生物制药产业发展简史与现状）

Up to now, the history of biopharmaceuticals can be divided broadly into six periods:

Stage 1:

During 1944—1975, knowledges and technologies related to genetically-engineered biotherapeutics have been gradually accumulated and shaped up.

The publication of work on the chemical nature of the substance inducing transformation of the pneumococcal types by Avery O.T. *et al.* in 1944 and the discovery of the double helical structure of DNA by Watson & Crick in 1953, marked the beginning of molecular biology, laying the foundation of modern biotechnology.

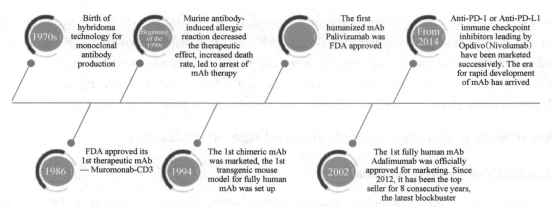

Fig. 1-4　The development course of antibody therapeutics.

Birth of Biotechnology

In 1972, Stanford University researcher Paul Berg and his colleagues integrated segments of λ phage DNA, as well as a segment of *E. coli* DNA containing the galactose operon, into the SV40 genome. He thereby created the first DNA molecule made of parts from different organisms. This type of molecule became known as "hybrid DNA" or "recombinant DNA". Among other things, Paul Berg's method opened the way to creating bacteria that produce substances used in medicines. That work led to the emergence of the recombinant DNA technology.

Biotechnology was born during a meeting at a Hawaiian delicatessen (熟食店) in 1972. The shop has long since been torn down, and there is no plaque to mark biotech's inception — but its legacy lives on. And the two pioneers who met there blazed (照耀) distinct career paths that have become well trodden.

Stanford medical professor Stanley Cohen and biochemist Herbert Boyer from the University of California, San Francisco, were in Honolulu to attend a meeting on plasmids, the ringlets (小圆圈) of DNA contained in bacteria. Cohen reported on the ability to introduce plasmid DNA into *Escherichia coli*, which allowed researchers to propagate and clone the plasmids in the bacteria. Boyer told the meeting about his work with a revolutionary enzyme called *Eco*RI that could cleave the double-stranded DNA molecule to produce single-stranded ends with identical termini.

Both saw the potential for combining the two discoveries into what would become genetic engineering. First, use *Eco*RI to slice both plasmid DNA and the DNA of choice. Then, with the identical DNA termini exposed, attach the DNA fragment to the plasmid DNA, and clone the whole in *E. coli*.

The two men first discussed collaboration at a deli (熟食店) near Waikiki Beach. Their chat over a late-night snack (小吃，加餐，零食，快餐) led to a scientific achievement that later rocked the world of science. Within a year, they had cloned DNA molecules made by splicing together DNA fragments of two different plasmids, thus creating recombinant DNA. The foundations for biotechnology were established.

1970s — The hybridoma technology is born for producing monoclonal antibody

In 1975, Kohler and Milstein created the monoclonal antibody hybridoma technique by fusing mouse myeloma cells with mouse spleen B lymphocytes immunized with sheep red blood cells, resulting in hybridoma cells that could both produce antibodies and proliferate indefinitely. This technological breakthrough not only creates a new era for the basic research of medicine and biology, but also provides a new tool for diagnosis, prevention and treatment of clinical diseases, and opens the prelude of antibody engineering.

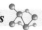

Stage 2:

During 1976—1988, new inventions and innovations made the genetically engineered technology more perfect and full-grown. Biotech companies gradually entered public view. Biotechnology and its related products have been gradually accepted.

Foundation of Genentech（基因泰克，基因工程科技公司）—— the start point of biotech industry

Boyer and Cohen chose different paths, both affected by concerns about the safety of recombinant DNA technology [which would lead in 1975 to the Asilomar conference, where scientists, ethicists, and journalists pondered the implications（可能的结果，影响）of genetic engineering].

While Cohen stayed in academia and defended recombinant DNA technology in US congressional hearings（国会听证会），Boyer saw the potential for profit. In South San Francisco in 1976, Boyer and venture-capitalist Robert Swanson set up Genentech, the world's first biotechnology company. The company's goal was to develop a new generation of therapeutics created from genetically engineered copies of naturally occurring molecules important in human health and disease.

In January 1976, 28-year-old venture capitalist Robert Swanson entered the picture. A successful cold-call（不请自来的推销）to Boyer's lab led to a couple of beers — and an agreement to start a pharmaceutical company. Investing $500 each, they capitalized a new business, Genentech, to seek practical uses for Boyer and Cohen's engineered proteins. Swanson raised money for staff and labs... Although the two confidently assert that it was the first biotech company, others clearly came before, including Cetus Corporation which was founded in 1971. The Swiss global health-care company F. Hoffmann-La Roche AG now completely owns Genentech after completing its purchase on March 26, 2009, for approximately $46.8 billion.

Pioneers at Genentech and their collaborators at the California Institute of Technology were the first to synthesize DNA in the lab. But they wanted to use *E. coli* as a factory to synthesize mammalian proteins. Proof of principle had been demonstrated earlier by Cohen and his colleagues at Stanford, when they used the bacteria to produce a functioning mouse-cell protein. The Genentech scientists eventually succeeded, producing a **human** hormone called somatostatin（生长激素抑制剂）in the bacteria — and so heralded （通报，预示……的来临）the era of commercial biotechnology. The production of insulin and growth hormone followed soon after.

In the fall of 1980, Genentech, Inc., became the overnight darling of Wall Street, raising over $38 million in its initial public stock offering. Lacking marketed products or substantial profit, the firm nonetheless saw its share price escalate from $35 to $89 in the first few minutes of trading, at that point the largest gain in stock market history. Coming at a time of economic recession and declining technological competitiveness in the United States, the event provoked banner headlines（通栏大标题）and ignited a period of speculative frenzy over biotechnology as a revolutionary means for creating new and better kinds of pharmaceuticals, untold profit, and a possible solution to national economic malaise（低迷）.

In the following years, a flood of biotech firms entered the scene. Harvard professor Walter Gilbert and Phillip Sharp at the Massachusetts Institute of Technology, now both Nobel laureates, set up Biogen （百健）in Geneva in 1978. Cetus, of Emeryville, California — founded in 1971 as a "bioengineering company" — made the push towards biotechnology and, within ten years, developed the polymerase chain reaction, which amplifies DNA. Biotech firm Amgen of thousand Oaks, California, started up in 1980 with less than 50 employees — it had more than 10 000 worldwide by the end of 2002.

The industry began with a focus on human proteins made in bacteria and on antibodies. It then moved on to immunological treatment for cancer, and small-molecule treatments for disease.

An early example of a biopharmaceutical medication is recombinant human insulin. In 1982, the Eli Lilly Corporation produced a human insulin that became the first approved genetically engineered pharmaceutical product. Without needing to depend on animals, researchers could produce genetically engineered insulin in unlimited supplies.

The bud of antibody technology began shooting out in 1986, when the first murine therapeutic antibody was licensed — in 1986, the first monoclonal antibody, Muromonab-CD3 monoclonal antibody, was approved by FDA. However, the sales of the murine antibody Orthoclone OKT3 haven't taken off.

Stage 3:

The biotechnology industry had been expanding during 1989—2000.

In the 1990s, there was a wave of neurobiology companies, followed by a wave of genomics companies.

New technologies have fueled the biotechnology fire. Hood and Applied Biosystems, the company he founded in 1981 in Foster City, California, came up with（提供，提出，拿出）the automated protein synthesizer, protein sequencer, DNA synthesizer, and DNA sequencer. The first three are what Hood calls "sophisticated plumbing" problems, as they just involved engineering（设计）a series of valves to mix the correct quantities of reagents. The last was more sophisticated; it needed the integration of biology, chemistry, engineering, and computer science.

In the early 1990s, mAb therapy hit a trough as mouse-derived antibodies induced allergic reactions in humans, reducing their efficacy and increased mortality. Monoclonal antibodies must be transformed into humanized or human antibodies if they are to have a foothold in competition and a wider application in medicine.

In order to resolve that issue, the companies focusing on research and development of antibody therapeutics at that time managed to sortie（出击，突围）out through **two strategies**. The first strategy focuses on antibody protein engineering and humanization. This **type** of monoclonal antibody can be divided into **two levels**. The first level is **Chimeric Antibody**: in which the constant area (of antibody) is replaced with the human amino acid sequence. Approximately 33% of the amino acid sequence of the chimeric monoclonal antibody protein is derived from mice, while the remaining 67% is from humans. The second level is **Humanized Antibody**, in which only a few regions that are specific to an antigen (CDR regions) are to be taken from a mouse antibody, and implanted into a human antibody. In a humanized monoclonal antibody, the sequence of human origin accounts for 90%. The second strategy of antibody therapeutics is fully human monoclonal antibody, here **two techniques**, **phage display** and **transgenic mice**, were used to approach the problem.

1994 was also a scientific milestone. The first human antibody transgenic mouse model was established in 1994, and PD-1 was discovered in 1992.

GenPharm and Cell Genesys（美国细胞基因系统工程公司）published high-impact papers in *Nature* and *Nature Genetics* almost at the same time, respectively, announcing the establishment of HumAb and XenoMouse technologies. The maturation of the XenoMouse technology platform was marked by the publication of the paper in Nature Genetics in February 1997. In June 1997, Ishida Gong（石田功）published his results in Nature Genetics. With chromosome fragments as the vector, antibody diversity reached its peak, *i.e.*, the limitation of transgenosis（基因转移）technology.

Meanwhile, the very first chimeric antibody Abciximab（阿昔单抗）was released in 1994. Abciximab (ReoPro®,Centocor, Eli Lilly) (chimeric), the second antibody drug, only became available in the United States, is an IgG1κFab anti-GPⅡb/Ⅲa. The chimeric monoclonal antibody (mAb) was approved by FDA in 1994 (8 years later than the first one), by Health Canada（加拿大卫生部）in 1996, and by TGACNZ in 2005. More than 2 million patients have been treated worldwide with Abciximab to prevent ischemic complications of percutaneous（经皮的，通过皮肤的）coronary interventions [angioplasty（血管成形术）and stent（血管支架）placement] in patients with myocardial infarction and other conditions since its approval by the FDA in 1994.

Reopro's success has greatly boosted the biologics industry's confidence in therapeutic monoclonal antibodies.

Researchers made their first clone of an animal, Dolly the Sheep, in 1996; her birth was announced on February 22, 1997. Dolly (July 5, 1996—February 14, 2003), a ewe（母羊）, was cloned at the Roslin Institute in Scotland. It was the first mammal to have been successfully cloned from an adult cell.

Rituxan（利妥昔单抗，美罗华，瑞图宣）**.** In 1997, the first humanized monoclonal antibody, actually an anti-CD20 monoclonal antibody drug, a chimeric (mouse/human) antibody against CD20, **Rituxan (Rituximab)**, was approved by the FDA. Its approval marks the beginning of a new era in the treatment of B-cell malignancies. Monoclonal antibody drugs have changed the way diseases are treated, especially in the field of cancer. Since the launching of Rituximab, a large number of monoclonal antibody drugs have entered the clinic.

Herceptin（赫赛汀）**.** In the treatment history of breast cancer and even cancer, the advent of **Herceptin (trastuzumab, 曲妥珠单抗)**, a humanized monoclonal antibody for treating breast cancer approved in **1998,** has epoch-making significance（划时代意义）— it is not only the first monoclonal antibody drug targeting oncogenic proteins in human history, but also the first molecular targeting drug for solid tumor therapy, opening the door for scientists to explore molecular targeting drugs for cancer. As the first monoclonal antibody drug targeting oncogenic proteins, Herceptin has benefited millions of breast cancer patients since it launched on the market. It has become a "lifesaving drug" for women with breast cancer, which is why herceptin's invention team won the Lasker Clinical Research Award in 2019, 21 years after its approval.

New technologies, meanwhile, continue to infuse（注入）the industry. Nanotechnology and pharmacogenomics, for example, are both areas of potential job growth. Gilbert sees 'lifestyle drugs' such as Viagra (FDA approved in March 1998) as the wave of the future, and companies such as Memory Pharmaceuticals (founded in 1997) in Montvale, New Jersey, are trying to develop drugs that enhance memory and attention. Such prospects seem a far cry（远距离,大不相同的，悬殊）from the ideas raised at that Hawaiian deli less than 30 years ago.

Stage 4:

After 2000, multinational pharmaceutical companies began to realize that macromolecular drugs would gradually replace small-molecule drugs and occupy the dominant position in the market.

During 2001—2010, with the completion of the Human Genome Project, and the maturation of antibody technology, drug development has entered the post-genome era. Reversed Genetics（反向遗传学）, bioinformatics, pharmacogenomics（药物基因组学）and nanobiotechnology became the essential approaches towards more precisely designed therapeutics, meanwhile prepared for the concept of fully human monoclonal antibody, the newest generation of therapeutic antibodies.

Researchers also became more integrated (综合的，融合的). Many biologists joined the chemists working for big drug companies, and technological needs opened the field up to researchers with skills outside biology. Such powerful technologies have changed the way biologists do science. "Big science", once unique to chemistry and physics, has entered biology. Now, researchers no longer have to start their gene search with a hypothesis — with whole genomes at their disposal (处理，支配), they can find a gene by doing a quick database search, and then use those data in a hypothesis-driven manner for some further discovery.

Although the proliferation (激增，涌现) of big science and genomic data sparked (引发) a revolution, firms that depended too much on the human genome have faltered (踌躇，犹豫，衰退). Celera of Rockville, Maryland, which sequenced a draft of the human genome, has shed jobs (裁员) in its effort to become a pharmaceutical company. And DoubleTwist of Oakland, California, which hoped to sell a "superior" annotation of the human genome, went bankrupt in 2002.

Although stocks in the industry languished in 2002, the industry itself did not. So small companies that are 3~5 years old are having trouble raising money at the exaggerated levels that they managed a few years ago. Promising new companies can still raise money, just in small amounts. But some downsizing by older biotechs may have been offset (抵挡，弥补) by new start-ups. The demand for pharmacogenomics and bioinformatics expertise continues to grow, along with the companies featuring them (以……为特色) — much more than the rest of the industry. With pharmaceutical firms now bigger and more marketing-driven than ever, biotech companies remain important engines of innovation.

In order to make **Humira®** (修美乐)(adalimumab, 阿达木单抗), the very first fully human monoclonal antibody approved in 2002, a technology called phage display to identify optimal CDRs was used, allowing for easy screening of the CDRs exhibiting the strongest antigen binding. Phage display technique makes it possible to produce genetically engineered antibodies while completely avoiding animal usage. Without needing to depend on animals, researchers could produce antibodies in unlimited supplies.

Following the FDA-approval of Vectibix® (维克替比)(panitumumab, 帕尼单抗，帕妥木单抗), the first fully human monoclonal antibody product with high EGFR-affinity (XenoMouse technology) in 2006, began the era of fully human monoclonal antibody, with no traces of mouse protein left at all. This is an important milestone, marking the first time that a fully human monoclonal antibody produced from mice has been approved for sale as a drug. Although transgenic mice came out late, their technical advantages were the most obvious.

Chromatin (Catumaxomab, 卡妥索单抗) was approved by EMA in 2009 for the treatment of EPCAM (表皮细胞黏附因子) positive malignant ascites (腹水), ovarian cancer, and gastric cancer. It was the landmark in the development of the **Triomab (三功能抗体) drugs**.

2009 is destined to be the year to change the structure of the world pharmaceutical industry. At that time, there have been four major mergers and acquisitions (并购) in the pharmaceutical industry, the mega-mergers, each of which has had far-reaching consequences.

Stage 5:

During 2011-2020, antibody has been entering the stage of full blossom. With the development of tumor immunology and genetic engineering, active specific immunotherapy with a vaccine that causes the body to kill the tumor(s) has become a new hotspot of tumor biotherapy. And we'd hit a turning point of a new gene therapy.

With the continuous improvement of the technology, the monoclonal antibody market has entered a period of rapid development. Since the invention of hybridoma technology, after more than 40 years of continuous improvement, the research, preparation and application of monoclonal antibody drugs have reached a relatively mature stage (Fig. 1-4). Nowadays, great progress has been made in the treatment of oncology, immune diseases and other fields, and the market size is expected to develop rapidly.

Perjeta (Pertuzumab, 帕妥珠单抗), a humanized monoclonal antibody indicated for the treatment of HER2-positive metastatic breast cancer, is the first in a new class of drugs — the human epidermal growth factor receptor (HER) dimerization inhibitors — approved for marketing (2012).

Ipilimumab（伊匹单抗，易谱利姆玛）, a fully human monoclonal antibody product originated from a scientific research cooperation starting in 1996, which targets cytotoxic T-lymphocyte antigen-4 (CTLA-4), was approved in 2011 by the US Food and Drug Administration (FDA)**, made it the first to move into clinical trials, the first approved immune checkpoint inhibitor for treating patients with advanced melanoma.**

Since 2014, anti-PD-1/L1 drugs such as Opdivo（欧狄沃）(**Nivolumab,** 纳武单抗) have been launched successively, and monoclonal antibodies have experienced rapid development.

Nivolumab, a fully human monoclonal antibody, was approved in July, 2014 in Japan — This milestone marks the emergence of cancer immunotherapy on the world stage, shining in the spotlight after a century of setbacks（挫折）.

Discovered in 1992, PD-1 is another brake that keeps the immune system from killing tumor cells. In a landmark paper published in Nature in 2002, it was reported that PD-L1 (the PD-1 receptor, identified in 1999) is expressed only on the surface of tumor cells and is one of the main mechanisms by which tumor cells escape from the host immune system. Then a project targeting the PD-1 pathway was launched the same year. Opdivo (Nivolumab), a next generation checkpoint inhibitor, originally called MDX-1106, was hidden deep in the pipeline at that time.

Then **Nivolumab** and pembrolizumab（派姆单抗）(Keytruda, a humanized monoclonal antibody), which target the programmed cell death receptor-1 (PD-1) signaling pathway, were developed quickly with ipilimumab（伊匹单抗）and gained rapid acceptance for multiple indications after demonstrating significant efficacy and safety advantages over standard treatments.

Cyramza® (Ramucirumab, 雷莫芦单抗) is a fully human monoclonal antibody (IgG1) developed for the treatment of solid tumors. It is directed against the vascular endothelial growth factor receptor 2 (VEGFR2). and specifically blocks downstream angiogenesis related pathways. The approval of Cyramza (in December 2014) is a landmark event in the history of immunotherapy.

Data shows that eight of the world's 10 best-selling drugs in 2019 were biologics. Among them, adalimumab, the first fully human monoclonal antibody approved in the United States in 2002, has topped the list for eight consecutive years since 2012, and is known as the "King of Medicine".

Cell therapy refers to products that treat or prevent diseases after human autologous（自体的）or allogeneic（同种异体的）cells are treated *in vitro*. The treated cells play a major therapeutic role.

Chimeric antigen receptor (CAR) T-cell therapy, one of cell therapy products, which first proposed in the late 1980s and has been in development for more than 30 years, has seen **explosive growth** since the launch of two CAR-T cell therapies in 2017 (Fig. 1-5). Following the approval of two CAR-T products, Yescarta and Kymriah, in 2017, the global CAR-T market grew from approximately $13 million in 2017 to approximately $734 million in 2019 and is expected to grow further to $4.7 billion in 2024.

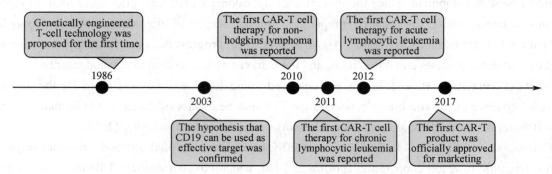

Fig. 1-5   The development course of CAR-T.

Tisagenlecleucel, the first CAR-T cell immunotherapy approved by the FDA, is a CD19-directed genetically modified autologous（自体的）T cell immunotherapy, or a CAR-T cell therapy for B-cell acute lymphoblastic leukemia. It was granted approval by FDA in August 2017 under the market name **Kymriah**.

Tisagenlecleucel is an immunocellular therapy that involves autologous T cells that are collected from each individual patient and genetically engineered to express a specific protein called a chimeric antigen receptor (CAR) that specifically target CD19 antigens. Modified T cells are infused back into the patient's body. These CD19-directed chimeric antigen receptors (CD19 CAR-T cells) direct the T cells to target and kill leukemia cells that express a specific antigen (CD19) on the cell surface. Tisagenlecleucel is the first CAR-T drug to be marketed, the first *in vivo* drug that would ideally not only not be metabolized but also expand in the body.

Luxturna. "As the first directly administered gene therapy drug approved (in 2017) in the United States, Luxturna (voretigene neparvovec-rzyl) is **a milestone for the scientific community**." It introduces a healthy VERSION of the RPE65 gene into patients with an inherited form of vision loss that may result in blindness, a disease caused by mutations in a specific gene, allowing them to produce a protein that functions normally and thus improves vision. FDA's approval of Luxturna becomes the first true gene therapy in the US market, marking the official arrival of the era of gene therapy, and further opening the door to the potential of gene therapies, marks another first in the field of gene therapy — both in how the therapy works and in expanding the use of gene therapy beyond the treatment of cancer to the treatment of vision loss, This milestone reinforces the potential of this breakthrough approach in treating a wide-range of challenging diseases.

Cablivi®. The world's first nano antibody drug Cablivi® (Caplacizumab/Caplaxizumab-YHDP), developed by Ablynx, was approved by THE EU EMA in 2018 for the treatment of rare blood diseases, indicating that the new form of nano antibody has officially entered the commercial market.

In April 2020, FDA Accelerated Approval for the first Trop-2-targeted agent Trodelvy (sacituzumab govitecan-hziy) in Previously-treated Metastatic Triple-Negative Breast Cancer, meanwhile approved Clinical Trial Application by China National Medical Products Administration（国家药品监督管理局）

to initiate China registration study of Sacituzumab Gaovitecan for the treatment of Metastatic Triple-Negative Breast Cancer.

Stage 6:

From 2021 on, precision medicine will continue to yield unusually brilliant results. Various vaccines came out to try their hands, taking advantage of the COVID-19 pandemic.

Advances in precision medicine continue to facilitate drug development, allowing diseases like dMMR endometrial cancer, lung cancer, and Alzheimer's to be subset into biomarker-defined populations appropriate for targeted therapies. With Jemperli, Rybrevant, and Aduhelm's successive approvals in April, May and June 2021, for the first time, patients with dMMR endometrial cancer, non-small cell lung cancer with EGFR exon 20 insertion mutations, and Alzheimer's will each have a targeted treatment option.

Jemperli (dostarlimab), a humanized monoclonal antibody, works by targeting the cellular pathway known as PD-1/PD-L1. Jemperli helps the body's immune system in its fight against cancer cells by blocking this pathway.

Rybrevant (amivantamab-vmjw) is the first fully-human bispecific antibody indicated for the treatment of adult patients with locally advanced or metastatic non-small cell lung cancer (NSCLC) with epidermal growth factor receptor (EGFR) exon 20 insertion mutations. It is EGF receptor-directed and MET receptor-directed.

The approval of Aduhelm (aducanumab), a recombinant, fully human anti-Aβ IgG1 monoclonal antibody, is the first therapy to target and affect the underlying disease process of Alzheimer's.

Chronology key events in genetically engineered pharmaceuticals are listed in Table 1-1.

Table 1-1 Chronology key events in genetically engineered pharmaceuticals

Year	Key events
1953	DNA structure proposed by James Watson and Francis Crick.
1960	Arthur Komberg synthesized DNA *in vitro*.
1970	Hamilton Smith and Kent Wilcox isolated the first restriction enzyme.
1971	The first biological engineering company, Cetus, founded.
1972	Paul Berg used a restriction enzyme to form a hybrid circular molecule.
1973	Stanley Cohen and Herbert Boyer developed DNA cloning and recombinant DNA.
1975	Asilomar Conference discussed the ethics of recombinant DNA research; In 1975, monoclonal antibodies were first generated using a hybridoma technique.
1976	Robert Swanson and Herbert Boyer found Genentech; Guidelines from the US National Institute of Health (NIH) prohibited some categories of recombinant DNA experiments.
1977	Genentech cloned the hormone somatostatin in bacteria, the first cloning of a protein using a synthetic recombinant gene, or the first successful expression of a human gene in bacteria; A human gene was first expressed in bacteria in 1977.
1978	Biogen（百健）founded, now the oldest independent biotech company; The recombinant human insulin was successfully expressed in *E. coli*.
1979	NIH recombinant DNA guidelines relaxed; Genentech cloned human growth hormone.

Fundamentals, Approaches and Breakthroughs in R & D Genetically Engineered Biotherapeutics

Year	Key events
1980	Amgen founded; Leroy Hood and Mike Hunkapiller developed protein sequencer; Fred Sanger and colleagues developed the shotgun method for sequencing genomes; Bayh-Dole Act passes, encouraging technology transfer; US Supreme Court decreed （颁布） that life forms are patentable.
1982	Recombinant vaccine against coccidiosis （抗球虫病疫苗）, 1st recombinant animal vaccine; Human insulin, the first biotechnology drug, hit the market, with the name Humulin.
1983	Kary Mullis invented the polymerase chain reaction.
1984	Chimeric antibody technology was established.
1985	Orthoclone OKT3 (muromonab-CD3) was licensed by the FDA to prevent renal transplant rejection, the first murine therapeutic antibody, the first therapeutic monoclonal antibody drug.
1986	US Environmental Protection Agency approved release of genetically altered tobacco, the first genetically engineered crop; The first recombinant vaccine (hepatitis B vaccine, Recombivax2HB) was marketed in the United States; The first biotech drug to treat tumor, interferon ALPHA 2A (IntronA), has been released in the United States.
1987	Susan Horvath, Mike Hunkapiller and Leroy Hood developed DNA synthesizer; The first genetically engineered product, recombinant tPA, expressed in animal cells (CHO), was approved by the U.S. FDA for the treatment of thrombotic diseases.
1988	Phillip Leder and Timothy Stewart were awarded patent for mouse breast-cancer model, the first patent given for a genetically altered animal.
1989	RECOMBINANT human erythropoietin (rhEPO) got FDA approval to market, which became the top-seller drug two years later for the treatment of anemia due to chronic renal failure and anemia after chemotherapy.
1993	The Biotechnology industry Organization (BIO) was formed.
1994	US Food and Drug Administration deemed the Flavr Savr, a genetically modified tomato, safe, thus bringing to market the first transgenic food product; ReoPro® （Abciximab, 阿昔单抗）, the first recombinant chimeric antibody, hit the market.
1997	Roslin Institute scientists cloned Dolly the sheep, the first mammal to be cloned successfully from an adult cell; Rituxan (Rituximab, 利妥昔单抗，美罗华，瑞图宣), the first therapeutic antibody for tumor therapy, was marketed; The first tissue-engineered cartilage substitute Carticel, came to market.
1998	Human embryonic stem cells were isolated and cultured successfully for the first time; Enbrel® (Etanercept), a dimeric fusion protein consisting of the extracellular ligand-binding portion of the human 75 kilodalton (p75) tumor necrosis factor receptor (TNFR) linked to the Fc portion of human IgG1, the best selling drug around the world to treat multiple inflammatory disease, was first approved in the US; The U.S. Food and Drug Administration (FDA) approved Herceptin (Trastuzumab), the first humanized antibody approved for the treatment of HER2 positive metastatic breast cancer; Basiliximab （巴昔单抗）, which is specifically indicated for the prophylaxis of acute renal graft rejection, was licensed by FDA and EMEA; The first antisense oligonucleotide drug (Vitravene) was marketed for the treatment of cytomegalovirus (CMV) retinitis （巨细胞病毒性视网膜炎） in patients with AIDS; Neupogen （Filgrastim 非格司亭） became the first biotech blockbuster drug (with annual sales in excess of $1 billion).
2000	The work draft of human genome has been plotted; Mylotarg (gemtuzumab ozogamicin) received accelerated approval, the first antibody-directed chemotherapy (ADC) that won regulatory approvals in the USA and Japan.

continued

Year	Key events
2001	The first targeted drugs has been (FDA) approved（靶向药物获准上市）； Gleevec（格列卫，matinib，伊玛替尼）was first approved by FDA to treat patients with advanced Philadelphia chromosome positive chronic myeloid leukemia, a blood and bone marrow disease linked to a genetic abnormality； Public and private teams publish draft versions of the human genome sequence.
2002	Over 200 000 jobs exist across 4000 biotech companies worldwide, according to analysts Ernst & Young； Humira®（修美乐®）(Adalimumab 阿达木单抗), the first fully human monoclonal antibody, was approved. Soon after it becomes Britain's first biotech blockbuster. The product had received marketing authorizations in the United States, European Union, or Japan for a total of more than 10 indications up to now. Furthermore, it is the first drug brought about by phage display technique.
2003	Somavert (pegvisomant), an analog of hGH, the only and very first drug designed and structurally altered to act as a GH receptor antagonist, has been approved by FDA (with 9 amino acid substitution and 4~6 PEG molecules covalently bounded).
2004	China approved the country's first genetic therapeutics, recombinant human p53 adenovirus injection； ERBITUX®（爱必妥）(cetuximab, 西妥昔单抗), a targeted therapy that targets and binds to the epidermal growth factor receptors (EGFR), got its initial U.S. Approval and European Union Approval.
2008	Melacine®（黑素瘤疫苗）, an allogeneic melanoma tumor cell lysate vaccine, the very first approved cancer vaccine in the world, has been approved in Canada.
2009	Catumaxomab (Removab®), a trifunctional, bispecific, hybrid, mouse-rat, monoclonal antibody (Triomab® technology) against human EpCAM and human CD3, was approved for marketing in Europe in April 2009, became the first bispecific antibody to attain regulatory approval.
2010	Denosumab, a fully human monoclonal antibody to RANK ligand [RANK-L]) was approved； The world's first therapeutic cancer vaccine, Provenge (sipuleucel T), has been approved by the US FDA, heralding a major breakthrough in the struggle to harness the immune system to fight tumors.
2011	Belatacept（贝拉西普）, a first-in-class immunosuppressant which can prevent the immune system rejecting new organs, was approved by the US FDA. the first costimulation blocker approved for the prophylaxis of organ rejection in adult patients receiving a kidney transplant； ADCETRIS（本妥昔单抗）was granted accelerated approval by the US FDA in August 2011 for relapsed Hodgkin lymphoma (HL) and sALCL and conditional marketing authorization by the European Commission in Octobel 2012 for relapsed or refractory HL and sALCL. It is the first new FDA-approved treatment for HL since 1977 and the first specifically indicated to treat ALCL； Ipilimumab, which targets cytotoxic T-lymphocyte antigen-4 (CTLA-4), was the first approved immune checkpoint inhibitor for treating patients with advanced melanoma.
2012	ABthrax（Raxibacumab，雷昔库单抗）was FDA approved. It is a human IgG1λ monoclonal antibody that binds the protective antigen (PA) component of *Bacillus anthracis* toxin, which is indicated for the treatment of adult and pediatric patients with inhalational anthrax due to *B. anthracis* in combination with appropriate antibacterial drugs, and for prophylaxis of inhalational anthrax when alternative therapies are not available or are not appropriate； Pertuzumab (anti-HER2), a humanized monoclonal antibody and the first in the class of agents called HER2 dimerization inhibitors, was FDA approved for people with HER2-Positive Metastatic Breast Cancer； FDA approved Bydureon® BCise™ (exenatide extended-release) injectable suspension, the first and only once-weekly medicine for adults with type 2 diabetes.
2013	Kadcyla（曲妥珠单抗）, the first antibody-drug conjugate (ADC) for treating HER2-positive metastatic breast cancer, got its initial U.S. Approval.

continued

Year	Key events
2014	BLINCYTO® (Blinatumomab), the first-in-class bispecific T cell engager (BiTE) therapeutic monoclonal antibody, was approved under the FDA's accelerated approval program, and indicated for the treatment of Philadelphia chromosome-negative relapsed or refractory B-cell precursor acute lymphoblastic leukemia (ALL); Cyramza (ramucirumab, 雷莫芦单抗), a recombinant human monoclonal antibody, was FDA approved for the treatment of advanced gastric or gastro-esophageal junction adenocarcinoma and metastatic non-small cell lung carcinoma, which marks an important milestone for patients with this difficult to treat disease, and later a series of indications. Cancer-drug Keytruda (pembrolizumab, 派姆单抗), the first approved drug that blocks a cellular pathway known as PD-1, which restricts the body's immune system from attacking melanoma cells, was FDA-approved. It is the first PD-1 inhibitor to hit the market. Soon after, it became a runaway best-seller; Bristol-Myers Squibb Announces Multiple Regulatory Milestones for Opdivo (Nivolumab, 纳武单抗). Opdivo, the first checkpoint immunotherapeutic agent to gain regulatory approval for Non-Small Cell Lung Cancer (NSCLC), a programmed death receptor-1 (PD-1) blocking antibody, Bristol-Myers Squibb's crown jewel, won initial FDA approval.
2015	Tremelimumab (替西木单抗, 曲美木单抗, 替西利姆单抗), a fully human monoclonal antibody specific for human cytotoxic T - lymphocyte - associated antigen 4, was approved as an orphan drug for the treatment of Malignant mesothelioma（间皮瘤）in the United States; Nucala (mepolizumab 美泊利单抗) gained approval in the EU as an add-on treatment of adults suffering from severe refractory eosinophilic asthma, which makes Nucala the first and only anti-interleukin-5 (IL-5) monoclonal antibody to be approved in the EU for the treatment of patients with severe refractory eosinophilic asthma; DARZALEX® (达拉他滨, 达雷木单抗), the first and first-in-class CD38-targeted monoclonal antibody, was approved based on its superiority to existing treatments; FDA approved first biosimilar product Zarxio (filgrastim-sndz).
2016	Atezolizumab（Tecentriq©）was FDA approved for use in the United States in 2016, hence became the first PD-L1 antibody ever approved.
2017	The U.S. Food and Drug Administration (FDA) granted Bavencio© （Avelumab） accelerated approval for both indications — metastatic MCC (March 2017) and urothelial（泌尿道上皮的）carcinoma (May 2017). Avelumab is a fully human anti-PD-L1 IgG1 lambda monoclonal antibody which specifically binds to PD-L1 and inhibits the interaction between PD-L1 and PD-1, promoting an immune response against cancer cells. It is the first FDA-approved treatment for metastatic MCC, a rare, aggressive form of skin cancer. Avelumab has more than 15 indications; Tisagenlecleucel, a CD19-directed genetically modified autologous T cell immunotherapy, or a CAR-T cell therapy for B-cell acute lymphoblastic leukemia, was granted approval by FDA. It is the first chimeric antigen receptor (CAR) T-cell immunotherapy approved by the FDA; The U.S. Food and Drug Administration approved Luxturna (voretigene neparvovec-rzyl), the first directly administered gene therapy approved by the U.S. FDA that targets a disease caused by mutations in a specific gene; Dupixent® (Dupilumab), the first and only biologic medicine approved for the treatment of adults suffering from atopic dermatitis (AD), received its first global approval in the USA.
2018	The U.S. Food and Drug Administration (FDA) has granted approval of Trogarzo™ (ibalizumab-uiyk) Injection, the first monoclonal antibody protein for HIV-1 therapy, the first HIV treatment approved with a new mechanism of action in more than 10 years, also the first long acting HIV drug; FDA approved Ultomiris (ravulizumab-cwvz/ALXN1210) for the treatment of adult patients with paroxysmal nocturnal hemoglobinuria (PNH, 阵发性睡眠性血红蛋白尿症), hence became the first and the only long-acting C5 complement inhibitor to get an approval for PNH; Gamifant (emapalumab-lzsg), which target interferon gamma (IFNγ), the first and only FDA-approved treatment for primary hemophagocytic lymphohistiocytosis (HLH, 嗜血细胞性淋巴组织细胞增多症) in patients with refractory, recurrent, or progressive disease or intolerance to conventional therapy, got its first approval; The European Commission has granted marketing authorization for Cablivi™ (caplacizumab) for the treatment of adults experiencing an episode of acquired thrombotic thrombocytopenic purpura (aTTP, 获得性血栓性血小板减少性紫癜), a rare blood-clotting disorder. Cablivi is the first therapeutic specifically indicated for the treatment of aTTP; FDA approved Fulphila (pegfilgrastim-jmbd), a leukocyte growth factor biosimilar to Neulasta (pegfilgrastim), a man-made form of granulocyte colony-stimulating factor (G-CSF), the first biosimilar to Neulasta.

continued

Year	Key events
2019	Developed a *de novo* computational approach for designing proteins (*e.g.*, Noeleukin2/15 mimics of interleukin-2) that recapitulate（重现）the binding sites of natural cytokines but are otherwise unrelated in topology or amino acid sequence; The European Medicines Agency and the US Food and Drug Administration approved ERVEBO® (Ebola Zaire Vaccine, Live), the first Ebola vaccine（埃博拉疫苗）.
2020	Immunomedics' Trodelvy, a first-in-class Trop-2 directed antibody-drug conjugate (ADC) that was granted accelerated approval, won FDA nod for triple-negative breast cancer; FDA approved **Inmazeb (atoltimab, maftivimab, and odesivimab-ebgn)**, a mixture of three monoclonal antibodies, as the first FDA-approved treatment for Zaire ebolavirus (Ebola virus) infection in adult and pediatric patients.
2021	Ad5-nCoV, or Recombinant novel coronavirus vaccine (adenovirus type 5 vector) (CanSinoBio) was approved in China by NMPA; FDA approved Jemperli (dostarlimab, 多塔利单抗) for treating patients with recurrent or advanced endometrial cancer whose cancers have a specific genetic feature known as dMMR; FDA approved Rybrevant (amivantamab-vmjw) as the first treatment for adult patients with non-small cell lung cancer whose tumors have specific types of genetic mutations: epidermal growth factor receptor (EGFR) exon 20 insertion mutations; FDA approved Aduhelm (aducanumab) for the treatment of Alzheimer's. This treatment option is the first therapy to target and affect the underlying disease process of Alzheimer's; FDA approved Rethymic for the treatment of pediatric patients with congenital athymia（无胸腺）, a rare immune disorder. Rethymic is the first thymus tissue product approved in the U.S.
2022	FDA approved Zynteglo (betibeglogene autotemcel), the first cell-based gene therapy [a customized treatment created using the patient's own cells (bone marrow stem cells) that are genetically modified to produce functional beta-globin (a hemoglobin component)] for the treatment of adult and pediatric patients with beta-thalassemia（地中海贫血）who require regular red blood cell transfusions.

1.1.2 Development of genetic engineering drugs in China（我国基因工程药物的发展）

The starting point of genetic engineering research in China is not behindhand. In 1982, the artificial synthesis, cloning and expression of the Leu-enkephalin（亮氨酸脑啡肽）gene were successfully realized in Shanghai. The first industrialized genetically engineered pharmaceutical product, recombinant interferon alpha 1b, began to appear on the market in 1993. China approved its first gene-therapy drug in 2003.

In the 21st century, China's **biotechnology has become a new economic growth point, in which** biologics industry has entered a stage of rapid development, and new biopharmaceutical enterprises are emerging constantly. As a strategic emerging industry, the biology industry became a powerful driving force for China's economic growth.

While China still lags behind the advanced western countries in terms of the development of the biologics industry, the scale of the Chinese biologics market has been growing rapidly in the past few years at a rate several times that of the global biologics market, with a compound annual growth rate of more than 20%. China has emerged as the second-largest pharmaceutical market in the world, where a growing patient population, significant unmet medical needs, new regulatory reforms and expanding reimbursement（补偿，报销）are driving demand for high quality, innovative medicines.

Up to now, about **600 (640) kinds** of biopharmaceuticals have received NMPA（National Medical Products Administration, 国家药品监督管理局）market approval, 86 are awaiting for NMPA approval, and nearly 1500 (1497) biologics are under clinical research in China, **according to the April 8, 2023 data on https://data.pharmacodia.com.** However, most of the above drugs are generic, so it is extremely urgent and important to develop novel genetically engineered pharmaceuticals with independent intellectual property rights. And most encouragingly, 4, 15, 17, 16 and 24 biologics were NMPA approved in 2017, 2018, 2019, 2020, and 2021 respectively. Within them, 1, 5, 4, 2 and 12 made their debut in China. And by the end of 2020, altogether there have been over a dozen of monoclonal antibodies approved were made in China. (截至 2020 年底, 国产上市单抗药物已达十几种) In 2020, the NMPA approved the first antibody drug conjugate, emmetastuzumab (Roche).

With the support of domestic innovation in drug R&D, domestic monoclonal antibody research and drug development have been **in full bloom** in recent years.

The revolutionary changes brought about by technologies such as gene editing and cell engineering have given new momentum to the long-term development of the biomedical industry. Moreover, with the patent expiration of many best-selling monoclonal antibody (Mab) therapeutics, biosimilars have also become hot topics in China monoclonal antibody R&D. In 2019, the first China-approved rituximab (利妥昔单抗) biosimilar HLX01 (Shanghai Hanlius Biotech Inc, 复宏汉霖) was approved to market, and the research on domestic biosimilars has made rapid progress.

Currently, there is no approved CAR-T product in the Chinese market, but the countdown (倒计时) has begun for the launch of CAR-T cell therapy product and new products are expected to be launched soon. As of August 30, 2020, the ClinicalTrails. gov database shows that there are about 390 clinical trials related to CAR-T therapy in China, among nearly 1100 worldwide, ranking the highest in terms of the number of projects. And about 160 clinical projects have been officially carried out, mainly focusing on the targets CD19, BCMA and Mesothelin (间皮素).

Progress in the development of COVID-19 vaccines

By the beginning of September 2020, according to incomplete statistics, 179 COVID-19 vaccine R&D projects are being carried out around the world in an orderly way, and 9 of them have entered clinical phase Ⅲ, among which four are in China, and the development of the COVID-19 vaccine is at the forefront. "The worldwide endeavor to create a safe and effective COVID-19 vaccine is bearing fruit. Almost two dozen vaccines have now been authorized around the globe; many more remain in development." according to the Regulatory Affairs Professionals Society (RAPS)'s statement (https://www.raps.org) on Oct. 15, 2021.

mRNA vaccine

Pharmaceutical and biotechnology companies in China have also stepped up to the development of vaccines of COVID-19. Several biotechnology companies have announced the development of mRNA vaccines against this coronavirus. Stemirna Therapeutics (斯微生物) (cooperating with Shanghai East Hospital of Tongji University), Abogen Biosciences Co., Ltd (艾博生物), RNAcure (蓝鹊生物), Zhuhai lifanda Biotechnology Co., Ltd (珠海丽凡达生物技术有限公司), and Shenzhen Institute of Advanced Technology are in the list.

DNA vaccine

A synthetic DNA-base COVID-19 vaccine, INO-4800, has been jointly developed by Advaccine Biopharmaceuticals Suzhou (艾棣维欣生物) and INOVIO Pharmaceuticals. Phase 1 clinical data showed promising immunogenicity and good safety and tolerability without serious side effects. Phase-2/3 trial has already began in.

1.1.3   Characteristics of genetically engineered pharmaceuticals production（基因工程制药的特点）

Compared with the traditional pharmaceutical industry, the outstanding advantages of genetically engineered pharmaceuticals production are as follows:

1. **By using genetically engineered techniques, physiologically active substances can be obtained which could not be obtained naturally, and therefore can be used clinically.** *e.g.*, **Human growth hormone（hGH or HGH）** is a peptide hormone that stimulates growth. It can be used to treat children's growth disorders (*e.g.*, idiopathic short stature) and adult growth hormone deficiency. Prior to its production by recombinant DNA technology, growth hormone used to treat deficiencies was extracted from the pituitary glands of cadavers. In 1985, unusual cases of Creutzfeldt-Jakob disease were found in individuals that had received cadaver-derived HGH ten to fifteen years previously. Based on the assumption that infectious prions causing the disease were transferred along with the cadaver-derived HGH, cadaver-derived HGH was removed from the market. In that same year, biosynthetic human growth hormone replaced pituitary-derived human growth hormone for therapeutic use in the U.S. and elsewhere, resolving the issue of limited supplies of HGH, hence putting an end to the potential hazard in the corresponding therapy .

2. **By using genetically engineered techniques, genes encoding active proteins and peptides can be expressed efficiently in microbes, cells and even animal bioreactors or plant bioreactors, so that the physiologically active proteins and peptides can be produced on a large scale which is not readily available before, hence guarantee the clinical requirement.** *E.g.*, biosynthetic human insulin（insulin human rDNA, INN）for clinical use is manufactured by recombinant DNA technology. Biosynthetic human insulin has increased purity when compared with extracted animal insulin, which in turn reduces antibody formation. The vast majority of insulin currently used worldwide is now biosynthetic recombinant "human" insulin or its analogues. Furthermore, researchers have succeeded in introducing the gene for human insulin into plants as another method of producing insulin ("biopharming") in safflower. This technique is anticipated to reduce production costs.

3. **By using genetically engineered techniques, a sufficient amount of physiologically active substances can be offered to further dig out more information on their structure, function and characteristics, therefore enlarging the application scope of these active substances.**

4. **By using genetically engineered techniques, more and more new physiologically active substances can be explored and developed.** *e.g.*, the best sellers Erythropoietin (EPO) and Granulocyte Colony-Stimulating Factor (G-CSF), and Nerve Growth Factor (NGF), the neurotrophic peptide.

5. **Genetic engineering techniques and protein engineering techniques can be used to modify endogenous physiological active substances, therefore the physiological activity may be further elevated.** When some endogenous physiological active substances have been used as drugs, they do not work as well as expected. If that is the case, structure modification may be a smart solution to help settle the issue. For instance, after the Cys125 of interleukin-2 has been replaced with Ser125 via protein engineering, the *in vivo* half-life of the resultant recombinant IL-2 Interking（洛金，英特康欣）is significantly prolonged, hence reducing the dosage and improving the efficacy.

6. **By using genetically engineered techniques, new physiologically active substances can be obtained, hence expanding sources of pharmaceuticals.** On the basis of comprehensively analyzing

the biosynthetic gene clusters of microbial secondary metabolites and their functions, novel organic compounds —"unnatural" natural products (or artificial natural products) — can be generated by combinatorial biology（组合生物学）and genetic manipulation for biological and pharmaceutical applications, laying a foundation for the invention of new drugs. For example, significant progress has been made towards creating novel erythromycin（红霉素）analogs (For more details, see section 1.2.7.). In addition, genetically engineered antibodies, recombinant immunotoxins are also belong to unnatural biomacromolecules. They are new classes of biotherapeutics genetically engineered.

Sophisticated technology has been used to create new protein sequences that are more potent, stable, and selective than natural or modified proteins. Neoleukin 2/15 is a computationally designed mimic of IL-2 that was *de novo* designed to avoid common side effects by providing no binding site for IL-2R α subunit. It has superior therapeutic activity to IL-2 in mouse models of melanoma and colon cancer, with reduced toxicity and undetectable immunogenicity. With only 14 percent the same amino acid sequence as human IL-2, Neo-2/15 conserves most of the properties of IL-2. It is currently being commercialized into a therapeutic.

1.1.4 Genetically engineered pharmaceuticals and human genome research and post genome research（基因工程药物与人类基因组、后基因组研究）

Human Genome Project

What is The Human Genome Project?

The Human Genome Project is one of the greatest research projects of human life science history. The **Human Genome Project (HGP)** is a global scientific research program created to understand the hereditary （遗传的，世代相传的）instructions that make each of us unique. The human genome refers to all the DNA sequences and structures necessary for the synthesis of proteins, polypeptide chains and RNAs in various human cells with functions, including the sum of all the genetic information carried by DNA on 23 pairs of human chromosomes, namely the sequence of 3 billion base pairs. **The HGP will create a vast resource of detailed scientific information about the structure, organization and function of human DNA.** Scientists at the *U.S. Department of Energy (DOE)* were the first to envision（预想，设想，展望，愿景）the project, in 1986, as a project to explore newly developing DNA analysis technologies. By 1988, the *National Institutes of Health (NIH)* joined the project and a joint effort（共同努力）was formally announced in 1990, officially starting the Human Genome Project. The Department of Energy's Human Genome Program and the National Institutes of Health's National Human Genome Research Institute (NHGRI) together coordinate the HGP. The HGP's original plan was a *three-billion-dollar 15-year project* that would be completed in 2005. However, through rapid technological advances, worldwide efforts on the project have greatly accelerated, changing the expected completion date to 2003 (making the project a 13-year endeavor). *Over 1 000* researchers, including *16* institutions across *6* nations (the United States, Great Britain, France, Germany, Japan and China), are involved with the HGP. Besides the HGP, there are numerous other programs and institutions involved in genome research. At least 18 countries have established Human Genome Research programs. Some of the larger programs are in Australia, Brazil, Canada, China, Denmark, European Union（欧洲联盟，欧盟）, France, germany, Israel, Italy, Japan, Korea, Mexico, Netherlands, Russia, Sweden, United Kingdom, and the

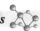

United States. Some developing countries are participating through studies of molecular biology techniques for genome research and studies of organisms that are particularly interesting to their geographical regions. The Human Genome Organisation (HUGO http://www.gene.ucl.ac.uk/hugo/) helps to coordinate international collaboration for the HGP.

The demands are great for a successful completion of the ambitious HGP goals. This effort includes working to develop a range of *new and innovative technologies*, including the establishment of a way to quickly and efficiently distribute the information to all scientists, physicians, and others worldwide so that the results may be rapidly used for the public good. In fact, this will lead to improved technology for biomedical research as an important byproduct of the HGP. From the beginning, it has been clearly recognized that acquiring and using genetic knowledge from the HGP will have significant implications（影响）for individuals and for society. The HGP is the first large scientific undertaking（事业，任务）to address（处理，解决）the *ethical, legal, and social issues* that may arise from the project. The US government also has a commitment（承诺，保证）to share the technology with the private sector（私营部分）. By licensing（许可，特许，发许可证给）technologies to private companies and awarding grants for innovative research, the project is motivating the biotechnology industry and promoting the development of new medical applications.

What are the overall goals of the HGP?

The Human Genome Project has several goals, which include *mapping*, *sequencing*, and *identifying* genes, *storing* and *analyzing* data, and *addressing* the ethical, legal, and social issues (ELSI) that may arise from the availability of personal genetic information. *Mapping* is the construction of a series of chromosome descriptions that depict the position and spacing（间距）of genes, which are on the DNA of chromosomes. ***The ultimate goal of the Human Genome Project is to decode, letter by letter, the exact sequence of all 3.2 billion nucleotide bases that make up the human genome.*** This means constructing *detailed genetic and physical maps of the human genome*. Besides determining the complete nucleotide sequence of human DNA, this includes locating the genes within the human genome. The HGP agenda also includes analyzing the genomes of several other organisms (including *E. coli*, the fruit fly, and the laboratory mouse) that are used extensively in research laboratories as model systems. Studying the genetic makeup of non-human organisms will help in understanding and deciphering the human genome.

Summary of basic HGP goals:

- *Identify* all estimated 50 000~100 000 genes in human DNA
- *Determine the sequence* of 3 billion chemical bases that make up human DNA
- Store information in databases
- Develop faster, more efficient *sequencing technologies*
- Develop tools for *data analysis*
- Map genomes of select *non-human* organisms
- Address *ethical, legal, and social issues* (ELSI) that may arise from the project

Development Course

Due to widespread international cooperation and advances in the field of genomics (especially in sequence analysis), as well as major advances in computing technology, a 'rough draft' of the genome was finished in 2000 [announced jointly by U.S. President Bill Clinton and the British Prime Minister（总

理，首相）Tony Blair on June 26, 2000], signifying human genome sequencing had entered the final stage of the comprehensive accomplishment. On July 7, 2000, the UCSC（University of California Santa Cruz，加州大学圣克鲁斯分校）Genome Bioinformatics Group released a first working draft on the web. The scientific community downloaded about 500 GB of information from the UCSC genome server in the first 24 hours of free and unrestricted access. By February 2001 Celera and the HGP scientists published details of their drafts. Special issues of *Nature* (which published the publicly funded project's scientific paper) and *Science* (which published Celera's paper) described the methods used to produce the draft sequence and offered analysis of the sequence. These drafts covered about 83% of the genome (90% of the euchromatic regions with 150 000 gaps and the order and orientation of many segments not yet established). According to *Nature*, February 15, 2001, only 1% of the human genome are protein-coding genes, and all together there are 26 500~30 000 genes. At the time of the joint publications（集体创作，合著出版物），press releases（新闻稿，通讯稿，新闻发布）announced that the project had been completed by both groups. An improved draft was announced upon the final sequencing mapping of the human genome on April 14, 2003, and the more complete draft was published, two years earlier than planned. Although this was reported to be 99% of the euchromatic human genome with 99.99% accuracy, a major quality assessment of the human genome sequence was published on May 27, 2004 indicating over 92% of sampling exceeded 99.99% accuracy which was within the intended goal. In May 2006, another milestone was passed on the way to completion of the project, when the sequence of the very last chromosome was published in *Nature*. Further analyses and papers on the HGP continue to occur.

Findings

Key findings of the draft (2001) and complete (2004) genome sequences include:

1. There are approximately 20 500 genes in human beings, the same range as in mice.

2. The human genome has significantly more segmental duplications（中段重复，大段区段性复制）(nearly identical, repeated sections of DNA) than had been previously suspected.

3. At the time when the draft sequence was published fewer than 7% of protein families appeared to be vertebrate-specific.

Accomplishment

The Human Genome Project was started in 1990 with the goal of sequencing and identifying all three billion chemical units in the human genetic instruction set（指令系统），finding the genetic roots of disease, and then developing treatments. It is considered a Mega Project（特大工程，特大项目）because the human genome has approximately 3.3 billion base pairs. With the sequence in hand, the next step was to identify the genetic variants that increase the risk for common diseases like cancer and diabetes.

Applications and proposed benefits

The sequencing of the human genome holds benefits for many fields, from molecular medicine to human evolution. The Human Genome Project, through its sequencing of the DNA, can help us understand diseases including: genotyping（基因型分型，基因型检测）of specific viruses to direct appropriate treatment; identification of mutations linked to different forms of cancer; the design of

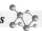

medication and more accurate prediction of their effects; advancement in forensic（法庭科学取证的）applied sciences; biofuels and other energy applications; agriculture, animal husbandry（饲养，饲养业），bioprocessing（生物工艺，通过生物物质配制法制造／处理）; risk assessment; bioarcheology（生物考古学），anthropology（人类学）and evolution. Another proposed benefit is the commercial development of genomics research related to DNA based products, a multibillion-dollar industry.

Developments

The work on interpretation and analysis of genome data is still in its initial stages. It is anticipated that detailed knowledge of the human genome will provide new avenues for advances in medicine and biotechnology. Clear practical results of the project emerged even before the work was finished. For example, a number of companies, such as Myriad Genetics, started offering easy ways to administer（给予）genetic tests that can show predisposition to a variety of illnesses, including breast cancer, hemostasis disorders（凝血异常），cystic fibrosis, liver diseases and many others. Also, the etiologies（病因学，病原学，致病源）for cancers, Alzheimer's disease and other areas of clinical interest are considered likely to benefit from genome information and possibly may lead in the long term to significant advances in their management.

There are also many tangible benefits for biologists. For example, a researcher investigating a certain form of cancer may have narrowed down his/her search to a particular gene. By visiting the human genome database on the World Wide Web, this researcher can examine what other scientists have written about this gene, including (potentially) the three-dimensional structure of its product, its function(s), its evolutionary relationships to other human genes, or to genes in mice or yeast or fruit flies, possible detrimental mutations, interactions with other genes, body tissues in which this gene is activated, and diseases associated with this gene or other datatypes. Further, a deeper understanding of the disease processes at the level of molecular biology may determine new therapeutic procedures. Given the established importance of DNA in molecular biology and its central role in determining the fundamental operation of cellular processes, it is likely that expanded knowledge in this area will facilitate medical advances in numerous areas of clinical interest that may not have been possible without them.

Whilst the project may offer significant benefits to medicine and scientific research, some authors have emphasized the need to address the potential social consequences of mapping the human genome. "Molecularizing disease and their possible cure will have a profound impact on what patients expect from medical help and the new generation of doctors' perception of illness."

Post-genome study — blazing a trail for novel pharmaceutical research and development

With the accomplishment of human genome sequencing, Post-Genome study has been launched, whose core is to decipher the functions of proteins encoded by the astronomical figure-like DNA information, as well as the regulatory functions of non-coding regions of human genome sequences.

Bioinformatics, functional genomics, especially proteomics and pharmacogenomics are closely related to the development of genetically engineered pharmaceuticals.

Through bioinformatics, new genes can be found and identified, and important disease-related genes can be confirmed through research on the functions and structures of the genes.

The human genome project was launched in 1990, although only 3% of the total DNA sequence had been analyzed, the study of the functional genome was already on the agenda and the post genomic era was already with us. The aim of the new era, the era of the proteomics, is to elucidate the expression, structure and function of all the proteins which are after all responsible for life's activities. The main techniques for the separation and identification of all the expressed proteins are two-dimentional gel electrophoresis, two-dimentional HPLC, mass spectrometry and bioinformatics. Proteome research is not only the major task in life sciences facing us in the 21st century, but also has far reaching implications（影响）in innovations for medicine, agriculture and industrial production.

The great achievement of Human Genome Research has brought the drug research and development into a new stage, which not only enables people to have an in-depth understanding of the disease mechanism and the relationship between drug-targets and disease proteins, and between drugs and disease proteins, so as to conduct（组织并实施）research on new drugs based on gene information, but also makes more gene drugs and/or genetically engineered pharmaceuticals keep emerging with the discovery of new genes.

Therefore, more and more new genetically engineered pharmaceuticals can be obtained through genetically engineered pharmaceutics. With the accomplishment of the draft human genome, a new round of gene research upsurge is underway around the world.

1.2 Development trend of genetically engineered pharmaceuticals （基因工程药物发展趋势）

In the early 1970s, the molecular biology revolution began to sweep the world. The year 1972 witnessed the born of recombinant DNA technology, which makes genetic engineering technology, the core of modern biotechnology, get rapid development.

The establishment of RECOMBINANT DNA technology in 1973 led directly to the birth of the first generation of biotechnology companies, with the main products of cytokine therapeutics and growth factor medications (protein medications).

In 1975, monoclonal antibody technology (hybridoma technology) was born, which gave birth to the second generation of biotechnology companies, with antibodies as their main products. The advantages of low toxicity and high specificity of monoclonal antibody drugs enable them to gradually replace traditional chemotherapy.

After 12 years of twists and turns since the establishment of HumAb and XenoMouse technologies in 1994, fully human monoclonal antibody drugs derived from transgenic mice were officially introduced. Ever since then, the technologies and products have been benefiting more and more patients around the world.

Biotech drugs, also called biopharmaceuticals, approved by the FDA was 13 from 1982 to 1989, 15 from 1990 to 1994, and 27 from 1995 to 1999, 43 from 2001 to 2005, 44 from 2006 to 2010, 78 from 2011 to 2015, 131 from 2016 to 2020, showing a rapid growth rate.

Before the year 2010, in the approved biopharmaceuticals in the United States, cytokines and other recombinant proteins took first place, while therapeutic monoclonal antibodies and vaccines are hotspots in the research of novel pharmaceuticals. Then the tide has turned. The year 2000 brought the R&D of monoclonal antibody therapeutics into a golden age, and thereafter antibody technologies gradually **grow to maturity**. Though the first therapeutic monoclonal antibody drug muromonab-CD3 was FDA-licenced in 1985, the harvest time of antibody therapeutics came after 2010. Among the biopharmaceuticals approved from 1995 to 1999, 15 (55.6%) were genetically engineered pharmaceuticals (recombinant proteins and antisense nucleic acids), and 7 (25.9%) were monoclonal antibodies and polyclonal antibodies. The number of antibodes therapeutics became 7 (16.3%), 10 (22.7%) and 26 (33.3%) during 2001-2005, 2006-2010 and 2011-2015 respectively, and soar to 77 (including 7 ADC) (58.8%) during 2016-2020.

Today's immune system-boosting cancer drugs are at the peak of their development thanks to several major mergers and acquisitions in 2009, which paved the way for the flourishment of fully human monoclonal antibodies today. By the year 2018, 23 fully human monoclonal antibodies have been approved worldwide with the maturity of the following technologies. Among them, 6 were generated by phage display technology, 17 by transgenic mouse technology, and 10 by Medarex technology and 5 by Abgenix technology.

The field of biologics is the most prone to becoming blockbuster products, and at present, biologics are truly the most marketable pharmaceutical products in the world.

At present (by April 8, 2023, according to **https://data.pharmacodia.com**), there are over 1500 (1571) biologics have been approved worldwide, and over 3700 (3745) kinds of biopharmaceuticals are under research and development, forming a huge high-tech industry and producing immeasurable social and economic benefits. There is no doubt that the 21st century is the century of life science, meanwhile the century of biotechnology.

In terms of the categories of biologics, **genetically engineered pharmaceuticals, the core of biopharmaceuticals, is** one of the most successful fields in the biotech industry, **also an important direction for new drug research and development.** It is of great significance in the aspects of prevention and control of major diseases endangering human health. They are mainly targeted at diseases such as tumors, infectious diseases, AIDS/HIV infections and related diseases, autoimmune diseases, organ transplantation, cardiovascular diseases, neurological disorders, respiratory diseases, diabetes, *etc*. Up to now, cancer becomes a chronic disease that can be controlled.

Despite all kinds of favorable policies and increasing financial input, facing the increasingly changeable external environment, the biologics industry will face both opportunities and challenges.

The medical and health industry is characterized by high investment, high risk, long cycle and high return, which requires huge financial support, especially the research and development of biological innovation new drugs.

The ever-increasing aging population, the high incidence of cancer, neuropsychiatric diseases and other diseases, result in increased demand for biologics; This has brought about great opportunities for the development of biologics. Furthermore, biotech companies are increasingly favored by the **global Capital market. From a technology innovation point of view,** the deep integration of **artificial intelligence (AI), big data, cloud computing** and other emerging technologies in the biomedical industry accelerates the innovation process of the biopharmaceutical industry; The growing maturity of biotechnology, such as gene editing and cell therapy, offers the possibility of cures for diseases such as tumors and neurological disorders.

The R&D of the next generation of computational design-driven drugs combines **AI** with biophysics for drug research and development and high-throughput experiments, explores the underlying logic of drug research and development from multiple dimensions by studying the interactions between proteins, resolves multi-level issues such as protein dynamic structure, free energy state and functional action mechanism, and focuses on early discovery of therapeutic drugs by characterizing **protein-protein interactions (PPI)**.

With the continuous improvement of biotechnology and residents' economic level, the domestic demand for biologics has been surging; With the vigorous support of the government to the biological industry, the market size of the biologics industry is expected to continue to maintain rapid growth.

Driven by such factors as technological innovation and residents' awareness of health care, the biologics market in China will expand rapidly in the future, and the market size is expected to reach more than 640 billion yuan in 2023.

The Future of Monoclonal Antibodies

It is difficult to predict what the future of antibody humanization will look like. Over time, the humanization process of mouse-derived antibodies has become much more sophisticated, with several companies **now** performing *in silico* optimization of CDRs for T-cell epitope avoidance to reduce immunogenicity. Yeast display is a new technology that in theory avoids some of the disadvantages of the phage display process for monoclonal antibody generation. Newer transgenic mice that have a fuller complement of human antibody genes are also being used to develop a new generation of fully human monoclonal antibodies.

Since the first ADC drug came into the market in 2000, ADC had been in the uneventful stages in the industry. Until 2019, FDA successively approved three ADC drugs (Polivy, PADCEV and Enhertu). On January 22, 2020, the China National Medical Products Administration (NMPA) officially approved the novel HER2-targeted agent Kadcyla® (Trastuzumab Emtansine), which ushered in the growth spurt period of ADC drugs that had been once stagnant.

CAR-T therapy

CAR-T therapy has a good therapeutic effect. It has the potential to become a first-line therapy, with huge market potential. With the continuous development of CAR-T technology, new technologies such as superb tumor-infiltrating T lymphocyte therapy and neoantigen-targeted T cell therapy are expected to break through the previous checkpoint in the treatment of solid tumors.

In addition, the R&D of generic CAR-T therapies could reduce costs and improve drug accessibility.

Vaccines, a special class of drugs

With the development of immunology, biochemistry, molecular microbiology and biotechnology, global vaccine development entered a stage of rapid development in the second half of the 20th century.

From the point of view of technical route and preparation process, vaccines can be divided into the following three generations: the first generation of vaccines (inactivated vaccines, attenuated vaccines, *etc*.); the second generation vaccines (subunit vaccines made from natural components of microorganisms and their products, and recombinant protein vaccines produced by recombining the genes of components that can elicit an immune response); and the third generation vaccine (nucleic acid vaccine represented by mRNA vaccines, DNA vaccines and recombinant viral vector vaccines).

Though the new generation vaccine R&D has the advantages of a shorter development cycle and higher generality (普遍性) of production platform, mRNA vaccine technology is not mature to be used in

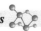

immune prophylaxis and therapy. As the representative of the new generation, the mRNA vaccine R&D needs to be further developed and improved in the aspects of mRNA stability, preparation technology and delivery technology. While DNA vaccine is temperature-stable and cold-chain free, and the DNA plasmid manufacture process allows for scalable manufacture of drug products (*e.g.*, through fermentation of *E. coli*). Therefore, in the near future, those generations of vaccines will coexist for quite sometime.

The Vaccine Administration Law enacted in 2019 is the world's first comprehensive vaccine management law, which further clarifies at the legal level the need to increase investment in vaccine research and development, and includes the development, production and storage of vaccines for disease prevention and control into the national strategy, thus creating a favorable environment for the development of the vaccine industry.

Influenced by the epidemic of the COVID-19, the research and development of the COVID-19 vaccine has improved the prosperity of the vaccine industry, the public has realized the importance of vaccination for disease prevention and control, the awareness and willingness for vaccination have increased, and the market demand for the vaccine is expected to further expand.

1.2.1 New mode of research & development of new type biopharmaceuticals（研发新型生物药物的新模式）

Until the late 20th century, drug discovery was largely based on the screening and detection of hundreds of thousands of chemical or natural molecules. The research & development process is time-consuming, and expensive, whereas success is usually happening serendipitously（偶然）. With the draft of the human genome completed ahead of schedule in June 2000, the era of the genome revolution, the third technological revolution after the industrial revolution and the computer revolution, has arrived. The rapid development in the burgeoning（迅速生长的）field of bioscience and bioengineering research, such as genomics, proteomics, bioinformatics, high-throughput screening, protein engineering, glycosylation engineering, and metabolic engineering, allows the rapid design and rapid discovery of new drugs (including proteins, nucleic acids and small-molecule drugs) on a rational basis, which accelerates the research & development of new biopharmaceuticals, especially genetically engineered pharmaceuticals, hence bringing about dramatically increased numbers of new biopharmaceuticals and new drug targets, and greatly elevated clinical effectiveness and drug safety in the recent decade.

Fig. 1-6 summarizes the process of research & development of new biopharmaceuticals. Biotechnology is the key to the discovery of biopharmaceuticals, and is used throughout the whole process of research & development of biopharmaceuticals, especially genetically engineered pharmaceuticals. The study of bioinformatics of human genome brings the understanding of human diseases into the molecular level and provides the basis for the discovery and confirmation of new drug targets. The research on the relationship between the structure and biological activity of functional proteins makes it possible to design new biopharmaceutical molecules. The new technology of genetic recombination is used to generate a biomolecular library, from which new bioactive molecules can be selected via high-throughput screening, and made into new biopharmaceuticals through research & development of downstream engineering. Furthermore, new dosage forms would make them more effective in the treatment.

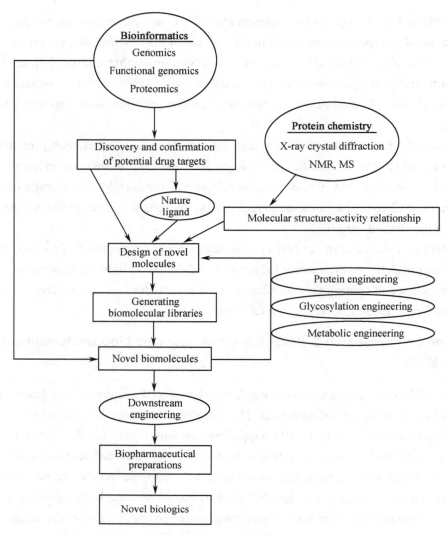

Fig. 1-6   Development process of new biopharmaceuticals.

The Post Genomic Era: what does it all mean?

Information may no longer be a bottleneck to understanding and tackling（着手处理，解决）complex genetic diseases such as cancer. For those who cut their research teeth（初试牛刀，初获经验）not so very long ago, before PCR was thought of by Kary Mullis, this is truly an amazing（令人惊异的）position to be in. To think that effective management of cancer is potentially just a time and money issue equation（制衡局面）, where new disease causation data needs to be converted into novel targeted or personalized therapies, how can we eliminate drug discovery economics as an overriding（高于一切的，最重要的）limiting factor?

For the past couple of decades, advances in genome sequencing and research have been exponential. Moreover, we are probably not seeing a plateau in these capabilities yet and even now we have literally hundreds of potential new targets in cancer alone to pursue new therapies. So what now must be done to speed up the translation of these targets into drugs?

One of the first issues is that many candidates are not directly 'drugable' and thus require additional searches downstream for drugable proteins. The second issue is that many putative new cancer targets are low in frequency, making them challenging to pick up by biotech and pharma （制药公司） until new information on their role in normal and disease biology is defined; especially if they can be placed in higher frequency cancer pathways. This is one area, therefore, that academia can have a major impact on by continuing to de-orphan these targets and perhaps even perform end-to-end （端对端的） drug discovery. Finally, new technologies are sorely （非常） needed to reduce the large amounts of time, money and attrition （磨损，消耗） associated with all stages of drug discovery and development, in particular those associated with performing large and unselected clinical trials.

Academia and industry must heavily invest in a post-genomics world; firstly to understand "what it all means", *i.e.*, decipher which genetic variations are consequential and which are merely random noise; secondly, design early and accurate diagnostic tests to enable potentially remedial therapies to be given before cancers become incurable; and thirdly, to have accurate and predictive models of human cancer, so that novel treatments can be developed quicker and directed to the patients most likely to respond. Such focused drug development will not only be faster and more likely to succeed, but also be more ethical to the patient, who has a better chance of entering into a worthwhile trial. To usher in （使开始，迎来，迎接） this new era of high-throughput functional genomics, predictive disease modelling and ultimately the design of rational clinical trials, scientists will need to be able to alter the DNA-sequence of a human cellular genome in a manner that is now routine and facile （易做到的，轻而易举的） in mice and other lower organisms.

Why are we moving towards "personalized" medicine?

Very few diseases are simple. They are either highly multi-factorial （多因子的） like cancer, and so require many different treatments tailored to the right patient; or they can be caused by a single agent, such as HIV or a bacterial infection, but it mutates over time; and thus requires doctors to keep rapid pace with a moving target. In the case of cancer it is both these things, which makes it such a challenge to manage. In the future, however, we will have the ability to rationally prescribe and adapt the right drug, drug combination, or drug dose, to each patient based on having a detailed understanding of their disease genetics, to far more effectively manage their disease.

This is, in essence, the concept of personalized medicine; a phenomenon that is already happening, but has a long way to go to realize its full potential. The principle issue is that there are currently nowhere （不存在的，没有的） near enough drugs in the personalized medicine toolbox to tailor to the right patients. The reality is we have only scratched （抓） the surface of "drugging" （用药于，给……用药） the cancer genome and will fail to do so in the present generation unless some hard decisions are made. Another issue is that an entirely new industry and service needs to be developed to provide early, routine and accurate diagnostic tests to support the development and tailoring of any future novel therapies, which has its own harsh economic models to deal with if performed outside of the established pharma industry. Finally, regulatory and healthcare agencies will need to foster these endeavors and ultimately be convinced of why this isn't going to cost them a lot more money. Wisdom would predict this will be true, given that it will enable us to move away from blanket （通用，不容例外，不加区分） or over-prescription （处方过量） of expensive new drugs, where we are again only at the tip of the iceberg right now.

The stark facts （极明显的事实） are that for every drug developed, approximately nine fail and the cost of these failures is ultimately passed on to the consumer. Combined with the approximate 10 years and $1 billion spent per drug to reach Phase Ⅲ and then fail, this is clearly an unsustainable situation moving forward into a more personalized, or segmented（分割，细分）, therapy world. There will be many reasons why drugs fail, but one that in principle can be fixed is to better understand which patients are more or less likely to respond. With the advent of clinical diagnostics and accurate models of human disease, new drugs in development or even already approved treatments, can increasingly be targeted to the "right" patient populations who possess unambiguous "biomarker" signatures（明显特征，识别标记）of response.

Disease models in early stage drug discovery

Coming now to applications of gene targeting and genetically-defined disease models, the first thing any drug developer has to do is to choose a specific target, preferably a good one given how long and expensive it is. However, prior to recent largescale, consortium（财团）-based, cancer genome profiling （扼要描述）efforts, choosing a "good" cancer target was very hard to qualify or quantitate in some way. All too often a "validated"（证实，验证，确认）target was simply one that another company was working on, but not too many as this would be overly（过度地，极度地）competitive. True disease validation was effectively minimal, with elevated expression or perceived pathway relevance typically being the best marker of cancer relevance, which is often misleading.

DNA-alterations (mutations and/or copy number gains or losses) in contrast, are unambiguous events and, if present in high enough frequency in a cancer type, are, more often than not, key drivers of the disease. Now we have a plethora of such information, several new issues actually arise: Firstly, most "cancer genes" are tumor suppressors, which are either inactivated or completely lost in tumors, and thus are unrealistic targets for small-molecules that are typically easier to design as inhibitors of protein function. Secondly, many gain-of-function（功能获得性，获得功能，功能的获得）"oncogenes" are also hard to drug, such as nonenzymatic transcription factors. Thirdly and of practical importance, most newly identified candidate cancer genes, including the drugable ones, have very low tumor mutation frequencies (often <5%), which could simply represent passenger "noise" in genetically unstable tumors. Due to all these factors, there is currently a heavy operational bias towards drugging signalling pathway kinases, which if directly implicated in disease progression can be highly effective, but are also subject to a rapid onset of resistance via compensatory signalling pathways or events. This may also be exacerbated （加重，使……恶化）by the typical cytostatic（抑制细胞生长的）nature（特点）seen for single agent pathway-targeted drugs.

All this represents a major challenge for the next wave of targeted drug discovery. In the conventional arena（舞台，竞技场）, we need to find more functionally characterized targets, *i.e.*, which of the many mutant genes are drivers vs（对，相对）passengers, and then determine which of these stack-up（层叠） into more frequent mutated pathways so that become viable（可行的）for drug developers. Here the ability to alter gene function positively and negatively will enable the dissection（解剖，详细查究）of their normal vs disease biology. Moreover, the pointed（明确的）search for key downstream effectors of undrugable genes will be significantly aided by simple "isogenic"（同基因的，等基因的）model systems, which will enable high-throughput expression profiling and siRNA screens to be performed. Such isogenic "X-MAN" (gene-X; Mutant And Normal) cell-lines are being created by Horizon Discovery（a UK biotechnology company）using rAAV, which comprised thousands of different disease models based on internal production and the establishment of 50 academic centers of excellence.

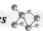

As well as feeding（注入，得到滋养）the conventional drug discovery process, X-MAN disease models can also be used in "chemical genetic" screens to identify new drugable targets that impact tumor-specific defects, especially those that are undrugable tumor suppressors. Moreover, if the compound libraries are chosen wisely, *i.e.*, *in vivo* validated compounds, perhaps even isolate drug candidates directly. Many examples of such "synthetically lethality"（杀伤力，致死性，致死率，致死现象）screens are now being described, the most notable and advanced of which is the toxic interaction of inhibiting PARP（poly-ADP-ribose polymerase，聚腺苷二磷酸-核糖聚合酶）activity in BRCA2-null cancers. This observation first gleaned from an isogenic BRCA-2 null mES cell system, is now being used to successfully treat BRCA-null breast cancer patients.

Disease models in later stages of drug discovery

In conventional drug discovery, once sufficient "ontarget"（正确的，准确的，精确的）chemistry has been obtained, sufficient ontarget biology is next addressed. The question then arises, however, what is sufficient on-target biology? One could argue that this should be the selective death of tumor cells harboring（怀有）specific cancer causing mutations given the direction we like to take as a field. At this stage, X-MAN disease models can be assayed for target patient-specific activity *in vitro* or in animal models, which often reveal phenotypes and drug effects that were unexpected. Moreover, if a target patient population is unknown, a wide range of patient-genotypes can be rapidly profiled prospectively（可能，潜在，预期）*in vitro* for those that are likely to respond the best. Together, these profiling tools will allow the design of smaller clinical trials centered on the patients most likely to respond, and if a drug fails here, it fails quickly rather than continuing for many years in larger trials, probably to the same result. The massive amounts of money saved can then be used to bring a wider set of next-generation targets and drugs into the same efficient process, allowing the best chance for single agents to show anticancer activity, and thus build a diverse enough drug portfolio（公文包，集，组合）to be mixed and matched in the right ways. This is ultimately where we will need to be to significantly impact cancer. Moreover, this strategy will form a sustainable biotechnology model moving forward.

Supporting this concept is AstraZeneca's Iressa (gefitinib), the first clear example of how knowing ahead of time which patients would respond (in this case mutant EGFR lung cancer patients) could have saved many development years and dollars. We also know now that in addition to primary "sensitivity biomarkers", one also needs to define other pre-existing, or treatment acquired alterations, that cause drug resistance. Here genome editing techniques can be used to create isogenic（同基因的）models that harbor defined combinations of disease causing and/or candidate drug resistance genes and then used to prospectively profile for potential resistance mechanisms.

As a landmark example of this approach, Horizon's co-founder Alberto Bardelli and research colleagues used X-MAN disease models harboring different K-Ras variants (G12V and G13D) to test whether they are both equally resistant to Cetuximab（西妥昔单抗）therapy. *In vitro* proliferation assays and xenografted tumors both demonstrated unambiguously that G13D and WT K-Ras containing cells were highly responsive to Cetuximab, whereas G12V containing cells were not. Subsequent sequence analysis of tumor samples taken from actual patients treated with Cetuximab confirmed this picture; and thus with follow-up prospective clinical trials, these data may lead to changes in the rules for prescribing EGFR targeted therapies in colon cancer, where currently patients carrying any K-Ras mutation are excluded from therapy. Isogenic models will also form the ideal tool to rationally find rational drug combinations to reverse （颠倒，倒转）resistance.

One final area where genetically-defined disease models will help both the later stages of drug development and the prescription of approved drugs is in the development of reliable diagnostic kits and platforms. Armed with isogenic gDNA, which can be mixed in fixed proportions to mimic the heterogenous nature of tumor samples, these will form the perfect precision standards to determine the performance envelope （安全性能范围）of emerging diagnostics （新型的诊断）and as patient-relevant controls for CLIA （chemiluminescent immunoassay, 化学发光免疫测定）labs running them.

Concluding remarks

Personalized therapies and diagnostics represent the logical direction for providing effective cancer therapy in the future and for the most part, the pharma industry has embraced these ideals; especially since healthcare reimbursers （偿还，报销）are moving to a system where they pay handsomely （慷慨地）for effective medicines and not at all for marginal ones. There is still a limit to how infrequent （罕见的，稀少的，不频发的）a target industry will currently tackle （处理）, so it is imperative for new functional genomics technologies and genetically defined disease models to connect the dots. Given the complexity of future clinical trials, pharmaceutical companies will probably continue the trend of focusing on late stage development and divesting （抛弃）early-stage research. Here, predictive and patient relevant disease models will enable the triage （分类，伤病员鉴别分类，病人筛选）of patients into more focused trials with greater certainty of a positive outcome and drug approval; and at earlier stages of drug discovery, will enable academia and biotechnology companies to increasingly feed （供给）validated （确证，验证）targets and drug candidates into pharma in a sustainable way. Finally, as a society, it would pay for us to explore ways to incentivize （激励）academia and industry to perform research on the wide diversity of rare cancer targets now presented to us, such as targeted translational funding （转化资金）for academia, early pre-approval from successful focused clinical trials and extended patent lifetimes for industry on any new "first-in-class" （首创的，创新的）drugs. These measures would stimulate in an entrepreneurial （企业家的，创业者的，中间商的）way the breadth （广度）of research and drugs we need; and once available, will likely have larger patient populations than anticipated once they are studied and combined in the right ways.

1.2.2 Human genome project and research and development of novel genetically engineered pharmaceuticals （人类基因组计划与基因工程新药的研发）

Although there are about 5 000 drugs on the market, the drug targets for the pharmaceutical industry are only about 500, among which 45% are cell membrane receptors, 28% are enzymes, the rest are hormones, ion channels, nuclear receptors and DNAs, and about 7% is unknown, therefore the discovery of targets become the main limiting factors in the process of new drug discovery. The Human Genome Project (HGP) has been changing the traditional drug discovery paradigm （范例，样式）, making a great impact on the discovery of new drugs.

The accomplishment of the draft human genome had helped discover new drug targets by at least one order of magnitude. Of the 30 000 to 40 000 genes predicted by Human Genome Research, about 3 000 to 10 000 are possible drug targets. Potential drug targets can be predicted via homology analysis by aligning and comparing the unknown DNA sequences with that of a known drug target, as well as by identifying genes with single nucleotide polymorphisms (SNP) markers, which is particularly important

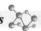

for the analysis of polygenic (多基因遗传的) diseases. As functional genomics and proteomics techniques have been developed rapidly, they have been applied in the confirmation of drug targets and the discovery of alternative approaches for drug action. For example, biochip technology (mainly refers to the DNA chip technology, also known as DNA microarray technology) can be used to compare gene expression patterns of different tissues/cells, study the differences in gene expression between the normal and pathological tissues, establish gene expression models of a model organism or host cell, set up models for pathogen gene expression, study the changes in gene expression after the drug acting on the cells. In addition, biochips can be used as a technology platform for ultra-high throughput drug screening, simultaneously detecting the change of the levels of tens of thousands of genes or proteins, hence playing an important role in the research of pharmacogenomics and toxicology, and widely used in drug R&D.

In addition, the human genome project opens up more possibilities for searching for new therapeutic genes. New genetically engineered therapeutics can be found directly from genome sequences. Almost as soon as the human genome project got started, many companies in the United States began taking the lead to develop genomic drugs. The human genome sciences (HGS，人类基因组科学公司) was one step ahead in this field. While seeking for potential drug targets from membrane proteins (including growth factor receptors, neurotransmitter receptors and cytokine receptors, *etc.*), it devoted to discovering secretory proteins (*i.e.*, hormones, growth factors and cytokines, *etc.*) as well, and managed to search & develop new genetically engineered therapeutics. A number of genetically engineered drugs were discovered and entered into clinical studies one after another (such as MPIF-1, KGF-2, VEGF-2, *etc.*) .

In 2000, HGS announced that its product B Lymphocyte Stimulator (BLyS，B 淋巴细胞刺激因子) had been approved by the US FDA as an orphan drug, with the main indication being Common Variable Immunodeficiency Disease (CVID，常见变异型免疫缺陷病). CVID patients cannot produce normal amounts of immunoglobulin, so they cannot resist the infection of bacteria, viruses, *etc*. The use of BLyS can help patients produce their own antibodies, which might protect them from infection.

BLyS is a human protein, a cytokine that belongs to the tumor necrosis factor (TNF) ligand family. This cytokine is expressed in B cell lineage cells, and acts as a potent B cell activator. It has been also shown to play an important role in the proliferation and differentiation of B cells. BLyS is one of the most important cytokines involved in the modulation of the immune system. As an immunostimulant, BLyS is necessary for maintaining normal immunity. An inadequate level of BLyS will fail to activate B cells to produce enough immunoglobulin and will lead to immunodeficiency. With the discovery of BLyS, effective treatment can be achieved toward a variety of serious diseases caused by B cell injury, such as immune deficiency, autoimmune disease and B cell tumor.

The R&D of these drugs integrates the latest advances in genomics, proteomics, bioinformatics, *etc*. The prospect of genomic medicine is terribly attractive given that 10 "blockbusters" out of the 2 000 secretory proteins known before the human genome project began to be developed. Though the fruits of the human genome project would be shared by all mankind, researching and developing gene therapeutic agents is protected by intellectual property laws. In November 1998, the United States Patent and Trademark Office (USPTO) granted Incyte (因塞特制药公司) the first patent of EST (expression sequence marker) in the company's history. Therefore, the exploitation, utilization and protection of genetic resources has become extremely urgent for all humanity, especially in developing countries.

DNA microarray/Biochip 生物芯片技术

A **DNA microarray** (also commonly known as DNA chip or biochip) is a collection of microscopic DNA spots attached to a solid surface. Scientists use DNA microarrays to make certain of the presence of particular genes in a biological sample, measure the expression levels of large numbers of genes simultaneously or to genotype multiple regions of a genome. Each DNA spot contains picomoles (10^{-12} moles) of a specific DNA sequence, known as *probes* (or *reporters* or *oligos*). These can be a short section of a gene or other DNA element that is used to hybridize a cDNA or cRNA (also called antisense RNA) sample (called *target*) under high-stringency conditions. Probe-target hybridization is usually detected and quantified by detection of fluorophore-, silver-, or chemiluminescence-labeled targets to determine relative abundance of nucleic acid sequences in the target（Fig. 1-7）.

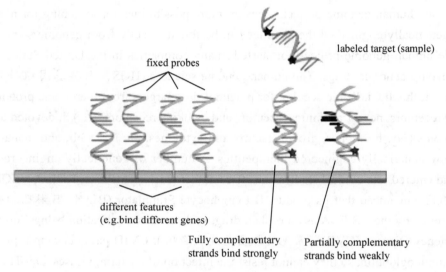

Fig. 1-7.　**Hybridization of the target to the probe.**

In molecular biology, **biochips** are essentially miniaturized（使小型化，使微型化）laboratories that can perform hundreds or thousands of simultaneous biochemical reactions. Biochips enable researchers to quickly screen large numbers of biological analytes for a variety of purposes, from disease diagnosis (identifying the underlying genetic cause of a particular disease to expedite appropriate care and support) to detection of bioterrorism（生物恐怖主义）agents.

Principle

The core principle behind microarrays is hybridization between two DNA strands, the property of complementary nucleic acid sequences to specifically pair with each other by forming hydrogen bonds between complementary nucleotide base pairs. A high number of complementary base pairs in a nucleotide sequence means tighter non-covalent bonding between the two strands. After washing off non-specific binding sequences, only strongly paired strands will remain hybridized. Fluorescently labeled target sequences that bind to a probe sequence generate a signal that depends on the hybridization conditions (such as temperature), and washing after hybridization. Total strength of the signal, from a spot (feature 模块), depends upon the amount of target sample binding to the probes present on that spot. Microarrays use relative quantitation in which the intensity of a feature is compared to the intensity of the same feature under a different condition, and the identity of the feature is known by its position.

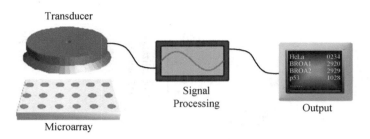

Fig. 1-8 Biochips are a platform that require, in addition to microarray technology, transduction and signal processing technologies to output the results of sensing experiments.

Fig. 1-8 shows the makeup of a typical biochip platform. The actual sensing component (or "chip") is just one piece of a complete analysis system. Transduction (转换) must be done to translate the actual sensing event (DNA binding, oxidation/reduction, *etc.*) into a format (格式，方式) understandable by a computer (voltage, light intensity, mass, *etc.*), which then enables additional analysis and processing to produce a final, human-readable output. The multiple technologies needed to make a successful biochip — from sensing chemistry, to microarraying (微阵列), to signal processing — require a true multidisciplinary approach, making the barrier to entry steep. One of the first commercial biochips was introduced by Affymetrix. Their "GeneChip" products contain thousands of individual DNA sensors for use in sensing defects, or single nucleotide polymorphisms (SNPs), in genes such as p53 (a tumor suppressor) and BRCA1 and BRCA2 (related to breast cancer). The chips are produced using microlithography techniques traditionally used to fabricate (制造) integrated circuits (集成电路) (see below).

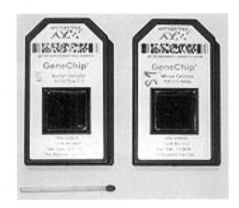

Two Affymetrix chips. A match is shown at bottom left for size comparison.

Uses and types

Many types of arrays exist and the broadest distinction is whether they are spatially arranged on a surface or on coded beads:

• The traditional solid-phase array is a collection of orderly microscopic "spots", called features, each with thousands of identical and specific probes attached to a solid surface, such as glass, plastic, or silicon biochip (commonly known as a *genome chip*, *DNA chip* or *gene array*). Thousands of these features can be placed in known locations on a single DNA microarray.

• The alternative bead array is a collection of microscopic polystyrene (聚苯乙烯) beads, each with a specific probe and a ratio of two or more dyes, which do not interfere with the fluorescent dyes used on the target sequence.

DNA microarrays can be used to detect DNA (as in comparative genomic hybridization), or detect RNA (most commonly as cDNA after reverse transcription) that may or may not be translated into proteins. The process of measuring gene expression via cDNA is called expression analysis or expression profiling (分析，概况) (Fig. 1-9).

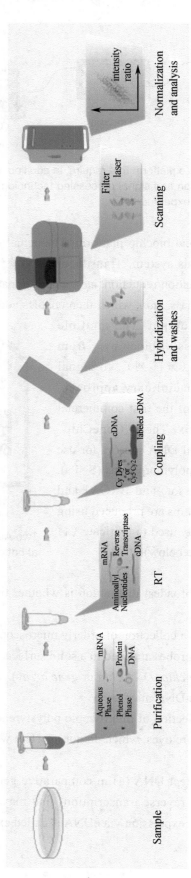

Fig. 1-9   The steps required in a microarray experiment.

Applications of DNA microarrays are listed in Table 1-2.

Table 1-2   Applications of DNA microarrays

Application or technology	Synopsis （概要，大纲）
Gene expression profiling	In an mRNA or gene expression profiling experiment the expression levels of thousands of genes are simultaneously monitored to study the effects of certain treatments, diseases, and developmental stages on gene expression. For example, microarray-based gene expression profiling can be used to identify genes whose expression is changed in response to pathogens or other organisms by comparing gene expression in infected to that in uninfected cells or tissues.
Comparative genomic hybridization	Assessing genome content in different cells or closely related organisms.
GeneID	Small microarrays to check IDs of organisms in food and feed (like GMO), mycoplasms （支原体） in cell culture, or pathogens for disease detection, mostly combining PCR and microarray technology.
Chromatin （染色质） immunoprecipitation on Chip (ChIP)	DNA sequences bound to a particular protein can be isolated by immunoprecipitating that protein (ChIP), these fragments can be then hybridized to a microarray [such as a tiling array （瓦片阵列，嵌合阵列）] allowing the determination of protein binding site occupancy throughout the genome. Example protein to immunoprecipitate are histone modifications (H3K27me3, H3K4me2, H3K9me3, *etc.*), Polycomb-group protein （多梳家族蛋白） (PRC2:Suz12, PRC1:YY1) and trithorax-group protein （三空腔结构蛋白质组） (Ash1) to study the epigenetic （表观遗传的，后生的） landscape or RNA Polymerase II to study the transcription landscape.
DamID （DNA 腺嘌呤甲基转移酶鉴定法，DNA adenine methyltransferase identification）	Analogously to ChIP, genomic regions bound by a protein of interest can be isolated and used to probe a microarray to determine binding site occupancy. Unlike ChIP, DamID does not require antibodies but makes use of adenine methylation near the protein's binding sites to selectively amplify those regions, introduced by expressing minute amounts of protein of interest fused to bacterial DNA adenine methyltransferase.
SNP detection	Identifying single nucleotide polymorphism （SNP，单核苷酸多态性） among alleles within or between populations. Several applications of microarrays make use of SNP detection, including Genotyping （基因型分型）, forensic analysis, measuring predisposition to disease, identifying drug-candidates, evaluating germline mutations in individuals or somatic mutations （体细胞突变） in cancers, assessing loss of heterozygosity （杂合性，异型接合性）, or genetic linkage （遗传连锁，基因连锁） analysis.
Alternative splicing detection	An *exon junction array* design uses probes specific to the expected or potential splice sites of predicted exons for a gene. It is of intermediate density, or coverage, to a typical gene expression array (with 1~3 probes per gene) and a genomic tiling array (with hundreds or thousands of probes per gene). It is used to assay the expression of alternative splice forms of a gene. Exon arrays have a different design, employing probes designed to detect each individual exon for known or predicted genes, and can be used for detecting different splicing isoforms.
Fusion genes microarray	A fusion gene microarray can detect fusion transcripts, *e.g.*, from cancer specimens. The principle behind this is building on the alternative splicing （选择性拼接） microarrays. The oligo design strategy enables combined measurements of chimeric transcript junctions with exon-wise measurements of individual fusion partners.
Tiling array	Genome tiling arrays consist of overlapping probes designed to densely represent a genomic region of interest, sometimes as large as an entire human chromosome. The purpose is to empirically detect expression of transcripts or alternatively spliced forms which may not have been previously known or predicted.

continued

Application or technology	Synopsis（概要，大纲）
Double-stranded B-DNA microarrays	Right-handed double-stranded B-DNA microarrays can be used to characterize novel drugs and biologicals that can be employed to bind specific regions of immobilized, intact, double-stranded DNA. This approach can be used to inhibit gene expression. They also allow for characterization of their structure under different environmental conditions.
Double-stranded Z-DNA microarrays	Left-handed double-stranded Z-DNA microarrays can be used to identify short sequences of the alternative Z-DNA structure located within longer stretches of right-handed B-DNA genes (*e.g.*, transcriptional enhancement, recombination, RNA editing). The microarrays also allow for characterization of their structure under different environmental conditions.
Multi-stranded DNA microarrays (triplex-DNA microarrays and quadruplex-DNA microarrays)	Multi-stranded DNA and RNA microarrays can be used to identify novel drugs that bind to these multi-stranded nucleic acid sequences. This approach can be used to discover new drugs and biologicals that have the ability to inhibit gene expression. These microarrays also, allow for characterization of their structure under different environmental conditions.

GMO—基因改造生物（genetically modified organism）

Protein biochip array and other microarray technologies

Microarrays are not limited to DNA analysis; protein microarrays, antibody microarray, chemical compound microarrays can also be produced using biochips. Randox Laboratories Ltd. launched Evidence, the first protein Biochip Array Technology analyzer in 2003. In protein Biochip Array Technology, the biochip replaces the ELISA [酶联免疫吸附测定(enzyme-linked immunosorbent assay)] plate or cuvette（透明小容器，小池，吸收池）as the reaction platform. The biochip is used to simultaneously analyze a panel of related tests in a single sample, producing a patient profile. The patient profile can be used in disease screening, diagnosis, monitoring disease progression or monitoring treatment. Performing multiple analyses simultaneously, described as multiplexing（多路技术），allows a significant reduction in processing time and the amount of patient sample required. Biochip Array Technology is a novel application of a familiar methodology, using sandwich, competitive and antibody-capture immunoassays. The difference from conventional immunoassays is that the capture ligands are covalently attached to the surface of the biochip in an ordered array rather than in solution.

In sandwich assays an enzyme-labeled antibody is used; in competitive assays an enzyme-labeled antigen is used. On antibody-antigen binding a chemiluminescence（化学发光）reaction produces light. Detection is by a charge-coupled device（CCD，电荷耦合装置/器件）camera. The CCD camera is a sensitive and high-resolution sensor able to accurately detect and quantify very low levels of light. The test regions are located using a grid pattern（网格图形，网格模式）then the chemiluminescence signals are analyzed by imaging software to rapidly and simultaneously quantify the individual analytes.

1.2.3 Discovery of drug target natural ligand and development of new drug（药物靶标天然配基的发现与新药的研发）

When a protein is affirmed to be a new therapeutic target, theoretically speaking, its natural ligand is exactly a new therapeutic candidate. Therefore, the study on the relationship between ligand-targetbinding propensity and biological activity can provide information for designing new biological molecules. The main methods of seeking natural ligands for therapeutic targets include mass spectrometry, yeast two-hybrid systems and display technology.

1.2.3.1 *Mass spectrometry*（质谱）

Treat the cell lysate with beads that have been fixed with therapeutic target molecules (such as receptors) to allow affinity binding to occur, then get rid of the impurity molecules that non-specifically bind to the beads, and finally elute（洗提，洗脱）the bound ligands with some specific solution. The specifically bound molecules were then hydrolyzed with protease and the resultant peptide segments were analyzed via mass spectrometry. A ligand cannot be identified directly by just knowing the molecular weight of the resultant peptide segment from protease hydrolysis, but the resultant peptide spectra can be compared with the hydrolyzed segment spectra of theoretically all possible proteins in a proteome to find the most matched sequences. The sensitivity of Mass spectra allows it to be successfully used to detect some components of a protein complex, such as nuclear pore complex of yeast, chloroplast of peal and protein components of the interchromatin granules (IG) of yeast.

1.2.3.2 *Two-hybrid screening*（双杂交系统）

Two-hybrid screening (also known as **yeast two-hybrid system** or **Y2H**) is a molecular biology technique used to discover **protein-protein interactions** (**PPIs**) and protein-DNA interactions by testing for physical interactions (such as binding) between two proteins or a single protein and a DNA molecule, respectively.

The premise behind the test is the activation of downstream reporter gene(s) by the binding of a transcription factor onto an upstream activating sequence（UAS，上游激活序列）. For two-hybrid screening, the transcription factor is split into two separate fragments, called the **binding domain (BD)** and **activating domain (AD)**. The BD is the domain responsible for binding to the UAS and the AD is the domain responsible for the activation of transcription. The Y2H is thus a protein-fragment complementation assay（蛋白质片段互补测定法）.

History

Pioneered by Stanley Fields and Ok-Kyu Song in 1989, the technique was originally designed to detect protein-protein interactions using the GAL4 transcriptional activator of the yeast *Saccharomyces cerevisiae*（酿酒酵母）. The GAL4 protein activated transcription of a protein involved in galactose（半乳糖）utilization, which formed the basis of selection. Since then, the same principle has been adapted to describe many alternative methods, including some that detect protein-DNA interactions or DNA-DNA interactions, as well as methods that use *Escherichia coli* instead of yeast.

Basic premise

The key to the two-hybrid screen is that in most eukaryotic transcription factors, the activating and binding domains are modular（模块化的，组件的，组合的）and can function in proximity to each other without direct binding. This means that even though the transcription factor is split into two fragments, it can still activate transcription when the two fragments are indirectly connected.

The most common screening approach is the **yeast two-hybrid assay**. This system often utilizes a **genetically engineered strain of yeast** in which the biosynthesis of certain nutrients (usually amino acids or nucleic acids) is lacking. When grown on media that lacks these nutrients, the yeast fail to survive. This mutant yeast strain can be made to incorporate foreign DNA in the form of plasmids. In yeast two-hybrid screening, separate bait and prey plasmids are simultaneously introduced into the mutant yeast strain.

A plasmid is engineered to produce **a protein product** in which **the DNA-binding domain (BD) fragment** is fused onto **a first protein** while another plasmid is engineered to produce **another protein product** in which **the activation domain (AD) fragment** is fused onto **a second protein** (Fig. 1-10). The protein fused to the BD may be referred to as the bait protein, and is typically a known protein the investigator is using to identify new binding partners. The protein fused to the AD may be referred to as the prey protein and can be either a single known protein or a library of known or unknown proteins. In this context, a library may consist of a collection of protein-encoding sequences that represent all the proteins expressed in a particular organism or tissue, or may be generated by synthesizing random DNA sequences. Regardless of the source, they are subsequently incorporated into the protein-encoding sequence of a plasmid, which is then transfected into the cells chosen for the screening method. This technique, when using a library, assumes that each cell is transfected with no more than a single plasmid and that, therefore, each cell ultimately expresses no more than a single member from the protein library.

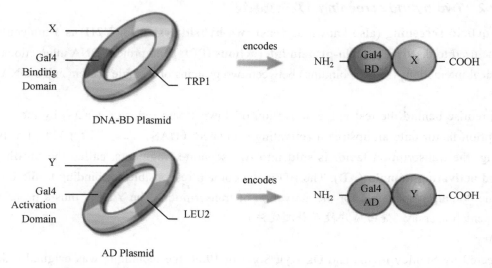

Fig. 1-10 Illustration of how fusion proteins create from the respective plasmids elaborately constructed.

If the bait and prey proteins interact (*i.e.*, bind), then the AD and BD of the transcription factor are indirectly connected, bringing the AD in proximity to the transcription start site and transcription of reporter gene(s) can occur. If the two proteins do not interact, there is no transcription of the reporter gene (Fig. 1-11). In this way, a successful interaction between the fused proteins is linked to a change in the cell phenotype.

Fixed domains

In any study, some of the protein domains, those under investigation, will be varied according to the goals of the study whereas other domains, those that are not themselves being investigated, will be kept constant. For example in a two-hybrid study to select DNA-binding domains, the DNA-binding domain, BD, will be varied while the two interacting proteins, the bait and prey, must be kept constant to maintain a strong binding between the BD and AD. There are a number of domains from which to choose the BD, bait and prey and AD, if these are to remain constant. In protein-protein interaction investigations, the BD may be chosen from any of many strong DNA-binding domains such as Zif268 （zinc finger protein 225，锌指蛋白 225）. A frequent choice of bait and prey domains are residues 263~352 of yeast Gal11P with a N342→V mutation and residues 58~97 of yeast Gal4, respectively. These domains can be used in both yeast- and bacterial-based selection techniques and are known to bind together strongly.

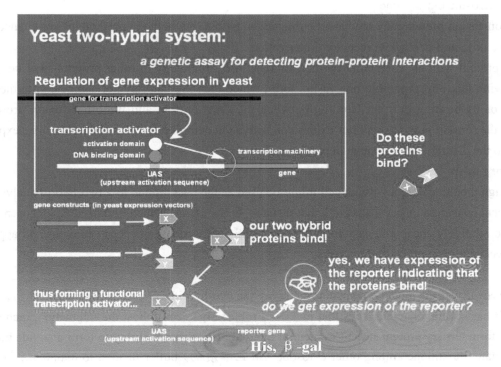

Fig. 1-11　Overview of two-hybrid assay, checking for interactions between two proteins, called here *Bait and Prey*. **A.** *Gal4* transcription factor gene produces two domain protein (*BD* and *AD*), which is essential for transcription of the reporter gene (*LacZ*). **B,C.** Two fusion proteins are prepared: *Gal4BD+Bait* and *Gal4AD+Prey*. None of them is usually sufficient to initiate the transcription (of the reporter gene) alone. **D.** When both fusion proteins are produced and Bait part of the first interact with Prey part of the second, transcription of the reporter gene occurs.

The AD chosen must be able to activate transcription of the reporter gene, using the cell′s own transcription machinery. Thus, the variety of ADs available for use in yeast-based techniques may not be suited to use in their bacterial-based analogues. The *herpes simplex* (单纯性疱疹) virus-derived AD, VP16 and yeast Gal4 AD have been used with success in yeast whilst a portion of the α-subunit of *E. coli* RNA polymerase has been utilized in *E. coli*-based methods.

Whilst powerfully activating domains may allow greater sensitivity towards weaker interactions, conversely, a weaker AD may provide greater stringency.

Recovery of protein information

Once the selection has been performed, the primary structure of the proteins which display the appropriate characteristics must be determined. This is achieved by retrieval (读取, 找回) of the protein-encoding sequences (as originally inserted) from the cells showing the appropriate phenotype.

Non-fusion proteins

A third, non-fusion protein may be co-expressed with two fusion proteins. Depending on the investigation, the third protein may modify one of the fusion proteins or mediate or interfere with their interaction.

Co-expression of the third protein may be necessary for modification or activation of one or both of the fusion proteins. For example *S. cerevisiae* (酿酒酵母) possesses no endogenous tyrosine kinase. If an investigation involves a protein that requires tyrosine phosphorylation, the kinase must be supplied in the form of a tyrosine kinase gene.

The non-fusion protein may mediate the interaction by binding both fusion proteins simultaneously, as in the case of ligand-dependent receptor dimerization.

For a protein with an interacting partner, its functional homology to other proteins may be assessed by supplying the third protein in non-fusion form, which then may or may not compete with the fusion-protein for its binding partner. Binding between the third protein and the other fusion protein will interrupt the formation of the reporter expression activation complex and thus reduce reporter expression, leading to the distinguishing change in phenotype.

Host organism

Although theoretically, any living cell might be used as the background to a two-hybrid analysis, there are practical considerations (考虑因素) that dictate (导致，影响) which is chosen. The chosen cell line should be relatively cheap and easy to culture and sufficiently robust (强健的) to withstand application of the investigative methods and reagents.

Yeast

S. cerevisiae was the model organism used during the two-hybrid technique's inception (起初，开始，开端). It has several characteristics that make it a robust organism to host the interaction, including the ability to form tertiary protein structures, neutral internal pH, enhanced ability to form disulfide bonds and reduced-state glutathione among other cytosolic (细胞溶质的) buffer factors, to maintain a hospitable (友好的，舒适的，适宜的) internal environment. The yeast model can be manipulated through non-molecular techniques and its complete genome sequence is known. Yeast systems are tolerant of diverse culture conditions and harsh chemicals that could not be applied to mammalian tissue cultures.

A number of yeast strains have been created specifically for Y2H screens, *e.g.*, Y187 and AH109, both produced by Clontech. Yeast strains R2HMet and BK100 have also been used.

E. coli

E. coli-based methods have several characteristics that may make them preferable (更好的，更可取的，更合意的) to yeast-based homologues. The higher transformation efficiency and faster rate of growth lends *E. coli* to (适用于，适宜于，有助于) the use of larger libraries (in excess of 10^8). A low false positive rate of approximately 3×10^{-8}, the absence of requirement for a nuclear localization signal (核定位信号) to be included in the protein sequence and the ability to study proteins that would be toxic to yeast may also be major factors to consider when choosing an experimental background organism.

It may be of note that the methylation (甲基化，甲基化作用) activity of certain *E. coli* DNA methyltransferase (甲基转移酶) proteins may interfere with some DNA-binding protein selections. If this is anticipated, the use of an *E. coli* strain that is defective for a particular methyltransferase may be an obvious solution.

Applications

Determination of sequences crucial for interaction

By changing specific amino acids through mutating the corresponding DNA base-pairs in the plasmids used, the importance of those amino acid residues in maintaining the interaction can be determined.

After using bacterial cell-based method to select DNA-binding proteins, it is necessary to check the specificity of these domains as there is a limit to the extent to which the bacterial cell genome can act as a sink (槽，容器) for domains with an affinity for other sequences (or indeed, a general affinity for DNA).

Drug and poison discovery

Protein-protein signaling interactions pose (introduce，提供) suitable therapeutic targets due to their specificity and pervasiveness (广泛性，普遍性). The random drug discovery approach uses compound banks that comprise random chemical structures, and requires a high-throughput method to test these structures in their intended target.

The cell chosen for the investigation can be specifically engineered to mirror (反映) the molecular aspect that the investigator intends to study and then used to identify new human or animal therapeutics or anti-pest agents.

Determination of protein function

By determination of the interaction partners of unknown proteins, the possible functions of these new proteins may be inferred (推断). This can be done using a single known protein against a library of unknown proteins or conversely, by selecting from a library of known proteins using a single protein of unknown function.

Zinc finger protein selection

To select zinc finger proteins (ZFPs) for protein engineering, methods adapted from the two-hybrid screening technique have been used with success. A ZFP is itself a DNA-binding protein used in the construction of custom DNA-binding domains that bind to a desired DNA sequence.

By using a selection gene with the desired target sequence included in the UAS, and randomizing (随机化，不规则分布，随机选择) the relevant amino acid sequences to produce a ZFP library, cells that host a DNA-ZFP interaction with the required characteristics can be selected. Each ZFP typically recognizes only 3~4 base pairs, so to prevent recognition of sites outside the UAS, the randomized ZFP is engineered into a 'scaffold' consisting of another two ZFPs of constant sequence. The UAS is thus designed to include the target sequence of the constant scaffold in addition to the sequence for which a ZFP is selected.

A number of other DNA-binding domains may also be investigated using this system.

Strengths and Weaknesses

Two-hybrid screens are low-tech; they can be carried out in any lab without sophisticated equipment. They can provide an important first hint for the identification of interaction partners. The assay is scalable (可扩展的), which makes it possible to screen for interactions among many proteins. Furthermore, it can be automated, and by using robots many proteins can be screened against thousands of potentially interacting proteins in a relatively short time. And yeast two-hybrid data can be of similar quality to data generated by the alternative approach of coaffinity purification (免疫沉淀法) followed by mass spectrometry (AP/MS). Meanwhile a high number of false positive (and false negative) identifications occur in the yeast two-hybrid screen of protein-protein interactions for some various reasons, earlier estimates were as high as 70%. The probability of generating false positives means that all interactions should be confirmed by a high confidence assay, for example co-immunoprecipitation (免疫共沉淀) of the endogenous proteins, which is difficult for large scale protein-protein interaction data. Hence the major role of two-hybrid screening is just digging out the essential first hint, though not accurate, but easy, quick, and high throughput.

1.2.3.3 *Phage display*（展示技术）

Phage display is a laboratory technique for the study of protein-protein, protein-peptide, and protein-DNA interactions that uses bacteriophages (viruses that infect bacteria) to connect proteins with the genetic information that encodes them. In this technique, a gene encoding a protein of interest is inserted into a phage coat protein gene, causing the phage to "display" the protein on its outside while containing the gene for the protein on its inside, resulting in a connection between genotype and phenotype（表型，显性）. These displaying phages can then be screened against other proteins, peptides or DNA sequences, in order to detect interaction between the displayed protein and those other molecules. In this way, large libraries of proteins can be screened and amplified in a process called *in vitro* selection, which is analogous to natural selection.

The most common bacteriophages used in phage display are M13 and fd filamentous phage（丝状噬菌体）, though T4, T7, and λ phage have also been used.

History

Phage display was first described by George P. Smith in 1985, when he demonstrated the display of peptides on filamentous phage by fusing the peptide of interest on to gene Ⅲ of filamentous phage. A patent by George Pieczenik claiming priority from 1985 also describes the generation of phage display libraries. This technology was further developed and improved by groups at the Laboratory of Molecular Biology with Greg Winter and John McCafferty, The Scripps Research Institute with Lerner and Barbas and the German Cancer Research Center with Breitling and Dübel for display of proteins such as antibodies for therapeutic protein engineering.

Principle

Like the two-hybrid system（双杂交系统）, phage display is used for the high-throughput screening of protein interactions. In the case of M13 filamentous phage display, the DNA encoding the protein or peptide of interest is ligated into the pⅢ or pⅧ gene, encoding either the minor or major coat protein, respectively. Multiple cloning sites are sometimes used to ensure that the fragments are inserted in all three possible reading frames so that the cDNA fragment is translated in the proper frame. The phage gene and insert DNA hybrid is then inserted [a process known as "transduction"（转导，转导作用）] into *Escherichia coli* (*E. coli*) bacterial cells such as TG1, SS320, ER2738, or XL1-Blue *E. coli*. If a "phagemid"（噬菌粒）vector is used (a simplified display construct vector) phage particles will not be released from the *E. coli* cells until they are infected with helper phage（辅助噬菌体）, which enables packaging of the phage DNA and assembly of the mature virions（病毒粒子，病毒体）with the relevant protein fragment as part of their outer coat on either the minor (pⅢ) or major (pⅧ) coat protein. By immobilizing a relevant DNA or protein target(s) to the surface of a microtiter plate（微量滴定板）well, a phage that displays a protein that binds to one of those targets on its surface will remain while others are removed by washing. Those that remain can be eluted, used to produce more phage (by bacterial infection with helper phage) and so produce a phage mixture that is enriched with relevant (*i.e.*, binding) phage. The repeated cycling of these steps is referred to as "panning" [（用淘盘）淘洗，淘金], in reference to the enrichment of a sample of gold by removing undesirable materials. Phage eluted in the final step can be used to infect a suitable bacterial host, from which the phagemids can be collected and the relevant DNA sequence excised（切除，切掉）and sequenced to identify the relevant, interacting proteins or protein fragments (Fig. 1-12).

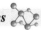

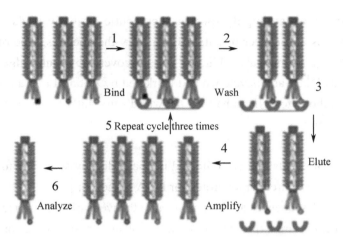

Fig. 1-12 The sequence of events that are followed in phage display screening to identify polypeptides that bind with high affinity to desired target protein or DNA sequence.

The use of a helper phage can be eliminated by using "bacterial packaging cell line" technology.

Applications

Applications of phage display technology include determination of interaction partners of a protein (which would be used as the immobilized phage "bait" with a DNA library consisting of all coding sequences of a cell, tissue or organism) so that the function or the mechanism of the function of that protein may be determined. Phage display is also a widely used method for *in vitro* protein evolution (also called protein engineering). As such（正因如此）, phage display is a useful tool in drug discovery. It is used for finding new ligands (enzyme inhibitors, receptor agonists and antagonists) to target proteins. The technique is also used to determine tumor antigens (for use in diagnosis and therapeutic targeting) and in searching for protein-DNA interactions using specially-constructed DNA libraries with randomized segments.

Competing methods for *in vitro* protein evolution include yeast display, bacterial display, ribosome display, and mRNA display.

Antibody maturation *in vitro*

The invention of antibody phage display revolutionized antibody drug discovery. Initial work was done by laboratories at the MRC Laboratory of Molecular Biology（英国剑桥分子生物实验室）(Greg Winter and John McCafferty), the Scripps Research Institute (Richard Lerner and Carlos F. Barbas) and the German Cancer Research Centre (Frank Breitling and Stefan Dübel). In 1991, The Scripps group reported the first display and selection of human antibodies on phage. This initial study described the rapid isolation of human antibody Fab that bound tetanus toxin（破伤风毒素）and the method was then extended to rapidly clone human anti-HIV-1 antibodies for vaccine design and therapy.

Phage display of antibody libraries has become a powerful method for both studying the immune response as well as a method to rapidly select and evolve human antibodies for therapy. Antibody phage display was later used by Carlos F. Barbas at the Scripps Research Institute to create synthetic human antibody libraries, a principle first patented in 1990 by Breitling and coworkers (Patent CA 2035384), thereby allowing human antibodies to be created *in vitro* from synthetic diversity elements.

Antibody libraries displaying millions of different antibodies on phage are often used in the pharmaceutical industry to isolate highly specific therapeutic antibody leads, for development into antibody drugs primarily as anti-cancer or anti-inflammatory therapeutics. One of the most successful was HUMIRA（修美乐）(adalimumab，阿达木单抗), discovered by Cambridge Antibody Technology （剑桥抗体技术公司）as D2E7 and developed and marketed by Abbott Laboratories（雅培公司，雅培制药）. HUMIRA, an antibody to TNF alpha, was the world's first fully human antibody, which achieved annual sales exceeding $1bn.

General protocol

Below is the sequence of events that are followed in phage display screening to identify polypeptides that bind with high affinity to desired target protein or DNA sequence:

1. Target proteins or DNA sequences are immobilized to the wells of a microtiter plate.

2. Many genetic sequences are expressed in a bacteriophage library in the form of fusions with the bacteriophage coat protein, so that they are displayed on the surface of the viral particle. The protein displayed corresponds to the genetic sequence within the phage.

3. This phage-display library is added to the dish（凹形容器）and after allowing the phage time to bind, the dish is washed.

4. Phage-displaying proteins that interact with the target molecules remain attached to the dish, while all others are washed away.

5. Attached phage may be eluted and used to create more phage by infection of suitable bacterial hosts. The new phage constitutes an enriched mixture, containing considerably less irrelevant phage (*i.e.*, non-binding) than were present in the initial mixture.

6. Steps 3 to 6 are optionally repeated one or more times, further enriching the phage library in binding proteins.

7. Following further bacterial-based amplification, the DNA within the interacting phage is sequenced to identify the interacting proteins or protein fragments.

Bioinformatics resources and tools

Databases and computational tools for mimotopes（模拟表位）have been an important part of phage display study. Databases, programs and web servers have been widely used to exclude target-unrelated peptides, characterize small molecules-protein interactions and map protein-protein interactions.

1.2.4 Construction of biomolecule libraries in the hope of searching out new drugs（构建生物分子库以发现新药）

The key technologies required to construct biomolecule libraries for screening include site-directed mutagenesis of proteins, DNA shuffling, and computer-aided *de novo* protein design, in addition to constructing combinatorial libraries for protein displaying as mentioned above.

1.2.4.1 Site-directed mutagenesis（定点突变）

Site-directed mutagenesis is a molecular biology method that is used to make specific and intentional changes to the DNA sequence of a gene and any gene products by using a PCR technique. Also called **site-specific mutagenesis** or **oligonucleotide-directed mutagenesis**, it is used for rapidly and efficiently improving the traits and characterization of target proteins coded by those site-directly mutated genes, and also for investigating the structure and biological activity of DNA, RNA, and protein molecules, as

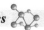

well as for protein engineering.

Site-directed mutagenesis is one of the most important techniques in the laboratory for introducing a mutation into a DNA sequence. However, with decreasing costs of oligonucleotide synthesis, artificial gene synthesis is now occasionally used as an alternative to site-directed mutagenesis.

History

Early attempts at mutagenesis using radiation or chemical mutagens were non-site-specific. Analogs of nucleotides and other chemicals were later used to generate localized point mutations, examples of such chemicals are aminopurine（氨基蝶呤）, nitrosoguanidine（亚硝基胍）, and bisulfite（亚硫酸氢盐）. Site-directed mutagenesis was achieved in 1973 in the laboratory of Charles Weissmann using a nucleotide analogue N^4-hydroxycytidine（N^4-羟基胞嘧啶核苷）, which induces transition（转变，转换）of GC to AT. These methods of mutagenesis, however, are constrained by the kinds of mutations they can achieve, and they are not as specific as later site-directed mutagenesis methods.

In 1971, Clyde Hutchison and Marshall Edgell showed that it is possible to produce mutants with small fragments of phage φX174 and restriction nucleases. Hutchison later produced with his collaborator Michael Smith in 1978, a more flexible approach to site-directed mutagenesis by using oligonucleotides in a primer extension method with DNA polymerase. For his part in the development of this process, Michael Smith later shared the Nobel Prize in Chemistry in October 1993 with Kary B. Mullis, who invented the polymerase chain reaction.

Basic mechanism

The basic procedure requires the synthesis of a short DNA primer. This synthetic primer contains the desired mutation and is complementary to the template DNA around the mutation site so it can hybridize with the DNA in the gene of interest. The mutation may be a single base change (a point mutation), multiple base changes, deletion, or insertion. The single-strand primer is then extended using a DNA polymerase, which copies the rest of the gene. The gene thus copied contains the mutated site, and is then introduced into a host cell as a vector and cloned. Finally, mutants are selected by DNA sequencing to check that they contain the desired mutation (Fig .1-13).

The original method using single-primer extension was inefficient due to a low yield of mutants. This resulting mixture contains both the original unmutated template as well as the mutant strand, producing a mixed population of mutant and non-mutant progenies. Furthermore, the template used is methylated while the mutant strand is unmethylated, and the mutants may be counter（反方向地，背道而驰地）- selected due to presence of mismatch repair（错配修复，失配校正）system that favors the methylated template DNA, resulting in fewer mutants. Many approaches have since been developed to improve the efficiency of mutagenesis.

Applications

Site-directed mutagenesis is used to generate mutations that may produce rationally designed proteins that have improved or special properties (*i.e.*, protein engineering).

Investigative tools — specific mutations in DNA allow the function and properties of a DNA sequence or a protein to be investigated in a rational approach.

1.2.4.2 *DNA shuffling*（DNA 洗牌技术）

DNA shuffling, also known as DNA random splicing technique, and sexual PCR, is a way to rapidly

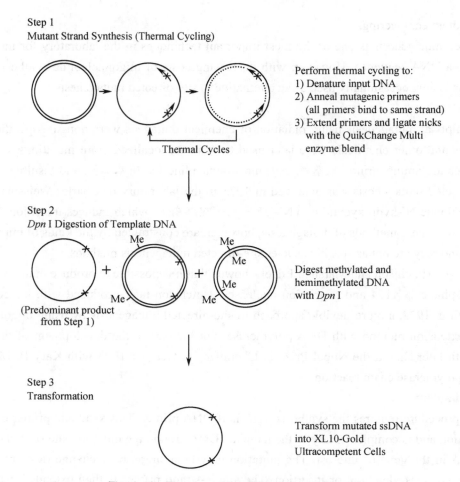

Fig. 1-13 Process of Site-directed mutagenesis.

propagate beneficial mutations in a directed evolution experiment. It is used to rapidly increase the size of DNA library，because it is a recombination between different DNA species with different mutations.

Procedure

First, DNase is used to fragment a set of parent genes into pieces of 50~100 bp in length. This is then followed by a polymerase chain reaction (PCR) without primers — DNA fragments with sufficient overlapping homologous sequence will anneal to each other and are then extended by DNA polymerase (Fig. 1-14).

Several rounds of this PCR extension are allowed to occur. After some of the DNA molecules reach the size of the parental genes, novel DNA mutants with a large number of random combinations can be obtained. These genes can then be amplified with another PCR, this time with the addition of primers that are designed to complement the ends of the strands. The primers may have additional sequences added to their 5′ ends, such as sequences for restriction enzyme recognition sites needed for ligation into a cloning vector.

It is possible to recombine portions of these genes to generate hybrids or chimeric forms with unique properties, which is called DNA shuffling. DNA shuffling offers the possibility of designing protein molecules artificially.

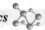

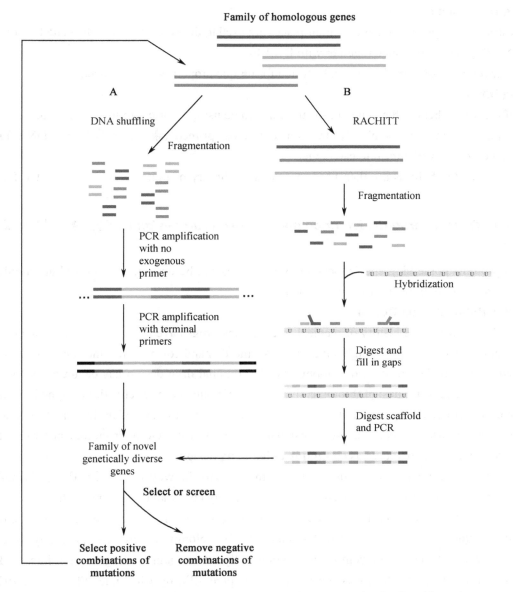

Fig. 1-14   Increasing genetic diversity by shuffling fragments of a family of homologous genes or a pool of randomly mutated sequences arising from a single gene.

(A) The "classical" DNA-shuffling strategy begins by fragmenting a pool of double-stranded parent genes with DNase I. Selection of small fragments by size fractionation maximizes the probability of multiple recombination events occurring, as the fragments cross-prime each other in a round of PCR amplification. The full-length, diversified products are then obtained by PCR amplification with terminal primers. (B) RACHITT begins with DNase I fragmentation and size fractionation of single-stranded DNA, and hybridization — in the absence of polymerase — to a complementary single-stranded scaffold (支架). Any overlapping fragments leave single-stranded overhangs that are trimmed down. The gaps between fragments are filled in; the fragments are then ligated, yielding a pool of full-length, diversified single strands hybridized to the scaffold. This scaffold, which is synthesized so as to include uracil (U), can be efficiently fragmented so as to preclude (排除) its amplification. With PCR, it is replaced by a new strand that is complementary to the diversified strand, and the whole is amplified.

Shuffling methods

Using restriction enzymes

1. Restriction enzymes that cut in similar places are used to digest members of the gene family

2. DNA fragments are joined together with DNA ligase

3. Large numbers of hybrids that can be tested for unique properties are produced

Using DNase 1

1. Different members of the gene family are fragmented using DNase 1 followed by PCR

2. During PCR different members of the family are cross-primed（杂交并互为引物）, DNA fragments with high homology will anneal to each other

3. The generated hybrids are then used to generate a library of mutants, which are tested for unique properties

1.2.4.3 *Rational drug design or computer-aided drug design*（合理药物设计或计算机辅助药物设计）

Small proteins possessing special secondary structures can be designed, optimized and produced by using the computer optimization screening method.

What is Rational Drug Design?

Throughout most of the history of medical science, new drugs have been discovered through a process of trial-and-error or simply through sheer luck. As the demand for new and more effective drugs has increased, a new method of drug development called rational drug design has begun to replace the old methods. In rational drug design, biologically active compounds are specifically designed or chosen to work with a particular drug target. This method often involves the use of molecular design software, which researchers use to create three-dimensional models of drugs and their biological targets. For this reason, the process is also known as **computer-aided drug design**.

Very few **pharmaceutical** products actually make it all the way（达到预定目标）through **drug** development, and sometimes the process can be an extremely costly and frustrating failure.

Older methods of developing new medications have several flaws that make drug discovery an expensive business. The easiest and fastest method of developing a new drug is simply to discover, through sheer luck, that a certain compound is biologically active against a drug target of interest. Perhaps the most famous such incident was the discovery of penicillin by Alexander Fleming in 1928. The microbiologist discovered the first antibiotic when some bacterial cultures he was working with became contaminated with a bactericidal fungus. Of course, this type of chance discovery does not happen very often, and luck is not something that drug companies rely on for the development of new medications.

The most common method used to develop new medications is a lengthy, large-scale process called combinatorial library screening. In this process, large numbers of chemical compounds are created and then screened for biological activity. If a given compound shows signs of interacting with a biological target, it receives further attention and might be developed into a new drug (Fig. 1-15). This process can take many years and enormous amounts of money, though, and even at the end of the development period, the drug might not be effective enough or safe enough for human use.

Rational drug design is a more streamlined process that requires careful consideration of the target of the drug as well as the drug itself. This method of drug design uses special equipment to examine the three-dimensional structure of a drug target and then find a compound that can interact with the target.

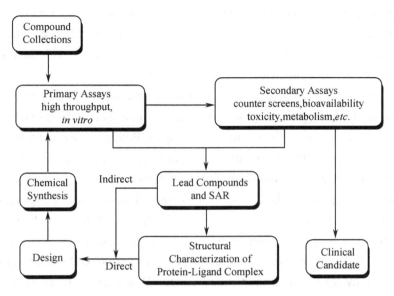

Fig. 1-15   Technique route of biomimetic affinity.

This process therefore requires significant knowledge of chemistry as well as biology, because chemical interactions between drugs and their targets are what determine whether a drug is biologically active.

Compounds can be located for testing in two ways. The first involves the use of combinatorial library screening. In this case, however, the process is streamlined because researchers using rational drug design methods will screen the library for compounds of a shape that is specific enough to interact with the drug target of interest. The second method involves the actual design of a compound that can interact with the target. This requires consideration of the chemical makeup of the compound and knowledge of what chemical groups the compound might require in order to be capable of interacting with the drug target.

Although design techniques for prediction of binding affinity are reasonably successful, there are many other properties, such as bioavailability, metabolic half-life, side effects, *etc.*, that first must be optimized before a ligand can become a safe and efficacious drug. These other characteristics are often difficult to predict with rational design techniques. Nevertheless, due to high attrition rates（损耗率）, especially during clinical phases of drug development, more attention is being focused early in the drug design process on selecting candidate drugs whose physicochemical properties are predicted to result in fewer complications during development and hence more likely to lead to an approved, marketed drug. Furthermore, *in vitro* experiments complemented with computation methods are increasingly used in early drug discovery to select compounds with more favorable ADME (absorption, distribution, metabolism, and excretion) and toxicological profiles（情况，简况）.

The first drug developed using a process of rational drug design was an antiviral drug called Relenza®（瑞乐砂）. This drug was designed to interact with an influenza（流感）protein called neuraminidase（神经氨酸酶）. Without this protein, the influenza virus cannot infect new cells; therefore treatment with the drug can shorten the duration of the illness. Other rationally designed drugs include HIV drugs such as ritonavir（利托那韦）and indinavir（茚地那韦）, both of which interact with viral proteins called proteases.

Target Validation and Rational drug discovery

A drug target, or biological target, is usually one of two types. The first type is a molecule in the human body that causes disease when it is defective in some way. The second is a molecule from a disease-causing microorganism. Drug development involves discovering or designing new chemical compounds that interact with these targets in a beneficial way, such as by interacting with cholesterol to remove it from the body or by interacting with a virus to cause its death.

A biomolecular target (most commonly a protein or nucleic acid) is a key molecule involved in a particular metabolic or signaling pathway that is associated with a specific disease condition or pathology or with the infectivity or survival of a microbial pathogen. Potential drug targets are not necessarily disease-causing but must by definition be, disease-modifying. In some cases, small molecules will be designed to enhance or inhibit the target function in the specific disease modifying pathway. Small molecules [for example receptor agonists, antagonists, inverse agonists, or modulators; enzyme activators or inhibitors; or ion channel openers (开放剂) or blockers] will be designed that are complementary to the binding site of target. Small molecules (drugs) can be designed so as not to affect any other important "off-target" (脱靶，偏离目标) molecules (often referred to as antitargets) since drug interactions with off-target molecules may lead to undesirable side effects. Due to similarities in binding sites, closely related targets identified through sequence homology have the highest chance of cross-reactivity and hence highest side effect potential.

Most commonly, drugs are organic small molecules produced through chemical synthesis, but biopolymer-based drugs (also known as biopharmaceuticals) produced through biological processes are becoming increasingly more common. In addition, mRNA-based gene silencing technologies may have therapeutic applications.

In contrast to traditional methods of drug discovery (known as forward pharmacology), which rely on trial-and-error (反复试验，尝试错误法) testing of chemical substances on cultured cells or animals, and matching the apparent effects to treatments, rational drug design (also called reverse pharmacology) begins with a hypothesis that modulation of a specific biological target may have therapeutic value. In order for a biomolecule to be selected as a drug target, two essential pieces of information are required. The first is evidence that modulation of the target will be disease-modifying. This knowledge may come from, for example, disease linkage studies that show an association between mutations in the biological target and certain disease states. The second is that the target is "druggable" (可成药的). This means that it is capable of binding to a small molecule and that its activity can be modulated by the small molecule.

Once a suitable target has been identified, the target is normally cloned and expressed. The expressed target is then used to establish a screening assay. In addition, the three-dimensional structure of the target may be determined.

Pharmaceutical drug design — lead screening, lead optimization

Pharmaceutical drug design includes synthetic versions of natural compounds along with entirely new **drugs**, and analysis of potential **pharmaceuticals** includes meticulous work to break down their components and understand how they function.

The search for small molecules that bind to the target is begun by screening libraries of potential drug compounds. This may be done by using the screening assay (a "wet screen"). In addition, if the structure of the target is available, a virtual screen (虚拟筛选) may be performed on candidate drugs. Ideally the candidate drug compounds should be "drug-like", *i.e.*, possess properties that are predicted to lead to oral bioavailability, adequate chemical and metabolic stability, and minimal toxic effects. Several methods are available to estimate drug-likeness such as Lipinski's Rule of Five（里宾斯基五规则）and a range of scoring methods such as lipophilic efficiency. Several methods for predicting drug metabolism have also been proposed in the scientific literature.

Due to the large number of drug properties that must be simultaneously optimized during the design process, multi-objective optimization（多目标优化）techniques are sometimes employed. Finally because of the limitations in the current methods for prediction of activity, drug design is still very much reliant on serendipity（好运，意外发现，意外发现珍奇事物的本领）and bounded rationality（有限理性）.

Computer-aided drug design

The most fundamental goal in drug design is to predict whether a given molecule will bind to a target and if so how strongly. Molecular mechanics（分子力学）or molecular dynamics（分子动力学）are most often used to predict the conformation of the small molecule and to model conformational changes in the biological target that may occur when the small molecule binds to it. Semi-empirical, *ab initio* quantum chemistry methods（量子化学从头计算方法）, or density functional theory（密度泛函理论）are often used to provide optimized parameters for the molecular mechanics calculations and also provide an estimate of the electronic properties (electrostatic potential, polarizability（极化性，极化度）, *etc.*) of the drug candidate that will influence binding affinity.

Molecular mechanics methods may also be used to provide semi-quantitative prediction of the binding affinity. Also, knowledge-based scoring function（计分函数，打分函数）may be used to provide binding affinity estimates. These methods use linear regression, machine learning, neural nets（神经网络）or other statistical techniques to derive predictive binding affinity equations by fitting experimental affinities to computationally derived interaction energies between the small molecule and the target.

Ideally, the computational method will be able to predict affinity before a compound is synthesized, and hence in theory, only one compound needs to be synthesized, saving enormous time and cost. The reality is that present computational methods are imperfect and provide, at best, only qualitatively accurate estimates of affinity. In practice it still takes several iterations（重复，反复）of design, synthesis, and testing before an optimal drug is discovered. Computational methods have accelerated discovery by reducing the number of iterations required and have often provided novel structures.

Drug design with the help of computers may be used at any of the following stages of drug discovery:

1. Hit（命中，碰撞，好运气，偶然发现，成功）identification using virtual screening (structure- or ligand-based design).

2. Hit-to-lead（先导化合物）optimization of affinity and selectivity (structure-based design, QSAR, *etc.*).

3. Lead optimization of other pharmaceutical properties while maintaining affinity.

In order to overcome the insufficient prediction of binding affinity calculated by recent scoring functions, the protein-ligand interaction and compound 3D structure information are used for analysis. For structure-based drug design, several post-screening analyses focusing on protein-ligand interaction have been developed for improving enrichment and effectively mining potential candidates:

- Consensus（一致性）scoring
- Cluster analysis（聚类分析，群类分析）

Types

There are two major types of drug design. The first is referred to as **ligand-based drug design** (indirect) and the second, **structure-based drug design** (direct). Drug discovery cycle highlighting both ligand-based and structure-based drug design strategies.

Ligand-based

Ligand-based drug design (or **indirect drug design**) relies on knowledge of other molecules that bind to the biological target of interest. These other molecules may be used to derive a pharmacophore（药效团，药效基团）model that defines the minimum necessary structural characteristics a molecule must possess in order to bind to the target. In other words, a model of the biological target may be built based on the knowledge of what binds to it, and this model in turn may be used to design new molecular entities that interact with the target. Alternatively, a quantitative structure-activity relationship (QSAR), in which a correlation between calculated properties of molecules and their experimentally determined biological activity, may be derived. These QSAR relationships in turn may be used to predict the activity of new analogs.

Structure-based

Structure-based drug design (or **direct drug design**) relies on knowledge of the three-dimensional structure of the biological target obtained through methods such as X-ray crystallography or NMR spectroscopy. If an experimental structure of a target is not available, it may be possible to create a homology model（同源模型）of the target based on the experimental structure of a related protein. Using the structure of the biological target, candidate drugs that are predicted to bind with high affinity and selectivity to the target may be designed using interactive graphics and the intuition of a medicinal chemist（药物化学家）. Alternatively, various automated computational procedures may be used to suggest new drug candidates.

Current methods for structure-based drug design can be divided roughly into three main categories. The first method is the identification of new ligands for a given receptor by searching large databases of 3D structures of small molecules to find those fitting the binding pocket of the receptor using fast approximate docking programs. This method is known as "**virtual screening**". A second category is *de novo* design of new ligands. *De novo* protein design, refers to the design of some *de novo* proteins (unnatural proteins) which possess certain structures and functions. In this method, ligand molecules are built up within the constraints of the binding pocket by assembling small pieces in a stepwise manner. These pieces can be either individual atoms or molecular fragments. The key advantage of such a method is that novel structures, not contained in any database, can be suggested. Because the second set of genetic codes that instruct protein production — the rule of protein folding — has not yet been fully deciphered, designing *de novo* proteins is still in its infancy. A third method is the optimization of known ligands by evaluating proposed analogs within the binding cavity (Fig. 1-16).

Binding site identification

Binding site identification is the first step in structure-based design. If the structure of the target or a sufficiently similar homolog is determined in the presence of a bound ligand, then the ligand should be observable in the structure, in which case the location of the binding site is trivial（无价值的，不重要的）. However, there may be unoccupied allosteric binding sites（变构结合点）that may be of interest. Furthermore, it may be that only apoprotein（脱辅基蛋白）(protein without ligand) structures are available and the reliable identification of unoccupied sites that have the potential to bind ligands with high affinity is non-trivial（重要的，有意义的）. In brief, binding site identification usually relies on identification of

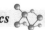

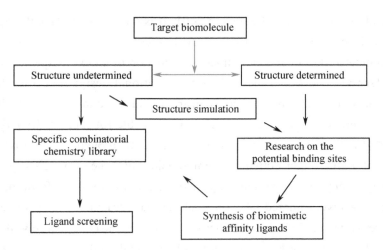

Fig. 1-16   Drug dicovery cycle.

concave surfaces on the protein that can accommodate drug sized molecules that also possess appropriate "hot spots"(hydrophobic surfaces, hydrogen bonding sites, *etc*.) that drive ligand binding.

Scoring functions

Structure-based drug design attempts to use the structure of proteins as a basis for designing new ligands by applying the principles of molecular recognition. Selective high affinity binding to the target is generally desirable since it leads to more efficacious（有效的，灵验的）drugs with fewer side effects. Thus, one of the most important principles for designing or obtaining potential new ligands is to predict the binding affinity of a certain ligand to its target (and known antitargets) and use the predicted affinity as a criterion for selection.

Examples

At present, only small proteins with certain secondary structures can be designed by using computer technology, such as carrying out a functional protein design, functional domain assembly, polypeptide mimicking, and small molecule design.

A particular example of rational drug design involves the use of three-dimensional information about biomolecules obtained from such techniques as X-ray crystallography and NMR spectroscopy. Computer-aided drug design, in particular, becomes much more tractable（易驾驭的）when there is a high-resolution structure of a target protein bound to a potent ligand. This approach to drug discovery is sometimes referred to as structure-based drug design. The first unequivocal example of the application of structure-based drug design leading to an approved drug is the carbonic anhydrase inhibitor（碳酸酐酶抑制剂）dorzolamide（多佐胺）, which was approved in 1995.

Another important case study in rational drug design is imatinib（伊马替尼）(sold under the brand name Gleevec among others). Gleevec is a small-molecule drug that has a similar structure to that of ATP, a tyrosine kinase inhibitor designed specifically to compete with ATP for binding to a site on BCR-ABL, which needs ATP to bind to signal the division of more white blood cells, that is characteristic for Philadelphia chromosome-positive leukemias [chronic myelogenous（骨髓性的）leukemia and occasionally acute lymphocytic（淋巴细胞的）leukemia]. Imatinib is substantially（很大程度地）different from previous drugs for cancer, as most agents of chemotherapy simply target rapidly dividing cells, not differentiating between cancer cells and other tissues. What is more, It is taken by mouth. Imatinib was approved for medical use in the United States in 2001. It is on the World Health Organization's List of Essential Medicines, the most effective and safe medicines needed in a health system.

The first fully automated design and experimental validation of a novel sequence for an entire protein was described by Dahiyat and Mayo in 1997. A computational design algorithm based on physical-chemical potential functions and stereochemical constraints was used to screen a combinatorial library of 1.9×10^{27} possible amino acid sequences and 1.1×10^{62} possible rotamer（旋转异构体）sequences for compatibility（兼容性，适应性）with the design target, a ββα protein motif based on the polypeptide backbone structure of a zinc finger domain 28 amino acid long. The designed sequence FSD-1, which has very low identity to any known protein sequence (*i.e.*, totally different from that of the zinc finger domain), forms a compact well-ordered（井然有序的）tertiary structure, which is in excellent agreement with the design target structure. FSD-1 is the shortest sequence consisting entirely of naturally occurring amino acids that folds to a well-ordered structure without metal binding, oligomerization（寡聚化）, or disulfide bond formation at that time.

The same group (Malakauskas and Mayo) also utilized an objective（客观存在的，真实的）computer algorithm to select some amino acid sequences that are optimal for a target fold. It was achieved by simultaneous optimization (considering multiple interactions simultaneously). Their redesign results in a hyperstable variant of the streptococcal protein G β1 domain (Gβ1), a seven-fold mutant that exhibits a melting temperature above 100℃, while retaining the wild-type protein's biological function — correctly-folding and human IgG-binding capacity.

1.2.5 Protein engineering and new drug research（蛋白质工程与新药研究）

Protein engineering

Protein engineering is the process of developing useful or valuable proteins. It is a young discipline, with much research taking place into the understanding of protein folding and recognition of protein design principles. It is also a product and services market, with an estimated value of $168 billion by 2017.

Protein engineering is the design of new enzymes or proteins with new or desirable functions. It is based on the use of recombinant DNA technology to change amino acid sequences. The first papers on protein engineeing date back to the early 1980s: in a review by Ulmer (1983), the prospects for protein engineering, such as X-ray crystallography, chemical DNA synthesis, and computer modeling of protein structure and folding, were discussed and the combination of crystal structure and protein chemistry information with artificial gene synthesis was emphasized as a powerful approach to obtain proteins with desirable properties. In a later review in 1992 by Gupta, protein engineering was mentioned as a highly promising technique within the frame of biocatalyst engineering to improve enzyme stability and efficiency in low water system (microaqueous organic solvents). Today, owing to the development of recombinant DNA technology and high-throughput screen techniques, protein engineering methods and applications are becoming increasingly important and widespread.

(1) Protein engineering is either transforming nature proteins or designing and synthesizing *de novo* proteins which possess some specific properties through recombinant DNA technology.

(2) Protein engineering has been developed on the basis of the disciplines of biochemistry, molecular biology, molecular genetics and so on, and integrates multiple disciplines of protein crystallography,

protein dynamics, protein chemistry and computer-aided design.

(3) The esssence of protein engineering is to transform certain kinds of proteins into novel mutant proteins to answer certain needs of mankind. The practice is based on the knowledge of the structure-function relationship of proteins, and usually through some elaborate molecular design.

(4) Protein engineering can improve the properties of natural proteins, and add some new properties to the natural proteins, such as improving thermal stability and/or antioxidant ability, changing the optimum pH, changing the clearance rate of protein, improving the catalytic efficiency of enzymes, facilitating proteins purification, adding new substrate specificities or coenzyme specificities to enzymes, acquiring some new antibody specificities, improving drug targeting specificities, hence pushing the research of proteins and enzymes into a new era.

Protein engineering approaches

Many different protein engineering methods are available today, owing to the rapid development in biological sciences, more specifically, recombinant DNA technology. There are two general strategies for protein engineering: rational protein design and directed evolution. These methods are not mutually exclusive (互相排斥的); researchers will often apply both.

In a review article by Antikainen and Martin (2005), the major protein engineering methods were described in detail. These methods were classified as rational methods that involve site-directed mutagenesis, random methods including random mutagenesis and evolutionary methods which involve "DNA shuffling".

Rational design is an effective approach when the structure and mechanisms of the protein of interest are well-known. In many cases of protein engineering, however, there is a limited amount of information on the structure and mechanisms of the protein of interest. Thus, the use of "evolutionary methods" that involve "random mutagenesis and selection" for the desired protein properties was introduced as an alternative approach. The application of random mutagenesis could be an effective method, particularly when there is limited information on protein structure and mechanism. The only requirement here is the availability of a suitable selection scheme that favors the desired protein properties. "Localized or region-specific random mutagenesis" is another technique that is a combination of rational and random approaches to protein engineering. It includes the simultaneous replacement of a few amino acid residues in a specific region, to obtain proteins with new specificities.

Rational design

The most classical method in protein engineering is the so-called "rational design" approach which involves "site-directed mutagenesis of proteins". Site-directed mutagenesis allows introduction of specific amino acids into a target gene.

In rational protein design, a scientist uses detailed knowledge of the structure and function of a protein to make desired changes. In general, this has the advantage of being inexpensive and technically easy, since site-directed mutagenesis methods are well-developed. However, its major drawback is that detailed structural knowledge of a protein is often unavailable, and, even when available, it can be very difficult to predict the effects of various mutations.

Computational protein design algorithms seek to identify novel amino acid sequences that are low in energy when folded to the pre-specified (预先设定的) target structure. While the sequence-conformation space that needs to be searched is large, the most challenging requirement for computational protein design is a fast, yet accurate, energy function that can distinguish optimal sequences from similar suboptimal （次优的，次最优的，未达最佳标准的）ones.

Directed evolution

Generally, directed evolution may be summarized as an iterative two-step process that involves the generation of protein mutant libraries, and high throughput screening processes to select for variants with improved traits.

In directed evolution, random (Random mutations can be introduced using either error-prone PCR, or site saturation mutagenesis. "Saturation mutagenesis" involves the replacement of a single amino acid within a protein with each of the natural amino acids, and provides all possible variations at that site.) or focused mutagenesis is applied to a protein to generate libraries of mutant proteins, and a selection regime （管理方式）is used to select variants harboring desired traits. Further rounds of mutation and selection are then applied. This method mimics natural evolution and, in general, produces superior results to rational design.

Mutants may also be generated using recombination of multiple homologous genes. An added process, termed DNA shuffling, mixes and matches pieces of successful variants to produce better results. Such processes mimic the recombination that occurs naturally during sexual reproduction （有性生殖）. In the DNA shuffling protocol, a group of genes each consisting of a double-stranded DNA and having relatively similar sequences is either obtained from various organisms or generated by error-prone PCR.

Digestion of these genes with DNaseI yields randomly cleaved small fragments, which are purified and reassembled by PCR, using an error-prone and thermostable DNA polymerase. The fragments themselves are used as PCR primers, which align （排成一条直线）and cross-prime each other. Thus, a hybrid DNA with parts from different parent genes is obtained.

Advantages of directed evolution are that it requires no prior structural knowledge of a protein, no prior knowledge of the protein structure and function relationship, and it is not necessary to be able to predict what effect a given mutation will have. Indeed, the results of directed evolution experiments are often surprising in that desired changes are often caused by mutations that were not expected to have some effect.

The drawback is that they require high-throughput screening, which is not feasible for all proteins. Large amounts of recombinant DNA must be mutated and the products screened for desired traits. The large number of variants often requires expensive robotic （自动操作的）equipment to automate the process. Further, not all desired activities can be screened for easily.

Nature has evolved a limited number of beneficial sequences. Directed evolution makes it possible to identify undiscovered protein sequences which have novel functions. This ability is contingent （依情况而变的）on the proteins ability to tolerate amino acid residue substitutions without compromising folding or stability.

Natural Darwinian evolution can be effectively imitated in the lab toward tailoring protein properties for diverse applications. While more conservative than direct selection from deep sequence space, redesign of existing proteins by random mutagenesis and selection/screening is a particularly robust method for optimizing or altering extant （现存的）properties. It also represents an excellent starting point for achieving more ambitious engineering goals. Allying experimental evolution with modern computational methods is likely the broadest, most fruitful strategy for generating functional macromolecules unknown to nature.

The main challenges of designing high quality mutant libraries have shown significant progress in the recent past. This progress has been in the form of better descriptions of the effects of mutational loads（突变负荷）on protein traits. Also computational approaches have shown great advances in reducing the innumerably large sequence space to more manageable screenable sizes, thus creating smart libraries of mutants. Library size has also been reduced to more screenable sizes by the identification of key beneficial residues using algorithms for systematic recombination. Finally a significant step forward toward efficient reengineering of proteins or peptides has been made with the development of more accurate statistical models and algorithms quantifying and predicting coupled mutational effects on protein functions.

Semi-Rational Design

Semi-rational design uses information about a proteins sequence, structure and function, in tandem with（同……合作）predictive algorithms. Together these are used to identify target amino acid residues which are most likely to influence protein function. Mutations of these key amino acid residues create libraries of mutant proteins that are more likely to have enhanced properties.

Advances in semi-rational enzyme engineering and *de novo* enzyme design provide researchers with powerful and effective new strategies to manipulate biocatalysts. Integration of sequence, and structure based approaches in library design has proven to be a great guide for enzyme redesign. Generally, current computational *de novo* and redesign methods do not compare to evolved variants in catalytic performance. Although experimental optimization may be produced using directed evolution, further improvements in the accuracy of structure predictions and greater catalytic ability will be achieved with improvements in design algorithms. Further functional enhancements may be included in future simulations（模拟）by integrating protein dynamics.

Biochemical and biophysical studies, along with the fine-tuning of predictive frameworks, will be useful to experimentally evaluate the functional significance of individual design features. Better understanding of these functional contributions will then provide feedback for the improvement of future designs.

Directed evolution will likely not be replaced as the method of choice for protein engineering, although computational protein design has fundamentally changed the way protein engineering can manipulate biomacromolecules. Smaller, more focused and functionally-rich libraries may be generated by using methods that incorporate predictive frameworks for hypothesis-driven protein engineering. New design strategies and technical advances have begun a departure（背离）from traditional protocols, such as directed evolution, which represents the most effective strategy for identifying top-performing candidates in focused libraries. Whole-gene library synthesis is replacing shuffling and mutagenesis protocols for library preparation. Also, highly specific low throughput screening assays are increasingly applied in place of monumental（庞大的）screening and selection efforts of millions of candidates. Together, these developments are poised to（准备就绪）take protein engineering beyond directed evolution and towards practical, more efficient strategies for tailoring biomacromolecules.

Peptidomimetics

Another important method that finds applications in protein engineering is peptidomimetics（模拟肽）Remove extra Space. It involves mimicking or blocking the activity of enzymes or natural peptides upon design and synthesis of peptide analogs that are metabolically stable. Peptidomimetics is an important approach for bioorganic and medical chemistry. It includes a variety of synthesis methods such as the use of a common intermediate, solid phase synthesis and combinatorial approaches.

Enzyme engineering

Enzyme engineering is the application of modifying an enzyme's structure (and, thus, its function) or modifying the catalytic activity of isolated enzymes to produce new metabolites, to allow new (catalyzed) pathways for reactions to occur, or to convert certain compounds into others (biotransformation 生物转化). These products are useful as chemicals, pharmaceuticals, fuel, food, or agricultural additives.

An *enzyme reactor* consists of a vessel containing a reactional medium that is used to perform a desired conversion by enzymatic means. Enzymes used in this process are free in the solution.

Examples of engineered proteins

Computing methods have been used to design a protein with a novel fold, named Top7, and sensors for unnatural molecules. The engineering of fusion proteins has yielded rilonacept (利纳西普), a pharmaceutical that has secured Food and Drug Administration (FDA) approval for treating cryopyrin-associated periodic syndrome (CAPS，隐热蛋白 - 相关周期综合征).

Another computing method, Iterative Protein Redesign and Optimization (IPRO，迭代蛋白质重新设计和优化), successfully engineered the switching of cofactor specificity of *Candida boidinii* xylose reductase (假丝酵母木糖还原酶). IPRO redesigns proteins to increase or give specificity to native or novel substrates and cofactors. This is done by repeatedly randomly perturbing the structure of the proteins around specified design positions, identifying the lowest energy combination of rotamers (旋转异构体，构象异构体), and determining whether the new design has a lower binding energy than prior ones.

Computation-aided design has also been used to engineer complex properties of a highly ordered nano-protein assembly. A protein cage, *E. coli* bacterioferritin (细菌铁蛋白) (EcBfr), which naturally shows structural instability and an incomplete self-assembly behavior by populating two oligomerization states, is the model protein in this study. Through computational analysis and comparison to its homologs, it has been found that this protein has a smaller-than-average dimeric interface (二聚交界面) on its two-fold symmetry axis (二次对称轴) due mainly to the existence of an interfacial water pocket centered on two water-bridged asparagine residues. To investigate the possibility of engineering EcBfr for modified structural stability, a semi-empirical computational method is used to virtually explore the energy differences of the 480 possible mutants at the dimeric interface relative to the wild-type EcBfr. This computational study also converges (聚集，集中) on the water-bridged asparagines. Replacing these two asparagines with hydrophobic amino acids results in proteins that fold into alpha-helical monomers and assemble into cages, as evidenced by circular dichroism and transmission electron microscopy. Both thermal and chemical denaturation confirm that, all redesigned proteins, in agreement with the calculations, possess increased stability. One of the three mutations shifts the population in favor of the higher order oligomerization state in solution as shown by both size exclusion chromatography and native gel electrophoresis.

In the future, more detailed knowledge of protein structure and function, and advances in high-throughput screening, may greatly expand the abilities of protein engineering. Eventually, even unnatural amino acids may be included, via newer methods, such as expanded genetic code, that allow encoding novel amino acids in genetic code.

1.2.5.1 *Insulin analog*（新型胰岛素）

An **insulin analog** is an altered form of insulin, different from any occurring in nature, but still available to the human body for performing the same action as human insulin in terms of glycemic（血糖的）control. Through genetic engineering of the underlying（表面下的）DNA, the amino acid sequence of insulin can be changed to alter its ADME (absorption, distribution, metabolism, and excretion) characteristics. Officially, the U.S. Food and Drug Administration (FDA) refers to these as "insulin receptor ligands", although they are more commonly referred to as insulin analogs.

These modifications have been used to create two types of insulin analogs: those that are more readily absorbed from the injection site and therefore act faster than natural insulin injected subcutaneously, intended to supply the bolus（大剂量，团）level of insulin needed at mealtime [prandial（膳食的，正餐的）insulin]; and those that are released slowly over a period of between 8 and 24 hours, intended to supply the basal level of insulin during the day and particularly at nighttime (basal insulin)（Fig. 1-17）. The first insulin analog approved for human therapy (insulin Lispro rDNA) was manufactured by Eli Lilly and Company.

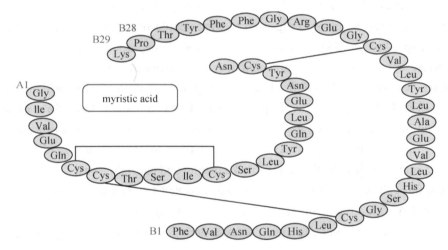

Fig. 1-17   Modification of insulin. C-terminal structure of insulin determines the tendency for dimerization. Left: Structure of insulin monomer, highlight the C-terminal fragment. Right: Formation of dimer through interaction of amino acid from C-terminal fragments. In Insulin lispro, the penultimate lysine and proline residues on the C-terminal end of the B-chain are reversed: B28Pro——B29Lys (Natural Insulin), B28Lys——B29Pro (Insulin lispro).

Insulin lispro (marketed by Eli Lilly and Company as "Humalog") is a fast acting insulin analog. It was first approved for use in the United States in 1996, making it the first insulin analog to enter the market.

Engineered through recombinant DNA technology, the penultimate lysine and proline residues on the C-terminal end of the B-chain are reversed. This modification does not alter receptor binding, but blocks the formation of insulin dimers and hexamers（Fig. 1-18）. This allowed larger amounts of active monomeric insulin to be immediately available（即时生效）for postprandial（餐后的）injections.

Insulin lispro has one primary advantage over regular insulin for postprandial glucose control. It has a shortened delay of onset, allowing slightly more flexibility than regular insulin, which requires a longer waiting period before starting a meal after injection. Both preparations should be coupled with a longer

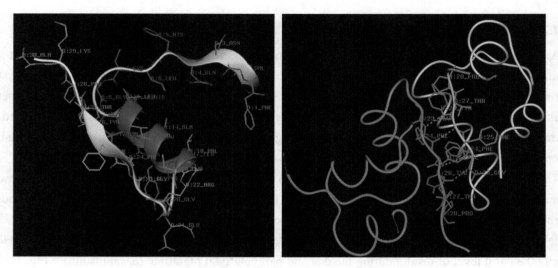

Fig. 1-18　Schematic diagram of long-acting insulin analogue.

acting insulin [*e.g.*, Insulin degludec (德谷胰岛素)] for good glycemic control.

Insulin lispro is an FDA approved drug used to treat people living with Type 1 diabetes or Type 2 diabetes. Insulin lispro has non-FDA labeled uses for d iabetic nephropathy (糖尿病肾病) prevention, diabetic neuropathy (糖尿病神经病变) prevention, and cardiovascular disease prevention.

Insulin aspart (诺和锐，门冬胰岛素) is another fast-acting insulin analog, which was marketed by Novo Nordisk (诺和诺德公司) as **NovoLog/NovoRapid**. It is a manufactured form of human insulin; where a single amino acid has been exchanged. This change helps the fast-acting insulin analog be absorbed quickly into the bloodstream. As a result, it starts working in minutes (the onset of action is approximately 15 minutes), which allows one to take insulin and eat right away.

It was created through recombinant DNA technology so that the amino acid, B28, which is normally proline, is substituted with an aspartic acid residue. This analog has increased charge repulsion, which prevents the formation of hexamers, to create a faster-acting insulin. **Insulin aspart** was expressed by yeast.

Insulin degludec (德谷胰岛素)

Insulin degludec (INN/USAN) is an ultralong-acting basal insulin analogue that was developed by Novo Nordisk under the brand name Tresiba.

Insulin degludec is a modified insulin that has one single amino acid deleted in comparison to human insulin, and is conjugated to hexadecanedioic acid (十六烷基二酸) via gamma-L-glutamyl (γ-L- 谷氨酰胺) spacer at the amino acid lysine at position B29. The addition of hexadecanedioic acid to lysine at the B29 position allows for the formation of multi-hexamers in subcutaneous tissues. This allows for the formation of a subcutaneous depot (仓库) that results in slow insulin release into the systemic circulation.

Insulin degludec is an ultra-long acting insulin that, unlike insulin glargine (甘精胰岛素), is active at a physiologic pH. It is administered via subcutaneous injection once daily to help control the blood sugar level of those with diabetes. Insulin degludec has an onset of action of 30~90 minutes (similar to insulin glargine and insulin detemir). There is no peak in activity, due to the slow release into systemic circulation. It has a duration of action that lasts up to 42 hours (compared to 18 to 26 hours provided by other marketed

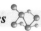

long-acting insulins such as insulin glargine and insulin detemir), making it a once-daily basal insulin, that is one that provides a base insulin level, as opposed to the fast- and short-acting bolus insulins.

Studies have shown that patients taking insulin degludec needed to take significantly smaller doses of basal insulin than those taking insulin glargine U100 while achieving similar blood glucose levels. Insulin degludec also has the ability to be mixed with other insulins, thereby improving glycemic control. This allows the creation of a novel formulation that retains the smooth control of a long-acting basal with rapid-acting mealtime control from insulin aspart. This 2-component insulin retains the ultralow risk characteristics of degludec with simultaneous mealtime coverage.

Insulin degludec received FDA approval on September 25, 2015 and marketing began on January 26, 2016.

1.2.5.2   *Creation of novel enzymes by mutagenesis* （通过突变获得新型酶）

Nucleoside analogs are widely used inhibitors of human herpesvirus（疱疹病毒）replication. The antiviral activity of these substances depends on metabolic activation by phosphorylation to their respective mono-, di- and triphosphates. The preferential initial phosphorylation to the nucleoside monophosphate by viral enzymes is one mechanism of selective antiviral activity.

Type I *herpes simplex* virus（单纯性疱疹病毒）'s thymidine kinase (HSV1-TK) has been the most investigated of such enzymes. It is non-toxic for eukaryotic cells and can specifically transform some nucleoside（核苷）analogs (NA) such as Acyclovir (ACV，阿昔洛韦), or Ganciclovir (GCV，更昔洛韦)（each of which lacks a hydroxyl group at the 3′-terminus), into monophosphorylated molecules, a transformation that cell-kinases cannot normally accomplish. These monophosphorylated nucleosides are then converted by cell enzymes into triphosphorylated nucleotides. The latter molecules can be incorporated into elongating DNA, hence blocking elongation and eventually kill dividing cells. This is a property that can be used for eliminating cancer cells or cells infected by HIV.

The experimental treatment is based on the introduction into tumor cells of a suicide gene coding for the *herpes simplex* virus type I thymidine kinase (HSV1-TK), through the intratumoral injection. Cells that transfected with the gene and express HSV1-TK become sensitive to GCV or ACV. GCV and ACV have no toxicity for normal cells, but kill cells expressing the HSV1-TK enzyme. Such toxicity is restricted to cells undergoing division.

The mechanism is that GCV or ACV can be transformed by viral thymidine kinase into a monophosphorylated form, which is subsequently converted by endogenous mammalian kinases to GCV or ACV diphosphate and triphosphate. The later competes with normal nucleotides for DNA replication in mammalian cells and causes a premature chain termination when incorporated into the replicating DNA, disrupts cellular proliferation, and causes cell death.

Researchers also sought to remodel the active site of HSV-1 TK to increase substrate specificity towards the guanosine（尿苷）nucleoside analogs GCV and ACV and concomitantly to decrease thymidine utilization.

Random sequence mutagenesis can be used to tailor HSV-1 TKs for gene therapy of cancers and for a wide variety of other applications. By random sequence mutagenesis, over one million variants of the HSV-1 TK gene have been created to identify mutants in *Escherichia coli* that exhibit heightened GCV and/or ACV sensitivity when expressed in mammalian cells. As a result, mutants were obtained with 2~6 amino acid substitutions that confer up to dozens of times of increase in GCV and ACV sensitivity to mammalian cells (Analysis of 3 drug-sensitive enzymes demonstrated that 1 produced stable mammalian cell transfectants（转染子）that are 43-fold more sensitive to ganciclovir and 20-fold more sensitive to acyclovir).

Besides, there is evidence that after intratumoral injection, it is only the tumor cells, but not the quiescent cells of the healthy tissue surrounding them, that express the HSV1-TK gene and can be destroyed by GCV. In addition, tumor cells that do not express the gene, but which are located in the immediate vicinity of the transduced（转导）cells, are also destroyed through a "bystander effect", also restricted to cells undergoing division. It is therefore not necessary for all the tumor cells to express HSV1-TK for all of them to be destroyed. Finally, preliminary data suggest that this localized tumoricidal activity may trigger a more general antineoplastic action, by facilitating a specific antitumor immune response.

1.2.6 Glycosylation engineering and new drug research （糖基化工程与新药研究）

Since the sequencing of the human genome revealed a surprisingly low number of 20 000~25 000 genes, more attention is being paid to post-transcriptional and post-translational events. N-glycosylation, the enzymatic coupling of glycans（聚糖，多糖，多聚糖）to specific asparagine residues of nascent polypeptide chains, is one of the most widespread post-translational modifications (PTM). The importance of glycosylation in generating proteome diversity is illustrated by several observations. First, the glycosylation machinery（装置）is encoded for by 1%~2% of the human genome. This includes all proteins that are in some way involved in the synthesis, modification, localization or binding of glycans. Second, about 50% of all human proteins are glycosylated. However, since glycosylation is not template-driven and combinatorial modification with different types and numbers of glycans is possible, each single glycoprotein is invariably（一贯地）present as a heterogeneous array（系列）of glycoforms (isoforms differing in the glycan chain structures), thus significantly increasing the diversity of the proteome. One could speculate that from an evolutionary point of view, in order to increase diversity and complexity, it is more beneficial to expand the "glycoproteome"（糖蛋白质组）rather than to increase the number of genes. Simply put, expansion of the glycome（糖组）with one oligosaccharide would double the potential size of the glycoproteome while maintaining genome size. However, doubling the proteome by introducing new genes and/or gene variants would significantly increase the size of the protein-coding part of the genome and, as such enhance the burden placed on the replication machinery to avoid unwanted mutations. Third, genetic defects in the glycosylation pathways cause a range of diseases. To date, more than 30 glycosylation synthesis-related disorders have been identified, mainly caused by defects in N- and O-linked glycosylation-related genes. The impact of these genetic defects is illustrated by the often high mortality rate and the broad range of phenotypes patients have, since all organs and basically the entire system is affected. Fourth, disease has been reported to alter the glycosylation profile （概况）of the organs or cell types affected. So not only can changes in glycosylation cause disease, variations in the glycosylation profile of proteins have been identified as disease markers as well.

Biopharmaceuticals are increasingly dominating the biopharmaceutical industry pipelines, and the current survey period has also been characterized by a continual rise in the market value of biopharmaceuticals. About 165 had gained approval up to about 2006, resulting in an estimated market size of some $70 billion (though data from various La Merie financial reports indicate that cumulative sales over 2014~2017 reached $651 billion, whereas total sales for 2017 alone reached $188 billion).

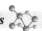

More than two-thirds of the estimated 2 500 biotech-based drugs that were in the pipelines (discovery phase, preclinical, or clinical trials) are glycoproteins. This makes glycosylation a critical factor in drug development that cannot be ignored by biopharmaceutical companies. Here we will focus our attention on N-linked glycosylation.

The central step of eukaryotic N-linked glycosylation takes place at the luminal（腔的）side of the endoplasmic reticulum (ER) membrane and involves the transfer of a tetradecaoligosaccharide to specific asparagine residues of nascent polypeptide chains. The process is catalyzed by a membrane protein complex, termed the oligosaccharyltransferase (OST). The Glc3Man9GlcNAc2 precursor is then further modified by a number of glycosidases（糖苷酶）and glycosyltransferases（糖苷转移酶）in the ER and the Golgi complex. The processing reactions that occur in the ER are highly conserved between lower and higher eukaryotes. In contrast, processing reactions taking place in the Golgi complex are species- and cell type-specific.

Besides promoting folding in the ER, the mere（仅仅的，只不过的）presence of N-glycans（聚糖，多糖）increases stability, solubility and resistance to proteases. Additionally, glycans affect circulation half-life, tissue distribution, and biological activity. Non-glycosylated versions of glycoproteins tend to be misfolded, rapidly cleared from the blood, and often show an altered biological activity. On the other hand, modification of glycoproteins with non-human oligosaccharides might result in undesired immunogenicity.

Due to its non-template driven nature, glycosylation typically leads to the synthesis of a heterogeneous（由不同成分形成的）collection of glycans. As a consequence, therapeutic glycoproteins are essentially produced as a mixture of individual pharmaceuticals, only differing in the identity of the attached glycans. Since N-glycans influence circulation half-life, tissue distribution, and biological activity, each glycoform has its own pharmacokinetic（药代动力学的）, pharmacodynamic（药效学的）and efficacy profile. The importance of glycosylation heterogeneity（异质性，异成分混杂）for the biopharmaceutical drug industry is illustrated by the fact that up to 80% of CHO cell-produced erythropoietin (EPO) is reportedly being discarded due to underglycosylation of the final product.

Therefore, it is no surprise that engineering of the N-glycosylation pathway of most currently used heterologous protein expression systems (bacteria, mammalian cells, insect cells, yeasts and plants) is actively pursued by several academic and industrial laboratories. These research efforts are in the first place directed at humanizing the N-glycosylation pathway and eliminating immunogenic glycotopes. Moreover, one wants to establish new structure-function relationships of different glycoforms, which helps to decrease the complexity of the N-glycan repertoire towards one defined N-glycan structure.

The desired glycoform profile of a biopharmaceutical glycoprotein may vary depending on the desired therapeutic effect (Table 1-3). Choosing the most suitable expression system for a particular glycoprotein is of critical importance since every system has its peculiarities.

At present, mammalian cell lines are the preferred system of choice for the production of therapeutic glycoproteins for intravenous injection and long circulation times due to their ability to modify proteins with complex-type sialylated（唾液酸化）N-glycans, which are glycoform profiles most closely to the requirements of medicinal use.

However, mammalian cells are not suitable for expressing all of the glycoproteins. Different mammalian cell expression system or different cell lines should be selected to achieve the optimal glycosylation.

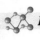

Table 1-3　The Most Suitable Expression System for a Particular Therapeutic Glycoprotein

Application	Desired N-glycan Features	Comment	Classical Expression System	Engineered Expression Systems	Example
Long circulation half-life intravenous injection	Multiantennary Terminal sialic acid	Exposed galactose, GlcNAc and mannose residues are efficiently recognized by lectins (植物凝集素) like the asialoglycoprotein (脱唾液酸蛋白) receptor (liver) and the mannose receptor (macrophages, dendritic cells,...) resulting in a drastically reduced plasma-half life. Terminal sialic acid residues efficiently shield these residues and consequently decrease the clearance rate from the blood significantly. For EPO, a direct correlation between sialic acid content and plasma half-life has been shown.	Mammalian cell lines, are currently the only expression system that can modify glycoproteins with multiantennary sialylated N-glycans	Glycoengineered *P. pastoris* strains and insect cell lines that can synthesize biantennary sialylated N-glycans have been created	Erythropoietin (Aranesp®; Epogen®; Procrit®; Eprex®; NeoRecormon®)
Short circulation half-life Intravenous injection	high mannose hybrid complex	Recognition of terminal mannose, galactose, GlcNAc and residues by lectin receptors will result in rapid clearance from the blood, with the notable exception of monoclonal antibodies.	Mammalian cell lines, bacteria, yeast	Glycoengineered yeast, insect cells and plants	Imaging reagents, antibodies for cancer treatment
Modulation of monoclonal antibody effector functions	Fc N-glycan (N297) of IgG—core fucosylation (盐藻糖基化) —Bisecting GlcNAc—terminal galactose	Different antibody glycoforms show different ADCC and CDC activity. The ability to produce antibody glycoforms with homogenous Fc N-glycosylation potentially allows ADCC and CDC tuning.	Mammalian cell lines	Glycoengineered *P. pastoris* strains, mammalian and insect cell lines, and plants	Anti-CD20 mAb Rituximab (Rituxan®; MabThera®)
Glycoconjugate vaccines Intramuscular injection	Bacterial O-antigen or capsular polysaccharide glycans	May be beneficial for increasing the immunogenicity of the injected protein.	Bacteria	Glycoengineered bacteria	Under development by GlycoVaxyn
Enzyme replacement therapy for lysosomal disorders	High mannose mannose-6-phosphate	Intravenously injected lysosomal enzymes with the correct glycosylation can be efficiently internalized via the mannose and the mannose-6-phosphate receptor.	Mammalian cell lines	Engineered yeast strains, plants and insect cells	Glucocerebrosidase (葡糖脑苷脂酶) (Cerezyme®) α-galactosidase A (Fabrazyme®)

Otherwise, one can modify a host cell line on its glycosylation characteristics through random mutation, or modify from a metabolic engineering point of view by using recombinant technology, such as coexpressing tPA with rat α-2, 6-sialyltransferase in CHO cells, which can make the sialic acid join the carbohydrate chain of the expressed tPA, connecting with 2,6-glycosidic bond, hence forming correct carbohydrate chain.

Furthermore, the glycosylation [including the degree of glycosylation, degree of branching of carbohydrate chains, degree of sialylation (唾液酸化) and sulfation, *etc.*] of glycoproteins expressed by mammalian cells is also affected by culture medium, culture conditions and other factors (such as the presence or absence of cytokines and hormone), *etc.* Sialidase and other glycosidase enzymes secreted or released by dead cells would degrade carbohydrate chains on the glycoprotein.

However, it is important to realize that cell lines in general use synthesized "mammalian" glycans, not "human" ones.

Insect cells have evolved to become a good alternative to mammalian cell cultures. Glycoengineering approaches have led to the construction of stable cell lines capable of synthesizing sialylated complex-type N-glycans. However, the presence of immunogenic glycotopes is still a major safety concern.

Bacteria are currently the preferred expression system for the production of heterologous proteins that are non-glycosylated or do not require posttranslational modifications for proper folding, stability, and/or activity. However, the discovery of the *C. jejuni* (空肠弯曲菌) N-glycosylation pathway and its functional transfer to *E. coli* were the first steps in the promising new field of bacterial glycoengineering.

Recent engineering efforts in the yeast *P. pastoris* have led to the construction of strains capable of modifying their glycoproteins with hybrid and complex type N-glycans. Since these strains produce relatively homogeneous glycosylation profiles they provide glycobiologists with a unique toolset for studying the structure-function relationship of N-glycans. Moreover, *Pichia* strains capable of producing sialylated N-glycans provide an alternative platform to mammalian cell culture.

Finally, transgenic plants are being evaluated as protein expression platforms as well. One of the major problems associated with plants is the modification of glycoproteins with immunogenic glycotopes. Transgenic plants with inactive β-1,2-xylosyltransferase (β-1,2- 木糖基转移酶) and α-1,3-fucosyltransferase (α-1,3- 岩藻糖转移酶) genes have recently been created. In the case of *Lemna minor* (无菌浮萍), this led to the homogeneous modification of an antibody with GlcNAc2Man3GlcNAc2 N-glycans. Also efforts to produce sialylated glycoproteins *in planta* (植物原位，植株原位) are underway.

So in R & D of glycoproteins, a lot of work should be done to determine the appropriate conditions for producing a homogeneous recombinant glycoprotein.

Future perspectives

Glycosylation pathway engineering is an active field of research both in academic and industrial research laboratories. Many challenges remain but great progress is being made. The engineering results in microorganisms also open the door to entirely novel ways of engineering the carbohydrates attached to recombinant glycoproteins. Therefore, the future of N-glycan engineering looks brighter than ever.

1.2.7 Metabolic engineering-combinatorial biology and new drug R&D （代谢工程 - 组合生物学与新药研发）

Metabolic engineering, also known as metabolic pathway engineering, is an applied discipline that uses the principles of molecular biology to systematically analyze the cell metabolic network, rationally design the cell metabolic pathway, and carry out genetic modification through recombinant DNA technology, so as to accomplish the modification of cell traits.

Through rational design for multi-step cascade in the process of cell metabolism and modification of cellular metabolic network, and using recombinant DNA technology to strengthen and/or inactivate, even rearrange relevant genes which control metabolic pathways, the production of natural products can be elevated, classical or *de novo* metabolic pathways can be modified or constructed on the basis of the combination of biology, in order to synthesize new products,

For genetically engineered pharmaceuticals, metabolic engineering is generally used to optimize the biological characteristics of recombinant cells, such as growth rate and tolerance toward adverse environmental conditions, and increase the yield and/or quality of recombinant protein products, such as genetic modification of host cells on glycosylation characteristics.

Metabolic engineering

Metabolic engineering is the practice of optimizing genetic and regulatory processes within cells to increase the cells' production of a certain substance. These processes are chemical networks that use a series of biochemical reactions and enzymes that allow cells to convert raw materials into molecules necessary for the cell's survival. Metabolic engineering specifically seeks to mathematically model these networks, calculate a yield of useful products, and pinpoint (准确指出，查明) parts of the network that constrain the production of these products. Genetic engineering techniques can then be used to modify the network in order to relieve these constraints. Once again this modified network can be modeled (做出……的模型) to calculate the new product yield.

The ultimate goal of metabolic engineering is to be able to use these organisms to produce valuable substances on an industrial scale in a cost effective (高性价比的，价格划算的) manner. Current examples include producing beer, wine, cheese, pharmaceuticals, and other biotechnology products.

Since cells use these metabolic networks for their survival, changes can have drastic effects on the cells' viability. Therefore, trade-offs (权衡，取舍) in metabolic engineering arise between the cells ability to produce the desired substance and its natural survival needs. Therefore, instead of directly deleting and/or overexpressing the genes that encode for metabolic enzymes, the current focus is to target the regulatory networks in a cell to efficiently engineer (操纵，引导) the metabolism.

History and applications of metabolic engineering

In the past, to increase the productivity of a desired metabolite, a microorganism was genetically modified by chemically induced mutation, and the mutant strain that overexpressed the desired metabolite was then chosen. However, one of the main problems with this technique was that the metabolic pathway for the production of that metabolite was not analyzed, and as a result, the constraints to production and relevant pathway enzymes to be modified were unknown.

In 1990s, a new technique called **metabolic engineering** emerged. This technique analyzes the metabolic pathway of a microorganism, and determines the constraints and their effects on the production of desired compounds. It then uses genetic engineering to relieve these constraints.

At the industrial scale, metabolic engineering is becoming more convenient and cost effective.

Metabolic engineering continues to evolve in efficiency and processes aided by breakthroughs in the field of synthetic biology. Researchers in synthetic biology optimize genetic pathways, which in turn

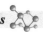

influence cellular metabolic outputs (产出, 产量) . Recent decreases in cost of synthesized DNA and developments in genetic circuits (遗传回路) help to influence the ability of metabolic engineering to produce desired outputs.

Metabolic flux analysis

Setting up a metabolic pathway for analysis

The first step in the process is to identify a desired goal to achieve through the improvement or modification of an organism's metabolism. Reference books and online databases are used to research reactions and metabolic pathways that are able to produce this product or result. These databases contain copious (丰富的, 很多的, 多产的) genomic and chemical information including pathways for metabolism and other cellular processes. Using this research, an organism is chosen that will be used to create the desired product or result. Considerations that are taken into account when making this decision are how close the organism's metabolic pathway is to the desired pathway, the maintenance costs associated with (与……有关系) the organism, and how easy it is to modify the pathway of the organism. *Escherichia coli* (*E. coli*) is widely used in metabolic engineering to synthesize a wide variety of products such as amino acids because it is relatively easy to maintain and modify. If the organism does not contain the complete pathway for the desired product or result, then genes that produce the missing enzymes must be incorporated into the organism.

Analyzing a metabolic pathway

The completed metabolic pathway is modeled mathematically to find the theoretical yield of the product or the reaction fluxes (反应通量) in the cell. A flux is the rate at which a given reaction in the network occurs. Simple metabolic pathway analysis can be done by hand (手工) , but most require the use of software to perform the computations. These programs use complex linear algebra (线性代数) algorithms (算法, 运算规则) to solve these models. To solve a network using the equation for determined systems shown below, one must input the necessary information about the relevant reactions and their fluxes. Information about the reaction [such as the reactants (反应物) and stoichiometry (化学计量学)] is contained in the matrices (矩阵) G_x and G_m. Matrices V_m and V_x contain the fluxes of the relevant reactions. When solved, the equation yields the values of all the unknown fluxes (contained in V_x).

$$V_x = -(G_x)^{-1} \times (G_m \times V_m)$$

Determining the optimal genetic manipulations

After solving for the fluxes of reactions in the network, it is necessary to determine which reactions may be altered in order to maximize the yield of the desired product. To determine what specific genetic manipulations to perform, it is necessary to use computational algorithms, such as OptGene or OptFlux. They provide recommendations for which genes should be overexpressed, knocked out, or introduced in a cell to allow increased production of the desired product. For example, if a given reaction is in a particularly low flux state and is limiting the amount of product, the software may recommend that the enzyme catalyzing this reaction should be overexpressed in the cell to increase the reaction flux. The necessary genetic manipulations can be performed using standard molecular biology techniques. Genes may be overexpressed or knocked out from an organism, depending on their effect on the pathway and the ultimate goal.

Experimental measurements

In order to create a solvable model, it is often necessary to have certain fluxes already known or experimentally measured. In addition, in order to verify the effect of genetic manipulations on the metabolic network (to ensure they align with the model), it is necessary to experimentally measure the fluxes in the network. To measure reaction fluxes, carbon flux measurements are made using carbon-13 isotopic labeling. The organism is fed a mixture that contains molecules where specific carbons are engineered to be carbon-13 atoms, instead of carbon-12. After these molecules are used in the network, downstream metabolites also become labeled with carbon-13, as they incorporate those atoms in their structures. The specific labeling pattern (模式) of the various metabolites is determined by the reaction fluxes in the network. Labeling patterns may be measured using techniques such as gas chromatography-mass spectrometry (GC-MS) along with computational algorithms to determine reaction fluxes.

Combinatorial biology（组合生物学）

In biotechnology, **combinatorial biology** is the creation of a large number of compounds (usually proteins or peptides) through technologies such as phage display. Similar to combinatorial chemistry, compounds are produced by biosynthesis rather than organic chemistry. This process was developed independently by Richard A. Houghten and H. Mario Geysen in the 1980s. Combinatorial biology allows the generation and selection of a large number of ligands for high-throughput screening.

These large numbers of peptides are generated and screened by physically linking a gene encoding a protein with a copy of this protein. This could involve the protein being fused to the M13 minor coat protein pⅢ, with the gene encoding this protein being held within the phage particle. Large libraries of phages with different proteins on their surfaces can then be screened through automated selection and amplification for a protein that binds tightly to a particular target（Fig. 1-19）.

Combinatorial biology and novel erythromycin analogs

The structures of complex polyketide（聚酮化合物）natural products, such as erythromycin, are programmed by multifunctional polyketide synthases (PKSs) that contain modular arrangements of functional domains. It is well established that the "modular" polyketide synthases (PKSs) (i) each are encoded by a cluster of contiguous（连续的，邻近的）genes and (ii) have a linear, modular organization of similar catalytic domains that both build and modify the polyketide backbone. Each module（模块）contains a set of three domains — a ketosynthase, an acyltransferase (AT), and an acyl carrier protein (ACP) — that catalyze a 2-carbon extension of the growing polyketide chain.

The remarkable structural diversity of polyketides is governed by the combinatorial possibilities of catalytic domains within each module, the sequence and number of modules, and the post-polyketide synthesis cyclization and "tailoring" enzymes that accompany the PKS genes. The natural polyketides thus far revealed represent only a small fraction of the combinatorial potential that might be realized from permutations（排列）of modules in a PKS. The direct correspondence between the catalytic domains of modules in a

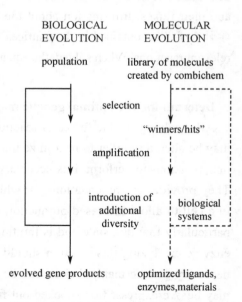

Fig. 1-19 Comparison of natural and synthetic selection processes for peptide generation.

PKS and the structure of the resulting biosynthetic product portends（预示，意味着）the possibility of modifying polyketide structure by modifying the domains of the modular PKS.

Although efforts were made successfully to chemically modify the existing functional groups of the macrolide（大环内酯物）ring of erythromycin, most of the ring remained inaccessible to chemical modification. After the discovery of the programmed nature of modular polyketide biosynthesis, genetic engineering strategies emerged for the production of novel polyketides.

Robert McDaniel *et al.* have engineered the erythromycin polyketide synthase genes to effect（实现）combinatorial alterations of catalytic activities in the biosynthetic pathway, generating a library of > 50 macrolides（大环内酯）that would be impractical to produce by chemical methods. By using **6-deoxyerythronolide B synthase（DEBS, 6-脱氧红霉内酯-B合成酶）**, the PKS that produces the macrolide ring of erythromycin, they have constructed a combinatorial library of polyketides. This was accomplished by substituting the ATs and β-carbon processing domains of DEBS with counterparts from the rapamycin（雷帕霉素）PKS (RAPS) that encode alternative substrate specificities and β-carbon reduction/dehydration activities. Engineered DEBS containing single, double, and triple catalytic domain substitutions catalyzed production of erythromycin macrolactones with corresponding single, double, and triple modifications.

Therefore, via genetic engineering, it is now feasible to contemplate（盘算）modifications of the chemically intractable（棘手的）sites of such molecules to produce hundreds or even thousands of new "unnatural" natural products. Such novel macrolides could in themselves provide the basis for new pharmaceuticals or could serve as scaffolds for new semisynthetic analogs.

1.2.8 Research on novel biopharmaceutical preparations（新型生物药物制剂的研究）

With the development of biologics, biomacromolecular drugs such as peptides, proteins, and nucleic acids keep emerging and are widely used in the treatment of various diseases. There are some common issues about these drugs. Including poor *in vivo* stability, a strong likeliness to be denatured and inactivated, and a greater likelihood to be removed from the blood circulation; therefore, it is needed to develop a non-injection-based drug delivery system which is safe, effective, and with high bioavailability, to apply the most effective means and approach to make biologics achieve and then act on every target sites or cells in the body. Therefore developing and improving biopharmaceutical preparation is the key to promoting the clinical application of biologics. At present, studies on the mechanism of absorption and transportation of macromolecular drugs, as well as various drug delivery systems, have become new hotspot issues, among which nasal administration, oral administration, pulmonary（肺的）inhalation and percutaneous（经由皮肤的）administration, *etc.* have made certain achievements and have entered into the stage of clinical application. For example, the salmon calcitonin（降钙素）nasal spray has been used in clinical practice for many years. Every year, 1.3 million US citizens use estradiol（雌二醇）transdermal patches. With the development of biological engineering, biomaterials, nanotechnology and pharmaceutical science, the research in the field of biopharmaceutical preparations will continue to be dug deeper and developed rapidly.

In short, the rapid development of genetic engineering pharmaceutical industry in the recent decades is based on the development of some fundamental disciplines, such as molecular biology, molecular genetics, molecular pathology, *etc.*, and backed by the development of some fundamental engineering disciplines, such as genetic engineering, cell engineering, fermentation engineering, enzyme engineering, and protein engineering. This industry, which combines the most advanced technologies, equipments and methods of modern biology, medicine, and pharmacy, has brought a revolution to the pharmaceutical industry. After research in biology entered the post-genome era, the accumulation of genomics and proteomics data and the application of high-throughput screening techniques in the process of researching and developing novel biopharmaceutical molecules will accelerate the process of discovering novel biologics, especially of genetically engineered therapeutics. Meanwhile, continually emerging new biotechnology, new downstream technology, new biopharmaceutical preparations, and new products in the field of genetic engineering pharmaceutics will bring a new revolution to the pharmaceutical industry. Genetically engineered therapeutics have become a mainstay of the biopharmaceutical industry in the 21st century. We should grasp the golden opportunity provided by the great achievement of the Human Genome Project for the R&D of novel genetically engineered therapeutics, and strive to research and develop biologics with our own intellectual property rights, so that the modern pharmaceutical industry centered on genetic engineering will truly become a sunrise industry in China.

Chapter 2
Basic Principles of Genetic Engineering
第 2 章　基因工程基本原理

2.1　The definition and history of genetic engineering（基因工程的定义及发展沿革）

2.1.1　The definition of genetic engineering（基因工程的定义）

Gene（基因）：A **gene** is a locus (or region) of DNA that encodes a functional RNA or protein product, and is the molecular unit of heredity. The transmission of genes to an organism's offspring is the basis of the inheritance of phenotypic traits. Most biological traits are under the influence of polygenes (many different genes) as well as the gene-environment interactions. Some genetic traits are instantly visible, such as eye color or number of limbs（肢）, and some are not, such as blood type, risk facton for specific diseases, or the thousands of basic biochemical processes that comprise life.

Genes can acquire mutations in their sequence, leading to different variants, known as alleles, in the population. These alleles encode slightly different versions of a protein, which cause different phenotype traits. Colloquial usage of the term "having a gene" (*e.g.*, "good genes," "hair color gene") typically refers to having a different allele of the gene. Genes evolve due to natural selection or survival of the fittest of the alleles.

The concept of a gene continues to be refined as new phenomena are discovered. For example, regulatory regions of a gene can be far removed from its coding regions, and coding regions can be split into several exons. Some viruses store their genome in RNA instead of DNA and some gene products are functional non-coding RNAs. Therefore, a broad, modern working definition of a gene is any discrete locus（基因座）of heritable, genomic sequence which affects an organism's traits by being expressed as a functional product or by regulation of gene expression.

Genetic engineering（基因工程）：**Genetic engineering**, also called **genetic modification**, is the modification of an organism's genome through biotechnology, *i.e.*, the direct manipulation of an organism's genome using biotechnology. It is a set of technologies used to change the genetic makeup of cells, including the transfer of genes within and across species boundaries to produce improved or novel organisms. New DNA may be inserted in the host genome by first isolating and copying the genetic material of interest using molecular cloning methods to generate a DNA sequence, or by synthesizing the DNA, and then inserting this construct into the host organism. Genes may be removed, or "knocked out", using a nuclease. Gene targeting is a different technique that uses homologous recombination to change an endogenous gene, and can be used to delete a gene, remove exons, add a gene, or introduce point mutations. Genetic engineering is the most important part of bioengineering.

An organism that is generated through genetic engineering is considered to be a genetically modified organism (GMO). The first kind of GMOs were bacteria in 1973 and GM mice were generated in 1974. Insulin-producing bacteria were commercialized in 1982 and genetically modified food has been sold since 1994. Glofish（荧光鱼，荧光热带鱼），the first kind of GMO designed as a pet, was first sold in the United States in December 2003.

Genetic engineering techniques have been applied in numerous fields including research, agriculture, industrial biotechnology, and medicine. Enzymes used in laundry（洗衣店，洗衣房）detergent and medicines such as insulin and human growth hormone are now manufactured in GM cells, experimental GM cell lines and GM animals such as mice or zebrafish are being used for research purposes, and genetically modified crops have been commercialized.

Definition

Genetic engineering alters the genetic make-up of an organism using techniques that remove heritable material or that introduce DNA prepared outside the organism either directly into the host or into a cell that is then fused or hybridized with the host. This involves using recombinant nucleic acid (DNA or RNA) techniques to form new combinations of heritable genetic material, followed by the incorporation of that material either indirectly through a vector system or directly through micro-injection（显微注射法），macro-injection（巨量注射法）and micro-encapsulation（微胶囊法）techniques.

Genetic engineering does not normally include traditional animal and plant breeding（育种），*in vitro* fertilization, induction of polyploid（多倍体，多倍性），mutagenesis（突变形成）and cell fusion techniques that do not use recombinant nucleic acids or a genetically modified organism in the process. However the European Commission has also defined genetic engineering broadly as including selective breeding and other means of artificial selection. Cloning and stem cell research, although not considered genetic engineering, are closely related and genetic engineering can be used within them. Synthetic biology is an emerging discipline that takes genetic engineering a step further by introducing artificially synthesized material from raw materials into an organism.

If genetic material from another species is added to the host, the resulting organism is called transgenic. If genetic material from the same species or a species that can naturally breed with（彼此可以配种）the host is used, the resulting organism is called cisgenic（同种基改）. Genetic engineering can also be used to remove genetic material from the target organism, creating a gene knockout organism. In Europe genetic modification is synonymous（同义的，同义突变的）with genetic engineering while in the United States of America it can also refer to conventional breeding methods. The Canadian regulatory system is based on whether a product has novel features regardless of method of origin. In other words, a product is regulated（规　定）as genetically modified if it carries some trait not previously found in the species whether it was generated using traditional breeding methods (*e.g.*, selective breeding, cell fusion（细胞融合），mutation breeding) or genetic engineering. Within the scientific community, the term *genetic engineering* is not commonly used; more specific terms such as *transgenic* are preferred.

2.1.2　History of genetic engineering（基因工程的发展沿革）

Humans have altered the genomes of species for thousands of years through selective breeding, or artificial selection as contrasted with natural selection, and more recently through mutagenesis. Genetic engineering as the direct manipulation of DNA by humans outside breeding and mutations has only existed since the 1970s. The term "genetic engineering" was first coined by Jack Williamson in his science fiction novel *Dragon's Island*, published in 1951 — one year before DNA's role in heredity was confirmed by Alfred Hershey and Martha Chase, and two years before James Watson and Francis Crick showed that the DNA molecule has a double-helix structure — though the general concept of direct genetic manipulation was explored in rudimentary（基本的，初步的）form in Stanley G. Weinbaum's science fiction story *Proteus Island*（普罗透斯岛）in 1936.

In 1972, Paul Berg created the first recombinant DNA molecules by combining DNA from the monkey virus SV40 with that of the lambda virus. In 1973, Herbert Boyer and Stanley Cohen created the first transgenic organism by inserting antibiotic resistance genes into the plasmid of the *E. coli* bacterium. A year later Rudolf Jaenisch created a transgenic mouse by introducing foreign DNA into its embryo, making it the world's first transgenic animal. These achievements led to concerns in the scientific community about potential risks from genetic engineering, which were first discussed in depth at the Asilomar Conference（艾西洛玛会议）in 1975. One of the main recommendations from this meeting was that government oversight（监管，照管）of recombinant DNA research should be established until the technology was deemed（认为）safe.

In 1976, Genentech, the first genetic engineering company, was founded by Herbert Boyer and Robert Swanson and a year later the company produced a human protein (somatostatin，生长抑素) in *E. coli*. Genentech announced the production of genetically engineered human insulin in 1978. In 1980, the U.S. Supreme Court in the *Diamond v. Chakrabarty* case ruled（规定）that genetically altered life could be patented. The insulin produced by bacteria, branded humulin, was approved for release by the Food and Drug Administration in 1982.

In the 1970s, graduate student Steven Lindow of the University of Wisconsin-Madison with D.C. Arny and C. D. Upper found a bacterium he identified as *Pseudomonas syringae*（*P. syringae*，丁香假单胞菌）that played a role in ice nucleation（成核，成核现象）, and in 1977 he discovered a mutant ice-minus strain（防霜负型突变型菌株）. Dr. Lindow (who is now a plant pathologist at the University of California-Berkeley) later successfully created a recombinant ice-minus strain. In 1983, a biotech company, Advanced Genetic Sciences (AGS) applied for U.S. government authorization to perform field tests with the ice-minus strain of *P. syringae* to protect crops from frost, but environmental groups and protestors delayed the field tests for four years with legal challenges（法律质疑）. In 1987, the ice-minus strain of *P. syringae* became the first genetically modified organism (GMO) to be released into the environment when a strawberry field and a potato field in California were sprayed with it. Both test fields were attacked by activist（积极分子，激进主义分子）groups the night before the tests occurred: "The world's first trial site attracted the world's first field trasher（捣毁者，故意破坏者，捣乱分子）".

The first field trials of genetically engineered plants occurred in France and the USA in 1986, tobacco plants were engineered to be resistant to herbicides（除草剂；除莠剂）. The People's Republic of China was the first country to commercialize transgenic plants, introducing a virus-resistant tobacco in

1992. In 1994, Calgene（卡尔基公司）attained approval to commercially release the Flavr Savr tomato, a tomato engineered to have a longer shelf life. In 1994, the European Union approved tobacco engineered to be resistant to the herbicide bromoxynil（溴草腈）, making it the first genetically engineered crop commercialized in Europe. In 1995, *Bacillus thuringiensis*（Bt，苏云金芽孢杆菌）potato was approved safe by the Environmental Protection Agency, after having been approved by the FDA, making it the first pesticide producing crop to be approved in the USA. In 2009, 11 transgenic crops were grown commercially in 25 countries, the largest of which by area grown were the USA, Brazil, Argentina, India, Canada, China, Paraguay and South Africa.

In 2010, scientists at the J. Craig Venter Institute created the first synthetic life form by adding a synthetic genome to an empty bacterial cell. The resulting bacterium was named Synthia（辛西娅，合成体，人造儿）. In 2014, a bacterium was developed that replicated a plasmid containing a unique（独特的）base pair, creating the first organism engineered to use an expanded genetic alphabet.

The greatest discoveries influencing the history of genetic engineering are described below in detail. The first experiment demonstrating DNA as genetic material is *S. pneumonia* **transformation**（肺炎链球菌的转化实验）.

2.1.2.1 *Bacterial transformation*（细菌转化实验）*(Avery, MacLeod, McCarty) 1940s*

DNA or Protein?

Clarification came during the first world war. During the war, hundreds of thousands of servicemen died from pneumonia, a lung infection caused by the bacterium *Streptococcus pneumoniae*. In the early 1920s, a young British army medical officer named Frederick Griffith began studying *Streptococcus pneumoniae* in his laboratory in the hopes of developing a vaccine against it. As so often happens in scientific research, Griffith never found what he was looking for (there is still no vaccine for pneumonia), but instead, he made one of the most important discoveries in the field of biology: a phenomenon he called "transformation." (Fig.2-1)

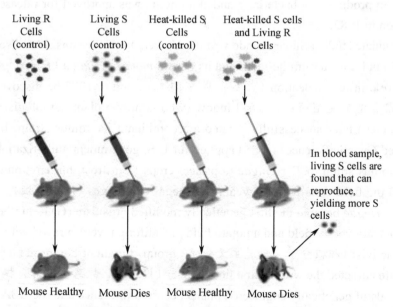

Fig. 2-1 Transformation of *Streptococcus pneumoniae* discovered by Frederick Griffith.

Dr. Griffith had isolated two strains of *S. pneumoniae*, one of which was pathogenic (meaning it causes sickness or death, in this case, pneumonia), and one of which was innocuous or harmless. The pathogenic strain looked smooth under a microscope due to a protective coat surrounding the bacteria and so he named this strain S, for smooth. The harmless strain of *S. pneumoniae* lacked the protective coat and appeared rough under a microscope, so he named it R, for rough.

Dr. Griffith observed that if he injected some of the S strain of *S. pneumoniae* into mice, they would get sick with the symptoms of pneumonia and die, while mice injected with the R strain did not become sick. Next, Griffith noticed that if he applied heat to the S strain of bacteria, then injected them into mice, the mice would no longer get sick and die. He thus hypothesized that excessive heat kills the bacteria, something that other scientists, including Louis Pasteur, had already shown with other types of bacteria.

However, Dr. Griffith didn't stop there — he decided to try something: he mixed living R bacteria (which are not pathogenic) with heat-killed S bacteria, then he injected the mixture into mice. Surprisingly, the mice got pneumonia infections and eventually died.

Dr. Griffith examined samples from these sick mice and found living S bacteria. This meant that either the S bacteria came back to life, an unlikely scenario (情况), or the live R strain was somehow "transformed" into the S strain. Thus, after repeating this experiment many times, Dr. Griffith named this phenomenon "transformation." This discovery was significant because it showed that organisms can somehow be genetically "re-programmed" into a slightly different version of themselves. One strain of bacteria, in this case the R strain of *S. pneumoniae*, can be changed into something else, presumably because of the transfer of genetic material from a donor, in this case the heat-killed S strain.

Scientists around the world began repeating this experiment, but in slightly different ways, trying to discover exactly what was happening. It became clear that, when the S bacteria are killed by heat, they break open and many substances are released. Something in this mixture can be absorbed by living bacteria, leading to a genetic transformation. But because the mixture contains protein, RNA, DNA, lipids, and carbohydrates, the question remained — which molecule is the "transforming agent?"

This question was examined in several ways, most famously by three scientists working at the Rockefeller Institute (now Rockefeller University) in New York, Oswald Avery, Colin MacLeod, and Maclyn McCarty. These scientists did almost exactly what Griffith did in his experiments but with the following changes. First, after heat-killing the S strain of bacteria, the mixture was separated into six test tubes. Thus, each of the test tubes would contain the unknown "transforming agent". A different enzyme was then added to each tube except one — the control — which received nothing. To the other five tubes, one of the following enzymes was added: RNase, an enzyme that destroys RNA; protease, an enzyme that destroys protein; DNase, an enzyme that destroys DNA; lipase, an enzyme that destroys lipids; or a combination of enzymes that break down carbohydrates. The theory behind this experiment was that if the "transforming agent" was, for example, protein — the transforming agent would be destroyed in the test tube containing protease, but no the others. Thus, whatever the transforming agent was, the liquid in one of the tubes would no longer be able to transform the *S. pneumonia* strains. When they did this, the result was both dramatic (引人注目的) and clear. The liquid from the tubes that received RNase, protease, lipase, and the carbohydrate-digesting enzymes was still able to transform the R strain of *S. pneumonia* into the S strain. However, the liquid that was treated with DNase completely lost the ability to transform the bacteria (Fig. 2-2).

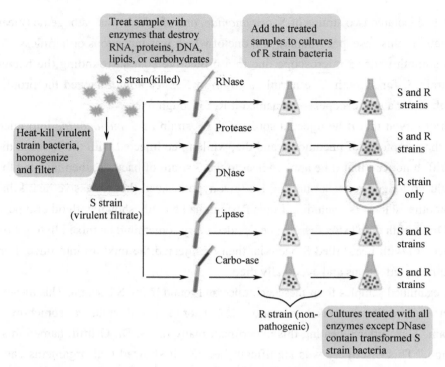

Fig. 2-2 Experiment done by Colin MacLeod, and Maclyn McCarty.

Thus, it was apparent that the "transforming agent" in the liquid was DNA. To further demonstrate this, the scientists took liquid extracted from heat-killed *S. pneumoniae* (S strain) and subjected it to extensive preparation and purification, isolating only the pure DNA from the mixture. This pure DNA was also able to transform the R strain into the S strain and generate pathogenic *S. pneumoniae*. These results provided powerful evidence that DNA, and not protein, was actually the genetic material inside of living cells.

2.1.2.2 *Hershey-Chase experiment on phage infection*（噬菌体感染实验）*(Hershey, Chase) 1952*

Despite this very clear result, some scientists remained skeptical and continued to think that proteins were likely（很可能的）the genetic molecule. Eight years after the famous Avery, MacLeod, and McCarty experiment was published, two scientists named Alfred Hershey and Martha Chase performed an entirely different type of genetic experiment. For their experimental system, they selected an extremely small virus called a bacteriophage (or just phage), which only infects bacterial cells. At that time, scientists knew that when these phage infect a bacterial cell, they somehow "reprogram" the bacterium to transform itself into a factory for producing more phage. They also knew that the phage itself does not enter the bacterium during an infection. Rather, a small amount of material is injected into the bacteria and this material must contain all of the information necessary to build more phages. Thus, this injected substance is the genetic material of the phage.

Hershey and Chase designed a very simple experiment to determine which molecule, DNA or protein, acted as the genetic material in phages. To do this, they made use of a technique called radioactive labeling. In radioactive labeling, a radioactive isotope of a certain atom is used and can be followed by tracking the radioactivity (radioactivity is very easily detected by laboratory instruments, even back in the 1940s, and remains a very common tool in scientific research). So, what Hershey and Chase did was to grow two batches of phage in their laboratory. One batch was grown in the presence of radioactive phosphorous. The element phosphorous is present in large amounts in DNA, but is not present in the proteins of bacteria and phage. Thus, this batch of phage would have radio-labeled DNA. The second batch of phage was grown in the presence of radioactive sulfur. Sulfur is an element that is often found in proteins, but never in DNA. Thus, the second batch of phage would have radio-labeled proteins (Fig.2-3).

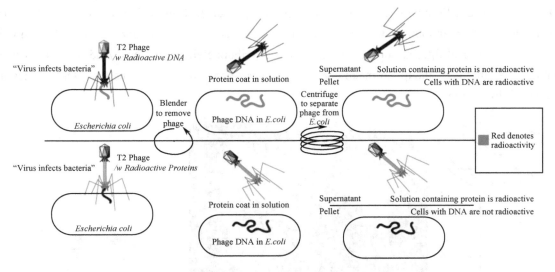

Fig. 2-3　Phage infection experiment.

Then, Hershey and Chase used these two batches of phage separately to infect bacteria and then measured where the radioactivity ended up. What they observed was that only those bacteria infected by phage with radiolabeled DNA became radioactive, bacteria infected by phage with radiolabeled protein did not. Thus Hershey and Chase concluded that it is DNA, and not protein, that is injected into the bacteria during phage infection and this DNA must be the genetic material that reprograms the bacteria.

The Blueprint of Life

Taken together, these experiments represented strong evidence that DNA is the genetic material. Other scientists later confirmed these result in many different kinds of experiments, including showing that eukaryotic, and even human cells can be "transformed" by the injection of DNA. The result of these findings was to convince the scientific and lay（外行的，非专业性的）communities that the molecule of heredity is indeed DNA. It turns out that the initial instincts of many scientists were exactly backward（落后的，相反地）：they assumed that protein was the genetic material of chromosomes and DNA merely provided structure. The opposite turned out to be true. The DNA molecule houses genetic information and proteins act as the structural framework of chromosomes.

The discovery that DNA was the "transforming agent" and the genetic component of human chromosomes was one of the greatest discoveries of science in the 20th century. However, the mechanism of how DNA codes for genetic information was initially a complete mystery and became the focus of intense scientific study. Still today, the study of how DNA functions comprises an entire discipline of science called molecular biology. Originally an offshoot of biochemistry, the field of molecular biology joins biologists, chemists, anthropologists, forensic（法医的）scientists, geneticists, botanists, and many others who are working to shed light onto（阐明）the immense complexity of DNA, the so-called blueprint of life.

2.1.2.3 *Watson and Crick-double helix model of DNA*（*Waston-Crick DNA*双螺旋模型）（*1953*）

As the 1950s began, both how proteins could be specified by instructions in the DNA and how this information can be inherited seemed completely mysterious.

In 1953, James Watson and Francis Crick predicted DNA double-helix structure, which immediately solve the mystery (Fig. 2-4).

On Feb.28, 1953, Francis Crick walked into the Eagle pub in Cambridge, England, and as James Watson later recalled, announced that "we had found the secret of life". Actually, they had. That morning, Watson and Crick had figured out the structure of deoxyribonucleic acid, DNA. And that structure — a "double helix" that can "unzip" to make copies of itself — confirmed suspicions that DNA carries life's hereditary information.

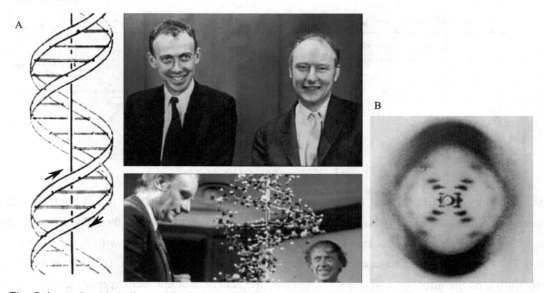

Fig. 2-4　A. Double helix model of DNA. The figure is purely diagrammatic. The two ribbons symbolize the two phosphate — sugar chains, and the horizontal rods the pairs of bases holding the chains together. The vertical line marks the fiber axis. B. Evidence for the structure of DNA. This photograph, taken by Rosalind Franklin, shows the X-ray diffraction pattern produced by wet DNA fibers. The cross pattern indicates a helical structure, and the strong spots at top and bottom correspond to a helical rise of 0.34 nm. The layer line spacing is one-tenth of the distance from the center to either of these spots, showing that there are 10 base pairs per repeat.

X-Ray Diffraction and the Structure of DNA

In 1951, James Watson, joined the lab and the two formed a close working relationship. They were convinced that the three-dimensional structure of a molecule known to play a role in passing genetic information — DNA — could be determined. They made models based on research done in several fields. Crick and Watson found the result of Rosalind Franklin's X-ray diffraction studies, and a final piece of the puzzle（拼图）was fitted（安装）. In 1953, they created a visual model of DNA.

Watson was shown this picture by Wilkins in early 1953. From the picture it was possible to calculate:

1) The distance between bases (0.34 nm)

2) The length of the period (3.4 nm)

3) The rise of the helix (36 degrees)

Building model

Therefore, knowing that DNA existed and contained four bases, a ribose (核糖) sugar and phosphate. Inspired by Pauling's successful attempts at building 3-D models of proteins, Crick and Watson believed this to be the correct way to proceed.

Bases

John Griffith, the mathematician nephew of Fred erick Griffith, calculated the attractive forces between "like" bases. Crick's idea was that since the bases were flat, perhaps they could be stacked on top of one another, and attracted that way. Griffith informed him that adenine attracted thymine and guanine attracts cytosine.

Chargaff's 1 : 1 Rule （Table 2-1）

Table 2-1   Chargaff's data

DNA source	Adenine	Thymine	Guanine	Cytosine
Calf Thymus	1.7	1.6	1.2	1.0
Beef Spleen	1.6	1.5	1.3	1.0
Yeast	1.8	1.9	1.0	1.0
Tubercle Bacillus	1.1	1.0	2.6	2.4

(From Vischer, Zamenhof and Chargaff, 1949, p. 433, and Chargaff *et al.*, 1949, p413).

Chargaff's rules state that DNA from any cell of all organisms should have a 1 : 1 ratio of pyrimidine and purine bases and, more specifically, that the amount of guanine is equal to cytosine and the amount of adenine is equal to thymine.

When Crick compared the bases that Griffiths had told him with Chargaff's data (Table 2-1), he realized that complementary base pairing could be the cause of the 1 : 1 rule.

Hydrogen bond

Watson and Crick thought that hydrogen bonding was too unstable to be responsible for replication. Crick also assumed that both tautameric (互变异构的) forms of the bases existed in the same DNA molecule, and that the proton could shift from one position to another, thus altering the sites for hydrogen bond formation.

The final model

This structure has two helical chains each coiled round the same axis.

Usual chemical assumptions, namely, that each chain consists of phosphate diester groups joining β-D-deoxyribofuranose residues with 3′, 5′ linkages.

Both chains follow right-handed helices, but owing to the dyad (一对，一双) the sequences of the atoms in the two chains run in opposite directions.

An angle of 36 degrees between adjacent residues in the same chain, so that the structure repeats after 10 residues on each chain, that is, after 34 nm. The distance of a phosphorus atom from the fiber axis is 1 nm.

As the phosphates are on the outside, cations have easy access to them.

The phosphates are negatively charged, and attract cations. The phosphates, being charged, are also hydrophilic.

For their outstanding work in discovering the double helical structure of DNA, Watson an Crick shared the 1962 Nobel Prize in Physiology or Medicine with Maurice Wilkins.

Widely regarded as one of the most important discoveries of the 20th century it has led the way to the mapping and deciphering of all the genes in the human chromosomes.

2.1.2.4 *Successfully decoding of the genetic code*（遗传密码的成功破译）

Nirenberg and Matthaei experiment in 1961—1964

The Nirenberg and Matthaei experiment was a scientific experiment performed on May 15, 1961 by Heinrich J. Matthaei in the research group of Marshall W. Nirenberg and Heinrich J. Matthaei. The experiment cracked the genetic code by using nucleic acid homopolymers to translate specific amino acids.

In the experiment, an extract from bacterial cells that could make protein even when no intact living cells were present was prepared. Adding an artificial form of RNA, polyuridylic acid（poly U, 多聚尿苷酸）, to this extract caused it to make an unnatural protein composed entirely of the amino acid phenylalanine (Phe). This showed that RNA controlled the production of specific types of protein (Fig.2-5).

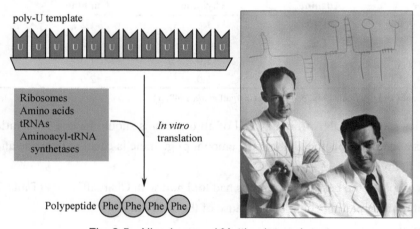

Fig. 2-5　Nirenberg and Matthaei experiment.

By 1959, experiments and analysis such as the Avery-MacLeod-McCarty experiment, the Hershey-Chase experiment, the Watson-Crick structure and the Meselson-Stahl experiment had shown DNA to be the molecule of genetic information. It was not known, however, how DNA directed the expression of proteins, or what role RNA had in these processes. Nirenberg teamed up with Heinrich J. Matthaei at the National Institutes of Health to answer these questions. They produced RNA comprised solely of uracil, a nucleotide that only occurs in RNA. They then added this synthetic poly-uracil RNA into a cell-free extract of *Escherichia coli* which contained the DNA, RNA, ribosomes and other cellular machinery for protein synthesis. They added DNase, which breaks apart the DNA, so that no additional proteins would be produced other than that from their synthetic RNA. They then added 1 radioactively labeled amino acid, the building blocks of proteins, and 19 unlabeled amino acids to the extract, varying the labeled amino acid in each sample. In the extract containing the radioactively labeled phenylalanine, the resulting protein was also radioactive. They realized that they had found the genetic code for phenylalanine: UUU (three uracil bases in a row) on RNA. This was the first step in deciphering the codons of the genetic code and the first demonstration of messenger RNA.

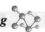

Nirenberg received great scientific attention for these experiments. Within a few years, his research team had performed similar experiments and found that three-base repeats of adenosine (AAA) produced the amino acid lysine, cytosine repeats (CCC) produced proline and guanine repeats (GGG) produced nothing at all. The next breakthrough came when Phillip Leder, a postdoctoral researcher in Nirenberg's lab, developed a method for determining the genetic code on pieces of tRNA (Fig. 2-6, Table 2-2). This greatly sped up the assignment of three-base codons to amino acids so that 50 codons were identified in this way. Khorana's experiments confirmed these results and completed the genetic code translation.

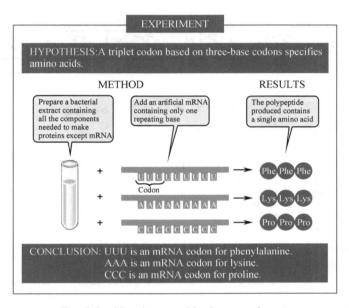

Fig. 2-6   Nirenberg and Leder experiment.

Table 2-2   Table of standard genetic code

First position (5′end)	Second position				Third position (3′end)
	U	C	A	G	
U	Phe	Ser	Tyr	Cys	U
	Phe	Ser	Tyr	Cys	C
	Leu	Ser	Stop	Stop	A
	Leu	Ser	Stop	Trp	G
C	Leu	Pro	His	Arg	U
	Leu	Pro	His	Arg	C
	Leu	Pro	Gln	Arg	A
	Leu	Pro	Gln	Arg	G
A	Ile	Thr	Asn	Ser	U
	Ile	Thr	Asn	Ser	C
	Ile	Thr	Lys	Arg	A
	Met	Thr	Lys	Arg	G
G	Val	Ala	Asp	Gly	U
	Val	Ala	Asp	Gly	C
	Val	Ala	Glu	Gly	A
	Val	Ala	Glu	Gly	G

2.1.2.5 *Lac operon of the model bacterium Escherichia coli (Francois Jacob, David Perrin, Carmen Sanchez and Jacques Monod)*（模式细菌大肠埃希菌的乳糖操纵子）*(1960)*

Francois Jacob, David Perrin, Carmen Sanchez and Jacques Monod proposed the operon concept for control of bacteria gene action. Jacob and Monod later proposed that a protein repressor blocks RNA synthesis of a specific set of genes, the *lac* operon, unless an inducer, lactose, binds to the repressor（Fig. 2-7）. With Lwoff, Jacob and Monod were awarded the Nobel Prize in Physiology or Medicine in 1965 due to their work on the lac operon.

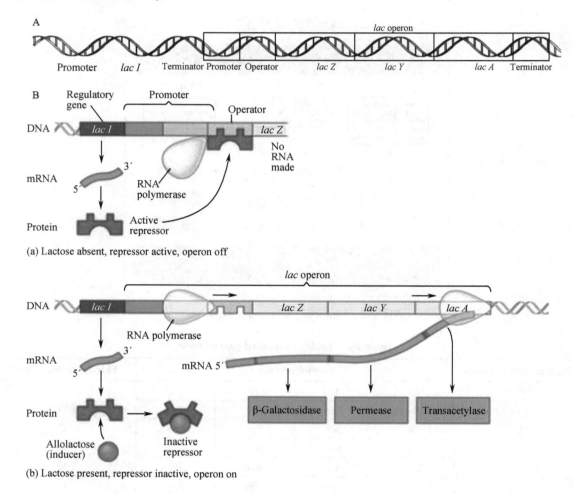

Fig. 2-7 Mechanism of *lac* operon induction. A. structure of *lac* operon. B. Top: The gene is essentially turned off. There is no allolactose to inhibit the *lac* repressor, so the repressor binds tightly to the operator, which obstructs the RNA polymerase from binding to the promoter, resulting in no *lacz, Y, A* mRNA transcripts. Bottom: The gene is turned on. Allolactose inhibits the repressor, allowing the RNA polymerase to bind to the promoter and express the genes, resulting in production of *lacz, Y, A*. Eventually, the enzymes will digest all of the lactose, until there is no allolactose that can bind to the repressor. The repressor will then bind to the operator, stopping the transcription of the *lacz, Y, A* genes.

The ***lac*** operon（lactose operon）is an operon required for the transport and metabolism of lactose in *Escherichia coli* and many other enteric bacteria. Although glucose is the preferred carbon source for most bacteria, the *lac* operon allows for the effective digestion of lactose when glucose is not available through the activity of β-galactosidase. Gene regulation of the *lac* operon was the first genetic regulatory mechanism to be understood clearly, so it has become a foremost（最好的，最重要的）example of prokaryotic gene regulation. This lactose metabolism system was used by François Jacob and Jacques Monod to determine how a biological cell knows which enzyme to synthesize (Fig. 2-8).

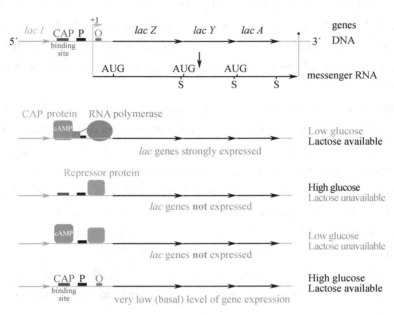

Fig. 2-8   The *lac* operon in detail: the *lac* operon and its control elements.

Bacterial operons are polycistronic transcripts that are able to produce multiple proteins from one mRNA transcript. In this case, when lactose is required as a sugar source for the bacterium, the three genes of the *lac* operon can be expressed and their subsequent proteins translated: *lac Z*, *lac Y*, and *lac A*. The gene product of *lac Z* is β-galactosidase that cleaves lactose, a disaccharide, into glucose and galactose. *lac Y* encodes β-galactoside permease（透性酶）, a transmembrane symporter（同向转运体）that pumps β-galactosides including lactose into the cell (Permease increases the permeability of the cell to β-galactosides). Finally, *lac A* encodes galactoside acetyltransferase, an enzyme that transfers an acetyl group from acetyl-CoA to β-galactosides.

Regulation

Specific control of the *lac* genes depends on the availability of the substrate lactose to the bacterium. The proteins are not produced by the bacterium when lactose is unavailable as a carbon source. The *lac* genes are organized into an operon; that is, they are oriented in the same direction immediately adjacent on the chromosome and are co-transcribed into a single polycistronic mRNA molecule. Transcription of all genes starts with the binding of the enzyme RNA polymerase (RNAP), a DNA-binding protein, which binds to a specific DNA binding site, the promoter, immediately upstream of the genes. Binding of RNA polymerase to the promoter is aided by the cAMP-bound catabolite activator protein (CAP, also known as the cAMP receptor protein). However, the *lac I* gene (regulatory gene for *lac* operon) produces a protein that blocks RNAP from binding to the promoter of the operon. This protein can only be removed when allolactose（异乳糖）binds to it, and inactivates it. The protein that is formed by the *lac I* gene is known as the *lac* repressor. The type of regulation that the *lac* operon undergoes is referred to as negative inducible, meaning that the gene is turned off by the regulatory factor (*lac* repressor) unless some molecule (lactose) is added. Because of the presence of the *lac* repressor protein, genetic engineers who replace the *lac Z* gene with another gene will have to grow the experimental bacteria on agar with lactose available on it. If they do not, the gene they are trying to express will not be expressed as the repressor protein is still blocking RNAP from binding to the promoter and transcribing the gene. Once the repressor is removed, RNAP then proceeds to transcribe all three genes (*lacZ Y A*) into mRNA. Each of the three genes on the mRNA strand has its own Shine-Dalgarno sequence, so the genes are independently translated. The DNA sequence of the *E. coli lac* operon, the *lacZ Y A* mRNA, and the *lac I* genes are available from GenBank.

The **first control mechanism** is the regulatory response to lactose, which uses an intracellular regulatory protein called the *lactose repressor* to hinder production of β-galactosidase in the absence of lactose. The *lac I* gene coding for the repressor lies nearby the *lac* operon and is always expressed (constitutive). If lactose is missing from the growth medium, the repressor binds very tightly to a short DNA sequence just downstream of the promoter near the beginning of *lac Z* called the *lac* operator. The repressor binding to the operator interferes with binding of RNAP to the promoter, and therefore mRNA encoding *Lac Z* and *Lac Y* is only made at very low levels. When cells are grown in the presence of lactose, however, a lactose metabolite called allolactose, made from lactose by the product of the *lacZ* gene, binds to the repressor, causing an allosteric shift（异构转变）. Thus altered, the repressor is unable to bind to the operator, allowing RNAP to transcribe the *lac* genes and thereby leading to higher levels of the encoded proteins.

The **second control mechanism** is a response to glucose, which uses the catabolite activator protein (CAP) homodimer to greatly increase production of β-galactosidase in the absence of glucose. Cyclic adenosine monophosphate (cAMP) is a signal molecule whose prevalence is inversely proportional to that of glucose. It binds to the CAP, which in turn allows the CAP to bind to the CAP binding site (a 16 bp DNA sequence upstream of the promoter on the left in Fig. 2-8, about 60 bp upstream of the transcription start site), which assists the RNAP in binding to the DNA. In the absence of glucose, the cAMP concentration is high and binding of CAP-cAMP to the DNA significantly increases the production of β-galactosidase, enabling the cell to hydrolyse lactose and release galactose and glucose.

However the lactose metabolism enzymes are made in small quantities in the presence of both glucose and lactose (sometimes called leaky expression) due to the fact that the *Lac I* repressor rapidly associates/ dissociates from the DNA rather than tightly binding to it, which can allow time for RNAP to bind and transcribe mRNAs of *lacZ,Y,A*. Leaky expression is necessary in order to allow for metabolism of some lactose after the glucose source is expended, but before *lac* expression is fully activated.

In summary:

➤ When lactose is absent then there is very little *Lac* enzyme production (the operator has *Lac* repressor bound to it).

➤ When lactose is present but a preferred carbon source (like glucose) is also present then a small amount of enzyme is produced (*Lac* repressor is not bound to the operator).

➤ When glucose is absent, CAP-cAMP binds to a specific DNA site upstream of the promoter and makes a direct protein-protein interaction with RNAP that facilitates the binding of RNAP to the promoter.

The experimental microorganism used by François Jacob and Jacques Monod was the common laboratory bacterium, *E. coli*, but **many of the basic regulatory concepts that were discovered by Jacob and Monod are fundamental to cellular regulation in all organisms**. The key idea is that proteins are not synthesized when they are not needed — *E. coli* conserves cellular resources and energy by not making the three Lac proteins when there is no need to metabolize lactose, such as when other sugars like glucose are available.

Use in molecular biology

The *lac* gene and its derivatives are amenable（经得起检验的）to use as a reporter gene in a number of bacterial-based selection techniques such as two hybrid analysis, in which the successful binding of a transcriptional activator（转录激活因子）to a specific promoter sequence must be determined.

The many *lac* fusion techniques which include only the *lac Z* gene are thus suited to X-gal plates or ONPG（邻硝基苯基 -β- 半乳糖苷）liquid broths.

2.1.2.6　*The discovery of restriction enzymes and the modification enzyme*（限制酶与修饰酶的发现）（*Werner Arber*）（*1962*）

A. Restriction enzymes

Restriction enzymes (bacterial enzymes that can break a chain of DNA in to two at a specific point) are used in genetic engineering.

Swiss biochemist Werner Arber was born in Granichen, Switzerland, and studied at the Swiss Federal Institute of Technology. In 1949, he left for Geneva to work on bacteriophages (viruses that attack and grow in bacteria). By 1962, Arber had conducted a series of experiments to show the genetic basis of 'host-induced' variation (the phenomenon by which a bacteriophage adapts to（使自己适应于）the particular strain of bacteria that it grows in).

In Arber's theory, certain bacterial strains were postulated to contain restriction enzymes which were able to cleave unprotected (bacteriophage) DNA. Furthermore, these restriction enzymes must have the ability to recognize a specific sequence of nucleotides within a bacteriophage DNA molecule in order not to destroy the bacteria's own DNA. These enzymes would protect bacteria from infection since bacteriophage DNA would be broken before it could replicate and destroy a cell.

In 1968, Arber and Linn demonstrated nuclease activity of *Eco*B restriction enzyme and Meselson and Yuan purified a similar enzyme from *E. coli* K. These were later classified as Type Ⅰ restriction enzymes, which cleave DNA at random positions, often far removed from the recognition site. In 1970, Smith and colleagues described the purification of the first Type Ⅱ restriction enzyme, HindⅡ, and the characterization of its recognition and cleavage site. Werner Arber, Hamilton O. Smith and Daniel Nathans shared the 1978 Nobel Prize in Physiology or Medicine for their discovery of restriction enzymes and their application to molecular genetics.

Because of the ability of these enzymes to cleave DNA at specific recognition sites, they have continued to play a fundamental role in cloning and DNA typing applications. Today such enzymes are routinely used by molecular biologists in genetic engineering to create pieces of DNA of a specified length.

B. Methylase

A methylase is an enzyme that attaches a methyl group to a molecule.

These are found in prokaryotes and eukaryotes. Bacteria use methylase to differentiate between foreign genetic material and their own, thus protecting their DNA from their own immune system. By placing a methyl group on a base of the recognition site of a restriction endonuclease, methylases prevent the enzyme from cleaving the bacterial DNA (Fig. 2-9).

There are methylases that can methylate DNA, RNA, proteins, or small molecules, for example, DNA methyltransferase, which methylates cytosine residues and adenine residues in DNA.

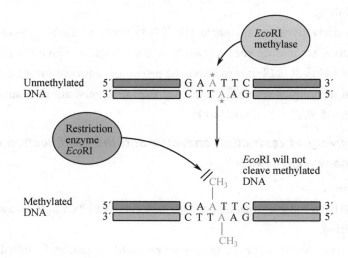

Fig. 2-9   How methylase works.

2.1.2.7   *Isolation of enzyme DNA ligase*（DNA 连接酶的分离）*(1967)*

In 1967, the enzyme DNA ligase was isolated. DNA ligase binds together strands of DNA. Its discovery, with the isolation of the first restriction enzyme in 1970, paved the way for the first recombinant DNA molecules to be created by Paul Berg in 1972. In the recombinant DNA process, ligase bonds the "sticky" ends of complementary DNA strands previously cut by a restriction enzyme.

2.1.2.8   *Discovery of reverse transcriptase*（逆转录酶的发现）（*Howard Temin, David Baltimore*）*(1970)*

Reverse transcriptases were discovered by Howard Temin at the University of Wisconsin-Madison （威斯康星大学麦迪逊分校）in virions of Rous sarcoma virus（RSV，呼吸道合胞病毒，劳斯肉瘤病毒）, and independently isolated by David Baltimore in 1970 at MIT（Massachusetts Institute of Technology 麻省理工学院）from two RNA tumor viruses: R-MLV（murine leukemia viruses）and RSV. Reverse transcriptase uses RNA as a template to synthesize a single-stranded DNA complement. This process establishes a pathway for genetic information flow from RNA to DNA. For their achievements, both shared the 1975 Nobel Prize in Physiology or Medicine (with Renato Dulbecco).

The idea of reverse transcription was very unpopular at first as it contradicted the **central dogma of molecular biology** which states that DNA is transcribed into RNA which is then translated into proteins. However, in 1970 when the scientists Howard Temin and David Baltimore both independently discovered the enzyme responsible for reverse transcription, named reverse transcriptase, the possibility that genetic information could be passed on in this manner was finally accepted.

2.1.2.9 Methods for sequencing DNA（DNA 测序方法）（Walter Gilbert and Fred erick Sanger）(1977)

Walter Gilbert and Fred erick Sanger independently developed methods to determine the exact sequence of DNA. Gilbert used the technique to determine the sequence of the operon of a bacterial genome. Sanger and colleagues used the technique to determine the sequence of all 5 375 nucleotides of the bacteriophage phi-X174, the first complete determination of the genome of an organism.

In 1975, together with Alan Coulson, Frederick Sanger published a sequencing procedure using DNA polymerase with radiolabeled nucleotides that he called the "Plus and Minus" technique. The procedure could sequence up to 80 nucleotides in one go and was a big improvement on what had gone before, but was still very laborious. Nevertheless, his group were able to sequence most of the 5 386 nucleotides of the single-stranded bacteriophage φ X174. This was the first fully sequenced DNA-based genome.

In 1977, Sanger and colleagues introduced the "dideoxy" chain-termination method for sequencing DNA molecules, also known as the "Sanger method". The same year, together with Allan Maxam, Gilbert published the procedures of another new DNA sequencing method using chemical methods developed by Andrei Mirzabekov. This was a major breakthrough and allowed long stretches of DNA to be rapidly and accurately sequenced.

With Paul Berg, Gilbert and Sanger were awarded the Nobel Prize in Chemistry in 1980. Gilbert and Sanger were recognized for their pioneering work in devising methods for determining the sequence of nucleotides in a nucleic acid. The new method was used by Sanger and colleagues to sequence human mitochondrial DNA (16 569 base pairs) and bacteriophage λ (48 502 base pairs). The dideoxy method was eventually used to sequence the entire human genome.

2.1.2.10 Discovery of plasmids（质粒的发现）

Plasmid

A plasmid is an extra-chromosomal DNA molecule separate from the chromosomal DNA which is capable of replicating independently of the chromosomal DNA. In many cases, it is circular and double-stranded. Plasmids usually occur naturally in bacteria, but are sometimes found in eukaryotic organisms (*e.g.*, the 2-micrometre-ring in *Saccharomyces cerevisiae*) (Fig. 2-10).

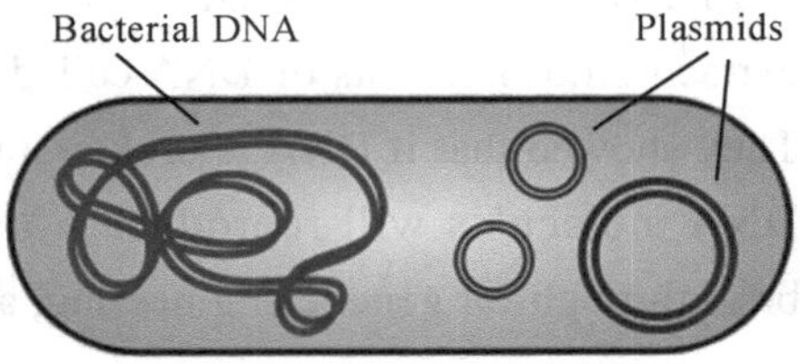

Plasmid size varies from 1 to over 1 000 kilobase pairs (kbp). The number of identical plasmids within a single cell can

Fig. 2-10 Illustration of a bacterium with plasmid enclosed showing chromosomal DNA and plasmids.

range anywhere from one to even thousands under some circumstances. Plasmids can be considered to be part of the mobilome, since they are often associated with conjugation, a mechanism of horizontal gene transfer（水平基因转移）.

The term plasmid was first introduced by the American molecular biologist Joshua Lederberg in 1952.

Plasmids are considered transferable genetic elements, or "replicons", capable of autonomous replication within a suitable host. Plasmids can be found in all three major domains（界）— Archea（古细菌）, Bacteria and Eukarya（真核生物）. Similar to viruses, plasmids are not considered a form of "life" as it is currently defined. Unlike viruses, plasmids are "naked" DNA and do not encode proteins necessary to encase (包装) the genetic material for transfer to a new host. Plasmid host-to-host transfer requires direct, mechanical transfer by "conjugation" or changes in host gene expression allowing the intentional uptake of the genetic element by "transformation". Microbial transformation with plasmid DNA is neither parasitic nor symbiotic (共生的) in nature, since each implies the presence of an independent species living in a commensal (共生的) or detrimental state with the host organism. Rather, plasmids provide a mechanism for horizontal gene transfer within a population of microbes and typically provide a selective advantage under a given environmental state. Plasmids may carry genes that provide resistance to naturally occurring antibiotics in a competitive environmental niche (生态位), or alternatively the proteins produced may act as toxins under similar circumstances. Plasmids also can provide bacteria with an ability to fix elemental nitrogen or to degrade recalcitrant (反抗的，难对付的) organic compounds which provide an advantage under conditions of nutrient deprivation (匮乏).

2.1.2.11   1st successful recombination and expression of DNA （DNA 的首次成功重组与表达）(Paul Berg, Stanley Norman Cohen) 1972—1973

The success of recombining DNA molecule and inserting it into bacterial cells initiated researches on genetic engineering.

Berg was the first one to construct a recombinant-DNA molecule, *i.e.,* a molecule which contains parts of DNA from different species. Berg has also used his method to analyze the chromosome of a virus in considerable details. (—Award Ceremony Speech of the Nobel Prize in Chemistry 1980)

Cohen's investigations in 1972, combined with those of Paul Berg and Herbert Boyer, led to the development of methods to combine and transplant (移植，迁移) genes. This discovery signaled the birth of genetic engineering and earned Cohen the National Medal of Science in 1988. He also co-authored (with Royston C. Clowes, Roy Curtiss III, Naomi Datta, Stanley Falkow and Richard Novick) a proposal for uniform (统一的) nomenclature for bacterial plasmids.

In 1973, Stanley Norman Cohen, Annie Chang, Robert Helling and Herbert Boyer showed that extrachromosomal bits of DNA called plasmids act as vectors for maintaining cloned genes in bacteria. They showed that if DNA is broken into fragments and combined with plasmid DNA, such recombinant DNA molecules will reproduce (复制) if inserted into bacterial cells. The discovery is a major breakthrough for genetic engineering, allowing for such advances as gene cloning and the modification of genes.

2.1.2.12   Development of polymerase chain reaction（PCR）(聚合酶链反应技术的发展)(Kary Mullis) 1983—1986

PCR is used to amplify target DNA many-fold. By **May 1983** Mullis synthesized oligonucleotide probes for a project at Cetus to analyze a sickle cell anemia mutation. Hearing of problems with their work, Mullis proposed an alternative technique based on Sanger's DNA sequencing method. Realizing the difficulty in making the Sanger method specific to a single location in the genome, Mullis then modified the idea to add a second primer on the opposite strand. Repeated applications of polymerase could lead to a chain reaction of replication for a specific segment of the genome — PCR.

Mullis began to test his idea later in **1983**, and repeated thermal cycling was included in experiments later that year. In **June 1984** on Cetus's annual meeting in Monterey (蒙特利), California, Mullis presented a poster on the production of oligonucleotides by his laboratory, and presented some of the results from his experiments with PCR.

In **September 1984** Tom White, vice president of Research at Cetus (and a close friend), pressured Mullis to take his idea to the group developing the genetic mutation assay. Together, they spent the following months designing experiments that could convincingly show that PCR is working on genomic DNA. In **November 1984** the amplification products were analyzed by Southern blotting（Southern 印迹法）, which clearly demonstrating increasing amount of the expected 110 bp DNA product. Having the first visible signal, the researchers began optimizing the process. In the **spring of 1985** the development group began to apply the PCR technique to other targets.

Also **early in 1985**, the group began using a thermostable DNA polymerase *Taq* (the enzyme used in the original reaction is destroyed at each heating step). *Taq* was found by Randy Saiki to support the PCR process several months later. (The use of *Taq* polymerase in PCR was announced by Henry Erlich at International Congress of Human Genetics in Berlin on **September 20, 1986**, and was published in early 1998.) This paved the way for dramatic improvements of the PCR method.

With patents submitted, work proceeded to report PCR to the general public and the scientific community. An abstract for an American Society of Human Genetics meeting in Salt Lake City was submitted in **April 1985**, and the first announcement of PCR was made there by Saiki in **October**. Details on the PCR process appeared on Science on **December 20, 1985**.

In **May 1986** Mullis presented PCR at the Cold Spring Harbor Symposium（专题研讨会）, and published a modified version of his original "idea" manuscript much later. The first non-Cetus report using PCR was submitted on **September 5, 1986**, indicating how quickly other laboratories began implementing the technique. The Cetus development group published their detailed sequence analysis of PCR products on **September 8, 1986**, and their use of ASO（Allele specific oligonucleotide，等位基因特异寡核苷酸）probes on **November 13, 1986**.

Mullis is awarded the Nobel Prize in Chemistry in 1993.

2.1.3 Applications of genetic engineering（基因工程的应用）

Genetic engineering has been playing vital roles in the development of life science. It has applications in medicine, research, industry and agriculture and can be used in a wide range of plants, animals and microorganisms.

Medicine

In medicine, genetic engineering has been used in manufacturing drugs, to create model animals and do laboratory research, and in gene therapy.

Manufacturing

Genetic engineering technology can be used to produce a large number of novel drugs for the prevention and treatment of serious human diseases. It has brought about a series of major technological transformations in the pharmaceutical industry, providing a brand-new way for the research and development of new medicine.

Genetic engineering is used to mass-produce insulin, human growth hormones, follistim (for treating infertility), human albumin（白蛋白，清蛋白）, monoclonal antibodies, antihemophilic factors（抗血友病的，抗血友病药）, vaccines and many other drugs. Mouse hybridomas, cells fused together to create monoclonal antibodies, have been humanized through genetic engineering to create human monoclonal antibodies. Genetically engineered viruses are being developed that can still confer immunity, but lack the infectious sequences.

Research

Genetic engineering is used to create animal models of human diseases. Genetically modified mice are the most common genetically engineered animal model. They have been used to study and model cancer (the oncomouse), obesity, heart disease, diabetes, arthritis, substance abuse, anxiety, aging and Parkinson's disease. Potential cures can be tested against these mouse models. Also genetically modified pigs have been bred with the aim of increasing the success of pig to human organ transplantation.

Gene therapy

Gene therapy is the genetic engineering of humans, generally by replacing defective genes with effective ones. This can occur in somatic (躯体的) tissue or germline (种系的) tissue. It provides a brand-new approach for the treatment of genetic diseases and major diseases.

Somatic (躯体的) gene therapy has been studied in clinical research in several diseases, including X-linked SCID (X 连锁重症联合免疫缺陷症), chronic lymphocytic leukemia (CLL, 慢性淋巴细胞性白血症), and Parkinson's disease. In 2012, Glybera (阿利泼金) became the first gene therapy treatment to be approved for clinical use in either Europe or the United States after its endorsement by the European Commission.

With regard to germline gene therapy, the scientific community has been opposed to attempts to alter genes in humans in inheritable ways using biotechnology since the technology was first introduced, and the caution has continued as the technology has progressed. With the advent of new techniques like CRISPR (clustered regularly interspaced short palindromic repeats, 成簇的有规律间隔的短回文重复序列), scientists urged a worldwide ban on clinical use of gene editing technologies to edit the human genome in a way that can be inherited in March 2015. In April 2015, Chinese researchers sparked (触发，激发) controversy when they reported results of basic research experiments in which they edited the DNA of non-viable (不能存活的) human embryos using CRISPR. In December 2015, scientists of major world academies (院校) called for a moratorium (暂停，中止) on inheritable human genome edits, including those related to CRISPR-Cas9 technologies.

There are also ethical concerns should the technology be used not just for treatment, but for enhancement, modification or alteration of human beings appearance, adaptability, intelligence, character or behavior. The distinction between cure and enhancement can also be difficult to establish. Transhumanists (超人类主义者) consider the enhancement of human desirable.

Genetic engineering is an important tool for natural scientists. Genes and other genetic information from a wide range of organisms are transformed into bacteria for storage and modification, creating genetically modified bacteria in the process. Bacteria are cheap, easy to grow, clone, multiply quickly, relatively easy to transform and can be stored at −80 ℃ almost indefinitely. Once a gene is isolated it can be stored inside the bacteria providing an unlimited supply for research.

Organisms are genetically engineered to discover the functions of certain genes. This could be the effect on the phenotype of the organism, where the gene is expressed or which of other genes it interacts with. These experiments generally involve loss of function, gain of function, tracking and expression.

➢ **Loss of function experiments**, such as in a gene knockout experiment, in which an organism is engineered to lack the activity of one or more genes. A knockout experiment involves the creation and

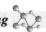

manipulation of a DNA construct *in vitro*, which, in a simple knockout, consists of a copy of the desired gene, which has been altered such that it is non-functional. Embryonic stem cells incorporate the altered gene, which replaces the already present functional copy. These stem cells are injected into blastocysts （囊胚，胚泡）, which are implanted into surrogate mothers. This allows the experimenter to analyze the defects caused by this mutation and thereby determine the role of particular genes. It is used especially frequently in developmental biology. Another method, useful in organisms such as Drosophila (fruit fly), is to induce mutations in a large population and then screen the progeny for the desired mutation. A similar process can be used in both plants and prokaryotes. Loss of function tells whether or not a protein is required for a function, but it does not always mean it′s sufficient, especially if a function requires multiple proteins and lose the said function if one protein is missing.

➢ **Gain of function experiments**, the logical counterpart of knockouts. These are sometimes performed in conjunction with knockout experiments to more finely establish the function of the desired gene. The process is much the same as that in knockout engineering, except that the construct is designed to increase the function of the gene, usually by providing extra copies of the gene or inducing synthesis of the protein more frequently. Gain of function is used to tell whether or not a protein is sufficient for a function, but it does not always mean it′s required. Especially when dealing with genetic/functional redundancy.

➢ **Tracking experiments**, which seek to gain information about the localization and interaction of the desired protein. One way to do this is to replace the wild-type gene with a 'fusion' gene, which is a juxtaposition （并列，并置） of the wild-type gene with a reporting element such as green fluorescent protein (GFP) that will allow easy visualization of the products of the genetic modification. While this is a useful technique, the manipulation can destroy the function of the gene, creating secondary effects and possibly calling into question the results of the experiment. More sophisticated techniques are now in development that can track protein products without mitigating （减轻，缓和） their function, such as the addition of small sequences that will serve as binding motifs to monoclonal antibodies.

➢ **Expression studies** aim to discover where and when specific proteins are produced. In these experiments, the DNA sequence before the DNA that codes for a protein, known as a gene′s promoter, is reintroduced into an organism with the protein coding region replaced by a reporter gene such as GFP or an enzyme that catalyzes the production of a dye. Thus the time and place where a particular protein is produced can be observed. Expression studies can be taken a step further by altering the promoter to find which pieces are crucial for the proper expression of the gene and are actually bound by transcription factor proteins; this process is known as promoter bashing （攻击启动子）.

Industrial

Using genetic engineering techniques one can transform microorganisms such as bacteria or yeast, or transform cells from multicellular organisms such as insects or mammals, with a gene coding for a useful protein, such as an enzyme, so that the transformed organism will overexpress the desired protein. One can manufacture mass quantities of the protein by growing the transformed organism in bioreactor equipment using techniques of industrial fermentation, and then purifying the protein. Some genes do not work well in bacteria, so yeast, insect cells, or mammalians cells, each a eukaryote, can also be used. These techniques are used to produce medicines such as insulin, human growth hormone, and vaccines, supplements such as tryptophan, aid in the production of food [chymosin （凝乳酶） in cheese making] and fuels. Other applications involving genetically engineered bacteria being investigated involve making the bacteria perform tasks outside their natural cycle, such as making biofuels, cleaning up oil spills (溢油，漂油，石油泄漏), carbon and other toxic waste and detecting arsenic (砷，砒霜) in drinking water. Certain genetically modified microbes can also be used in biomining (生物采矿) and bioremediation (生物整治，生物除污，生物降解), due to their ability to extract heavy metals from their environment and incorporate them into compounds that are more easily recoverable.

Experimental, lab scale industrial applications

In materials science, a genetically modified virus has been used in an academic lab as a scaffold for assembling a more environmentally friendly lithium-ion battery (锂离子电池).

Bacteria have been engineered to function as sensors by expressing a fluorescent protein under certain environmental conditions.

Agriculture

Bt-toxins present in peanut leaves protect it from extensive damage caused by European corn borer larvae (欧洲玉米螟幼虫).

One of the best-known and controversial applications of genetic engineering is the creation and use of genetically modified crops or genetically modified organisms, such as genetically modified fish, which are used to produce genetically modified food and materials with diverse uses. There are four main goals in generating genetically modified crops.

The first goal, and the first to be realized commercially, is to provide protection from environmental threats, such as cold (in the case of ice-minus bacteria), or pathogens, such as insects or viruses, and/ or resistance to herbicides (除草剂). There are also fungal and virus resistant crops developed or in development. They have been developed to make the insect and weed management of crops easier and can indirectly increase crop yield.

The second goal in generating GMOs is to modify the quality of produce (农产品) by, for instance, increasing the nutritional value or providing more industrially useful qualities or quantities. The Amflora potato, for example, produces a more industrially useful blend of starches. Cows have been engineered to produce more protein in their milk to facilitate cheese production. Soybeans and canola (芥花籽，菜籽) have been genetically modified to produce more healthy oils.

The third goal consists of driving the GMO to produce materials that it does not normally make. One example is "pharming" (农业医药), which uses crops as bioreactors to produce vaccines, drug intermediates, or drug themselves; the useful product is purified from the harvest and then used in the standard pharmaceutical production process. Cows and goats have been engineered to express drugs and other proteins in their milk, and in 2009 the FDA approved a drug produced in goat milk.

The fourth goal in generating GMOs, is to directly improve yield by accelerating growth, or making the organism more hardy (for plants, by improving salt, cold or drought tolerance). Some agriculturally important animals have been genetically modified with growth hormones to increase their size.

The genetic engineering of agricultural crops can increase the growth rates and resistance to different diseases caused by pathogens and parasites. This is beneficial as it can greatly increase the production of food sources with the usage of fewer resources that would be required to host the world's growing populations. These modified crops would also reduce the usage of chemicals, such as fertilizers and pesticides, and therefore decrease the severity and frequency of the damages produced by these chemical pollution.

Ethical and safety concerns have been raised around the use of genetically modified food. A major safety concern relates to the human health implications of eating genetically modified food, in particular whether toxic or allergic reactions could occur. Gene flow into related non-transgenic crops, off target effects on beneficial organisms and the impact on biodiversity are important environmental issues. Ethical concerns involve religious issues（宗教问题）, corporate（公司的）control of the food supply, intellectual property（知识产权）and the level of labeling needed on genetically modified products.

2.2   The main research content of genetic engineering（基因工程的主要研究内容）

The whole process of genetic engineering is divided into the following stages (Fig. 2-11)：

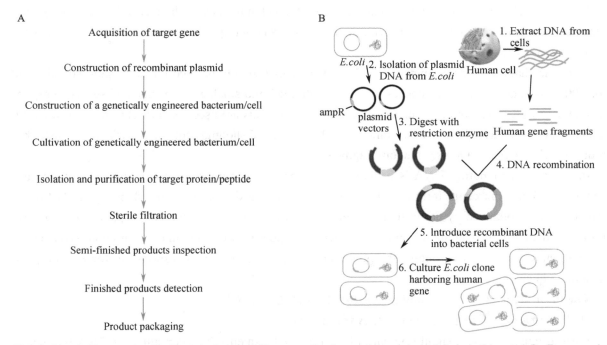

Fig. 2-11   A. Processes in the production of a genetically engineered protein/peptide and B. Panoramic technical procedures of genetical engineering.

2.2.1   Acquiring target genes carrying genetic information（获得具有遗传信息的目的基因）

2.2.1.1   *Shotgun cloning*（鸟枪克隆法）

Shotgun cloning (also known as the shotgun method) is a method to duplicate genomic DNA. The DNA to be cloned is cut using a restriction enzyme or by randomly using a physical method to smash the DNA into small pieces. These fragments are then taken together and cloned into a vector. The original DNA can be either genomic DNA (whole genome shotgun cloning) or a clone such as a YAC (yeast artificial chromosome) that contains a large piece of genomic DNA needing to be split into fragments.

If the DNA needs to be in a certain cloning vector, but the vector can only carry small amounts of DNA, then the shotgun method can be used. More commonly, the method is used to generate small fragments of DNA for sequencing. DNA sequence can be generated at about 600 bases at a time. The sequencing can always be primed with known sequence from the vector and the approach of shotgun cloning followed by DNA sequencing from both ends of the vector is called shotgun sequencing.

Shotgun sequencing was initially used to sequence small genomes such as that of the cauliflower mosaic virus (花椰菜花叶病毒，CMV). More recently, it has been applied to more complex genomes, including the human genome. Usually this involves creating a physical map and a contig (片段重叠群，line of overlapping clones) of clones containing a large amount of DNA in a vector such as a YAC, which are then shotgun clone into smaller vectors and sequenced. A whole genome shotgun approach has been used to sequence the mouse, fly and human genomes by the private company Celera. This involves shotgun cloning the whole genome and sequencing the clones without creating a physical map. It is faster and cheaper than creating a physical gene map and sequencing clones one by one.

Shotgun sequencing

In genetics, shotgun sequencing, also known as shotgun cloning, is a method used for sequencing long DNA strands. It is named by analogy with the rapidly-expanding, quasi-random (拟随机) firing pattern of a shotgun.

Since the chain termination method of DNA sequencing can only be used for fairly short strands (100 to 1 000 base pairs), longer sequences must be subdivided into smaller fragments, and subsequently re-assembled to give the overall sequence. Two principal methods are used for this: chromosome walking, which progresses through the entire strand, piece by piece, and shotgun sequencing, which is a faster but more complex process, and uses random fragments.

In shotgun sequencing, DNA is broken up randomly into numerous small segments, which are sequenced using the chain termination method to obtain reads. Multiple overlapping reads for the target DNA are obtained by performing several rounds of this fragmentation and sequencing. Computer programs then use the overlapping ends of different reads to assemble them into a continuous sequence.

Shotgun sequencing was one of the precursor technologies that was responsible for enabling full genome sequencing.

The basic steps of shotgun cloning (鸟枪克隆法的基本步骤)

(1) Preparation of target genomic DNA fragments

Basic principles: There should be partially overlapped sequence between adjacent DNA fragments; The DNA fragments would be uniform in size.

Concerning the separation and purification of eukaryotic genomic DNA, protease digestion and organic phase extraction are usually used to remove proteins, lipids and other macromolecules. Fragmentation of genomic DNA is mainly carried out by physical shearing and/or restriction enzymes digestion.

(2) Full-length cloning of exogenous DNA fragments

The appropriate vector should be chosen and linked to the exogenous DNA fragment.

The commonly used vectors are plasmids, phages, cosmids and YACs. The maximum lengths of DNA fragments that can be cloned into these vectors (capacity of a vector) are about 10, 23, 45, and 1000 kb respectively. The main parameter for performing vector selection is genome size, that is, the length of genomic DNA sequence. For example, when constructing the genomic library of an organism with a relatively small genome size such as *E. coli* (4.6×10^6 kb), satisfactory results can be obtained just by using plasmid vectors: a gene library consisting of 5 000 DNA fragments could represent a full *E. coli*

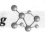
genome sequence when counting at an average length of 5 kb for each DNA fragment. Phages, cosmids and YACs are usually chosen as clonal vectors when constructing large fragment genome libraries. By means of transformation or transduction, recombinant DNA molecules containing different DNA fragments would be introduced into recipient cells hence obtaining a set of clones containing all the DNA sequences of a specific organism.

(3) Selection of expected recombinant

There are many ways helping us screen and identify clones containing some specific genes from numerous clones of the gene library, most of them are based on hybridization probing.

Hybridization probing is an experimental method using DNA or RNA fragments that are complementary to the target gene sequence as probes to find the DNA fragments containing the target genes by means of molecular hybridization.

The gene library can be rapidly screened by *in situ* hybridization or *in situ* immunoassay. Generally, a three-step or even a two-step screening method can be adopted to accomplish the screening of the full-length gene library in a short period of time. The procedure is as follows:

◇ Firstly, high-density plates were prepared, with 5 000~10 000 colonies or phage plaques densely distributed on each plate, then *in situ* hybridization was carried out;

◇ Solid agar was removed from the area of the original plate with positively hybridized clones corresponding to the spot on the photographic film, and then washed and diluted with fresh medium;

◇ The diluent is then spread on the plates once more so that each plate contains only 200~500 identifiable colonies or plaques;

◇ The same probe is used for a second round of hybridization until the desired recombinant clone was accurately selected.

2.2.1.2 *Artificial synthesis of target gene*（人工合成目的基因）

Several approaches are adopted in order to synthesize target gene artificially. They are:

(1) Enzymatic method（酶促方法）

Messenger RNAs (mRNA) encoded by the gene of interest are extracted from tissue of an organism with a higher expression of them, then act as templates to direct the synthesis of complementary DNAs (cDNA), catalyzed by reverse transcriptase. Then the resulting cDNAs are processed to be double strands DNAs (dsDNA) by DNA polymerase I.

Reverse transcriptase is used also to create cDNA libraries from mRNA. The commercial availability of reverse transcriptase greatly improved knowledge in the area of molecular biology, along with other enzymes, it allows scientists to clone, sequence, and characterize RNA.

Reverse transcriptase has also been employed in insulin production. By introducing eukaryotic mRNA for insulin production along with reverse transcriptase into bacteria, the mRNA can be reverse transcribed into cDNA, and the latter, in turn, integrated into the prokaryotic genome. Large amounts of insulin can then be created, sidestepping the need to harvest pig pancreas and other such traditional sources. Directly inserting eukaryotic DNA into bacteria would not work because it carries introns, so would not translate successfully using the bacterial ribosomes. Processing in the eukaryotic cell during mRNA production removes these introns to provide a suitable template. Reverse transcriptase converted this edited RNA back into DNA so it could be incorporated in the genome.

(2) Chemical synthesis（化学合成法）

The premise of using chemical synthesis is that the nucleotide sequence of the gene is known. The DNA fragments obtained by synthesis are usually short. Longer fragments can be obtained by ligating those short ones by DNA ligase.

(3) Polymerase Chain Reaction（聚合酶链反应，PCR）

The premise of using PCR-based approaches is that the nucleotide sequence of the gene is known, and the primers are designed according to the sequence. Then the target gene is obtained by PCR amplification.

In research to apply the polymerase chain reaction technique to RNA, reverse transcriptase is commonly used. This technique is called reverse transcription polymerase chain reaction (RT-PCR). The classical PCR technique can be applied only to DNA strands, but, with the help of reverse transcriptase, RNA can be transcribed into DNA, thus making PCR analysis of RNA molecules possible.

2.2.1.3 *New approaches for screening genes interested*（筛选目的基因的新方法）

A. Enrichment of encoding sequences（编码序列富集法）

Magnetic bead capture of expressed sequences encoded within large genomic segments

Magnetic bead capture utilizes biotin-streptavidin magnetic bead technology to isolate cDNAs rapidly from large genomic intervals, giving several thousand-fold enrichment of the selected cDNAs. The technique can allow parallel analysis of several large genomic segments of varying complexities and can be applied to the isolation of expressed sequences from various tissue sources.

Introduction

The isolation of rare human transcripts as cDNA clones can be fraught with（充满，带有，预示着）problems due to cDNA abundance and sequence complexity consideration. These can be summarized by the following approximations: it has been estimated that about 10 000 genes are expressed in a given human cell type at levels that may be as high as 200 000 mRNA molecules per cell or less than one mRNA per cell, with approximately one third of the genes being expressed at 1~10 molecules per cell. The complexity of sequences is thus within manageable limits, but the variation in abundance classes （种类）dictates that at least several hundred thousand clones must be screened to have a reasonable chance of finding a particular low abundance transcript. This problem is further exacerbated when a complex tissue is used as a source for cDNAs. In this case, numerous cell types exist, each containing widely varying transcript abundance classes. It is therefore unlikely that a conventional cDNA library of approximately one million cDNA clones will adequately represent all the transcripts that are expressed in such tissue, since it will probably not contain the lower abundance cDNAs. One approach that can be taken to surmount these obstacles is to attempt an approximate normalization of cDNA abundance classes using cDNA reassociation（重新组合，重新关联）methods, so that fewer clones need to be constructed and screened. An alternative strategy is to devise methods for rapidly screening very large numbers of primary cDNA. The hybridization selection schemes are capable of rapidly screening and may also result in some level of abundance normalization. The immediate application of these techniques is for the detection of coding regions within large regions of genomic DNA.

Identifying coding sequences within large genomic clones adds additional complications to those already mentioned above. On average, only 3% of the genomic DNA will be homologous to a cDNA and this homology may be very patchy due to the presence of introns. In addition, the repetitive elements within the genomic DNA are also present in a substantial proportion of the target cDNA population. As a result, the use of very large genomic clones in conventional screening schemes usually results in very poor signal to noise ratios and consequently is not very reproducible. Thus, by methodologies back then the task of identifying coding sequences is significantly difficult even when the region of interest is only 20~40 kb, and becomes truly daunting (使人畏缩的) when the region is a megabase in length.

Several techniques have been devised that are targeted at the identification of coding regions in human genomic DNA and seek to address the aforementioned problems. These methods can be roughly divided into two types: methods that are based upon the transcription of a genomic region either in a somatic cell hybrid, or within an artificial construct, and the subsequent detection of conserved transcriptional or processing sequences; and hybridization based schemes. Among the latter group, a method called **direct selection** was reported, which is based upon hybridizing an entire population of cDNAs to a genomic clone or genomic contig. These genomic clones are either in the form of yeast artificial chromosome clones or are within cosmid contigs. In 1991, Lovett M *et al.* have developed a strategy for the rapid enrichment and identification of cDNAs encoded by large genomic regions. The basis of this "direct selection" scheme is the hybridization of an entire library of cDNAs to an immobilized genome clone. The hybridizing cDNAs are eluted and then amplified using the polymerase chain reaction. Data indicated that one round of hybridization selection can enrich a low abundance cDNA (1 clone in 10^6) by approximately 1 000-fold and that new low abundance cDNAs can be rapidly isolated and identified by this method.

Since approximately 3%~5% of cDNAs contain repetitive elements, these must be blocked or eliminated from the hybridization prior to the selecton step. The blocked cDNAs are hybridized to the YAC and specific cDNAs are eluted after post-hybridization washing. The eluted cDNAs are then amplified and can be either cloned using restriction sites in the end linker or used in additional selection cycles.

In 1992, the same research group had modified the cDNA enrichment strategy by hybridizing biotinylated genomic DNA to cDNA probes in solution and subsequently capturing the hybridized complexes using streptavidin-coated magnetic beads, which allow the rapid and reproducible isolation of low abundance cDNAs encoded by large genomic clones. Biotinylated, cloned genomic DNAs are hybridized in solution with amplifiable cDNAs. The genomic clones and attached cDNAs are captured on streptavidin-coated magnetic beads, the cDNAs are then eluted and amplified. All of the selected cDNAs were initially present at very low abundance and were enriched by as much as 100 000-fold in two cycles of enrichment. This modified selection technique should be readily applicable to the isolation of many candidate disease loci as well as the derivation or detailed transcription maps across large genomic regions.

Steps

(1) Preparation of cDNA: Polyadenylated RNA was isolated by oligo (dT) cellulose chromatography and double stranded cDNA was synthesized from this RNA. Double stranded cDNA was digested with *Mbo*I, followed by phenol/chloroform extraction and ethanol precipitation. The cDNA was resuspended and ligated to a linker-adaptor oligonucleotide (*Mbo* linker I). Unligated linker-adaptor was removed by passage over a primerase column. Note that the *Mbo* linker I contains a frequently cutting restriction enzyme (*i.e.*, an *Eco*RI) recognition site for subsequent cloning steps.

(2) Preparation of genomic DNAs: Yeast chromosomes were prepared and electrophoresed on a

contour-clamped homogeneous electric field (CHEF) gel（等高锁状同源电场凝胶电泳）and the YAC containing the corresponding target gene was excised and purified using Geneclean Ⅱ. YAC DNA was digested with *Mbo* Ⅰ and ligated to a second oligonucleotide linker/adaptor (*Mbo* linker Ⅱ).

(3) The YAC DNA and cDNA samples were then separately amplified by PCR using the relevant primer for each linker/adaptor. In each case, the smaller oligonucleotide constituted the primer and each primer was only capable of priming its cognate linker. In the case of the YAC DNA, a 5′ biotinylated primer was used in the amplification.

(4) Blocking repeats within the cDNA.

(5) Hybridization: After repeats within the cDNAs were blocked, the cDNA was hybridized to the biotinylated YAC DNA in solution.

(6) Capture: The YAC DNA plus bound cDNAs were captured on streptavidin-coated magnetic beads. Then the beads were removed from the solution using a magnet, and subject to washing, elution, neutralization and desalting. For secondary cycles of enrichment, those amplified eluted cDNA was recycled through the above process, including the repeat blocking step.

Technical considerations

Fig. 2-12 shows schematically the general procedure involved in magnetic bead capture of cDNAs encoded from large genomic insert clones. The modification of biotinylating genomic DNA coupled with very high-affinity binding with streptavidin-coated paramagnetic beads provides better control of solution hybridization conditions compared to the kinetics of filter hybridization. The strength and stability of the biotin-streptavidin coupling allows DNA manipulations, such as thermal denaturation and elution of annealed cDNAs or relative ease in changing buffers and wash solutions. This ensures a flexible system where preblocking, hybridization and washing can be performed easily. In addition, the beads are of equal size (monodispersed) and thus they follow uniform kinetics when subjected to a magnetic field.

The biotin can be introduced into the genomic clones by photobiotinylation or nick-translation where, in both cases, biotin is incorporated randomly along the length of the DNA. An alternative way is to use a biotinylated primer during an *in vitro* PCR amplification reaction. The latter method has the advantage of tagging each amplified DNA strand at the 5′ end with only one biotin molecule, which can prevent any possible steric hindrance with *Taq* polymerase during PCR or with cDNA probes during hybridization.

The genomic DNA used for capturing cDNAs can be from any genomic source. However enrichment with cosmid DNA seems to work more efficiently than with YACs as during the gel-purification of the latter, YACs often comigrate with degraded, higher molecular weight yeast chromosomes that harbor tandem（串联的）ribosomal sequences. This has led to interesting enrichment artefacts（假象，人为现象）where researchers often find that 30~60 percent of the clones from the enriched sublibrary from YACS contain ribosomal sequences.

A key aspect of the methodology is that the technique is amenable to the parallel analysis of several large genomic segments of varying complexities in isolating expressed sequences from various tissue sources. As both genomic clones and cDNA probes are amplified by the polymerase chain reaction (PCR), the method provides another substantial advantage in that only a small quantity of starting materials is required. Specific transcripts found in low abundance can be enriched several thousand fold with an associated decrease in nonspecific, ubiquitous transcripts.

Magnetic bead capture of cDNAs constitutes a powerful tool for the isolation of cDNAs encoded

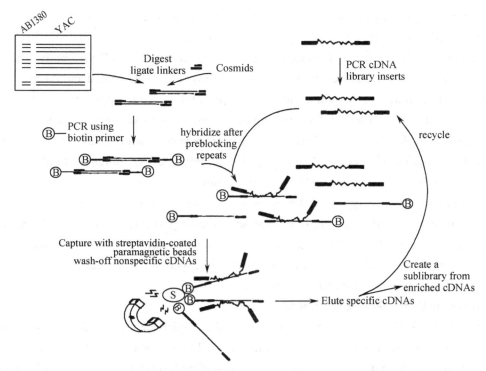

Fig. 2-12 General scheme for magnetic bead capture of expressed cDNAs from cosmids and YACs. Pools of miniprep cosmid DNA or of pulsed-field gel purified YAC genomic DNA are digested with four-base cutters and ligated to linkers. In place of restriction enzyme digestion, genomic DNA can also be sonicated and blunt-ended. The linkered genomic segments are PCR-amplified using a 5'-biotinylated primer whose sequence matches one of the linker arms. cDNA library inserts are PCR-amplified using vector primers and hybridized at high stringency to the biotinylated genomic fragments after suppression of repetitive sequences. The biotinylated genomic-cDNA complexes are captured using streptavidin-coated paramagnetic beads and the unbound, nonspecific cDNAs are washed off. The captured cDNAs are eluted and PCR-amplified. The PCR products are digested with *Eco*R1 and subcloned as a region-specific sublibrary. To increase selectivity, the captured cDNA material is recycled through a second enrichment. In a representative study, the minimal set of 8 overlapping YACS that spans the 2.2-Mb Huntington disease(HD) candidate interval from D4S126 to D4S98 was used either individually or combined together as a pool. The YACs ranged in size from 200 to 600 kb and were deemed to contain only chromosome 4 sequences. In addition, a pool of 17 arrayed cosmids that spans the region from D4S43 to D4S98 (approximately 550 kb) was used to capture cDNAs. Inserts from a commercially available random-primed, fetal brain cDNA library in λ-ZAP were amplified using T3 and T7 vector primers.

from large genomic regions. The technique is highly efficient and can be applied to many sources of cDNA and genomic clone pools in parallel. Furthermore, the method tends to normalize transcript levels, with a greater enrichment of rare messages than abundant ones. Several potential limitations, as well as possible solutions, are associated with this method. First, the resulting small insert sublibrary necessitates screening a full-length cDNA library to obtain full-length transcripts. The time involved in rescreening, however, can be cut substantially by screening random-primed cDNA libraries. Alternatively, the insert size of the enriched cDNAs can be preserved by direct cloning of the PCR products. Second, genomic clones that contain region-specific low-copy repeats can cause a significant number of enriched cDNAs to contain these repeat sequences. Once identified, however, a running catalogue of（一系列，一连串）these repeats can be used to pre-screen the sublibrary or can be incorporated as blocking agents in future magnetic bead capture experiments. Likewise, artefactually selected ribosomal cDNA clones can be pre-screened with ribosomal DNA probes. Third, since the methodology is based on hybridization by sequence homology, pseudogenes and members of multigene families may also be enriched. However, these can be sorted through by further mapping or sequencing of the enriched cDNAs. Last, in order to capture all encoded cDNAs from a given region, it would be ideal to use a cDNA library representing all possible transcribed human sequences. In this regard, it is possible to use pooled and normalized libraries from multiple tissue sources and from various developmental stages to approach (逐渐接近) such a complete cDNA library. One approach for sampling from many tissues, would be to employ multiplexing (多路技术) strategies, in which mixtures of cDNA libraries from various sources are 'tagged" with different end linkers. Combination of large YAC contigs and multiplexed cDNA libraries should be particularly powerful, allowing for the selection of cDNAs from a number of tissues at once.

The development of these types of strategies should lead to insights into gene distribution, the determination of tissue specific transcription maps across large genomic regions, and the rapid isolation of cDNAs, including candidate cDNAs for many disease-related genes across extensive portions of the human genome. And it is anticipated that this technique will expedite the process of finding the proverbial (谚语的) needle in a haystack for many disease loci.

B. Island rescue PCR (岛屿获救 PCR 法)

Island rescue PCR (IRP) is a PCR-based method developed for rapid and efficient generation of probes from YACS or cosmids that can be used for cDNA library screening. The method is based upon the observation that the 5′ ends of many genes are associated with (G+C)-rich regions called CpG islands. In IRP, the YAC of interest is digested with a restriction enzyme that recognizes sequences of high CpG content, and vectorette (小载体，人造载体) linkers are ligated to the cleaved ends. The PCR is used to amplify the region extending from the cleaved restriction enzyme site to the nearest SINE (Alu) repeat. In many cases this product contains sequences from the 5′ end of the associated gene. cDNA clones isolated with these products are then verified by mapping them back to the original YAC. The method allows rapid screening of human genomic whose fragment sizeis larger than 500 kb insert in one experiment, is tolerant of contaminating yeast sequences, and can also be applied to cosmid pools.

An important step in the understanding and accurate diagnosis of human inherited diseases is isolation of the causal gene (致病基因) from the chromosomal region targeted by positional cloning (定位克隆) studies. The limited resolution of genetic studies usually necessitates the cloning of large genomic regions. Once the candidate interval has been cloned in yeast artificial chromosomes (YACS) and/or cosmids, the challenge is to then identify coding regions within these largely uncharacterized genomic clones. The identification of transcripts from large genomic regions cloned in yeast artificial chromosomes (YACS) or cosmds continues to be a critical and often rate-limiting step in positional cloning of human disease genes. A common conventional strategy involves screening small unique genomic fragments from the region for evolutionary conservation. More recent advances allow the isolation of exons by virtue of 5′ and 3′ splice acceptor sites (exon trapping，外显子捕获), enrichment for coding sequences by magnetic bead capture, and direct screening of cDNA libraries by gel-purified YAC DNA or cosmids. However, all of these methods require DNA free of host sequences and are often difficult to apply to YACs.

Island rescue PCR was then developed (Fig. 2-13A) that generates high-quality exon-enriched probes from genomic DNA derived directly from YAC inserts. CpG islands are targeted by the presence of an *Eag* I , *Sac* II , or *BssH* II site. Since, on the average, each of these enzymes is expected to cut 1.2 times within an island, most islands should be accessible.

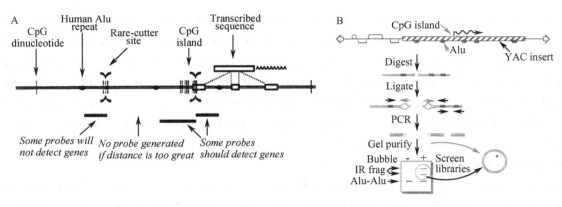

Fig. 2-13   Concept and strategy for the IRP method. (A) CpG islands are markers for the 5′ ends of many genes, whereas SINE(Alu) repeats tend to be scattered throughout the genome, occurring on average every 3 kb. Probes extending away from CpG islands(spanning to the nearest Alu sequence) should allow one to isolate genes associated with the CpG island. (B) In IRP, human genomic DNA in the form of a crude liquid YAC preparation is digested with rare-cutter enzymes(which target CpG islands). Vectorette("bubble") linkers are ligated onto the restricted ends, allowing PCR to be driven by a single primer. PCR is performed under conditions to favor amplification through (G+C)-rich regions, in the presence of Alu and bubble primers. The vectorette primer is identical in sequence to an internal region of noncomplementarity within the vectorette linkers. Products are separated by agarose gel electrophoresis, and unique bands (compared to an Alu primer-only lane) are isolated, labeled, and used to probe cDNA libraries. Alternatively, the entire bubble-linker and Alu primer PCR can be labeled and used as probe.

CpG islands differ from bulk genomic DNA by being relatively (G+C)-rich (>60%) and having a high concentration (10~20 times above average) of the CpG dinucleotide. CpG islands are often associated with transcribed sequences. In a study of 375 genes in the GenBank data base, it was found that virtually all widely expressed ("housekeeping") genes and 40% of tissue-specific genes are associated with CpG islands. Of the tissue-specific genes that lack CpG islands, many have shorter stretches (<100 bp) of (G+C)-rich sequence and may still contain a rare-cutter site (稀有切点). In a similar study of the GenBank/EMBL data base, it was estimated that 55.9% of all genes are associated with CpG islands. Additionally, the vast majority of islands (>80%) extend into 5′ flanking regions of the associated genes. Island rescue products, therefore, not only allow the rapid and efficient conversion of YAC inserts into usable probes but also potentially favor the isolation of the 5′ ends of genes, which are otherwise often difficult to clone. Overall, 78% of the IRP probes overlap a predicted exon.

The strategy for island rescue PCR (IRP) is outlined in Fig. 2-13B. Liquid YAC DNA is digested with a rare-cutter enzyme. Vectorette linkers are ligated to the restriction fragments, generating the genomic template. Using primers specific for Alu repeats (5′ Alu primer) as well as the vectorette primer, the genomic template is amplified by PCR. Products are analyzed by agarose gel electrophoresis. Island rescue fragments are then labeled as probe for cDNA library screening. The optimization of conditions to drive the PCR across (G+C)-rich genomic regions is rather an important aspect for this method.

The technique generates probes from crude YAC DNA that extend from rare-cutter sites (predominantly found in CpG islands) to Alu repeats. The method is rapid and efficient, allowing one to generate probes in less than a day that are suitable for direct screening of cDNA libraries.

IRP can serve as a useful complement to the repertoire of gene cloning methods. This method exploits selective criteria distinct from those used in other strategies and therefore gives one access to a different subset of transcribed sequences. This method is expected to target the 5′ ends of genes, which are typically the most difficult to isolate by conventional means; this bias necessitates the use of high-quality random primed cDNA libraries for screenings. Genes that lack CpG islands within 2 kb of an Alu repeat will be missed by the method, although this shortcoming can be partially reduced through the use of mutiple enzymes and long-range PCR. IRP therefore complements the search for transcribed sequences by quickly isolating some genes in the region of interest, while more exhaustive methods will often be needed to completely characterize the interval.

C. Zoo blot（动物园印迹法）

Advances in molecular techniques have made it feasible to search any segment of cloned DNA for expressed genes even if the nature of the gene products is not defined. Thus, genes that are of interest and whose chromosomal location is known can be identified and characterized. This has been a particularly fruitful approach for finding human disease-causing genes, even with the limitations imposed by available human pedigrees（背景，出身，血统，家谱）.

Unique/low copy sequences are evenly spaced along the cloned DNA. It is proved that most of the unique/low copy sequences studied are evolutionarily conserved, and most of the conserved sequences studied are expressed. Even for mammals evolutionarily distant from each other share conserved coding sequences. In general, hybridization signals tend to become weaker as evolutionary distance increases. They can be used as probes to search for conserved sequences in Southern blots from a variety of mammalian species.

The majority of the unique/low copy sequences were found to have homologues among humans and other species due to their conservation during evolution, so the genes of other species with known sequences can be used to fish out the target gene from the human genome library or cDNA library (already constructed). This method is very convenient and reliable to extract useful genes from the gene library. If there is a gene with high homology with that of other species, it can be used as a probe. Similarly, a member of a gene family with known sequence can also be used to fish out unknown members by taking advantage of the sequence similarity among members of the gene family.

To carry out such "zoo blots", some regions which had been subjected to closer scrutiny and well-characterized should be chosen as hybridization probes, then Southern blots hybridization and washing performed on DNAs from various mammals: rodents (rat and Chinese hamster), mink（貂）, cat, *etc*., and human under moderately high stringency.

Thus, "zoo blots" is a strategy searching for expressed genes in any segment of cloned DNA: identifying unique/low copy sequences that were homologous across species.

The finding of interspecific sequence homology was expected to be useful because in general the segments which comprise entire gene sequences evolve differently. If genes have important biological functions, their sequences should be expected to be conserved in evolution. Thus, any sequences that are conserved across species might represent coding exons of genes. Protein-coding and regulatory regions are conserved in evolution because of their functional constraints, whereas introns and non-regulatory regions diverge rapidly. Thus, sequence divergence in introns and intergenic sequences between different species will increase in proportion to the time since the two species split apart from a common ancestor.

Sequences with no functional significance will diverge to the point where residual homology cannot be detected by Southern blot hybridization. In "zoo blot" analyses, mouse and mammals other than rodents are, in practice, distant enough to permit distinguishing coding and non-coding sequences by Southern hybridization.

The detection of message in this "zoo blot" analysis largely depends on its tissue distribution.

D. Functional cloning（功能克隆法）

Functional cloning is a molecular cloning technique that relies on prior knowledge of the encoded protein's sequence or function for gene identification. In this assay, a genomic or cDNA library is screened to identify the genetic sequence of a protein of interest. Expression cDNA libraries may be screened with antibodies specific for the protein of interest or may rely on selection via the protein function. Historically, the amino acid sequence of a protein was used to prepare degenerate oligonucleotides which were then probed against the library to identify the gene encoding the protein of interest. Once candidate clones carrying the gene of interest are identified, they are sequenced and their identity is confirmed. This method of cloning allows researchers to screen entire genomes without prior knowledge of the location of the gene or the genetic sequence.

This technique can be used to identify genes that encode similar proteins from one organism to another. Similarly, this technique can be paired with metagenomic（宏基因组的）libraries to identify novel genes and proteins that perform similar functions, such as the identification of novel antibiotics by screening for β-lactamase activity or selecting for growth in the presence of penicillin.

Experimental workflow

The workflow of a functional cloning experiment (Fig. 2-14) varies depending on the source of genetic material, the extent of prior knowledge of the protein or gene of interest and the ability to screen for the protein function. In general, a functional cloning experiment consists of four steps: ① sample collection; ② library preparation; ③ screening or selection and ④ sequencing.

Sample collection

Genetic material is collected from a particular cell type, organism

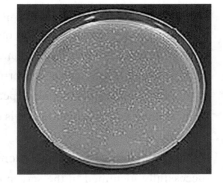

Genomic library in *Saccharomyces cerevisiae*（酿酒酵母）host.

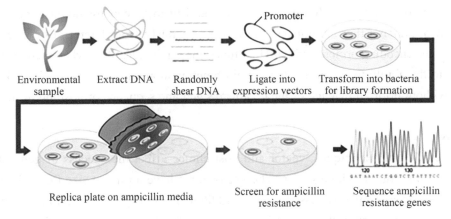

Fig. 2-14　Workflow for utilizing selection in a functional cloning experiment. Here only genes providing ampicillin resistance are selected.

or environmental sample relevant to the biological question. In functional cloning, mRNA is commonly isolated and cDNA is prepared from the isolated mRNA (RNA extraction). In certain circumstances genomic DNA may be isolated, particularly when environmental samples are used as the source of genetic material.

Library preparation

If the starting material is genomic DNA, the DNA is sheared to produce fragments of appropriate length for the vector of choice. The DNA fragments or cDNA are then treated with restriction endonucleases and ligated to a plasmid or chromosomal vectors. In the case of assays that screen for the protein or for its function, an expression vector is used to ensure that the gene product is expressed. The vector choice will depend on the origin of the DNA or cDNA to ensure proper expression and to ensure that the encoded gene will fall within the limits of the vector's insert size.

The choice of host is important to ensure that the codon usage will be similar to the donor organism. The host will also need to guarantee that the proper post-translational modifications and protein folding will occur to enable proper functioning of the expressed proteins.

Screening or selection

The method of screening the prepared genomic or cDNA libraries for the gene of interest is highly variable depending on the experimental design and biological question. One method of screening is to probe colonies via Southern blotting with degenerate oligonucleotides prepared from the amino acid sequence of the query protein. In expression libraries, the protein of interest can be identified by screening with an antibody specific for the query protein via Western blotting to identify colonies carrying the gene of interest. In other circumstances, a specific assay can be used to screen or select for the protein's activity. For example, genes conferring antibiotic resistance can be selected by growing the colonies of the library on media containing a specified antibiotic. Another example is screening for enzymatic activity by incubating with a substrate that is catalyzed to a colorimetric compound that can easily be visualized.

Sequencing

The final step of functional cloning is to sequence the DNA or cDNA from the clones that were successfully identified in the screen or selection step. The sequence can then be annotated and used for downstream applications, such as protein expression and purification for industrial applications.

Advantages

The advantages of functional cloning include the ability to screen for novel genes with desired applications in organisms that cannot be cultured, particularly from bacterial or viral specimens. Additionally, genes encoding proteins with related functions can be identified when there is low sequence similarity due to the ability to screen for the protein function alone. Functional cloning allows for gene identification without prior knowledge of the organism's genome sequence or position of the gene within the genome.

Limitations

As with other cloning techniques, vector and host choice affect the success of gene identification via functional cloning due to cloning bias. The vector must have an insert size that will accommodate the entire DNA sequence of the expressed protein. Additionally, in expression vectors the promoters and terminators must function within the chosen host organism. The host choice may affect transcription and translation due to differing codon usage, transcriptional and translational machinery or post-translational modifications within the host.

Other limitations include the labor-intensive library preparation and potential screens which can be both expensive and time-consuming.

Applications

Determining homology in the environment

Metagenomics（宏基因组）is one of the largest fields that commonly uses functional cloning. Metagenomics studies all the genetic material from a specific environmental sample, such as the gut microbiome（微生物组，微生物群系）or lake water. Functional libraries are created that contain DNA fragments from the environment. As the original bacterium that a DNA sequence originated from cannot be easily detected, creating metagenomic functional libraries possesses advantages. Less than 1% of all bacteria are easily cultured in the lab, leaving a large percentage of bacteria that cannot be grown. By using functional libraries, the gene functions of unculturable bacteria can still be studied. Furthermore, these uncultured microbes provide a source for the discovery of novel enzymes with biotechnological applications. Some novel proteins that have been discovered from marine environments include enzymes such as proteases, amylases, lipases, chitinases, deoxyribonucleases and phosphatases（磷酸酶）.

Determining homology in a known species

There are situations in which it is imperative to determine if a gene homolog from one source is present in another organism. For example, identification of novel DNA polymerases for polymerase chain reactions (PCR) which synthesize DNA molecules from deoxyribonucleotides. While human polymerase optimally works at 37 ℃ (98.6 ℉), DNA does not denature until 94~98 ℃ (201~208 ℉). This poses a problem as at these temperatures the human DNA polymerase would denature during the denaturation step of the PCR reaction resulting in a non-functioning polymerase protein and a failed PCR. To combat（防止）this a DNA polymerase from a thermophile（嗜热菌）, or bacteria that grows at high temperatures, could be used. An example is *Taq* polymerase which comes from the thermophilic bacterium *Thermus aquaticus*. One could set up a functional cloning screen to find homologous polymerases that have the added advantage of being thermostable at high temperatures.

With this in mind, 3173 Polymerase, another polymerase enzyme, now commonly used in RT-PCR reactions was discovered using the above theory. In RT-PCR reactions, two separate enzymes are commonly used. The first is a retroviral reverse transcriptase to convert RNA to cDNA. The second is a thermostable DNA polymerase to amplify the target sequence. 3173 Polymerase is able to perform both enzymatic functions resulting in a better option for RT-PCR. The enzyme was discovered using functional cloning from a viral host originally found in Octopus hot springs (93 ℃) in Yellowstone National Park.

Human health applications

One of the ongoing challenges of treating bacterial infections is antibiotic resistance which commonly arises when patients do not take their full treatment of medication and hence allow bacteria to develop resistance to antibiotics over time. To understand how to combat antibiotic resistance it is important to understand how the bacterial genome is evolving and changing in healthy individuals with no recent usage of antibiotics to provide a baseline. Using a functional cloning-based technique, DNA isolated from human microflora were cloned into expression vectors in *Escherichia coli*. Afterwards, antibiotics were applied as a screen. If a plasmid contained a gene insert that provided antibiotic resistance the cell survived and was selected on the plate. If the insert provided no resistance, the cell died and did not form a colony. Based on selection of cell colonies that survived, a better picture of genetic factors contributing to antibiotic resistance were pieced together. Most of the resistance genes that were identified were previously unknown. By using a functional cloning-based technique one is able to elucidate genes giving rise to antibiotic resistance to better understand treatment for bacterial infections.

E. Construction of cDNA library（构建 cDNA 文库）

Expressed sequence tag

In genetics, an **expressed sequence tag** (**EST**) is a short sub-sequence of a cDNA sequence, it represents a small part of an intact gene. ESTs may be used to identify gene transcripts, and are instrumental（起重要作用）in gene discovery and in gene-sequence determination. The identification of ESTs has proceeded rapidly, with approximately 74.2 million ESTs available in public databases (*e.g.*, GenBank 1 January 2013, all species).

Expressed sequence tags (ESTs) are single-pass reads (of approximately 20~2 000 bp in database, with an average length of 360 ± 120 bp, mostly 200~800 bp) generated from randomly selected clones from cDNA libraries. Since they represent the expressed portion of a genome, ESTs have proven to be extremely useful for purposes of gene identification and verification of gene prediction. They therefore represent a low-cost alternative to full genome sequencing.

An EST is derived through one-shot sequencing of a cloned cDNA. EST sequencing is a large-scale sampling and sequencing of all cDNA clones present in a library. The cDNAs used for EST generation are typically individual clones from a cDNA library. The resulting sequence is a relatively low-quality fragment whose length is limited by current technology to approximately 500 to 800 nucleotides. The ESTs represent portions of expressed genes. They may be represented in databases as either cDNA/mRNA sequence or as the reverse complement of the mRNA, the template strand.

ESTs have become a tool to refine the predicted transcripts for those genes, which lead to the prediction of their protein products and ultimately of their function. Moreover, the situation in which those ESTs are obtained (tissue, organ, disease state — *e.g.*, cancer) gives information on the conditions in which the corresponding gene is acting. ESTs contain enough information to permit the design of precise probes for DNA microarrays that then can be used to determine the gene expression.

The process of generating ESTs

The process of generating ESTs starts with the initial purification of pools of mRNAs from either a whole organism or specific tissues. mRNAs are isolated on the basis of their 3′ poly-A tails (hence their restriction to eukaryotes) and reverse transcribed to create libraries of cDNAs cloned into an appropriate vector. Individual clones from these libraries are then selected (typically at random) and subjected to a single sequencing reaction using universal primers that can be associated with either end of the insert. For each clone, single-pass sequencing of both ends (5′ and/or 3′) of insert. Downstream of the sequencing reaction, a number of sophisticated bioinformatics pipelines have been developed that process the raw sequence read to remove low-quality sequence information and contaminating vector sequence. The resultant high-quality trimmed sequence is then deposited（储存）in the specialized dbEST database. At each stage of this process, a number of strategic decisions must be made according to the objectives of the EST project. These include the source and number of clone libraries to generate ESTs, the sequencing technology itself and the software to employ for sequence processing.

Usage

A major goal for most EST projects is to identify functions associated with identified sequences.

ESTs can also be used to provide a snapshot of gene expression in the material from which they are derived. The study of expression patterns of genes across a range of cell types, life cycle stages, or environmental conditions has proved to be extremely useful for understanding gene functions.

Although ESTs can themselves be used for expression analyses, they are more commonly employed in their gene discovery role allowing the design and construction of novel microarray platform. ESTs have proved to be a cheap and effective tool for gene discovery across a variety of scales. Many small projects have been initiated to provide a first glimpse of genes that an organism may be expressing at critical stages of their life cycles. EST were successfully involved in drug target and gene discovery. cDNA expression libraries can be constructed from life cycle stages that are critical for establishment of some certain parasite infection and cDNA clones were subject to random expressed sequence tag analysis. The identification of some genes of interest along with structural and housekeeping genes by homology searches against the GenBank database allows researchers to recognize novel targets for antiparasitics — agents and/or vaccines.

EST, as a molecular tag of the region where the expression gene is located, is particular in its highly conserved sequence, which make it more likely to traverse the restriction between lineages（谱系）and species than those tags derived from non-expressed sequences (*i.e.*, AFLP, RAPD, SSR), hence ESTs are rather useful in comparing the genomic linkage maps and qualitative trait information between distantly related species. While if some DNA sequence is not available for a target species, a corresponding EST from other species can be used instead for genetic mapping of beneficial genes, so as to accelerate the transformation of corresponding information among species.

The role of EST is shown in (1) genetic maps and physical maps used to construct the genome; (2) acting as probes for radioactive hybridization; (3) positional cloning; (4) searching for new genes; (5) acting as molecular markers; (6) studying the polymorphism of biological populations; (7) studying the function of genes; (8) aiding in drug development, variety improvement; (9) promoting the development of gene chips and other aspects.

ESTs are indispensible for gene stucture, prediction, gene discovery and genome mapping: (a) Provide experimental evidence for the position of exons; (b) Provide regions coding for potentially new proteins; (c) Characterization of splice variants and alternative polyadenylation.

ESTs also provide an alternative to full-length cDNA sequencing. Since all ESTs generated from the same cDNA clone correspond to a single gene, while using the cDNA clone information and the 5′ and 3′ reads information, clusters can be joined. Therefore, sequences of multiple ESTs can reconstitute a full-length cDNA.

Both *cons*（反对论）and *pros*（赞成的意见）exist for the application of EST. *Cons* include (a) Low quality data; (b) Native databases; (c) 3′ ends are heavily represented; (d) Bad/no annotation; and (e) Gene indices. *Pros* include (a) Fast & cheap (automated techniques); (b) Indispensable for gene structure prediction, gene discovery and genome mapping; meanwhile (c) There are still some efforts to be made to improve the present situation: a) Normalized database; b) Good annotation; c) Improvements (pre-processing clustering assembling); d) ORESTE（俄瑞斯忒斯）; e) Emerging Gene indices（HUGO, ENSEMBL）.

Furthermore, ESTs are still the tool of choice for rapid exploration of the transcriptomes of various species, especially with large genomes. Besides, ESTs could form a very solid basis for evolutionary studies.

History

In 1979, teams at Harvard and Caltech extended the basic idea of making DNA copies of mRNAs *in vitro* to amplifying a library of such in bacterial plasmids. In 1991, Adams and co-workers coined the term EST and initiated more systematic sequencing as a project (starting with 600 brain cDNAs).

Sources of data and annotations

dbEST

dbEST is a division of GenBank established in 1992. As for GenBank, data in dbEST is directly submitted by laboratories worldwide and is not curated.

EST contigs

Because of the way ESTs are sequenced, many distinct expressed sequence tags are often partial sequences that correspond to the same mRNA of an organism. In an effort to reduce the number of expressed sequence tags for downstream gene discovery analyses, several groups assembled expressed sequence tags into EST contigs. Example of resources that provide EST contigs include: TIGR gene indices, Unigene, and STACK.

Constructing EST contigs is not trivial and may yield artifacts (contigs that contain two distinct gene products). When the complete genome sequence of an organism is available and transcripts are annotated, it is possible to bypass contig assembly and directly match transcripts with ESTs. This approach is used in the TissueInfo system (see below) and makes it easy to link annotations in the genomic database to tissue information provided by EST data.

Tissue information

High-throughput analyses of ESTs often encounter similar data management challenges. A first challenge is that tissue provenance（出处，起源）of EST libraries is described in plain English in dbEST. This makes it difficult to write programs that can unambiguously determine that two EST libraries were sequenced from the same tissue. Similarly, disease conditions for the tissue are not annotated in a computationally friendly manner. For instance, cancer origin of a library is often mixed with the tissue name (*e.g.*, the tissue name "glioblastoma" indicates that the EST library was sequenced from brain tissue and the disease condition is cancer). With the notable exception of cancer, the disease condition is often not recorded in dbEST entries. The TissueInfo project was started in 2000 to help with these challenges. The project provides curated data (updated daily) to disambiguate（消除……含糊意义）tissue origin and disease state (cancer/non cancer), offers a tissue ontology（本体论）that links tissues and organs by "is part of" relationships (*i.e.*, formalizes knowledge that hypothalamus is part of brain, and that brain is part of the central nervous system) and distributes open-source（源代码开放的）software for linking transcript annotations from sequenced genomes to tissue expression profiles calculated with data in dbEST.

F. Application of differential display（差异显示技术的应用）

Differential display（DDRT-PCR，差异显示技术）

In eukaryotes, life processes either in an individual's growth, development, aging, death, or in tissue's differentiation and apoptosis, a cell's response to various biological and physicochemical factors,

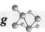

essentially involve selective gene expression. About 30 000 different genes exist in higher organisms, but only 10% of these genes are actually expressed in any cell of an organism. These genes are expressed in an orderly way following the time order and space order. This way of expression is genes' differential expression, which includes newly appeared gene expression and gene expression with differences in the expression level. The characteristics exhibited by various organisms is mainly caused by differences in gene expression. Since the change of gene differential expression is the core mechanism for regulating cell life activities, the comparison of differences in gene expression in the same kind of cells under different physiological conditions or in different growth stages can provide important information for analysis of life activities.

Differential display（DDRT-PCR）（传统 mRNA 差异显示技术）

Differential display (also referred to as **DDRT-PCR** or **DD-PCR**) is a laboratory technique that allows a researcher to compare and identify changes in gene expression at the mRNA level between two or more eukaryotic cell samples. It was the most commonly used method to compare expression profiles of two eukaryotic cell samples in the 1990s. Traditional mRNA differential display technology (DDRT PCR) is based on the structure poly A tail (polyA), which is seated on 3′ end of mRNA, and possessed by the vast majority of eukaryotic cells. An oligomeric nucleotide containing oligo (dT), as a primer, can be used to reverse transcribe different mRNA into cDNA.

First all the RNA in each sample is reverse transcribed using a set of 3′ "anchored primers" (having a short sequence of deoxythymidine nucleotides at the end) to create a cDNA library for each sample, followed by PCR amplification using arbitrary 3′ primers for cDNA strand amplification together with anchored 3′ primers for RNA strand amplification, identical to those used to create the library; about forty arbitrary primers is the optimal number to transcribe almost all of the mRNA. The resulting transcripts are then separated by electrophoresis and visualized, so that they can be compared (Fig. 2-15).

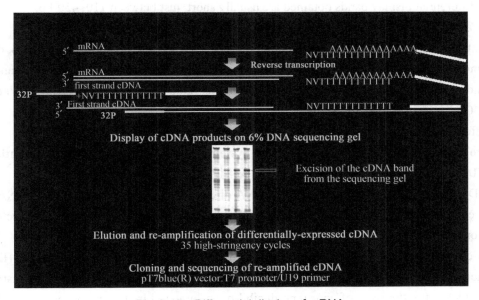

Fig. 2-15　Differential display of mRNA.

History

The method was first published in *Science* in 1992. Liang P and Pardee, founders of the method, deduced that besides AA, only 12 possibilities exist within the 2 bases preceding the starting point of poly A sequence. They designed and synthesized 12 kinds of downstream primer based on this finding, with a general formula of 5′-T11MN, and named them 3′-anchored primers. In order to amplify the mRNA sequences of all possibilities within 500 bp upstream polyA, they designed 20 kinds of random primers of 10 bp long at the 5′ end of mRNA. Upon PCR amplification, such constructed primers can produce about 20 000 DNA bands, in which every band represents a specific mRNA species, and that number generally covers all mRNAs expressed in a certain development stage in a certain cell type. DNAs are recovered from the stripes of differential expression, amplified to the required amount, then Southern blotting, Northern blotting or direct sequencing is carried out, in order to identify and analyze those differential stripes, and eventually obtain the target gene which has been differentially expressed.

In the mid-2000s, differential display was superseded by quantitative PCR, DNA microarrays analyses.

Although there are many advantages that exist for mRNA differential display technology (DDRT PCR):

(1) It is quick and easy to operate;

(2) It is possible to identify mRNA with low abundance due to utilization of PCR amplification technique;

(3) It is possible to compare the differences of gene expression between mRNA samples from different sources.

While some problems still exist in practical operation, mainly manifested as:

(1) Too many differential bands appears, false positive rate reaches about 70%, and there is great tendency towards mRNA with high copy numbers.

(2) From the differential display bands, it is difficult to know which gene has been studied and which one is an unknown.

(3) The differential display bands obtained are usually short, just between 110~450 bp.

(4) PCR amplification based on poly A primer is suitable only for eukaryotes.

Besides, the method was prone to error due to different mRNAs migrated into single bands, differences in less abundant mRNAs getting drowned by more abundant mRNAs, sensitivity to small changes in cell culture conditions, and a tendency to amplify 3′ fragments rather than full mRNAs, and the necessity to use about 300 primers to catch all the mRNA.

Thus differential displaying technique has been being refined since set up in 1992.

The second generation of differential display system — Restriction fragment differential display PCR（RFDD-PCR）（第二代差异显示系统——限制性酶切片段差异显示）

In RFDD-PCR, researchers do not amplify cDNA directly, instead they firstly digest cDNA by using restriction enzyme and then add on both sides of the cDNA fragments with special connectors before amplification (Fig. 2-16).

A series of special adaptors and primers are utilized in RFDD-PCR amplification system. High degree of reproducibility can be acquired due to the utilization of specific PCR primers and downstream PCR reactions, which settle the issue of poor reproducibility encountered in the first generation of differential display.

Since poly A is not used as primer for PCR amplification in the RFDD-PCR technique, this system is suitable for both prokaryotic and eukaryotic systems.

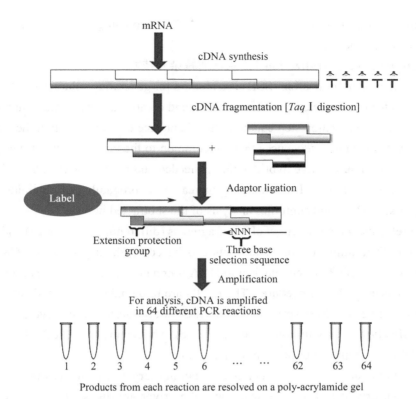

Fig. 2-16   Mechanism of restriction fragment differential display PCR
（RFDD-PCR）（限制性酶切片段差异显示原理）.

In the first generation of differential display system, the downstream primer binds specifically with poly A tail, therefore most of the differential expression sequence corresponds to 3′-untranslated region can be identified. While in RFDD-PCR, a restriction enzyme is adopted which give priority to cut translated sequence (*i.e.*, *Taq* I), hence prioritizes displaying coding region. Therefore RFDD-PCR is more suitable for functional analysis of the downstream region.

When a differential display gene is obtained by using RFDD-PCR, check with the network display FIT, then researchers can find out which gene has been studied and which gene is unknown. These data would direct further study.

In RFDD-PCR, consensus gene expression spectrum can be produced with highly stringent PCR conditions, emphasizing on and displaying coding region. It is useful for both prokaryotic and eukaryotic RNA, and greatly eliminate the false positive.

Subtractive hybridization and suppression subtractive hybridization （消减杂交技术和抑制性消减杂交技术）

Subtractive hybridization（消减杂交技术）

In higher eukaryotes, biological processes such as cellular growth and organogenesis（器官形成）are mediated by programs of differential gene expression. Subtractive cDNA hybridization has been a powerful approach to identify and isolate cDNAs of differentially expressed genes. Numerous cDNA subtraction methods have been reported. In general, they involve hybridization of cDNA from one population (tester/tracer) to excess of mRNA (cDNA) from other population (driver) and then separation of the unhybridized fraction (target) from hybridized common sequences. The latter step is usually accomplished by hydroxylapatite（羟基磷灰石）chromatography, avidin-biotin binding, or oligo (dT)$_{30}$-latex（乳胶）beads.

Suppression subtractive hybridization（抑制性消减杂交技术）

Suppression subtractive hybridization (SSH) is a method for generating subtracted cDNA libraries. It is based primarily on a technique called suppression PCR, and combines normalization and subtraction in a single procedure. The normalization step equalizes the abundance of cDNAs within the target population, and the subtraction step excludes sequences that are common to the target and the driver populations. As a result only one round of subtractive hybridization is needed and the subtracted library is normalized in the abundance of different cDNAs. It dramatically increases the probability of obtaining low-abundance differentially expressed cDNA and simplifies analysis of the subtracted library.

SSH is used to selectively amplify target cDNA fragments (differentially expressed) and simultaneously suppress nontarget DNA amplification. The method is based on the suppression PCR effect — long inverted terminal repeats (LITR) when attached to DNA fragments can selectively suppress amplification of undesirable sequences in PCR procedures. The LITRs are to be linked to the ends of the tester sample to form stable panhandle-like loop structures in each denaturation-annealing cycle. Consequently, no exponential amplification occurs in non-target sequences. The suppression PCR effect was applied in chromosome walking and rapid amplification of cDNA ends.

In subtractive hybridization, a DNA specimen containing target sequences is termed tester and that used for comparison, driver. In SSH, the tester and the driver are digested with a frequently cutting restriction endonuclease, and the tester fragments are ligated with an oligonucleotide adapter. Then the tester and the driver are combined at 1:30, denatured by heating, and hybridized under the conditions providing for the restoration of the double-stranded structure by single-stranded DNA fragments similar in sequence. The subtraction method overcomes the problem of differences in mRNA abundance by incorporating a hybridization step that normalizes (equalizes) sequence abundance of target cDNAs in the subtracted population — combining normalization and suppression PCR steps in a single cycle. It eliminates any intermediate step(s) for physical separation of ss and ds cDNAs, requires only one subtractive hybridization round. As a result of this procedure (subtractive hybridization proper), only tester-specific fragments form molecules suitable for subsequent PCR amplification. This makes it possible to increase the content of differentially presented sequences more than three orders of magnitude — rare differentially expressed transcripts have been reported to be enriched by 1 000-fold to 5 000-fold.

Procedure of SSH and its characteristics

The procedure of SSH is generally divided into six steps, including: ① synthesis of tester/driver cDNAs; ② digestion by a four-base cutting restrictive enzyme; ③ separation of the tester cDNA into two samples, followed by the step of two different suppression-adapter ligations; ④ two successive subtractive hybridization; ⑤ PCR amplification of target sequences; and ⑥ construction of the subtracted library. The schematic representation of SSH is shown in Fig. 2-17.

It should be emphasized that two sequential hybridizations are typically performed in each procedure of SSH to guarantee the enrichment and normalization of target fragments with differential expressions.

In the first hybridization step, two tester samples linked with adaptors 1 and 2 were mixed with a large excess of drivers and denatured separately. The ends of the adaptors are designed without phosphate groups, so that only the longer strand of each adaptor can be covalently attached to the 5′-ends of the

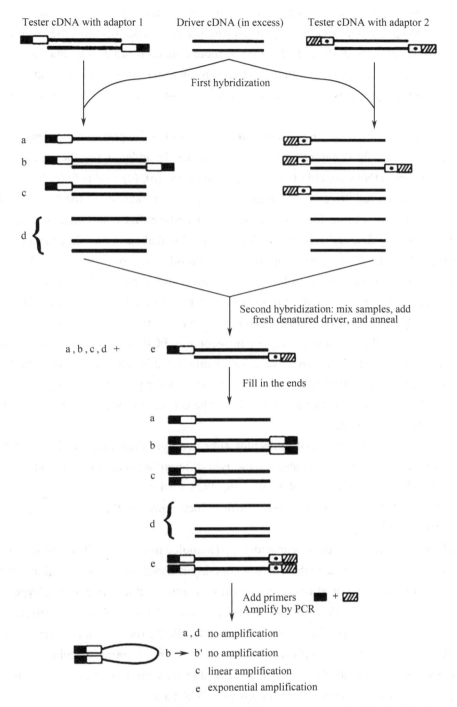

Fig. 2-17   Scheme of the SSH method. Solid lines represents the *Rsa* I digested tester or driver cDNA. Solid boxes represent the outer part of the adaptor 1 longer strand and corresponding PCR primer P1 sequence. Shaded boxes represent the outer part of the adaptor 2 longer strand and corresponding PCR primer P2 sequence. Clear boxes represent the inner part of the adaptors and corresponding nested PCR primers PN1 and PN2. Note that after filling in the recessed 3′ ends with DNA polymerase, types a, b, and c molecules having adapter 2 are also present but are not shown.

cDNA. They are then subjected to limited renaturation to generate types (a), (b), (c), and (d) molecules in each sample. The ss cDNA tester fraction (a) is normalized/equalized — concentrations of high and low abundance cDNAs become roughly equal. Normalization occurs because the reannealing process generating homo-hybrid cDNAs (b) is faster for the more abundant molecules, due to the second order kinetics of hybridization. Consequently, the ss cDNAs in the tester fraction (a) are significantly enriched in cDNAs for differentially expressed genes, as "common" non-target cDNAs form heterohybrids (c) with the driver.

During the second hybridization, the two primary hybridization samples without denaturing are mixed together, and then the freshly denatured driver is synchronously added. Only the remaining normalized and subtracted ss tester cDNAs are able to reassociate and form (b), (c), and new (e) hybrids. Addition of a second portion of denatured driver at this stage further enriches fraction (e) for differentially expressed genes. The newly formed (e) hybrids have an important feature that distinguishes them from hybrids (b) and (c) formed during first and second hybridizations. This feature is that they have different adaptor sequences at their 5′-ends. One is from sample 1 and the other is from sample 2. The two sequences allow preferential amplification of the subtracted and normalized fraction (e) using PCR and a pair of primers. For each subtraction, two PCR amplifications were performed. The primary PCR was conducted using PCR primers P1 and P2, which corrrespond to the outer part of the adaptor 1 and 2, respectively. Some of the products are then used as a template in secondary PCR, with the PCR primers replaced with nested PCR primers PN1 and PN2, respectively. To accomplish this selective amplification, an extension reaction is performed to fill in the sticky ends of the molecules for primer annealing before the initiation of the PCR procedure. The second hybridization should be carried out over a longer period to ensure that all cDNAs became double stranded.

Summarizing the entire population of molecules after two hybridizations, five kinds of products exist in the mixture, among which (e) molecules having two different adaptor sequences at their 5′-ends that will allow exponential amplification in the following PCR cycles — only the remaining equalized and subtracted ss tester cDNAs can form type (e) hybrids, which represent the differentially expressed genes between the tester and driver.

Exponential amplification can only occur with type (e) molecules — no PCR reactions can be expected in type (a) and (d) molecules because they do not contain primer-binding sites. Double-strand molecules of type (c), with only one adaptor at one end, can only be amplified at a linear rate. Type (b) molecules contain the same LITRs on both ends and thus form stable "panhandle-like" structures after each denaturation-annealing PCR step. The resulting "panhandle-like" structure cannot serve as a template for exponential PCR, preventing (b)'s amplification in PCR reaction — intramolecular annealing of longer adaptor sequences is both highly favored and more stable than intermolecular annealing of the much shorter PCR primers, which is the so-called suppression PCR effect.

So after these two successive nested PCR, those upregulated genes in testers can be obtained and used for constructing a subtracted library. Working on the same theory, reverse SSH (switching the samples used as tester and driver) can find out the down-regulated genes in former testers.

SSH is an efficient PCR-based subtractive hybridization method for detecting the differentially expressed genes at the mRNA level. Furthermore, standard SSH procedure can be modified to increase the possibility of identifying quantitatively regulated transcripts between the tester and driver cDNA

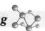

populations. Under standard conditions, the driver cDNA would have eliminated most of the common sequences between the tester and driver cDNA samples during the first hybridization step. However, quantitatively different cDNA species may still remain in the tester populations. To further eliminate common sequences, excess fresh driver cDNA needs to be added to the samples in the second hybridization step, thereby further subtracting quantitatively different but common sequences between the tester and driver populations.

SSH is a high throughput gene expression analysis method and its ability to identify differentially expressed genes lies on the facts that it is: irrespective of the expression level, can be performed in the absence of sequence information, eliminates the need for physical separation of single- and double-stranded molecules, allows for the equalization of the abundance of mRNA sequences within the target population and suitable for detection of rare transcripts, while combining high level enrichment, low background, easy handling and relatively low cost. The feasibility of using the uncloned substracted cDNA mixture as a hybridization probe makes this technique versatile and powerful.

The SSH technique is applicable to many molecular genetic and positional cloning studies for the identification of disease, developmental, tissue-specific, or other differentially expressed genes. Furthermore, SSH can also be applied in drug discovery for identifying pathways representing new possible targets, verifying the potential effect achieved by drugs modulating.

Subtractive hybridization allows enrichment in tester-specific sequences only when the corresponding fragments of two species differ in nucleotide sequences by at least 20%~25%.

2.2.1.4 *Reformation of genes already existed* (对已发现基因的改造)

Based on the studies of function associated regions in a gene, novel gene functions can be explored and reconfirmed by using techniques such as genetic modification and site-directed mutagenesis, so as to improve the stability of the products to be expressed from the target gene, and their half-lives *in vivo*, their biological activities, to reduce their effective dose or improve their expression, and/or to reduce the toxicity and immunogenicity. The main strategies for molecular designing of biotherapeutics through protein engineering are as follows: Some key amino acid residues of a physiologically active protein are to be replaced by mutagenesis; By adding, deleting or exchanging some peptide segments, structural domains or oligosaccharide chains on a peptide, a protein or a glycoprotein molecule, its activities can be modulated, suitable glycoforms can be generated, new biological functions can be created; When two genetically engineered biotherapeutics which are functionally complement with each other are fused at the gene level, the effect of such merit combination is not only the simple addition of the functions derived from the original therapeutics, but also the emergence of new pharmacological effects from the resulting chimeric macromolecules; Post-modification of the expressed products can also make improvement in the pharmacological effects of the protein engineered biotherapeutics.

Saturation mutagenesis or deep mutational scanning

When a protein or a peptide was found to possess some specific functions, one would assume that the replacement of some of the amino acids on the protein/peptide would affect its activity, efficiency or other properties. Some of the variations might have beneficial effects. The saturation mutagenesis or deep mutational scanning approach, where every amino acid is individually mutated to every other amino acid, is of great value to search out novel therapeutic proteins/peptides with improved properties. When the amino acid sequence of a satisfactory protein/peptide was determined, the gene coding for it can be ligated to a vector and subject to a normal genetic transformation or an alternative solution as usual.

In vitro molecular evolution

An attractive alternative to sequencing and site-directed mutagenesis is to accumulate beneficial mutations in sequential rounds of random mutagenesis or by a novel recombination approach, following a "directed evolution" strategy. Directed evolution has been proven useful in and important for modifying gene, creating novel functional protein, as well as enhancing enzyme performance in 'non-natural' environments and acquiring new features never required by nature, provided an efficient selection or screening method can be found to channel (引导，导向) the protein or enzyme's evolution towards the desired properties. A significant advantage of this approach over "rational" design methods is that neither structural information nor a mechanistic road-map are required to guide the directed evolution experiment. New functions can be engineered by introducing and recombining mutations, followed by subsequent testing of each variant for the desired new function. For instance, available natural enzyme resources are being tailored to fulfil increasing demands for new biocatalysts.

A range of methods are available for mutagenesis, and these can be used to introduce mutations at single sites, targeted regions within a gene or randomly throughout the entire gene. In addition, a number of different methods are available to allow recombination of point mutations or blocks of sequence space with little or no homology. With the development of DNA *in vitro* molecular evolution technology, remarkable achievements have been made in fundamental theory, medical research and modification of industrial enzyme.

Sequential rounds of error-prone PCR mutagenesis and screening is one effective method by which this can be accomplished. The accumulation of amino acid substitutions in an enzyme can result in significant improvements in performance, particularly for features not optimized under selective pressure. A directed evolution strategy was applied to subtilisin E (枯草杆菌蛋白酶 E) in *Bacillus subtilis* (枯草杆菌) by Frances H. Arnold from California Institute of Technology, involving sequential generations of polymerase chain reaction (PCR) random mutagenesis and screening to the serine protease subtilisin E to enhance total activity in aqueous dimethylformamide. She was awarded the Nobel Prize in Chemistry in 2018 for her team's pioneer work on "directed evolution of enzymes" in 1993.

Pharmaceutical synthesis can benefit greatly from the catalytic selectivity gains associated with enzyme evolution. **Savile *et al.*** applied a directed evolution approach to modify an existing transaminase enzyme so that it recognized a complex ketone in place of its smaller native substrate, and could tolerate the high temperature and organic cosolvent (助溶剂) necessary to dissolve this ketone. This biocatalytic reaction improved the production efficiency of sitagliptin (西他列汀) that treats diabetes. The resultant biocatalysts showed broad applicability toward the synthesis of chiral amines that previously were accessible only via resolution (拆分).

Since DNA and RNA molecules with specific binding or catalytic activities can be isolated from complex mixtures of random sequences using an iterative selection and amplification process, Keefe and Szostak developed a procedure that allows *in vitro* directed evolution of proteins. Hereby mRNA is covalently linked with its encoded protein product via a puromycin (嘌呤霉素) molecule during *in vitro* translation. The peptidyl-puromycin mRNA molecule can be screened for biochemical function of the protein (phenotype), whereas the RNA portion (genotype) serves as a tag to identify, amplify and mutate the selected protein species. Using this approach, the authors constructed an mRNA-peptide display library of 6×10^{12} proteins each containing 80 random amino acids — only a fraction of the theoretically possible sequence space of $20^{80} = 10^{104}$ protein species of that length. Based on the occurrence of functional proteins recovered before mutagenesis, the frequency of functional proteins in the initial random library was estimated to be 1 in 10^{11}, which is sufficient to allow discovery of functional proteins in sequence space by a stochastic (随机的) process. The experimental success and the small fraction of sequence space occupied by functional proteins together tend to favor evolutionary approaches over *de novo* design in the development of novel proteins with therapeutic or industrial utility.

2.2.2 Selecting gene vector to construct recombinant DNA（选择基因载体获得重组 DNA）

In molecular cloning, a vector is a DNA molecule used as a vehicle to artificially carry foreign genetic material into another cell, where it can be replicated and/or expressed. A vector containing foreign DNA is termed recombinant DNA. The four major types of vectors are plasmids, viral vectors, cosmids, and artificial chromosomes. Of these, the most commonly used vectors are plasmids. Common to all engineered vectors are an origin of replication, a multicloning site, and a selectable marker.

The vector itself is generally a DNA sequence that consists of an insert (transgene) and a larger sequence that serves as the "backbone" of the vector. The purpose of a vector which transfers genetic information to another cell is typically to isolate, multiply, or express the insert in the target cell. Vectors called expression vectors (expression constructs) specifically are for the expression of the transgene in the target cell, and generally have a promoter sequence that drives expression of the transgene. Simpler vectors called transcription vectors are only capable of being transcribed but not translated: they can be replicated in a target cell but not expressed, unlike expression vectors. Transcription vectors are used to amplify their insert.

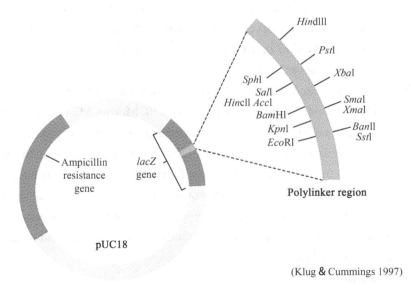

(Klug & Cummings 1997)

2.2.3 Introducing recombinant DNA into host cells（将重组 DNA 分子导入宿主细胞）

Insertion of a vector (a non-viral DNA) into the target cell is usually called **transformation**（转化）for bacterial cells and non-animal eukaryotic cells, **transfection**（转染）for animal cells, although insertion of a viral vector (virus mediated gene transfer) into eukaryotic cells is often called **transduction** （转导）. Electroporation, microinjection and gene gun are also used for introducing recombinant DNA into host cells.

Transformation (genetics)

In molecular biology, transformation is the genetic alteration of a cell resulting from the direct uptake and incorporation of exogenous genetic material (exogenous DNA) from its surroundings through the cell membrane(s). Transformation occurs naturally in some species of bacteria, but it can also be effected （实现）by artificial means in other cells. For transformation to happen, bacteria must be in a state of competence, which might occur as a time-limited response to environmental conditions such as starvation and cell density.

"Transformation" may also be used to describe the insertion of new genetic material into nonbacterial cells, including animal and plant cells; however, because "transformation" has a special meaning in relation to animal cells, indicating progression to a cancerous state, the term should be avoided for animal cells when describing introduction of exogenous genetic material. Introduction of foreign DNA into eukaryotic cells is often called "transfection".

History

Transformation was first demonstrated in 1928 by British bacteriologist Frederick Griffith. Griffith discovered that a strain of *Streptococcus pneumoniae* could be made virulent after being exposed to heat-killed virulent strains. Griffith hypothesized that some "transforming principle" from the heat-killed strain was responsible for making the harmless strain virulent. In 1944 this "transforming principle" was identified as being genetic by Oswald Avery, Colin MacLeod, and Maclyn McCarty. They isolated DNA from a virulent strain of *S. pneumoniae* and using just this DNA were able to make a harmless strain virulent. They called this uptake and incorporation of DNA by bacteria "transformation". The results of Avery *et al.* 's experiments were at first skeptically received by the scientific community and it was not until the development of genetic markers and the discovery of other methods of genetic transfer (conjugation in 1947 and transduction in 1953) by Joshua Lederberg that Avery's experiments were accepted. For more details, see section 2.1.2.1.

It was originally thought that *Escherichia coli*, a commonly used laboratory organism, was refractory （不感受的，不反应的）to transformation. However, in 1970, Morton Mandel and Akiko Higa showed that *E. coli* may be induced to take up DNA from bacteriophage λ without the use of helper phage after treatment with calcium chloride solution. Two years later in 1972, Stanley Cohen, Annie Chang and Leslie Hsu showed that $CaCl_2$ treatment is also effective for transformation of plasmid DNA. The method of transformation by Mandel and Higa was later improved upon by Douglas Hanahan. The discovery of artificially induced competence in *E. coli* created an efficient and convenient procedure for transforming bacteria which allows for simpler molecular cloning methods in biotechnology and research, and it is now a routinely used laboratory procedure.

Methods and mechanisms

Definitions

Bacterial transformation may be referred to as a stable genetic change brought about by the uptake of naked DNA (DNA without associated cells or proteins) to increase DNA quantity; competence refers to the state of being able to take up exogenous DNA from the environment. There are two forms of transformation and competence: natural and artificial.

Natural transformation

Natural transformation is a bacterial adaptation for DNA transfer that depends on the expression of numerous bacterial genes whose products appear to be responsible for this process. In general, transformation is a complex, energy-requiring developmental process. In order for a bacterium to bind, take up and recombine exogenous DNA into its chromosome, it must become competent, that is, enter a special physiological state. Competence development in *Bacillus subtilis* requires expression of about 40 genes. The DNA integrated into the host chromosome is usually (but with rare exceptions) derived from another bacterium of the same species, and is thus homologous to the resident（常驻的）chromosome. The capacity for natural transformation appears to occur in a number of prokaryotes, and thus far 67 prokaryotic species (in seven different phyla) are known to undergo this process.

Competence for transformation is typically induced by high cell density and/or nutritional limitation, conditions associated with the stationary phase（静止期，稳定期）of bacterial growth.

Transformation, as an adaptation for DNA repair

Competence is specifically induced by DNA damaging conditions. For instance, transformation is induced in *Streptococcus pneumoniae* by the DNA damaging agents mitomycin C（丝裂霉素 C）(a DNA crosslinking agent) and fluoroquinolone（氟喹诺酮）(a topoisomerase inhibitor that causes double-strand breaks). In *B. subtilis*, transformation is increased by UV light, a DNA damaging agent. In *Helicobacter pylori*（幽门螺杆菌）, ciprofloxacin（环丙沙星）, which interacts with DNA gyrase（旋转酶，促旋酶）and introduces double-strand breaks, induces expression of competence genes, thus enhancing the frequency of transformation. Using *Legionella pneumophila*（嗜肺军团菌）, Charpentier *et al*. tested 64 toxic molecules to determine which of these induce competence. Of these only six, all DNA damaging agents, caused strong induction. These DNA damaging agents were mitomycin C (which causes DNA interstrand crosslinks), norfloxacin（诺氟沙星）, ofloxacin（氧氟沙星）and nalidixic acid（萘啶酸，萘啶酮酸）(inhibitors of DNA gyrase that cause double-strand breaks), bicyclomycin（双环菌素）(causes single- and double-strand breaks), and hydroxyurea (induces DNA base oxidation). UV light also induced competence in *L. pneumophila*. Charpentier *et al*. suggested that competence for transformation probably evolved as a DNA damage response.

Natural competence

About 1% of bacterial species are capable of naturally taking up DNA under laboratory conditions; more may be able to take it up in their natural environments. DNA material can be transferred between different strains of bacteria, in a process that is called horizontal gene transfer. Some species upon cell death release their DNA to be taken up by other cells, however transformation works best with DNA from closely related species. These naturally competent bacteria carry sets of genes that provide the protein machinery to bring DNA across the cell membrane(s). The transport of the exogeneous DNA into the cells may require proteins that are involved in the assembly of type Ⅳ pili and type Ⅱ secretion system, as well as DNA translocase（移位酶）complex at the cytoplasmic membrane.

Due to the differences in structure of the cell envelope between Gram-positive and Gram-negative bacteria, there are some differences in the mechanisms of DNA uptake in these cells, however most of them share common features that involve related proteins. The DNA first binds to the surface of the competent cells on a DNA receptor, and passes through the cytoplasmic membrane via DNA translocase.

Only single-stranded DNA may pass through, the other strand being degraded by nucleases in the process. The translocated single-stranded DNA may then be integrated into the bacterial chromosomes by a RecA-dependent process. In Gram-negative cells, due to the presence of an extra membrane, the DNA requires the presence of a channel formed by secretins（分泌素，肠促胰液素）on the outer membrane. Pilin （菌毛蛋白）may be required for competence, but its role is uncertain. The uptake of DNA is generally non-sequence specific, although in some species the presence of specific DNA uptake sequences may facilitate efficient DNA uptake.

Artificial competence

Artificial competence can be induced in laboratory procedures that involve making the cell passively permeable to DNA by exposing it to conditions that do not normally occur in nature. Typically the cells are incubated in a solution containing divalent cations (often calcium chloride) under cold conditions, before being exposed to a heat pulse (heat shock).

It has been found that growth of Gram-negative bacteria in 20 mM Mg^{2+} reduces the number of protein-to-lipopolysaccharide bonds by increasing the ratio of ionic to covalent bonds, which increases membrane fluidity, facilitating transformation. The role of lipopolysaccharides here are verified from the observation that shorter O-side chains are more effectively transformed — perhaps because of improved DNA accessibility.

The surface of bacteria such as *E. coli* is negatively charged due to phospholipids and lipopolysaccharides on its cell surface, and the DNA is also negatively charged. One function of the divalent cation therefore would be to shield the charges by coordinating the phosphate groups and other negative charges, thereby allowing a DNA molecule to adhere to the cell surface.

DNA entry into *E. coli* cells is through channels known as zones of adhesion or Bayer's junction（接合点）, with a typical cell carrying as many as 400 such zones. Their role was established when cobalamine （钴胺素，氰钴胺素，维生素 B_{12}）(which also uses these channels) was found to competitively inhibit DNA uptake. Another type of channel implicated in DNA uptake consists of poly(HB):poly P:Ca. In this poly(HB) is envisioned to wrap（缠绕）around DNA (itself a polyphosphate), and is carried in a shield formed by Ca^{2+} ions.

It is suggested that exposing the cells to divalent cations in cold condition may also change or weaken the cell surface structure, making it more permeable to DNA. The heat-pulse is thought to create a thermal imbalance across the cell membrane, which forces the DNA to enter the cells through either cell pores or the damaged cell wall.

Yeast

Most species of yeast, including *Saccharomyces cerevisiae*, may be transformed by exogenous DNA in the environment. Several methods have been developed to facilitate this transformation at high frequency in the lab.

Yeast cells may be treated with enzymes to degrade their cell walls, yielding spheroplasts（原生质球）. These cells are very fragile but take up foreign DNA at a high rate.

Exposing intact yeast cells to alkali cations such as those of cesium（铯）or lithium（锂）allows the cells to take up plasmid DNA. Later protocols adapted this transformation method, using lithium acetate, polyethylene glycol, and single-stranded DNA. In these protocols, the single-stranded DNA preferentially binds to the yeast cell wall, preventing plasmid DNA from doing so and leaving it available for transformation.

Practical aspects of transformation in molecular biology

The discovery of artificially induced competence in bacteria allow bacteria such as *Escherichia coli* to be used as a convenient host for the manipulation of DNA as well as expressing proteins. Typically plasmids are used for transformation in *E. coli*. In order to be stably maintained in the cell, a plasmid DNA molecule must contain an origin of replication, which allows it to be replicated in the cell independently of the replication of the cell's own chromosome.

The efficiency with which a competent culture can take up exogenous DNA and express its genes is known as transformation efficiency and is measured in colony forming unit (cfu) per μg DNA used. A transformation efficiency of 1×10^8 cfu/μg for a small plasmid like pUC19 is roughly equivalent to 1 in 2 000 molecules of the plasmid used being transformed.

In calcium chloride transformation, the cells are prepared by chilling cells in the presence of Ca^{2+} (in $CaCl_2$ solution), making the cell become permeable to plasmid DNA. The cells are incubated on ice with the DNA, and then briefly heat-shocked (*e.g.*, at 42℃ for 30~120 seconds) (Fig. 2-18). This method works very well for circular plasmid DNA. Non-commercial preparations should normally give 10^6 to 10^7 transformants per microgram of plasmid; a poor preparation will be about 10^4/μg or less, but a good preparation of competent cells can give up to ~10^8 colonies per microgram of plasmid. Protocols, however, exist for making supercompetent cells that may yield a transformation efficiency of over 10^9. The chemical method, however, usually does not work well for linear DNA, such as fragments of chromosomal DNA, probably because the cell's native exonuclease enzymes rapidly degrade linear DNA. In contrast, cells that are naturally competent are usually transformed more efficiently with linear DNA than with plasmid DNA.

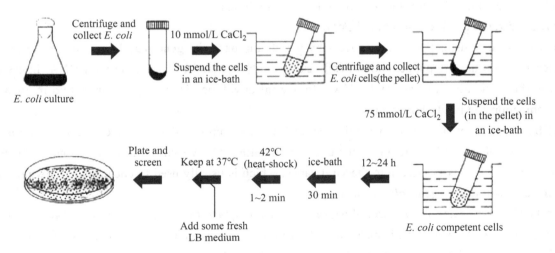

Fig. 2-18   Transformation induced by $CaCl_2$ (钙诱导的转化).

The transformation efficiency using the $CaCl_2$ method decreases with plasmid size, and electroporation therefore may be a more effective method for the uptake of large plasmid DNA.

Transduction (genetics) 〔转导〕

Transduction is the process by which DNA is transferred from one bacterium to another by a virus. More generally, **transduction** is the process by which genetic material, *e.g.*, DNA or siRNA, is inserted into a cell by a virus. It also refers to the process whereby (凭此) foreign DNA is introduced into another cell via a viral vector. Transduction does not require physical contact between the cell donating the DNA and the cell receiving the DNA (which occurs in conjugation), and it is DNase resistant (transformation is susceptible to DNase). Transduction is a common tool used by molecular biologists to stably introduce a foreign gene into a host cell's genome. Transduction was discovered by Norton Zinder and Joshua Lederberg at the University of Wisconsin-Madison in 1951.

When bacteriophages (viruses that infect bacteria) infect a bacterial cell, their normal mode of reproduction is to harness (利用) the replicational, transcriptional, and translational machinery of the host bacterial cell to make numerous virions, or complete viral particles, including the viral DNA or RNA and the protein coat.

Lytic and lysogenic (temperate) cycles

Transduction happens through either the lytic cycle or the lysogenic cycle. If the lysogenic cycle is adopted, the phage chromosome is integrated (by covalent bonds) into the bacterial chromosome, where it can remain dormant for thousands of generations. If the lysogen is induced (by UV light for example), the phage genome is excised from the bacterial chromosome and initiates the lytic cycle, which culminates (使达到高潮) in lysis of the cell and the release of phage particles. The lytic cycle leads to the production of new phage particles which are released by lysis of the host.

Transduction as a method for transferring genetic material

The packaging of bacteriophage DNA has low fidelity and small pieces of bacterial DNA, together with the bacteriophage genome, may become packaged into the bacteriophage genome. At the same time, some phage genes are left behind in the bacterial chromosome.

There are generally three types of recombination events that can lead to this incorporation of bacterial DNA into the viral DNA, leading to two modes of recombination.

Generalized transduction (普遍性转导)

Generalized transduction is the process by which any bacterial gene may be transferred to another bacterium via a bacteriophage, and typically carries only bacterial DNA and no viral DNA. In essence, this is the packaging of bacterial DNA into a viral envelope. This may occur in two main ways, recombination and headful packaging.

If bacteriophages undertake the lytic cycle of infection upon entering a bacterium, the virus will take control of the cell's machinery for use in replicating its own viral DNA. If by chance bacterial chromosomal DNA is inserted into the viral capsid which is usually used to encapsulate the viral DNA, the mistake will lead to *generalized transduction*.

If the virus replicates using "headful packaging", it attempts to fill the nucleocapsid (核衣壳蛋白，核蛋白壳，病毒粒子) with genetic material. If the viral genome results in spare capacity (备用容量，闲置的生产能力), viral packaging mechanisms may incorporate bacterial genetic material into the new virion.

The new virus capsule now loaded with part bacterial DNA continues to infect another bacterial cell. This bacterial material may become recombined into another bacterium upon infection.

When the new DNA is inserted into this recipient cell it is thought to have one of three fates：

(1) The DNA will be absorbed by the cell and be recycled for spare parts (备件).

(2) If the DNA was originally a plasmid, it will re-circularize inside the new cell and become a plasmid again.

(3) If the new DNA matches with a homologous region of the recipient cell's chromosome, it will

exchange DNA material similar to the actions in bacterial recombination.

Specialized transduction （局限性转导）

Specialized transduction is the process by which a *restricted*（有限的，很小的）set of bacterial genes is transferred to another bacterium. The genes that get transferred (donor genes) depend on where the phage genome is located on the chromosome. Specialized transduction occurs when the prophage excises imprecisely from the chromosome so that bacterial genes lying adjacent to the prophage are included in the excised DNA. The excised DNA is then packaged into a new virus particle, which then delivers the DNA to a new bacterium, where the donor genes can be inserted into the recipient chromosome or remain in the cytoplasm, depending on the nature of the bacteriophage.

When the partially encapsulated（封装）phage material infects another cell and becomes a "prophage" (is covalently bonded into the infected cell's chromosome), the partially coded prophage DNA is called a "heterogenote"（杂基因子，异基因子，异基因）.

Example of specialized transduction is λ phages in *Escherichia coli* discovered by Esther Lederberg.

Medical Applications

- Resistance to anti-biotic drugs
- Correcting genetic diseases by direct modification of genetic errors

Some vector-free methods include：**electroporation, microinjection** and **gene gun.**

Electroporation （电融合 / 电穿孔）

Electroporation is formation of transient holes in cell membranes using electric pulses of high field strength, this allows DNA to enter cells such as bacteria.

Electroporation, or **electropermeabilization**, is a microbiology technique in which an electrical field is applied to cells in order to increase the permeability of the cell membrane, allowing chemicals, drugs, or DNA to be introduced into the cell. In microbiology, the process of electroporation is often used to transform bacteria, yeast, or plant protoplasts by introducing new coding DNA. If bacteria and plasmids are mixed together, the plasmids can be transferred into the bacteria after electroporation. Several hundred volts across a distance of several millimeters are typically used in this process. Afterwards, the cells have to be handled carefully until they have had a chance to divide, producing new cells that contain reproduced plasmids. This process is approximately ten times more effective than chemical transformation.

Electroporation is also highly efficient for the introduction of foreign genes into tissue culture cells, especially mammalian cells. For example, it is used in the process of producing knockout mice, as well as in tumor treatment, gene therapy, and cell-based therapy. The process of introducing foreign DNA into eukaryotic cells is known as transfection. Electroporation is highly effective for transfecting cells in suspension using electroporation cuvettes. Electroporation has proven efficient for use on tissues *in vivo*, for in utero（子宫）applications as well as in ovo（卵）transfection. Adherent cells（贴壁细胞）can also be transfected using electroporation, providing researchers with an alternative to trypsinizing（使胰蛋白酶化）their cells prior to transfection.

Laboratory practice

Electroporation is performed with **electroporators**（电转化仪，电穿孔仪）, purpose-built appliances which create an electrostatic field（静电场）in a cell solution. The cell suspension is pipetted（用移液器吸取）into a glass or plastic cuvette which has two aluminum electrodes on its sides (Fig. 2-19A). For

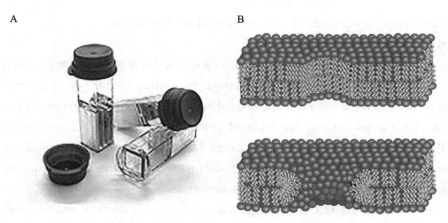

Fig. 2-19 A. Cuvettes for electroporation. These are plastic with aluminum（铝的）electrodes and a blue lid. They hold a maximum of 400 μl. B. Schematic（示意图）showing the theoretical arrangement of lipids in a hydrophobic pore (top) and a hydrophilic pore (bottom).

bacterial electroporation, typically a suspension of around 50 microliters is used. Prior to electroporation, this suspension of bacteria is mixed with the plasmid to be transformed. The mixture is pipetted into the cuvette, the voltage and capacitance（电容，电流容量）are set, and the cuvette is inserted into the electroporator. The process requires direct contact between the electrodes and the suspension. Immediately after electroporation, one milliliter of liquid medium is added to the bacteria (in the cuvette or in an Eppendorf tube), and the tube is incubated at the bacteria's optimal temperature for an hour or more to allow recovery of the cells and expression of the plasmid, followed by bacterial culture on agar plates.

The success of the electroporation depends greatly on the purity of the plasmid solution, especially on its salt content. Solutions with high salt concentrations might cause an electrical discharge（放电）[known as arcing（电弧作用）], which often reduces the viability of the bacteria. For a further detailed investigation of the process, more attention should be paid to the output impedance（阻抗）of the porator device（穿孔装置）and the input impedance of the cells suspension (*e.g.*, salt content).

Since the cell membrane is not able to pass current (except in ion channels), it acts as an electrical capacitor（电容器）. Subjecting membranes to a high-voltage electric field results in their temporary breakdown, resulting in pores that are large enough to allow macromolecules (such as DNA) to enter or leave the cell.

Drug and gene delivery

Electroporation can also be used to help deliver drugs or genes into the cell by applying short and intense electric pulses that transiently permeabilize cell membrane, thus allowing transport of molecules otherwise not transported through a cellular membrane. This procedure is referred to as electrochemotherapy when the molecules to be transported are chemotherapeutic agents or gene electrotransfer when the molecule to be transported is DNA. Scientists from Karolinska Institutet（卡罗林斯卡医学院）and the University of Oxford use electroporation of exosomes（外来体）to deliver siRNAs, antisense oligonucleotides, chemotherapeutic agents and proteins specifically to neurons after inject them systemically (in blood). Because these exosomes are able to cross the blood brain barrier this protocol could solve the issue of poor delivery of medications to the central nervous system and cure Alzheimer's, Parkinson's disease and brain cancer among other diseases.

Physical mechanism

Electroporation allows cellular introduction of large highly charged molecules such as DNA which would never passively diffuse across the hydrophobic bilayer core. This phenomenon indicates that the mechanism is the creation of nm-scale water-filled holes in the membrane. Although electroporation and dielectric breakdown (介质击穿，介电击穿) both result from application of an electric field, the mechanisms involved are fundamentally different. In dielectric breakdown the barrier material is ionized, creating a conductive pathway. The material alteration is thus chemical in nature. In contrast, during electroporation the lipid molecules are not chemically altered but simply shift position, opening up a pore which acts as the conductive pathway through the bilayer as it is filled with water.

Electroporation is a dynamic phenomenon that depends on the local transmembrane voltage at each point on the cell membrane. It is generally accepted that for a given pulse duration and shape, a specific transmembrane voltage threshold exists for the manifestation of the electroporation phenomenon (from 0.5 V to 1 V). This leads to the definition of an electric field magnitude threshold (强度极限) for electroporation (E_{th}). That is, only the cells within areas where $E \geqslant E_{th}$ are electroporated. If a second threshold (E_{ir}) is reached or surpassed, electroporation will compromise the viability (生存能力) of the cells, *i.e.*, irreversible electroporation (IRE).

Electroporation is a multi-step process with several distinct phases. First, a short electrical pulse must be applied. Typical parameters would be 300~400 mV for < 1 ms across the membrane [note the voltages used in cell experiments are typically much larger because they are being applied across large distances to the bulk solution so the resulting field across the actual membrane is only a small fraction of the applied bias (外来偏压)]. Upon application of this potential the membrane charges like a capacitor through the migration of ions from the surrounding solution. Once the critical field (临界场，临界电场) is achieved there is a rapid localized rearrangement in lipid morphology. The resulting structure is believed to be a "pre-pore" since it is not electrically conductive but leads rapidly to the creation of a conductive pore. Evidence for the existence of such pre-pores comes mostly from the "flickering" (忽隐忽现的，闪现) of pores, which suggests a transition between conductive and insulating states. It has been suggested that these pre-pores are small (~3 Å) hydrophobic defects. If this theory is correct, then the transition to a conductive state could be explained by a rearrangement at the pore edge, in which the lipid heads fold over to create a hydrophilic interface (Fig.2-19). Finally, these conductive pores can either heal, resealing the bilayer or expand, eventually rupturing it. The resultant fate depends on whether the critical defect size was exceeded which in turn depends on the applied field, local mechanical stress (机械应力) and bilayer edge energy.

Microinjection

Microinjection is the use of a glass micropipette (微量吸移管) to inject a liquid substance at a microscopic or borderline (边界的) macroscopic level. The target is often a living cell but may also include intercellular space. Microinjection is a simple mechanical process usually involving an inverted microscope with a magnification power of around 200 × [though sometimes it is performed using a dissecting (解剖的) stereomicroscope at 40~50 × or a traditional compound upright microscope (复合立式显微镜) at similar power to an inverted model].

For processes such as cellular or pronuclear injection (前核显微注射) the target cell is positioned under the microscope and two micromanipulators (显微操纵器) — one holding the pipette (移液管，

吸移管）and one holding a microcapillary needle usually between 0.5 and 5 μm in diameter (larger if injecting stem cells into an embryo) — are used to penetrate the cell membrane and/or the nuclear envelope. In this way the process can be used to introduce a vector into a single cell. Microinjection can also be used in the cloning of organisms, in the study of cell biology and viruses, and for treating male subfertility（生殖能力低下）through **intracytoplasmic sperm injection [ICSI**, *"IK-see"*（卵母细胞）胞浆内单精子注射]（Fig. 2-20）.

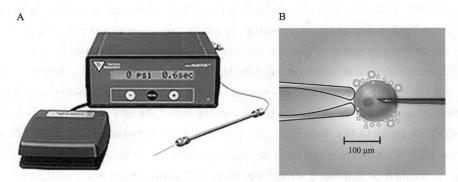

Fig. 2-20　A. A microinjection controller designed by Tritech Research for controlling the pressure applied to a hollow glass needle with a microscopic tip, placed in a brass needle holder, to regulate the delivery of substances like DNA into cells, stem cells into embryos, and sperm into eggs. B. Diagram of the intracytoplasmic sperm injection of a human egg. Micromanipulator on the left holds egg in position while microinjector on the right delivers a single sperm cell.

History

The use of microinjection as a biological procedure began in the early twentieth century, though even through the 1970s it was not commonly used. By the 1990s, its use had escalated significantly and it is now considered a common laboratory technique, along with vesicle fusion（囊泡融合）, electroporation, chemical transfection, and viral transduction, for introducing a small amount of a substance into a small target.

Basic types

There are two basic types of microinjection systems. The first is called a *constant flow system* and the second is called a *pulsed flow system*. In a constant flow system, which is relatively simple and inexpensive though clumsy and outdated, a constant flow of a sample is delivered from a micropipette and the amount of the sample which is injected is determined by how long the needle remains in the cell. This system typically requires a regulated pressure source, a capillary holder, and either a coarse or a fine micromanipulator. A pulsed flow system, however, allows for greater control and consistency（一致性）over the amount of sample injected: the most common arrangement for **ICSI** injection includes an Eppendorf "Femtojet" injector coupled with an Eppendorf "InjectMan", though procedures involving other targets usually take advantage of much less expensive equipment of similar capability. Because of its increased control over needle placement and movement and in addition to the increased precision over the volume of substance delivered, the pulsed flow technique usually results in less damage to the receiving cell than the constant flow technique. However, the Eppendorf line, at least, has a complex user interface（用户界面）and its particular system components are usually much more expensive than those necessary to create a constant flow system or than other pulsed flow injection systems.

Pronuclear injection（前核显微注射）

Pronuclear injection is a technique used to create transgenic organisms by injecting genetic material into the nucleus of a fertilized oocyte（卵母细胞）. This technique is commonly used to study the role of genes using mouse animal models.

Pronuclear injection in mice

The pronuclear injection of mouse sperm is one of the two most common methods for producing transgenic animals (along with the genetic engineering of embryonic stem cells). In order for pronuclear injection to be successful, the genetic material (typically linear DNA) must be injected while the genetic material from the oocyte and sperm are separate（单独的，分开的，各自的）(*i.e.*, the pronuclear phase). In order to obtain these oocytes, mice are commonly superovulated（使超数排卵）using gonadotrophins（促性腺激素）. Once plugging (mating plug 交配塞) has occurred, oocytes are harvested from the mouse and injected with the genetic material. The oocyte is then implanted（移植，着床）in the oviduct（输卵管）of a pseudopregnant（假孕）animal. While efficiency varies, 10%~40% of mice born from these implanted oocytes may contain the injected construct. Transgenic mice can then be bred to create transgenic lines.

Gene gun

Gene gun, also referred to as particle bombardment（轰击）, microprojectile（微粒）bombardment, or biolistics（基因枪）. A **gene gun** or a **biolistic** particle **delivery system**, is a device used in biolistic transfection, a process used to introduce genetic material to cells through the use of tiny DNA-coated particles fired at high velocity into a cluster of cells. The inserted genetic material are termed transgenes（转入基因，输异基因）. The payload is an elemental particle（基本粒子）of a heavy metal coated with plasmid DNA. Particles of gold or tungsten（钨）are coated with DNA and then shot into young plant cells or plant embryos (Fig. 2-21). Some genetic material will stay in the cells and transform them. This technique is often simply referred to as **bioballistics** or **biolistics**. The transformation efficiency is lower than in Agrobacterium-mediated transformation, but most plants can be transformed with this method.

With a gene gun, a "bullet" is made from some microcarriers, such as particles of gold or tungsten, which have been coated with exogenous DNA. Based on momentum（动量，动力，冲量）transfer, the bullet is fired into a petri dish with a sampling of cells, and the particles introduce the DNA to the cells, for gene transfer or temporary expression of proteins. While some of the cells may not survive the process, the remaining cells can be used in a variety of ways. The new genetic material also includes a marker which makes it easy to identify cells which have been successfully penetrated with the material.

Several different types of gene gun are available to researchers, sold by companies which specialize in scientific supplies, and some labs have devised their own to meet specific needs to address perceived shortcomings with commercial products.

The gene gun got its name because originally it was the bullet's launching（发射）from of a gun was used as the source of impulse, but now gene guns are mostly driven by the air pressure. The concept of the gene gun was introduced in the 1980s, as researchers were looking for new ways to introduce genetic material into the cells they studied. Gene guns were originally developed for use with plant cells (plant transformation), although they can also be used in animal cells.

Gene guns are used in laboratory settings to conduct research, develop new products, and tag samples of materials. This device is able to transform almost any type of cell, including plants, and is not limited

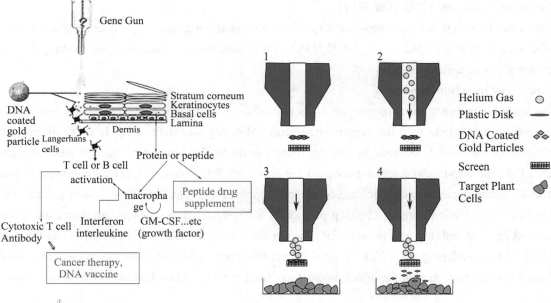

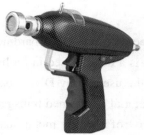

Fig. 2-21 A gene gun is used for injecting cells with genetic information, it is also known as biolistic particle delivery system. Gene guns can be used effectively on most cells but are mainly used on plant cells. **Step 1** The gene gun apparatus is ready to fire. **Step 2** When the gun is turned on and the helium (氦) flows through. **Step 3** The helium moving the disk (圆盘) with DNA coated particles toward the screen. **Step 4** The helium having pushed the particles moving through the screen and moving to the target cells to transform the cells.

to genetic material of the nucleus: it can also transform organelles (细胞器), including plastids (质体, 成形粒, 色素体). As with other pieces of lab equipment, gene guns are constantly being modified and refined to make them more useful.

Application

Gene guns are so far mostly applied for plant cells. However, there is much potential use in humans and other animals as well. Using a gene gun, a researcher can introduce new DNA to force a cell to produce proteins it wasn't making before (*e.g.*, gene gun can be used to deliver pharmaceutical DNA into tissue & cells, so that the DNA can express the corresponding pharmaceutical protein to achieve the goal of treating and/or preventing diseases). Gene guns have been used extensively in the genetic modification of crops to introduce genes which make crops more resistant to drought, increase the nutritional value of crops, or allow herbicides to be used safely around crops. Gene guns have also been used experimentally to deliver genetic vaccines, and to introduce DNA into animal cells for the purpose of tagging them for microscopy or for genetic engineering of such cells.

Gene gun design

The gene gun was originally a Crosman air pistol (气手枪) modified to fire dense tungsten (钨) particles. It was invented by John C Sanford, Ed Wolf and Nelson Allen at Cornell University, and Ted Klein of DuPont, between 1983 and 1986. The original target was onions (chosen for their large cell size) and it was used to deliver particles coated with a marker gene. Genetic transformation was then proven when the onion tissue expressed the gene.

The earliest custom（定制的，定做的）manufactured gene guns (fabricated by Nelson Allen) used a 22 caliber（口径）nail gun（射钉枪）cartridge（弹药筒）to propel an extruded（挤压过模子成型，压制的）polyethylene cylinder (bullet) down a 22 cal. Douglas barrel. A droplet（小滴，微滴）of the tungsten powder and genetic material was placed on the bullet and shot down the barrel at a lexan（勒克森聚碳酸酯纤维）"stopping" disk with a petri dish（有盖培养皿）below. The bullet welded（焊牢，使结合）to the disk and the genetic information blasted（猛攻，轰击）into the sample in the dish with a doughnut effect (devastation in the middle, a ring of good transformation and little around the edge). The gun was connected to a vacuum pump and was under vacuum while firing. The early design was put into limited production by a Rumsey-Loomis (a local machine shop then at Mecklenburg Rd in Ithaca, NY, USA). Later the design was refined by removing the "surge tank"（缓冲槽）and changing to nonexplosive propellants（推进剂）. DuPont added a plastic extrusion（压制品）to the exterior to visually improve the machine for mass production to the scientific community. Biorad contracted with Dupont to manufacture and distribute the device. Improvements include the use of helium propellant and a multi-disk-collision delivery mechanism. Other heavy metals such as gold and silver are also used. Gold may be favored because it has better uniformity（均匀性）than tungsten and tungsten can be toxic to cells, but its use may be limited due to availability and cost.

Biolistic construct design

A construct is a piece of DNA inserted into the target's genome, including parts that are intended to be removed later. All biolistic transformations require a construct to proceed and while there is great variation among biolistic constructs, they can be broadly sorted into two categories: those which are designed to transform eukaryotic nuclei, and those designed to transform prokaryotic-type genomes such as mitochondria, plasmids or plastids.

Those meant to transform prokaryotic genomes generally have the gene or genes of interest, at least one promoter and terminator sequence, and a reporter gene, which is a gene used to ease detection or removal of those cells which didn't integrate the construct into their DNA. These genes may each have their own promoter and terminator, or be grouped to produce multiple gene products from one transcript, in which case binding sites for translational machinery should be placed between each to ensure maximum translational efficiency. In any case the entire construct is flanked by regions called border sequences which are similar in sequence to locations within the genome, this allows the construct to target itself to a specific point in the existing genome.

Constructs meant for integration into a eukaryotic nucleus follow a similar pattern except that: the construct contains no border sequences because the sequence rearrangement that prokaryotic constructs rely on rarely occurs in eukaryotes; and each gene contained within the construct must be expressed by its own copy of a promoter and terminator sequence.

Though the above designs are generally followed, there are exceptions. For example, the construct might include a Cre-Lox system to selectively remove inserted genes; or a prokaryotic construct may insert itself downstream of a promoter, allowing the inserted genes to be governed by a promoter already in place and eliminating the need for one to be included in the construct.

Advantages

Biolistics has proven to be a versatile method of genetic modification and it is generally preferred to engineer transformation-resistant crops, such as cereals（谷类，谷物）. Notably, *Bt* maize（转 Bt 基因抗虫玉米）is a product of biolistics. Plastid（胚痕）transformation has also seen great success with particle bombardment when compared to other current techniques, such as *Agrobacterium* mediated transformation, which have difficulty targeting the vector to and stably expressing in the chloroplast（叶绿体）. In addition, there are no reports of a chloroplast silencing a transgene inserted with a gene gun. Additionally, with only one firing of a gene gun, a skilled technician can generate two transformed organisms. This technology has even allowed for modification of specific tissues *in situ*, although this is likely to damage large numbers of cells and transform only some, rather than all, cells of the tissue.

Limitations

However, biolistics introduces the construct randomly into the target cells. Thus the altered DNA sequences may be transformed into whatever genomes are present in the cell, be they nuclear, mitochondrial, plasmid or any others, in any combination, though proper construct design may mitigate（减轻，规避）this. Another issue is that the gene inserted may be overexpressed when the construct is inserted multiple times in either the same or different locations of the genome. This is due to the ability of the constructs to give and take genetic information from other constructs, causing some to carry no transgene and others to carry multiple copies; the number of copies inserted depends on both how many copies of the transgene an inserted construct has, and how many were inserted. Also, because eukaryotic constructs rely on illegitimate recombination（异常重组，非常规重组，不正常重组）, a process by which the transgene is integrated into the genome without similar genetic sequences, and not homologous recombination, which inserts at similar sequences, they cannot be targeted to specific locations within the genome.

2.2.4 Selection and screening of the clone containing the target gene（鉴定带有目的基因的克隆）

Because transformation usually produces a mixture of relatively few transformed cells and an abundance of non-transformed cells, a method is necessary to select for the cells that have acquired the plasmid. The plasmid therefore requires a selectable marker such that those cells without the plasmid may be killed or have their growth arrested. Antibiotic resistance is the most commonly used marker for prokaryotes. The transforming plasmid contains a gene that confers resistance to an antibiotic that the bacteria are otherwise sensitive to. The mixture of treated cells is cultured on media that contain the antibiotic so that only transformed cells are able to grow. Another method of selection is the use of certain auxotrophic（有营养缺陷的，营养缺陷体的）markers that can compensate（补偿，赔偿）for an inability to metabolize certain amino acids, nucleotides, or sugars. This method requires the use of suitably mutated strains that are deficient in the synthesis or utility of a particular biomolecule, and the transformed cells are cultured in a medium that allows only cells containing the plasmid to grow.

In a cloning experiment, a gene may be inserted into a plasmid used for transformation. However, in such experiment, not all the plasmids may contain a successfully inserted gene. Additional techniques may therefore be employed further to screen for transformed cells that contain plasmid with the insert. Reporter genes can be used as markers, such as the lacZ gene which codes for β-galactosidase used in **blue-white screening**. This method of screening relies on the principle of α-complementation, where a fragment of the lacZ gene (lacZα) in the plasmid can complement another mutant lacZ gene (lacZΔM15) in the cell. Both genes by themselves produce non-functional peptides, however, when expressed together, as when a plasmid containing lacZα is transformed into a lacZΔM15 cells, they form a functional β-galactosidase. The presence of an active β-galactosidase may be detected when cells are grown in plates containing X-gal, forming characteristic blue colonies. However, the multiple cloning site, where a gene of interest may be ligated into the plasmid vector, is located within the lacZα gene. Successful ligation therefore disrupts the lacZα gene, and no functional β-galactosidase can form, resulting in white colonies. Cells containing successfully ligated insert can then be easily identified by its white coloration from the unsuccessful blue ones.

Other commonly used reporter genes are green fluorescent protein (GFP), which produces cells that glow green under blue light, and the enzyme luciferase（荧光素酶）, which catalyzes a reaction with luciferin（荧光素）to emit light. The recombinant DNA may also be detected using other methods such as nucleic acid hybridization with radioactive RNA probe, while cells that expressed the desired protein from the plasmid may also be detected using immunological methods.

1. Insertional inactivation （插入失活筛选法）

Insertional inactivation is the inactivation of a gene by inserting a fragment of DNA into the middle of its coding sequence (Fig. 2-22). This technique is used in recombinant DNA engineering to disable expression of a gene.

The fundamental of insertional inactivation lies in that, when an exogenous gene (or DNA fragment) is inserted within a gene, the gene would lose its original function. Any future products from the inactivated gene will not work because of the extra codes added to it. An example is the use of pBR322, which has genes that respectively encode polypeptides that confer resistance to ampicillin and tetracycline antibiotics. Hence, when a genetic region of pBR322 coding for resistance to those antibiotics is interrupted by insertion, the gene function (*e.g.*, resistance to specific antibiotics) would be lost while new gene function would be gained.

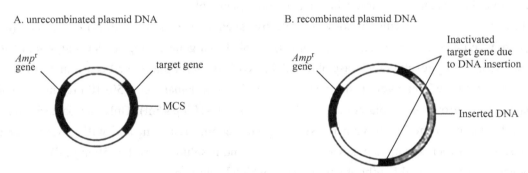

Fig. 2-22   Sketch diagram of insertional inactivation.

Insertional inactivation of antibiotic resistance genes （抗性基因插入失活筛选法）

One of the commonly used recombinant screening methods was designed according to the principle of insertional inactivation of antibiotic resistance genes. For example, the *Tet*^R gene and *Amp*^R (**Amp resistance**, a term for resistance to the antibiotic ampicillin, which is used as a selectable marker in bacterial transformation) gene on DNA of a nonrecombinant plasmid pBR322 (Fig. 2-23) are normal, with a phenotype of Ap^rTc^r. A recipient bacterium carrying this kind of plasmid will grow on an agar plate containing both tetracycline and ampicillin. While if a foreign gene fragment has been inserted within the *Tet*^R gene, leading to its inactivation, then the phenotype will be switched to Ap^rTc^s. A strain containing this kind of plasmid

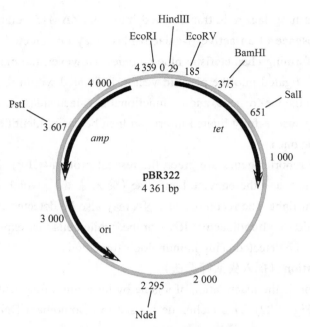

Fig. 2-23   Vector map of pBR322.

can only survive on a plate containing ampicillin, but will die on one which contains tetracycline.

Antibiotic resistance is an important tool for genetic engineering. By constructing a plasmid that contains an antibiotic-resistance gene as well as the gene being engineered or expressed, a researcher can ensure that, when bacteria replicate, only the individual cells that carry the plasmid survive. This ensures that the gene being manipulated passes along when the bacteria replicate.

In general, the most commonly used antibiotics in genetic engineering are "older" antibiotics. These include: ampicillin, kanamycin, tetracycline, and chloramphenicol.

Kanamycin is used in molecular biology as a selective agent most commonly to isolate bacteria (*e.g.*, *E. coli*) which have taken up genes (*e.g.*, of plasmids) coupled to a gene coding for **kanamycin resistance** [primarily Neomycin phosphotransferase II (**NPT II/Neo**)]. Bacteria that have been transformed with a plasmid containing the kanamycin resistance gene are plated on kanamycin (50~100 μg/ml) containing agar plates or are grown in media containing kanamycin (50~100 μg/ml). Only the bacteria that have successfully taken up the kanamycin resistance gene become resistant and will grow under these conditions. As a powder, kanamycin is white to off-white and is soluble in water (50 mg/ml).

Tetracycline (tc) is a broad family of antibiotics to which bacteria have evolved resistance. Tetracycline is used in cell biology as a selective agent in cell culture systems. It is toxic to prokaryotic and eukaryotic cells and selects for cells harboring the bacterial *tet*^{r} gene, which encodes a 399-amino-acid, membrane-associated protein. This protein actively exports tetracycline from the cell, rendering cells harboring this gene more resistant to the drug. The yellow crystalline powder can be dissolved in water (20 mg/ml) or ethanol (5 mg/ml), and is routinely used at 10 mg/L in cell culture. In cell culture at 37℃ (99℉), it is stable for days, with a half-life of approximately 24 hours.

The expression of tc resistance genes is regulated by **Tet Repressor Protein**, called **TetR.** TetR is used in artificially engineered gene regulatory networks because of its capacity for fine regulation. In the absence of tc, basal expression of TetR is very low, but expression rises sharply in the presence of even a minute quantity of tc through a positive feedback mechanism. TetR is present in the widely used *E. coli* cloning vector pBR322.

Chloramphenicol acetyltransferase (or **CAT**) is a bacterial enzyme (EC 2.3.1.28) that detoxifies the antibiotic chloramphenicol and is responsible for **chloramphenicol resistance** in bacteria. This enzyme covalently attaches an acetyl group from acetyl-CoA to chloramphenicol, which prevents chloramphenicol from binding to ribosomes. A histidine residue, located in the C-terminal section of the enzyme, plays a central role in its catalytic mechanism.

Insertional inactivation of lac z gene: Blue white screen

The blue-white screen is a molecular technique that allows for the detection of successful ligations in vector-based gene cloning. DNA of interest is ligated into a vector. The vector is then transformed into competent cell（感受态细胞）(bacteria). The competent cells are grown in the presence of X-gal. If the ligation was successful, the bacterial colony will be white; if not, the colony will be blue. This technique allows for the quick and easy detection of successful ligation, without the need to individually test each colony. An example of such a vector is the artificially reconstructed plasmid pUC19.

Molecular Mechanism

Cloning, alongside（与……一起）PCR, is one of the most common techniques in molecular biology. Blue white screening makes this procedure less time and labor intensive by allowing for the screening of successful cloning reactions through the color of the bacterial colony.

The molecular mechanism for blue/white screening is based on a genetic engineering of the lac operon in the *Escherichia coli* laboratory strain serving as a host cell combined with a subunit（亚基）complementation achieved with the cloning vector. The vector (*e.g.*, pBluescript) encodes the α subunit of LacZ protein with an internal multiple cloning site (MCS), while the chromosome of the host strain encodes the remaining Ω subunit to form a functional β-galactosidase enzyme. The MCS can be cleaved by different restriction enzymes so that the foreign DNA can be inserted within the lacZα gene, thus disrupting the production of functional β-galactosidase. The chemical required for this screen is X-gal, a colorless modified galactose sugar that is metabolized by β-galactosidase to form an insoluble product (5-bromo-4-chloroindole) which is bright blue, and thus functions as an indicator. Isopropyl β-D-1-thiogalactopyranoside (IPTG, 异丙基-β-D-1-硫代半乳糖苷), which functions as the inducer of the Lac operon, can be used in some strains to enhance the phenotype, although it is with many common laboratory strains unnecessary. The hydrolysis of colorless X-gal by the β-galactosidase causes the characteristic blue color in the colonies; it shows that the colonies contain vector without insert. White colonies indicate insertion of foreign DNA and loss of the cells' ability to hydrolyze the marker (Fig. 2-24).

Bacterial colonies in general, however, are white, and so a bacterial colony with no vector at all will also appear white. These are usually suppressed by the presence of an antibiotic in the growth medium. A resistance gene on the vector allows successfully transformed bacteria to survive despite the presence of the antibiotic.

The correct type of vector and competent cells are important considerations when planning a blue white screen.

It is also important to understand the lac operon is regulated by cAMP levels and the binding of cAMP to CAP（catabolite activator protein，降解物激活蛋白）. This CAP-cAMP complex promotes the binding of RNA polymerase to the lac promoter, which leads to transcription of the lac genes (For more

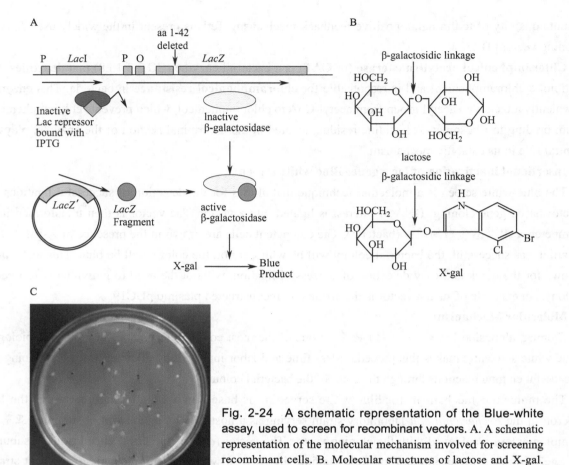

Fig. 2-24   A schematic representation of the Blue-white assay, used to screen for recombinant vectors. A. A schematic representation of the molecular mechanism involved for screening recombinant cells. B. Molecular structures of lactose and X-gal. C. A petri dish with blue and white colonies on it.

details, see section **2.1.2.5**). cAMP levels are regulated by the cell's incorporation（混合，揉合）of glucose. Since most bacteria preferentially utilize glucose even in the presence of lactose, the lac genes will only be turned on when glucose levels drop low enough to allow the CAP-cAMP complex to form.

2. Enzyme-Linked Immunoabsorbent Assay（ELISA，酶联免疫吸附试验）

The **enzyme-linked immunosorbent assay (ELISA)** (/i'laɪzə/, /ˌiː'laɪzə/) is a test that uses antibodies and color change to identify a substance.

ELISA is a popular format of "wet-lab" type analytic biochemistry assay that uses a solid-phase **enzyme immunoassay (EIA)** to detect the presence of a substance, usually an antigen, in a liquid sample or wet sample.

The ELISA has been used as a diagnostic tool in medicine and plant pathology, as well as a quality-control check in various industries.

Antigens from the sample are attached to a surface. Then, a further specific antibody is applied over the surface so it can bind to the antigen. This antibody is linked to an enzyme, and, in the final step, a substance containing the enzyme's substrate is added. The subsequent reaction produces a detectable signal, most commonly a color change in the substrate.

Performing an ELISA involves at least one antibody with specificity for a particular antigen. The sample with an unknown amount of antigen is immobilized on a solid support [usually a polystyrene（聚苯乙

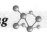

烯）microtiter plate（微量滴定板，酶标反应板）] either non-specifically (via adsorption to the surface) or specifically (via capture by another antibody specific to the same antigen, in a "sandwich" ELISA). After the antigen is immobilized, the detection antibody is added, forming a complex with the antigen. The detection antibody can be covalently linked to an enzyme, or can itself be detected by a secondary antibody that is linked to an enzyme through bioconjugation（生物偶联）. Between each step, the plate is typically washed with a mild detergent solution to remove any proteins or antibodies that are non-specifically bound. After the final wash step, the plate is developed（使显影）by adding an enzymatic substrate to produce a visible signal, which indicates the quantity of antigen in the sample.

Of note, ELISA can perform other forms of ligand binding assays instead of strictly "immuno" assays, though the name carried the original "immuno" because of the common use and history of development of this method. The technique essentially requires any ligating（连接）reagent that can be immobilized on the solid phase along with a detection reagent that will bind specifically and use an enzyme to generate a signal that can be properly quantified. In between the washes, only the ligand and its specific binding counterparts remain specifically bound or "immunosorbed" by antigen-antibody interactions to the solid phase, while the nonspecific or unbound components are washed away. Unlike other spectrophotometric （光谱光度测量的）wet lab assay formats where the same reaction well (*e.g.*, a cuvette) can be reused after washing, the ELISA plates have the reaction products immunosorbed on the solid phase which is part of the plate, and so are not easily reusable.

Principle

As an analytic biochemistry assay, ELISA involves detection of an "analyte" (*i.e.*, the specific substance whose presence is being quantitatively or qualitatively analyzed) in a liquid sample by a method that continues to use liquid reagents during the "analysis" (*i.e.*, controlled sequence of biochemical reactions that will generate a signal which can be easily quantified and interpreted as a measure of the amount of analyte in the sample) that stays liquid（保持液态）and remains inside a reaction chamber or well needed to keep the reactants contained; It is opposed to "dry lab" that can use dry strips（试纸条）— and even if the sample is liquid (*e.g.*, a measured small drop), the final detection step in "dry" analysis involves reading of a dried strip by methods such as reflectometry（反射计，反射测量术，反射测定法）and does not need a reaction containment chamber to prevent spillover（溢出）or mixing between samples.

As a heterogenous assay, ELISA separates some component of the analytical reaction mixture by adsorbing certain components onto a solid phase which is physically immobilized. In ELISA, a liquid sample is added onto a stationary solid phase with special binding properties and is followed by multiple liquid reagents that are sequentially added, incubated and washed followed by some optical change (*e.g.*, color development by the product of an enzymatic reaction) in the final liquid in the well from which the quantity of the analyte is measured. The qualitative "reading" usually based on detection of intensity of transmitted light by spectrophotometry, which involves quantitation of transmission of some specific wavelength of light through the liquid (as well as the transparent bottom of the well in the multiple-well plate format). The sensitivity of detection depends on amplification of the signal during the analytic reactions. Since enzyme reactions are very well known amplification processes, the signal is generated by enzymes which are linked to the detection reagents in fixed proportions to allow accurate quantification — thus the name "enzyme linked".

The analyte is also called the ligand because it will specifically bind or ligate to a detection reagent, thus ELISA falls under the bigger category of ligand binding assays. The ligand-specific binding reagent is "immobilized", *i.e.*, usually coated and dried onto the transparent bottom and sometimes also side wall of a well (the stationary "solid phase"/"solid substrate" here as opposed to solid microparticle/ beads that can be washed away), which is usually constructed as a multiple-well plate known as the "ELISA plate". Conventionally, like other forms of immunoassays, the specificity of antigen-antibody type reaction is used because it is easy to raise an antibody specifically against an antigen in bulk as a reagent. Alternatively, if the analyte itself is an antibody, its target antigen can be used as the binding reagent.

Experimental principle:

The enzyme is linked to the antibody (antigen) by the labeling technology, hence the corresponding antigen (antibody) in the sample to be tested can react specifically with the enzyme-labeled antibody (antigen). This method can be used for qualitative and quantitative analysis of samples to be tested. Actually, those enzyme conjugates are used in conjunction with a substrate, whether colorimetric （比 色 的）, fluorogenic, or chemiluminescent to create a detectable signal. The substrate is converted from a non-detectable soluble to a detectable usually insoluble form. When the corresponding substrate is encountered, the enzyme can catalyze and decompose the substrate with high efficiency and specificity to produce colored products. According to the shade of color, or the absorbance value, one can determine whether there is a specific antigen (antibody) in the sample (qualitatively) and its concentration (quantitatively). This method is a microassay technique widely used in biomedical field, simultaneously having the advantages of microscale, specificity, high efficiency, economy and simplicity.

Types

Currently, there are many enzyme-linked immunoassay (EIA) methods, which can be categorized into the following types according to different detection goals:

Direct method — used to determine antigens

Indirect method — used to determine antibodies

Double antibody sandwich method — mainly used for the determination of macromolecular antigens

Competitive inhibition method — mainly used for the determination of small molecule antigens

Direct ELISA

The steps of direct ELISA (Fig. 2-25) follows the mechanism below:

• A buffered solution of the antigen to be tested for is added to each well of a microtiter plate, where it is given time to adhere to the plastic through charge interactions.

• A solution of nonreacting protein, such as bovine serum albumin or casein, is added to well (usually 96-well plates) in order to cover any plastic surface in the well which remains uncoated by the antigen.

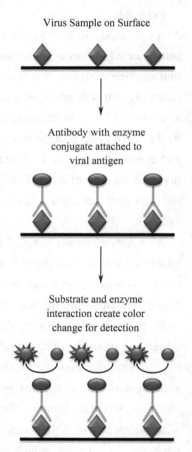

Virus Sample on Surface

Antibody with enzyme conjugate attached to viral antigen

Substrate and enzyme interaction create color change for detection

Fig. 2-25　Direct ELISA diagram.

- The primary antibody with an attached (conjugated) enzyme is added, which binds specifically to the test antigen coating the well.

- A substrate for this enzyme is then added. Often, this substrate changes color upon reaction with the enzyme.

- The higher the concentration of the primary antibody present in the serum, the stronger the color change. Often, a spectrometer is used to give quantitative values for color strength.

The enzyme acts as an amplifier; even if only few enzyme-linked antibodies remain bound, the enzyme molecules will produce many signal molecules. Within common-sense limitations, the enzyme can go on producing color indefinitely, but the more antibody is bound, the faster the color will develop. A major disadvantage of the direct ELISA is the method of antigen immobilization is not specific; when serum is used as the source of test antigen, all proteins in the sample may stick to the microtiter plate well, so small concentrations of analyte in serum must compete with other serum proteins when binding to the well surface. The sandwich or indirect ELISA provides a solution to this problem, by using a "capture" antibody specific for the test antigen to pull it out of the serum's molecular mixture.

ELISA may be run in a qualitative or quantitative format. Qualitative results provide a simple positive or negative result (yes or no) for a sample. The cutoff (截止点，划界点) between positive and negative is determined by the analyst and may be statistical. Two or three times the standard deviation (error inherent in a test) is often used to distinguish positive from negative samples. In quantitative ELISA, the optical density (OD) of the sample is compared to a standard curve, which is typically a serial dilution of a known-concentration solution of the target molecule. For example, if a test sample returns an OD of 1.0, the point on the standard curve that gave OD = 1.0 must be of the same analyte concentration as the sample.

The use and meaning of the names "direct ELISA" and "indirect ELISA" differs in the literature and on web sites depending on the context of the experiment. When the presence of an antigen is analyzed, the name "direct ELISA" refers to an ELISA in which only a labeled primary antibody is used, and the term "indirect ELISA" refers to an ELISA in which the antigen is bound by the primary antibody which then is detected by a labeled secondary antibody. In the latter case a sandwich ELISA is clearly distinct from an indirect ELISA. When the "primary" antibody is of interest, *e.g.*, in the case of immunization analyses, this antibody is directly detected by the secondary antibody and the term "direct ELISA" applies to a setting with two antibodies.

"Indirect" ELISA

The steps of "indirect" ELISA follows the mechanism below:

① A buffered solution of the antigen to be tested for is added to each well of a microtiter plate, where it is given time to adhere to the plastic through charge interactions.

② A solution of non-reacting protein, such as bovine serum albumin or casein, is added to block any plastic surface in the well that remains uncoated by the antigen.

③ Next the primary antibody is added, which binds specifically to the test antigen that is coating the well. This primary antibody could also be in the serum of a donor to be tested for reactivity towards the antigen.

④ Afterwards, a secondary antibody is added, which will bind the primary antibody. This secondary antibody often has an enzyme attached to it, which has a negligible effect on the binding properties of the antibody.

⑤ A substrate for this enzyme is then added. Often, this substrate changes color upon reaction with the enzyme. The color change shows that secondary antibody has bound to primary antibody, which strongly implies that the donor has had an immune reaction to the test antigen. This can be helpful in a clinical setting, and in R&D.

⑥ The higher the concentration of the primary antibody that was present in the serum, the stronger the color change. Often a spectrometer is used to give quantitative values for color strength.

Sandwich ELISA

A "sandwich" ELISA is used to detect sample antigen. The steps are:

① A surface is prepared to which a known quantity of capture antibody is bound.

② Any nonspecific binding sites on the surface are blocked.

③ The antigen-containing sample is applied to the plate, and captured by antibody.

④ The plate is washed to remove unbound antigen.

⑤ A specific antibody is added, and binds to antigen [hence the "sandwich": the Ag is stuck（动不了的）between two antibodies]. This primary antibody could also be in the serum of a donor to be tested for reactivity towards the antigen.

⑥ Enzyme-linked secondary antibodies are applied as detection antibodies that also bind specifically to the antibody's Fc region (nonspecific).

⑦ The plate is washed to remove the unbound antibody-enzyme conjugates.

⑧ A chemical is added to be converted by the enzyme into a color or fluorescent or electrochemical signal.

⑨ The absorbency or fluorescence or electrochemical signal (*e.g.*, current) of the plate wells is measured to determine the presence and quantity of antigen.

The image in Fig. 2-26 includes the use of a secondary antibody conjugated to an enzyme, though, in the technical sense, this is not necessary if the primary antibody is conjugated to an enzyme (which would be direct ELISA). However, the use of a secondary-antibody conjugate avoids the expensive process of creating enzyme-linked antibodies for every antigen one might want to detect. By using an enzyme-linked antibody that binds the Fc region of other antibodies, this same enzyme-linked antibody can be used in a variety of situations. Without the first layer of "capture" antibody, any proteins in the sample (including serum proteins) may competitively adsorb to the plate surface, lowering the quantity of antigen immobilized. Use of the purified specific antibody to attach the antigen to the plastic eliminates a

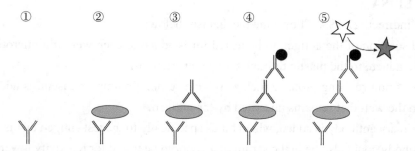

Fig. 2-26 A sandwich ELISA. ①Plate is coated with a capture antibody; ②sample is added, and any antigen present binds to capture antibody; ③detecting antibody is added, and binds to antigen; ④enzyme-linked secondary antibody is added, and binds to detecting antibody; ⑤substrate is added, and is converted by enzyme to detectable form.

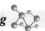

need to purify the antigen from complicated mixtures before the measurement, simplifying the assay, and increasing the specificity and the sensitivity of the assay. A sandwich ELISA used for research often need validation because of the risk of false positive results.

Competitive ELISA

A third use of ELISA is through competitive binding. The steps for this ELISA are somewhat different from the first two examples:

1. Unlabeled antibody is incubated in the presence of its antigen (sample).

2. These bound antibody/antigen complexes are then added to an antigen-coated well.

3. The plate is washed, so unbound antibodies are removed. (The more antigen in the sample, the more Ag-Ab complexes are formed and so there are less unbound antibodies available to bind to the antigen in the well, hence "competition".)

4. The secondary antibody, specific to the primary antibody, is added. This second antibody is coupled to the enzyme.

5. A substrate is added, and remaining enzymes elicit a chromogenic or fluorescent signal.

6. The reaction is stopped to prevent eventual saturation of the signal.

Some competitive ELISA kits include enzyme-linked antigen rather than enzyme-linked antibody. The labeled antigen competes for primary antibody binding sites with the sample antigen (unlabeled). The less antigen in the sample, the more labeled antigen is retained in the well and the stronger the signal.

Commonly, the antigen is not first positioned（小心放置）in the well.

For the detection of HIV antibodies, the wells of microtiter plate are coated with the HIV antigen. Two specific antibodies are used, one conjugated with enzyme and the other present in serum (if serum is positive for the antibody). Cumulative competition occurs between the two antibodies for the same antigen, causing a stronger signal to be seen. Sera to be tested are added to these wells and incubated at 37℃, and then washed. If antibodies are present, the antigen-antibody reaction occurs. No antigen is left for the enzyme-labeled specific HIV antibodies. These antibodies remain free upon addition and are washed off during washing. Substrate is added, but there is no enzyme to act on it, so positive result shows no color change.

Common ELISA formats are compared in Fig. 2-27, while mechanisms of various ELISA types are shown in Fig. 2-28.

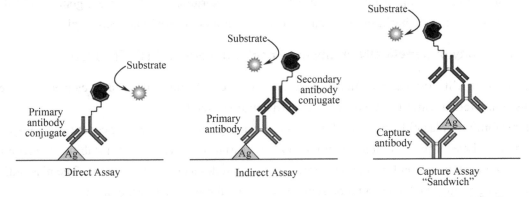

Fig. 2-27 Common ELISA formats. In the assay, the antigen of interest is immobilized by direct adsorption to the assay plate or by first attaching a capture antibody to the plate surface. Detection of the antigen can then be performed using an enzyme-conjugated primary antibody (direct detection) or a matched set of unlabeled primary and conjugated secondary antibodies (indirect detection).

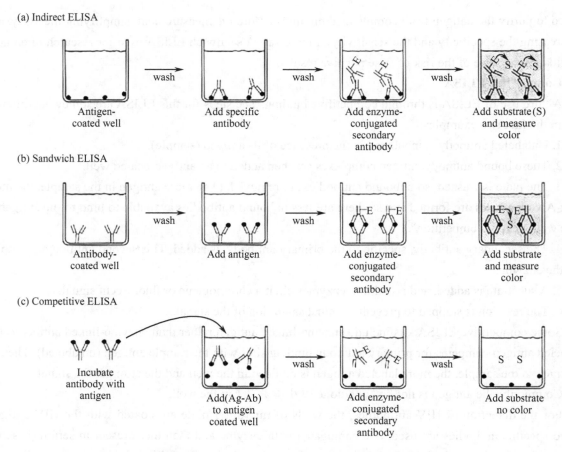

Fig. 2-28 Illustration of mechanisms of various ELISA types.

2.2.5 Amplification of the target gene and acquisition of the target product （目的基因的扩增及获得目的产物）

After affirmation of the presence of the target gene in the host bacterium/cell, it can then be amplified by simply proliferation of the recombinant bacterium/cell. If the cloning vector is not an expression vector, the cloned target gene should be extracted and cloned into an appropriate expression vector, and the latter in turn be introduced into an appropriate host bacterium/cell. The target gene would then be expressed in a new genetic background, then a special target product could be recovered.

2.2.6 Instability of genetically engineered bacteria （基因工程菌的不稳定性）

Plasmid instability indicates difficulties in maintainance of intact plasmid(s) caused by defect(s). transmission, internal rearrangements, and losses (deletion) of the DNA.

The instability of plasmids introduced into bacteria through gene engineering constitutes a major issue for the potential use of the recombinant strain on an industrial scale. The plasmid stability of recombinant strains is an essential criteria for high level fermentation and deserves more attention. The plasmid(s) of a genetically engineered bacteria should be stably maintained for at least 25 generations .

2.2.6.1 Plasmid instability （质粒的不稳定性）

Plasmid instability often occurs during passaging of genetically engineered bacteria. Plasmid instability falls into segregational plasmid instability and structural plasmid instability. This instability is characterized either by total plasmid loss due to defective distribution in the daughter cells (segregational instability) or by a modification in the plasmid DNA structure (structural instability) caused by a deletion, insertion or rearrangement.

The most common form of plasmid instability for genetically engineered bacteria is segregational plasmid instability. Segregational plasmid instability refers to the phenomenon that a certain proportion of genetically engineered bacterial daughter-cells do not contain any plasmid. This phenomenon is mainly related to two factors: one is the frequency of which the plasmid-containing strain produces daughter-cells that do not contain any plasmid. The plasmid lose rate is related with the type(s) of the host strain, the properties of the plasmid and the culture conditions. The second is the difference between the specific growth rates of these two strains. Since there should be a difference in growth rate between plasmid-harboring cells and plasmid-free ones, and the strain which has its plasmid lost generally has a growth advantage in a non-selective medium. In general, an increase in the expression level of a recombinant gene and the subsequent accumulation of the gene product is a serious burden to the host microorganism, which significantly reduces the growth rate and put the plasmid-bearing cell at a disadvantage compared to a plasmid-free counterpart. Once the plasmid is lost leaving some plasmid-free cells, the ratio of plasmid-harboring to plasmid-free cells will rapidly decline over time in culture medium, so that the plasmid-free strains can replace the plasmid-bearing conterpart as the dominant strain during cultivation, which can seriously affect the production rate of exogenous gene products.

The structural plasmid instability is caused by the loss of DNA segment(s) from plasmid(s), rearrangement, base substitution or base deletion, some cells may lose their ability to produce the cloned biomaterial due to genetic rearrangement of the structural gene (*trp*A1) while maintaining their antibiotic resistance. Cells under the expression condition are supposed to show more structural instability. The spontaneous deletion of plasmids is related to homologous recombination between short positive repeat sequences in plasmids. Plasmids with two tandem promoters are more likely to be missing. Loss may also occur between two sites without homology. The culture conditions may also influence the structural plasmid instability.

Amongst the factors influencing segregational plasmid instability, the culture conditions of the host cells are of primary importance. It has been shown that plasmid stability may be affected by temperature, pH, aeration, composition of the culture medium, incubation time and dilution rate.

Plasmid stability analysis method is as follows: appropriately dilute the sample of genetically engineered bacteria in liquid culture medium, uniformly spread on culture medium agar plate which does not contain antibiotics, culture for 10~12 h, then randomly select 100 colonies to inoculate on the culture medium plate containing the corresponding antibiotics matching with the antibiotics resistance gene, culture for 10~12 h, then count the number of colonies. Each sample should be repeated three times to calculate the ratio, which reflects the stability of the plasmid, called **plasmid stability** (ST).

2.2.6.2   *Methods for improving plasmid stability* （提高质粒稳定性的方法）

In order to improve the stability of genetically engineered bacteria, the following principal approaches can be adopted.

1. Choose the right bacterial host

The genetic characteristics of host bacteria have great influence on the stability of plasmids. The stability of plasmids is affected by the specific growth rate of the host bacteria, the characteristics of the gene recombination system, and whether there are homologous sequences on chromosome with plasmids and/or exogenous genes.

2. Select the appropriate vector

Genetically engineered bacteria with low copy number plasmid vectors have a higher frequency of producing daughter cells with no plasmids, so increasing the number of plasmids copies can improve the plasmid stability of genetically engineered bacteria of this type. On the contrary, genetically engineered bacteria containing high copy number plasmid vectors have lower frequency of producing plasmid-free daughter cells. But the specific growth rate of plasmid-harboring bacteria is significantly lower than that of the plasmid-free bacteria, due to the existence of a large number of exogenous plasmids. As soon as the plasmid-free bacterium is formed, it can quickly replace the plasmid containing bacteria as dominant strain. Therefore, further lifting the copy-number of bacterium of this kind can aggravate the negative growth potential of plasmid-harboring strain, which is unfavorable towards plasmid stability. For the same engineered strain, plasmid copy number can be changed through varying the specific growth rate. Ryan *et al.* reported the effect of specific growth rate on plasmid copy number and plasmid stability.

Plasmid copy number decreased at high specific growth rate, but plasmid stability increased significantly.

3. Selective pressure

Selective pressure, such as antibiotics, is a common method to improve the plasmid stability in the cultivation of engineered bacteria. When the recombinant plasmid containing the antibiotic resistance gene is transferred into the host cell, the genetically engineered bacteria acquire resistance. The addition of appropriate amount of corresponding antibiotics into the culture medium during fermentation can inhibit the growth of plasmid-loss bacteria, eliminate the effect of segregational instability of recombinant plasmid and improve the fermentation productivity. It is useless adding antibiotics selective pressure for plasmid structural instability. Adding antibiotics is undesirable for mass production — the production cost would increase when a large amount of antibiotics are used. In addition, some antibiotics can only maintain a certain period of time when they are easily hydrolyzed and inactivated.

4. Control of multi-stages cultivation

The higher the exogenous gene expression level, the more unstable the recombinant plasmid. When some plasmid instability occur due to highly efficient expression of foreign genes, it may be a worthwhile option to consider some fermentation process controlled in stages, *i.e.*, in the growth stage, repress the exogenous gene from expressing, avoid the issue plasmid instability caused by the heterogenous gene expression from occurring, let the plasmid pass on stably. Only when a disired bacteria density is achieved, the repression should be relieved or an induction made to express the exogenous genes. Since exogenous gene expression has not taken place in the first stage, the specific growth rate difference between recombinant bacteria and plasmid-loss bacteria was reduced, and the stability of plasmid was increased. Whereas in continuous culture, multistage cultivation can be considered, such as growth of bacteria in the first stage to maintain the stability of the recombinant bacteria, and expression of exogenous protein in the second stage.

5. Control of cultivation conditions

The culture conditions of engineered bacteria have a great effect on the stability and expression

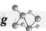

efficiency of their plasmids. The change of culture conditions has a great effect on the specific growth rate of *E. coli*, and the specific growth rate of genetically engineered bacteria, has in turn a great effect on the stability of their plasmids. Therefore, improving the specific growth rate is helpful to improve the plasmid stability.The specific growth rate of genetically engineered bacteria is related to culture environment, such as temperature, dissolved oxygen, pH, concentrations of limited nutrient and harmful metabolites, *etc*. Since the plasmid-harboring (gene) recombinant bacteria respond slower to the fermentation environment change than that of plasmid-free host strain, the specific growth rate of the two types of bacteria could change through changing culture conditions.

The environmental parameters that can be adjusted are medium components, culture temperature, pH and dissolved oxygen concentration. Some genetically engineered bacteria have high plasmid stability in a composite medium — composite medium containing organic nitrogen sources such as yeast extract, peptone, which is nutrient-rich, provides essential amino acids and other substances for microbial growth, hence microbes grow faster in a composite medium than in a minimal medium. The main reason for decline in the proportion of recombinant strains of recombinant bacteria in a minimal medium is the differences in growth rate between recombinant strains and host strain. While in a composite medium, the decline results from the co-participation of differences in specific growth rate and the probability of plasmid loss.

Cultivating genetically engineered bacteria needs to maintain a certain pH and dissolved oxygen level, the cause of poor stability of genetically engineered bacteria in low dissolved oxygen environment is that lack of oxygen restricts energy supply hence a high dissolved oxygen is needed during fermentation. And by using the method of intermittent oxygen supply or by the method of changing dilution rate can improve the stability of the plasmids. With the increase of specific growth rate, the successive passage number of *E. coli* which totally reserve the recombinant plasmid increases.

6. Immobilization

Immobilization can improve the stability of recombinant *E. coli*. After immobilization of gene recombinant *Escherichia coli*, plasmid stability and target gene product yield would be greatly improved. Selective pressure such as antibiotics, amino acids, are commonly used means to stabilize plasmid, but it is difficult to apply such selective pressure in mass production. When immobilization is adopted, this selective pressure could be eliminated. Satisfied stability is shown in various host bacteria and various plasmids using this immobilization system.

2.3 Major operating techniques in genetic engineering（基因工程的主要操作技术）

There are many techniques and approaches adopted in genetic engineering research, which have been developing rapidly in recent years. Here we describe only three of the most fundamental techniques — **Polymerase Chain Reaction**, **DNA sequencing** and **Construction of gene library**.

2.3.1 Polymerase chain reaction（PCR，聚合酶链反应）

The **polymerase chain reaction (PCR)** is a process used in molecular biology to amplify a single copy or a few copies of a piece of DNA across several orders of magnitude, generating thousands to millions of copies of a particular DNA sequence.

Developed in 1983 by Kary Mullis, PCR is now a common and often indispensable technique used in medical and biological research labs for a variety of applications. These include DNA cloning for sequencing, DNA-based phylogeny（种系发生）, or functional analysis of genes; the diagnosis of hereditary diseases; the identification of genetic fingerprints [used in forensic sciences and paternity testing（亲子鉴定）]; and the detection and diagnosis of infectious diseases. In 1993, Mullis was awarded the Nobel Prize in Chemistry along with Michael Smith for his work on PCR.

The method relies on thermal cycling, consisting of cycles of repeated heating and cooling of the reaction for DNA melting and enzymatic replication of the DNA. Primers (short DNA fragments) containing sequences complementary to the target region along with a DNA polymerase, which the method is named after, are key components to enable selective and repeated amplification. As PCR progresses, the DNA generated is itself used as a template for replication, setting in motion（发动）a chain reaction in which the DNA template is exponentially amplified. PCR can be extensively modified to perform a wide array of（一大批）genetic manipulations.

Almost all PCR applications employ a heat-stable DNA polymerase, such as *Taq* polymerase [an enzyme originally isolated from the bacterium *Thermus aquaticus*（栖热水生菌）]. This DNA polymerase enzymatically assembles a new DNA strand from DNA building-blocks, the nucleotides, by using single-stranded DNA as a template and DNA oligonucleotides (also called DNA primers), which are required for initiation of DNA synthesis. The vast majority of PCR methods use thermal cycling, *i.e.*, alternately heating and cooling the PCR sample through a defined series of temperature steps.

In the first step, the two strands of the DNA double helix are physically separated at a high temperature in a process called DNA melting（DNA 解链）. In the second step, the temperature is lowered and the two DNA strands become templates for DNA polymerase to selectively amplify the target DNA. The selectivity of PCR results from the use of primers that are complementary to the DNA region targeted for amplification under specific thermal cycling conditions.

2.3.1.1 Basic principle of PCR technology（PCR 技术的基本原理）

PCR principles and procedure

PCR amplifies a specific region of a DNA strand (the DNA target). Most PCR methods typically amplify DNA fragments of between 0.1 and 10 kilo base pairs (kbp), although some techniques allow for amplification of fragments up to 40 kbp in size. The amount of amplified product is determined by the available substrates in the reaction, which become limiting as the reaction progresses.

A basic PCR set up requires several components and reagents. These components include:

- *DNA template* that contains the DNA region (target) to amplify
- Two *primers* that are complementary to the 3′ (three prime) ends of each of the sense and anti-sense strand of the DNA target
- *Taq polymerase* or another DNA polymerase with a temperature optimum at around 70℃
- *Deoxynucleoside triphosphates* (dNTPs, sometimes called "deoxynucleotide triphosphates"; nucleotides containing triphosphate groups), the building-blocks from which the DNA polymerase synthesizes a new DNA strand
- *Buffer solution*, providing a suitable chemical environment for optimum activity and stability of the DNA polymerase

- *Bivalent cations*, magnesium or manganese（锰）ions; generally Mg^{2+} is used, but Mn^{2+} can be used for PCR-mediated DNA mutagenesis, as higher Mn^{2+} concentration increases the error rate during DNA synthesis

- *Monovalent cation* potassium ions

The PCR is commonly carried out in a reaction volume of 10~200 μl in small reaction tubes (0.2~0.5 ml volumes) in a thermal cycler. The thermal cycler heats and cools the reaction tubes to achieve the temperatures required at each step of the reaction (Fig. 2-29). Many modern thermal cyclers make use of the Peltier effect（培尔蒂埃效应，珀尔帖效应，热电致冷）, which permits both heating and cooling of the block holding the PCR tubes simply by reversing the electric current. Thin-walled reaction tubes permit favorable thermal conductivity to allow for rapid thermal equilibration. Most thermal cyclers have heated lids to prevent condensation at the top of the reaction tube. Older thermocyclers lacking a heated lid require a layer of oil on top of the reaction mixture or a ball of wax inside the tube.

Procedure

Typically, PCR consists of a series of 20~40 repeated temperature changes, called cycles, with each cycle commonly consisting of 2~3 discrete temperature steps, usually three (Fig. 2-29). The cycling is

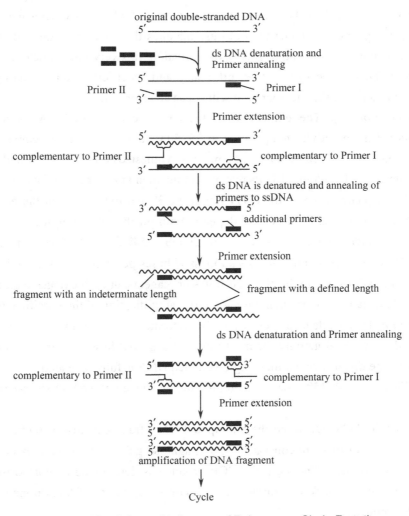

Fig. 2-29   Schematic diagram of Polymerase Chain Reaction.

often preceded by a single temperature step at a high temperature (＞90℃), and followed by one hold at the end for final product extension or brief storage. The temperatures used and the length of time they are applied in each cycle depend on a variety of parameters. These include the enzyme used for DNA synthesis, the concentration of divalent ions and dNTPs in the reaction, and the melting temperature (T_m) of the primers.

- *Initialization step* (Only required for DNA polymerases that require heat activation by hot-start PCR.): This step consists of heating the reaction to a temperature of 94~96℃ (or 98℃ if extremely thermostable polymerases are used), which is held for 1~9 minutes.

- *Denaturation step*: This step is the first regular cycling event and consists of heating the reaction to 94~98℃ for 20~30 seconds. It causes the melting of the DNA template by disrupting the hydrogen bonds between complementary bases, yielding single-stranded DNA molecules.

- *Annealing step*: The reaction temperature is lowered to 50~65℃ for 20~40 seconds allowing annealing of the primers to the single-stranded DNA template. This temperature must be low enough to allow for hybridization of the primer to the strand, but high enough for the hybridization to be specific, *i.e.*, the primer should only bind to a perfectly complementary part of the template. If the temperature is too low, the primer could bind imperfectly. If it is too high, the primer might not bind. Typically the annealing temperature is about 3~5℃ below the Tm of the primers used. Stable DNA-DNA hydrogen bonds are only formed when the primer sequence very closely matches the template sequence. The polymerase binds to the primer-template hybrid and begins DNA formation. It is very vital to determine the annealing temperature in PCR. This is because in PCR, efficiency and specificity are affected by the annealing temperature. An incorrect annealing temperature will cause an error in the test.

- *Extension/elongation step*: The temperature at this step depends on the DNA polymerase used; *Taq* polymerase has its optimum activity temperature at 75~80℃, and commonly a temperature of 72℃ is used with this enzyme. At this step the DNA polymerase synthesizes a new DNA strand complementary to the DNA template strand by adding dNTPs that are complementary to the template in 5′ to 3′ direction, condensing the 5′-phosphate group of the dNTPs with the 3′-hydroxyl group at the end of the nascent (extending) DNA strand. The extension time depends both on the DNA polymerase used and on the length of the DNA fragment to amplify. As a rule-of-thumb（经验法则，约略的估计）, at its optimum temperature, the DNA polymerase polymerizes a thousand bases per minute. Under optimum conditions, *i.e.*, if there are no limitations due to limiting substrates or reagents, at each extension step, the amount of DNA target is doubled, leading to exponential (geometric) amplification of the specific DNA fragment.

- *Final elongation*: This single step is occasionally performed at a temperature of 70~74℃ (this is the temperature needed for optimal activity for most polymerases used in PCR) for 5~15 minutes after the last PCR cycle to ensure that any remaining single-stranded DNA is fully extended.

- *Final hold*: This step at 4~15℃ for an indefinite time may be employed for short-term storage of the reaction.

To check whether the PCR generated the anticipated DNA fragment [also sometimes referred to as the amplimer（扩增引物）or amplicon（扩增子）], agarose gel electrophoresis is employed for size separation of the PCR products. The size(s) of PCR products is determined by comparison with a DNA ladder (a molecular weight marker), which contains DNA fragments of known size, run on the gel alongside the PCR products.

PCR stages

The PCR process can be divided into three stages:

➤ *Exponential amplification*: At every cycle, the amount of product is doubled (assuming 100% reaction efficiency). The reaction is very sensitive: only minute quantities of DNA need to be present.

➤ *Leveling off stage*: The reaction slows as the DNA polymerase loses activity and as consumption of reagents such as dNTPs and primers causes them to become limiting.

➤ *Plateau*: No more product accumulates due to exhaustion of reagents and enzyme.

Optimization

In practice, PCR can fail for various reasons, in part due to its sensitivity to contamination causing amplification of spurious（假的，似是而非的）DNA products. Because of this, a number of techniques and procedures have been developed for optimizing PCR conditions. Contamination with extraneous（外来的，无关的）DNA is addressed（处理）with lab protocols and procedures that separate pre-PCR mixtures from potential DNA contaminants. This usually involves spatial separation of PCR-setup areas from areas for analysis or purification of PCR products, use of disposable plasticware（塑料制品）, and thoroughly cleaning the work surface between reaction setups. Primer-design techniques are important in improving PCR product yield and in avoiding the formation of spurious products, and the usage of alternate buffer components or polymerase enzymes can help with amplification of long or otherwise problematic regions of DNA. Addition of reagents, such as formamide（甲酰胺）, in buffer systems may increase the specificity and yield of PCR. Computer simulations of theoretical PCR results (Electronic PCR) may be performed to assist in primer design.

Limitations

DNA polymerase is prone to error, which in turn causes mutations in the PCR fragments that are made. Additionally, the template DNA can also be mutated（变异）during PCR due to nonspecific binding of primers. Furthermore, prior information on the sequence is necessary in order to generate the primers.

2.3.1.2 *Thermostable PCR polymerase*（耐热 *PCR* 聚合酶）

The Klenow fragment

In the early 1980s, Kary Mullis was working at Cetus Corporation on the application of synthetic DNAs to biotechnology. He was familiar with the use of DNA oligonucleotides as probes for binding to target DNA strands, as well as their use as primers for DNA sequencing and cDNA synthesis. In 1983, he began using two primers, one to hybridize to each strand of a target DNA, and adding DNA polymerase to the reaction. This led to exponential DNA replication, greatly amplifying the amounts of DNA between the primers. The enzyme originally used in the polymerase chain reaction (PCR) process was the large (Klenow) fragment of the DNA Polymerase I from *E. coli*.

However, after each round of replication the mixture needs to be heated above 90℃ to denature the newly formed DNA, allowing the strands to separate and act as templates in the next round of amplification. This heating step also inactivates the DNA polymerase that was in use before the discovery of *Taq* polymerase, the Klenow fragment. The thermal stability of Klenow fragment is poor.

Taq polymerase（*Taq* DNA 聚合酶）— Another Pol I family enzyme

Another prokaryotic cellular (but non-*E. coli*) DNA polymerase of interest is ***Thermus aquaticus* DNA polymerase,** or *Taq* polymerase (pronounced; tack poll-im-er-aze), which is often abbreviated to "*Taq*

Pol" (or simply "*Taq*"). ***Taq* polymerase** /ˌtæk ˈpɒlɨməreɪz/ is a thermostable DNA polymerase named after the thermophilic bacterium *Thermus aquaticus*（栖热水生菌）from which it was originally isolated by Thomas D. Brock in 1965. It is frequently used in polymerase chain reaction (PCR).

Taq polymerase's utility for PCR stems from the fact that *Taq* polymerase is extremely heat stable and can tolerate the high temperatures required to melt duplex DNA during PCR cycling. This is because *T. aquaticus* lives in hot springs and hydrothermal vents（热液喷口）and thus must be able to replicate its DNA at very high temperatures, in some cases above the TM of the duplex.

Taq polymerase (94 kDa protein) is truly extremely heat stable. *Taq* polymerase was identified as an enzyme able to withstand the protein-denaturing conditions (high temperature) required during PCR, still functional even after continuous incubation at temperature of 95℃. Therefore it replaced the DNA polymerase from *E. coli* originally used in PCR. *Taq*'s optimum temperature for activity is 75~80℃, with a half-life of greater than 2 hours at 92.5℃, 40~45 minutes at 95℃ and 9 minutes at 97.5℃. The structural basis of this heat stability is still unclear.

Taq polymerase is a relatively processive enzyme, even though it is not known to associate with a clamp. It can replicate a 1 000 base pair strand of DNA in less than 10 seconds at 72℃. How this is achieved is also not clear, but it is not a replicative polymerase. *Taq* pol is related to Pol I and like Pol I it has an intrinsic 5′ → 3′ exonuclease activity.

One of *Taq*'s drawbacks is its lack of 3′ to 5′ exonuclease proofreading activity and is therefore error-prone, resulting in relatively low replication fidelity. Originally its error rate was measured at about 1 in 9 000 nucleotides. The remaining two domains act in coordination, via coupled domain motion. Some thermostable DNA polymerases have been isolated from other thermophilic bacteria and archaea, such as *Pfu* DNA polymerase, possessing a proofreading activity, and are being used instead of (or in combination with) *Taq* for high-fidelity amplification.

Taq makes DNA products that have A (adenine) overhangs at their 3′ ends. This may be useful in TA cloning, whereby a cloning vector (such as a plasmid) that has a T (thymine) 3′ overhang is used, which complements with the A overhang of the PCR product, thus enabling ligation of the PCR product into the plasmid vector.

Taq polymerase in PCR

The application of the thermotolerant DNA polymerase (*Taq* DNA polymerase) had greatly simplified the PCR operation, and hence brought it into the practical stage. Use of the thermostable *Taq* enables running the PCR at high temperature (~60℃ and above), which facilitates high specificity of the primers and reduces the production of unspecific products, such as primer dimer. Furthermore, use of the thermostable polymerase eliminates the need for having to add new enzyme to the PCR tube in each round of the reaction during the thermocycling process. A single closed tube in a relatively simple machine can be used to carry out the entire process. Thus, the use of *Taq* polymerase was the key idea that made PCR applicable to a large variety of molecular biology problems concerning DNA analysis.

Pfu DNA polymerase

***Pfu* DNA polymerase** is an enzyme found in the hyperthermophilic archaeon（古细菌）*Pyrococcus furiosus*（强烈火球菌）, where it functions to copy the organism's DNA during cell division. In the laboratory setting, *Pfu* is used to amplify DNA in the polymerase chain reaction (PCR), where the enzyme serves the central function of copying a new strand of DNA during each extension step.

Proofreading ability of *Pfu* polymerase

Pfu DNA polymerase has superior thermostability and proofreading properties compared to *Taq* DNA polymerase. Unlike *Taq* DNA polymerase, *Pfu* DNA polymerase possesses 3′ to 5′ exonuclease proofreading activity, meaning that as the DNA is assembled from the 5′ end to 3′ end, the exonuclease activity immediately removes nucleotides misincorporated at the 3′ end of the growing DNA strand. Consequently, *Pfu* DNA polymerase-generated PCR fragments will have fewer errors than *Taq*-generated PCR inserts.

Commercially available *Pfu* typically results in an error rate of 1 in 1.3 million base pairs and can yield 2.6% mutated products when amplifying 1 kb fragments using PCR. However, *Pfu* is slower and typically requires 1~2 minutes per cycle to amplify 1 kb of DNA at 72℃. Using *Pfu* DNA polymerase in PCR reactions also results in blunt-ended PCR products.

Pfu DNA polymerase is hence superior to *Taq* DNA polymerase for techniques that require high-fidelity DNA synthesis, but can also be used in conjunction with *Taq* polymerase to obtain the fidelity of *Pfu* with the speed of *Taq* polymerase activity.

2.3.1.3 *Primer design* (引物设计)

Good primer design is essential for a successful PCR reaction. There are many factors to take into account when designing the optimal primers for one's gene of interest. Here are some tips to consider when designing primers. The important design considerations described below are a key to specific amplification with high yield.

PCR Primer Design Guidelines

(1) Primer Length: Primers should be at least 18 nt long. In general, a length of 18~30 nucleotides for primers is good. It is generally accepted that the optimal length of PCR primers is 18~22 bp. This length is long enough for adequate specificity and short enough for primers to bind easily to the template at the annealing temperature. Oligonucleotide synthesis has become very inexpensive, so if adding a base or two will improve things, by all means, do it!

(2) Primer Melting Temperature: Primer Melting Temperature (T_m) by definition is the temperature at which one half of the DNA duplex will dissociate to become single stranded and indicates the duplex stability. The melting temperature (T_m) of the primers is generally 52~75℃.

The GC content of the sequence gives a fair indication of the primer T_m. It is calculated using the nearest neighbor thermodynamic theory, a much superior method for estimating it, which is considered the most recent and best available.

Formula for primer T_m calculation:

Melting Temperature T_m (K)=$\{\Delta H/ \Delta S + R \ln (C)\}$, or Melting Temperature T_m (℃) = $\{\Delta H/ \Delta S + R \ln (C)\}-273.15$ where

ΔH (kcal/mole) : H is the **Enthalpy**. Enthalpy is the amount of heat energy possessed by substances. ΔH is the change in Enthalpy. In the above formula the ΔH is obtained by adding up all the di-nucleotide pairs enthalpy values of each nearest neighbor base pair.

ΔS (kcal/mole) : S is the amount of disorder a system exhibits, called **Entropy**. ΔS is change in Entropy. Here it is obtained by adding up all the di-nucleotide pairs entropy values of each nearest neighbor base pair. An additional salt correction is added as the Nearest Neighbor parameters were obtained from DNA melting studies conducted in 1 M Na$^+$ buffer and this is the default condition (默认 状态) used for all calculations.

ΔS (salt correction) = ΔS (1M NaCl) + $0.368 \times N \times \ln ([Na^+])$

Where N is the number of nucleotide pairs in the primer (primer length −1).

[Na$^+$] is salt equivalent in mM.

[Na$^+$] calculation:

[Na$^+$] = Monovalent ion concentration + $4 \times$ free Mg^{2+}.

If the T_m of your primer is very low, try to find a sequence with more GC content, or extend the length of the primer a little.

Primer Pair Tm Mismatch Calculation: The two primers of a primer pair should have closely matched melting temperatures for maximizing PCR product yield. The difference of 5℃ or more can lead no amplification.

(3) Primer Annealing Temperature: The annealing temperature used during PCR should be 10 to 15℃ less than the T_m.

The primer melting temperature is the estimate of the DNA-DNA hybrid stability and critical in determining the annealing temperature. Too high T_a will produce insufficient primer-template hybridization resulting in low PCR product yield. Too low T_a may possibly lead to non-specific products caused by a high number of base pair mismatches. Mismatch tolerance is found to have the strongest influence on PCR specificity.

$T_a = 0.3 \times T_m$ (primer) $+ 0.7 T_m$ (product) −14.9

where,

T_m (primer) = Melting Temperature of the primers

T_m (product) = Melting temperature of the product

Optimum Annealing Temperature (T_a Opt): The formula of Rychlik is most respected. It usually results in good PCR product yield with minimum false product production.

T_a Opt $= 0.3 \times (T_m$ of primer$) + 0.7 \times (T_m$ of product$)$ −14.9

where

T_m of primer is the melting temperature of the less stable primer-template pair

T_m of product is the melting temperature of the PCR product.

(4) GC Content: The GC content (the number of G′s and C′s in the primer as a percentage of the total bases) of primer should be 40%~60%. It is best to aim for the GC content to be in the range of 45%~55%, with the 3′ of a primer ending in C or G to promote binding.

Strive to use approximately equal numbers of each nucleotide type, and avoid long runs of the same nucleotide, and have a balanced distribution of GC-rich and AT-rich domains.

(5) GC Clamp (夹) : The presence of G or C bases within the last five bases from the 3′ end of primers (GC clamp) helps promote specific binding at the 3′ end due to the stronger bonding of G and C bases. More than 3 G′s or C′s should be avoided in the last 5 bases at the 3′ end of the primer.

The 3′ end is the end which extends. Try to make the last two nucleotides some combination of Cs and As, as neither wobbles. This increases specificity.

If you are forced to have a small amount of self-complementarity at this end, such as (5′)...GT (3′), where the T can wobble pair with the G, by all means avoid any 5′ self-complementarity. The primer-

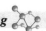

dimers which form can then reanneal to each other at their new 3′ ends, which are complements of the original self-complementary 5′ ends. These form ever increasing primer multimers with each cycle!

(6) Primer Secondary Structures: Presence of the primer secondary structures produced by intermolecular or intramolecular interactions can lead to poor or no yield of the product. They adversely affect primer template annealing and thus the amplification. They greatly reduce the availability of primers to the reaction.

i) Hairpins: It is formed by intramolecular interaction within the primer and should be avoided. Optimally a 3′ end hairpin with a ΔG of −2 kcal/mol and an internal hairpin with a ΔG of −3 kcal/mol is tolerated generally.

```
      ┌─ GTGT
      │   │
   A  │   │
      └─ TGCAGCAT
```

ΔG definition: The Gibbs Free Energy G is the measure of the amount of work that can be extracted from a process operating at a constant pressure. It is the measure of the spontaneity (自发性) of the reaction. The stability of hairpin is commonly represented by its ΔG value, the energy required to break the secondary structure. Larger negative value for ΔG indicates stable, undesirable hairpins. Presence of hairpins at the 3′ end most adversely affects the reaction.

$$\Delta G = \Delta H - T\Delta S$$

Try to avoid regions of secondary structure.

ii) Self Dimer: A primer self-dimer is formed by intermolecular interactions between the two (same sense) primers, where the primer is homologous to itself. Generally a large amount of primers are used in PCR compared to the amount of target gene. When primers form intermolecular dimers much more readily than hybridizing to target DNA, they reduce the product yield. Optimally a 3′ end self-dimer with a ΔG of −5 kcal/mol and an internal self-dimer with a ΔG of −6 kcal/mol is tolerated generally.

iii) Cross Dimer: Primer cross dimers are formed by intermolecular interaction between sense and antisense primers, where they are homologous. Optimally a 3′ end cross dimer with a ΔG of −5 kcal/mol and an internal cross dimer with a ΔG of −6 kcal/mol is tolerated generally.

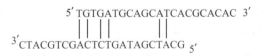

(a) Avoid intra-primer homology (more than 3 bases that complement within the primer) or inter-primer homology (forward and reverse primers having complementary sequences). These circumstances can lead to self-dimers or primer-dimers instead of annealing to the desired DNA sequences.

(b) Avoid internal hairpin structures, especially those which engulf the 3′ end.

(c) Never design a primer with 3′ self-complementarity, such as (5′)...GATC (3′). Such primers will anneal to each other, forming primer-dimers, which become useless end-products of the reaction.

(7) Avoid Template Secondary Structure: A single stranded Nucleic acid sequences is highly unstable and fold into conformations (secondary structures). The stability of these template secondary structures depends largely on their free energy and melting temperatures (T_m). Consideration of template secondary structures is important in designing primers, especially in qPCR. If primers are designed on a secondary structures which is stable even above the annealing temperatures, the primers are unable to bind to the template and the yield of PCR product is significantly affected. Hence, it is important to design primers in the regions of the templates that do not form stable secondary structures during the PCR reaction. A suitable software helps determine the secondary structures of the template and design primers avoiding them.

(8) Repeats: A repeat is a di-nucleotide occurring many times consecutively and should be avoided because they can misprime. For example: ATATATAT. A maximum number of di-nucleotide repeats acceptable in an oligo is 4 di-nucleotides. Hence, try to avoid runs of 4 or more of dinucleotide repeats.

(9) Runs（顺串）: Primers with long runs of a single base should generally be avoided as they can misprime. For example, AGCGGGGGATGGGG has runs of base "G" of value 5 and 4. A maximum number of runs accepted is 4 bp.

Hence, try to avoid runs of 4 or more of one base.

(10) 3′ End Stability: It is the maximum ΔG value of the five bases from the 3′ end. An unstable 3′ end (less negative ΔG) will result in less false priming.

(11) Avoid Cross Homology（避免与非扩增区存在同源性）: To improve specificity of the primers it is necessary to avoid regions of homology. Primers designed for a sequence must not amplify other genes in the mixture. Commonly, primers are designed and then a suitable software can be used to test the specificity. Then regions of cross homology would be avoided in designing primers. The software will identify regions significant cross homologies in each template and avoid them during primer search. Homology shared between primers and non-amplified regions should be less than 70%, and homology between 8 consecutive complementary base pairs should be avoided.

(12) Degenerate primer（简并引物） If a primer nucleotides sequence is deduced from an amino acid sequence, degenerate primer mixture should be added to the PCR reaction system, and Hot Start activation approaches may avoid mismatches and non-specific amplifications caused by degeneracy.

(13) Primer Design using Software

➢ A number of primer design tools are available that can assist in PCR primer design for new and experienced users alike. These tools may reduce the cost and time involved in experimentation by lowering the chances of failed experimentation.

➢ Primer Premier follows all the guidelines specified for PCR primer design. Primer Premier can be used to design primers for single templates, alignments, degenerate primer design, restriction enzyme analysis, contig analysis and design of sequencing primers.

➢ The guidelines for qPCR primer design vary slightly. Software such as AlleleID and Beacon Designer can design primers and oligonucleotide probes for complex detection assays such as multiplex assays, cross species primer design, species specific primer design and primer design to reduce the cost of experimentation.

➢ PrimerPlex is a software that can design primers for Multiplex PCR and multiplex SNP genotyping assays.

Other design key points for Primer Pair Design

(1) Typically, 3 to 4 nucleotides are added 5′ of the restriction enzyme site in the primer to allow for efficient cutting.

(2) If you are using the primers for mutagenesis, try to have the mismatched bases towards the middle

of the primer.

(3) If you are using the primers for cloning, cartridge purification（小柱提纯）is recommend as a minimum level of purification.

Nested primers（嵌套式引物）

Nested （嵌套） primers are regular primers that are just chosen within a DNA sequence that has been previously amplified. Nested primers are used to increase the specificity of an amplification or to reamplify the product of a PCR reaction that did not yield enough material. They are called nested because they are chosen within the target sequence of another set of primers.

Nested PCR

Nested PCR refers to a pair of PCRs run in series each with a pair of primers flanking the same sequence. Nested PCR is a variation of the polymerase chain reaction (PCR), in that two pairs (instead of one pair) of PCR primers are used to amplify a fragment. The first pair of PCR primers amplify a fragment similar to a standard PCR. However, a second pair of primers called nested primers (as they lie within the first fragment) bind inside the first PCR product fragment to allow amplification of a second PCR product which is shorter than the first one (Fig. 2-30).

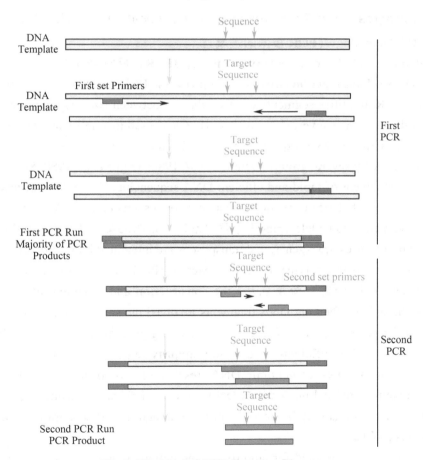

Fig. 2-30   Nested PCR Reaction Diagram.

The technique, because it uses four specific primers, rather than two, has greater specificity than regular PCR. For if the wrong PCR fragment was amplified, the probability is quite low that the region would be amplified a second time by the second set of primers. Thus, Nested PCR is a very specific PCR amplification. It can also yield detectable product in cases where simple PCR fails to do so.

Steps of the Nested PCR

Step One: The DNA target template is bound by the first set of primers shown in blue. The primers may bind to alternative, similar primer binding sites that give multiple products however only one of these PCR products give the intended sequence (multiple products not shown).

Step Two: PCR products from the first PCR reaction are subjected to a second PCR run however with a second new set of primers shown in red.

As these primers are nested within the first PCR product, they make it very unlikely that non-specifically amplified PCR product would contain binding sites for both sets of primers. This nested PCR amplification ensures that the PCR product from the second PCR amplification has little or no contamination from non-specifically amplified PCR products from alternative primer target.

Nested RT-PCR: This term refers to a nested PCR reaction that is initiated with cDNA that has been reverse transcribed from RNA.

Semi-nested PCR: Similar to a nested PCR except that in the second PCR one of the primers is a primer that was used in the first PCR.

2.3.1.4 *New progress in PCR technology and its application*（*PCR*技术的新进展及其应用）

Progress in PCR technology（PCR 技术的进展）

1. Inverse polymerase chain reaction (Inverse PCR，IPCR，反向 PCR）

Inverse polymerase chain reaction (Inverse PCR): **Inverse PCR** is a variant of the polymerase chain reaction. Standard PCR amplifies segments of DNA that lie between two inward-pointing primers. By contrast, inverse (also known as inverted or inside-out) PCR is used to amplify and clone unknown DNA that flanks one end of a known DNA sequence and for which no primers are available. The technique was developed independently by several groups (Ochman *et al*. 1988; Triglia *et al*. 1988; Silver and Keerikatte 1989), well before the advent of rapid and efficient DNA sequencing. These days, sequencing would in most cases be the method of choice to characterize an unknown segment of DNA. However, inverse PCR is still used extensively for rapid allelotyping［等位（基因）谱测定及变异普查］and to determine the locations at which retroviruses, transgenes, and transposons are integrated into genomes.

Prior to the invention of the polymerase chain reaction (PCR), the acquisition of a specific DNA fragment usually entailed（必需，必须包括）the construction and screening of DNA libraries, and the traditional "walking" into flanking DNA fragments involved the successive probing of libraries with clones obtained in the prior screening. These time-consuming procedures could be replaced by IPCR. Because IPCR can be used to efficiently and rapidly amplify regions of unknown sequence flanking any identified segment of cDNA or genomic DNA, researchers do not need to construct and screen DNA libraries to obtain additional unidentified DNA sequence information using this technique. Some recombinant phage or plasmids may be unstable in bacteria and amplified libraries tend to lose them. IPCR eliminates this problem.

Inverse PCR (IPCR) was designed for amplifying anonymous flanking genomic DNA regions. The technique involves digestion of source DNA (a preparation of DNA containing the known sequence and its flanking region) by a restriction enzyme, circulation of individual restriction fragments by intramolecular ligation, and amplification using oligonucleotides that prime the DNA synthesis directed away from the core region of a known sequence, *i.e.*, opposite of the direction of primers used in normal or standard PCR (Fig. 2-31).

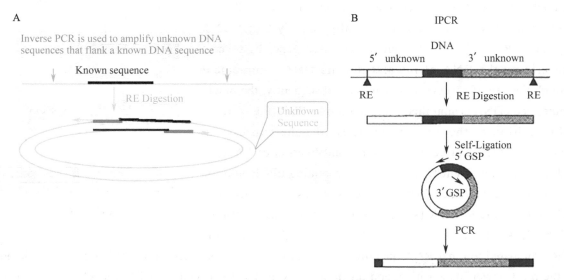

Fig. 2-31   A. Sketch map of IPCR. Diagram of IPCR for genomic DNA cloning. B. The procedure consists of four steps: genomic DNA isolation, restriction enzyme digestion(RE digestion), circularization of double-stranded DNA, and amplification of reverse DNA fragment. The black and open bars represent the known and unknown sequence regions of double-stranded cDNA, respectively. RE: restriction enzyme site; GSP: gene-specific primer.

(1) A target region with an internal section of known sequence and unknown flanking regions is identified.

(2) Genomic DNA is digested into fragments of a few kilobases by a usually low-moderate frequency (6~8 base) cutting restriction enzyme.

(3) Under low DNA concentrations, self-ligation is induced to give a circular DNA product.

(4) PCR is carried out as usual, with primers complementary to sections of the known internal sequence.

Finally the sequence is compared with the sequence available in the data base.

Inverse PCR is especially useful for the determination of insert locations. For example, various retroviruses and transposons（转座子，转位子）randomly integrate into genomic DNA. To identify the sites where they have entered, the known, "internal" viral or transposon sequences can be used to design primers that will amplify a small portion of the flanking, "external" genomic DNA. The amplified product can then be sequenced and compared with DNA databases to locate the sequence that has been disrupted.

2. Reverse transcription polymerase chain reaction（RT-PCR，反转录 PCR）

Reverse transcription polymerase chain reaction (RT-PCR) is one of many variants of polymerase chain reaction (PCR). This technique is commonly used in molecular biology to detect RNA expression. RT-PCR is often confused with real-time polymerase chain reaction (qPCR) by students and scientists alike. However, they are separate and distinct techniques. While RT-PCR is used to qualitatively detect gene expression through creation of complementary DNA (cDNA) transcripts from RNA, qPCR is used to quantitatively measure the amplification of DNA using fluorescent probes. qPCR is also referred to as quantitative PCR, quantitative real-time PCR, and real-time quantitative PCR.

Although RT-PCR and the traditional PCR both produce multiple copies of particular DNA isolates through amplification, the applications of the two techniques are fundamentally different. Traditional PCR is used to exponentially amplify target DNA sequences. RT-PCR is used to clone expressed genes by reverse transcribing the RNA of interest into its DNA complement through the use of reverse transcriptase. Subsequently, the newly synthesized cDNA is amplified using traditional PCR (Fig. 2-32).

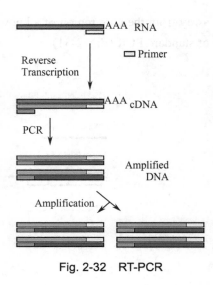

Fig. 2-32   RT-PCR

In addition to the qualitative study of gene expression, quantitative PCR can be utilized for quantification of RNA, in both relative and absolute terms, by incorporating qPCR into the technique. The combined technique, described as quantitative RT-PCR or real-time RT-PCR (sometimes even quantitative real-time RT-PCR), is often abbreviated as qRT-PCR, RT-qPCR, or RRT-PCR. Compared to other RNA quantification methods, such as Northern blot, qRT-PCR is considered to be the most powerful, sensitive, and quantitative assay for the detection of RNA levels. It is frequently used in the expression analysis of single or multiple genes, and expression patterns for identifying infections and diseases.

History

Since its introduction in 1977, Northern blot had been used extensively for RNA quantification despite its shortcomings: (a) time-consuming technique, (b) requires a large quantity of RNA for detection, and (c) quantitatively inaccurate in the low abundance of RNA content. However, the discovery of reverse transcriptase during the study of viral replication of genetic material led to the development of RT-PCR, which has since displaced Northern blot as the method of choice for RNA detection and quantification.

RT-PCR has risen to become the benchmark (衡量基准) technology for the detection and/or comparison of RNA levels for several reasons: (a) it does not require post PCR processing, (b) a wide range ($>10^7$-fold) of RNA abundance can be measured, and (c) it provides insight into both qualitative and quantitative data. Due to its simplicity, specificity and sensitivity, RT-PCR is used in a wide range of applications from experiments as simple as quantification of yeast cells in wine to more complex uses as diagnostic tools for detecting infectious agents such as the avian flu virus.

Principles

In RT-PCR, the RNA template is first converted into a complementary DNA (cDNA) using a reverse transcriptase. The cDNA is then used as a template for exponential amplification using PCR. RT-PCR is currently the most sensitive method of RNA detection available. The use of RT-PCR for the detection of RNA transcript has revolutionized the study of gene expression in the following important ways:

- Made it theoretically possible to detect the transcripts of practically any gene
- Enabled sample amplification and eliminated the need for abundant starting material that one faces when using Northern blot analysis
- Provided tolerance for RNA degradation as long as the RNA spanning the primer is intact

One-step RT-PCR vs. two-step RT-PCR

When quantifying mRNA, real-time RT-PCR can be performed as either a one-step reaction, where the entire reaction from cDNA synthesis to PCR amplification is performed in a single tube, or as a two-step reaction, where reverse transcription and PCR amplification occur in separate tubes (Fig. 2-33). There are several *pros* and *cons* associated with each method. One-step real-time RT-PCR is thought to minimize experimental variation because both enzymatic reactions occur in a single tube. However, this method uses an RNA starting template, which is prone to rapid degradation if not handled properly. Therefore, a one-step reaction may not be suitable in situations where the same sample is assayed on several occasions over a period of time. One-step protocols are also reportedly less sensitive than two-step protocols.

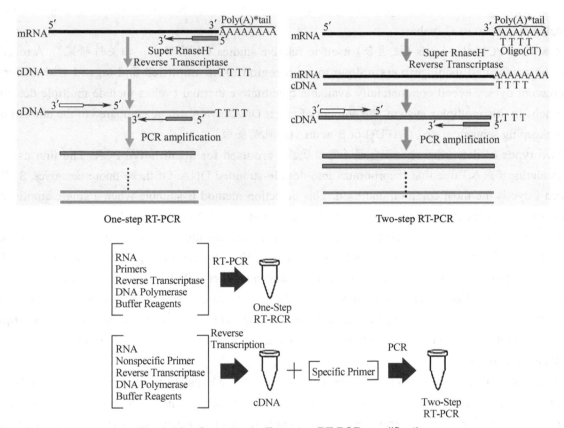

Fig. 2-33   One-step vs Two-step RT-PCR amplification.

Two-step real-time RT-PCR separates the reverse transcription reaction from the real-time PCR assay, allowing several different real-time PCR assays on dilutions of a single cDNA. Because the process of reverse transcription is notorious for its highly variable reaction efficiency, using dilutions from the same cDNA template ensures that reactions from subsequent assays have the same amount of template as those assayed earlier. Data from two-step real-time RT-PCR is quite reproducible with Pearson correlation coefficients ranging from 0.974 to 0.988. A two-step protocol may be preferred when using a DNA binding dye (such as SYBR Green I) because it is easier to eliminate primer-dimers through the manipulation of melting temperatures (Tms). However, two-step protocols allow for increased opportunities of DNA contamination due to more frequent sample handling.

3. Quantitative PCR（定量 PCR）

With the development of thermal cyclers incorporating fluorescent detection, PCR has a new, innovative application. In routine PCR, the critical result is the final quantity of amplicon（扩增子）generated after the process. Real-time or Quantitative PCR and RT-PCR use the linearity of DNA amplification to determine absolute or relative amounts of a known sequence in a sample. By using a fluorescent reporter in the reaction, it is possible to measure DNA generation.

In quantitative PCR, DNA amplification is monitored at each cycle of PCR. When the DNA is in the log linear phase of amplification, the amount of fluorescence increases above the background. The point at which the fluorescence becomes measurable is called the Threshold cycle (C_T，临界循环次数) or crossing point. By using multiple dilutions of a known amount of standard DNA, a standard curve can be generated of log concentration against C_T. The amount of DNA or cDNA in an unknown sample can then be calculated from its C_T value.

Real time PCR also lends（使适合）itself to relative studies（比较研究，相关性研究）. A reaction may be performed using primers unique to each region to be amplified and tagged with different fluorescent dyes. Several commercially available quantitative thermal cyclers include multiple detection channels. In this multiplex system, the amount of target DNA/cDNA can be compared to the amount of a housekeeping sequence, *e.g.*, GAPDH or β-actin（β- 肌动蛋白）.

Two types of detection chemistries（化学反应）are used for quantitative PCR. The first uses an intercalating（嵌入）dye that incorporates into double-stranded DNA. Of these fluorescent dyes, SYBR® Green I dye is the most common one used. This detection method is suitable when a single amplicon is being studied, as the dye will intercalate into any double-stranded DNA generated.

The second detection method uses a primer or oligonucleotide specific to the target of interest, as in TaqMan® probes, Molecular Beacons™（分子信标）, or Scorpion primers（蝎形引物）. The oligonucleotide is labeled with a fluorescent dye and quencher（淬灭剂）. The oligonucleotide itself has no significant fluorescence, but fluoresces either when annealed to the template (as in molecular beacons) or when the dye is clipped from the oligo during extension (as in TaqMan probes). Multiplex PCR is possible by using dyes with different fluorescent emissions（发射）for each primer.

Basic principles

Quantitative PCR is carried out in a thermal cycler with the capacity to illuminate each sample with a beam of light of a specified wavelength and detect the fluorescence emitted by the excited fluorophore（荧光团，荧光基团）. The thermal cycler is also able to rapidly heat and chill samples, thereby taking advantage of（利用）the physicochemical properties of the nucleic acids and DNA polymerase.

The PCR process generally consists of a series of temperature changes that are repeated 25~40 times. These cycles normally consist of three stages: the first, at around 95℃, allows the separation of the nucleic acid's double chain; the second, at a temperature of around 50~60℃, allows the binding of the primers with the DNA template; the third, at between 68~72℃, facilitates the polymerization carried out by the DNA polymerase. Due to the small size of the fragments the last step is usually omitted in this type of PCR as the enzyme is able to increase their number during the change between the alignment stage and the denaturing stage. In addition, some thermal cyclers add another short temperature phase lasting only a few seconds to each cycle, with a temperature of, for example, 80℃, in order to reduce the noise caused by the presence of primer dimers when a non-specific dye is used. The temperatures and the timings used

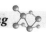

for each cycle depend on a wide variety of parameters, such as: the enzyme used to synthesize the DNA, the concentration of divalent ions and deoxyribonucleotides (dNTPs) in the reaction and the bonding temperature of the primers.

4. PCR single-strand conformation polymorphism（PCR-SSCP，DNA 单链构象多态性 PCR）

The nucleotide sequences of DNAs in humans are not identical in different individuals. Nucleotides substitutions have been estimated to occur every few hundred base pairs in human genome. Nucleotide sequence polymorphism has been detected as **restriction fragment length polymorphism** (RFLP). RFLP analysis of family members has been used to construct a genetic linkage map of the human genome, and this analysis has also revealed the chromosomal locations of genetic elements involved in hereditary disease such as Huntington disease, adult polycystic kidney disease（多囊性肾病）, cystic fibrosis, Alzheimer's disease, and Duchenne muscular dystrophy（杜氏肌营养不良）. Thus prenatal diagnosis of diseases such as cystic fibrosis is possible with RFLP probes.

Although RFLPs are very useful for distinguishing two alleles at chromosomal loci, they can be detected only when DNA polymorphisms are present in the recognition sequences for the corresponding restriction endonucleases or when deletion or insertion of a short sequence is present in the region detected by a particular probe.

When the single-strand conformation polymorphism (SSCP) technique is used to efficiently detect any small alteration in PCR-amplified products, the combination of methods is called **PCR single-strand conformation polymorphism** (PCR-SSCP).

Single-strand conformation polymorphism (SSCP), is defined as conformational difference of single-stranded nucleotide sequences of identical length as induced by differences in the sequences under certain experimental conditions. This property allows sequences to be distinguished by means of gel electrophoresis, which separates fragments according to their different conformations.

Polymerase chain reaction single-strand conformation polymorphism (PCR-SSCP) is a simple method that allows one to rapidly determine whether there are sequence differences between relatively short stretches of DNA. Coupled with sequence analysis, SSCP is an extremely useful method for both identifying and characterizing genetic polymorphisms and mutations. The theory of SSCP is that the primary sequence and the length of a single stranded DNA fragment determine its conformation when it is resolved in a nondenaturing polyacrylamide gel. Even single-base differences can cause different secondary conformations and thus result in different migration rates of the DNA strands. Radioactive nucleotides are incorporated into the DNA strands by PCR, making it possible to detect the DNA by autoradiography. Hence polymerase chain reaction-single strand conformational polymorphism (PCR-SSCP) is a simple and powerful technique for identifying sequence changes in amplified DNA. SSCP has been widely used to identify mutations in host genes such as *p53* and in viruses, such as simian immuno-deficiency virus (SIV), during the course of infection. SSCP has been used to identify and characterize polymorphisms in a variety of genes and was effective in characterizing alleles of linked（连锁的）genes present in individual sperm.

Technical progress in the determination of DNA sequence has resulted in an enormous amount of DNA sequence data, with technical innovations such as the polymerase chain reaction (PCR) accelerating the rate of increase of this data. This combination of data and techniques makes it possible now to exploit sequence differences between individuals. Such studies not only can answer biological questions, but also have potential clinical use in the diagnosis of cancer and hereditary diseases. Making comparative studies between individuals inevitably deals with a large number of samples, thus the methods employed in such studies should be simple.

One such method is PCR-single-strand conformation polymorphism (SSCP) analysis. Here, the target sequence is first labeled and amplified simultaneously by the PCR of the genomic DNA or cDNA using labeled substrates. The PCR product is then denatured and resolved (解离，分析) by polyacrylamide gel electrophoresis, and mutations are detected as altered mobility of separated single strands in the autoradiogram. Thus, the overall procedures are rapid and simple. The mutation can be characterized further by eluting the mutated allele from the gel used for autoradiography and amplifying again for sequence determination.

Principle

Electrophoretic mobility of a particle in a gel is sensitive to both its size and shape. In non-denaturing conditions, single-stranded DNA has a folded structure that is determined by intramolecular interactions, and therefore, by its sequence. In SSCP analysis, a mutated sequence is detected as a change of mobility in polyacrylamide gel electrophoresis caused by its altered folded structure. Kanazawa *et al.* described fragments of cloned mutated F1-ATPase gene of *Escherichia coli* that move anomalously in strand separation gel electrophoresis. It may seem that only limited sequence changes can cause detectable structural change of the molecule. However, it was found that because of its high resolving power, polyacrylamide gel electrophoresis can distinguish most conformational changes caused by subtle sequence differences such as one base substitution in a several-hundred-base fragment. At present, it is not possible to predict the shift of electrophoretic mobility induced by the mutation. Conversely, measurement of the mobility of directionally mutated sequences may provide an empirical approach to the prediction of higher-order structure of single-stranded nucleic acids. In PCR-SSCP analysis, changes in several hundred bases are detected, in contrast to some other techniques in which changes in relatively short (a few to 20-base) sequences are detected. Thus, PCR-SSCP analysis is much more sensitive to the replication errors that occur during the PCR. However, theoretical calculations based on the recent estimation of error rate of *Thermus aquaticus* (*Taq*) DNA polymerase indicate that such errors contribute to at most several percent of the final amplified fragment several hundred bases long. In addition to this, since the errors can be assumed to occur randomly, any particular erroneous sequence will never become a significant subpopulation if the PCR is started from the usual concentration of genomic DNA (more than 10^4 molecules per reaction). If, however, the reaction is started from a much smaller number (*e.g.*, 10) of molecules, errors in the early cycles of amplification can produce erroneous bands in the PCR-SSCP analysis. In such cases, confirmation by independent reaction is necessary.

Basic Information

Single-Strand Conformation Polymorphism (SSCP) Analysis

The SSCP process involves PCR amplification of the target fragment, denaturation of the double-stranded PCR product with heat and formamide (or other denaturants for example, sodium hydroxide, urea and methylmercury hydroxide) and electrophoresis on a non-denaturing polyacrylamide gel. During electrophoresis ssDNA fragments fold into a three-dimentional shape depending on their primary sequence. The electrophoretic mobility μ is affected by the shape of the folded, single stranded molecules. Even if the difference in the sequence between the wild-type sample (Normal DNA N) and the examined fragment (Mutated M) is just a single nucleotide, a unique electrophoretic mobility will be adopted (Fig. 2-34).

The SSCP method is based on the observation that under non-denaturing conditions, single stranded DNA (ssDNA) fragments fell into unique conformation determined by their primary sequence whose steric structures are stabilized by intramolecular interactions. As a consequence, even a single base alteration can result in a conformational change, which can be detected by the altered mobility of the single-stranded DNA molecule in SSCP. Unfortunately, no adequate theoretical model exists for predicting the three-dimentional structure assumed (呈现) by a single stranded DNA fragment of known nucleotide sequence under a given set of condition. Therefore, for

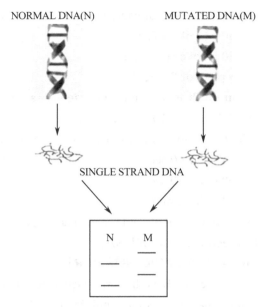

Fig. 2-34   Concise presentation of SSCP method.

each ssDNA fragment, the number of stable conformations, which give rise to bands of different mobility during SSCP electrophoresis, must be determined experimentally under rigorously controlled conditions.

Several parameters have been empirically found to affect the sensitivity of SSCP analysis. Among them are (i) type of mutation; (ii) size of DNA fragment; (iii) G and C content fragment; (iv) content of polyacrylamide or other gel matrix composition; (v) gel size and potential; (vi) gel temperature during electrophoresis; (vii) DNA concentration; (viii) run time of the electrophoresis; (ix) buffer composition, including ionic strength and pH; and (x) buffer additives, such as glycerol or sucrose.

5. Asymmetric PCR (不对称 PCR)

Asymmetric PCR is a PCR in which the predominant product is a single-stranded DNA, as a result of unequal primer concentrations.

As asymmetric PCR proceeds, the lower concentration primer is quantitatively incorporated into double-stranded DNA. The two templates would be amplified equally during the first 12 cycles. Then the lower concentration primer would be exhausted hence the production of its amplified product dwindles down to almost nothing. Meanwhile the higher concentration primer continues to prime synthesis, but only of its strand. From this point on the amplified product (*i.e.*, single-stranded DNA) accumulates linearly. In this way a great amount of single-stranded DNA (ssDNA) would be produced, and can be sequenced directly without cloning.

Asymmetric primer ratios are typically 50 : 1 to 100 : 1.

Procedure

① Pick a phage plaque and place in 100 μl TE or scrape a fresh colony of a bacterial transformant of choice and place in 50 μl of TE/TX100 in a microcentrifuge tube.

② Heat the tube for 10 min at 95℃.

③ Centrifuge at maximum speed for several minutes in a microcentrifuge to pellet cell debris. Collect the supernatant.

④ Add the following components in a PCR tube:

5 μl of phage or bacterial extract (from Step 3)

50 μM of dNTPs

50 pmol of Primer 1

1 pmol of Primer 2

in 1 × PCR Reaction Buffer to give a final reaction volume of 50 to 100 μl

2.5 Units of *Taq* polymerase

⑤ Run 30 to 35 cycles in a thermocycler using the following PCR program

95℃ for 60 sec

60℃ for 30 sec

72℃ for 2 min

⑥ Run a small aliquot on an agarose gel to analyze for single-stranded DNA (see Protocol on Agarose Gel Electrophoresis of DNA).

6. Multiplex PCR（多重 PCR）

Multiplex PCR is the term used when more than one pair of primers is used in a PCR. It is a PCR strategy that enables the amplification of multiple DNA targets in one run. The goal of multiplex PCR is to amplify several segments of target DNA simultaneously and thereby to conserve template DNA, save time, and minimize expense. This technique often requires extensive optimization because having multiple primer pairs in a single reaction increases the likelihood of primer-dimers and other nonspecific products that may interfere with the amplification of specific products. In addition, the concentrations of individual primer pairs often need to be optimized since different multiplex amplicons are often amplified with differing efficiencies, and multiple primer pairs can compete with each other in the reaction.

Multiplex RT-PCR (also referred to as relative RT-PCR) is used for genetic screening, microsatellite analysis, and other applications where it is necessary to amplify several products in a single reaction. This PCR technique is used in gene diagnosis to amplify and hence detect multitudinous（极多的，无数的）disease-related genes. It is commonly used for the semi-quantitative analysis of gene expression levels when defining tissue-restricted gene expression patterns. Typically, multiplex RT-PCR is performed to determine the changes in expression level of a gene in a series of tissue types, throughout stages of development or cellular differentiation, or after specific experimental treatments. Multiplex RT-PCR is also commonly used to examine the expression patterns of a series of related genes and to look at various regions of a large message for mutation analysis.

Since Multiplex PCR is the simultaneous amplification of multiple regions within one DNA template with multiplex pairs of primers, it is necessary to ensure that no primer-dimers formed between multiple pairs of primers, and each primer is highly specific towards the corresponding target template region.

Multiplex RT-PCR is a time and reagent saving amplification technique in which multiple primer sets are used to amplify multiple specific targets simultaneously from the same sample.

The difficulty of multiplex PCR does not lie in the complexity of its working principle and operation step, but the **multiplex primer design** (MPD). Some softwares have been developed automating the design of multiplex PCR primers, allowing an iterative design approach. The application can be quickly retooled（重新装配）to enable shift in targeted genes as new genetic evidence emerges.

7. Immuno-PCR（免疫 PCR）

Immuno-PCR（IPCR，免疫-PCR）is an **antigen detection system** developed since 1991, which is sensitive and specific. It is a polymerase chain reaction version resembling Capture-PCR. It detects specific antibody-DNA conjugates with high sensitivity.

The basic principle of Immuno-PCR is similar to that of enzyme-linked immunosorbent assays (ELISA) and of immunoenzymic staining test (IEST). The difference lies in that the marker is a plasmid DNA rather than an enzyme, and it is antigen-antibody-linker-DNA conjugate that forms as an intermediate, and (it is) via PCR amplification of reporter DNA that whether there is a specific antigen can be identified (Fig. 2-35).

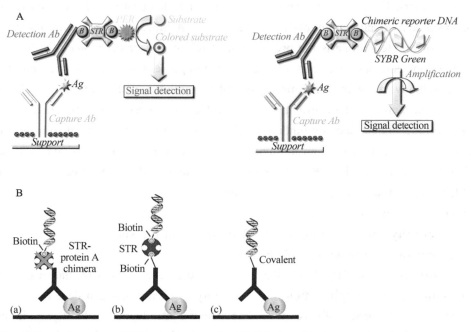

Fig. 2-35 Illustration of immuno-PCR. **A.** Replace the ELISA detection system (based on an enzyme) by a DNA reporter. **B.** The reagents employed in IPCR assays range from a protein A-STR fusion protein (a), which can be used as connector between biotinylated DNA and the Fc region of IgG, to a combination of STR, biotinylated IgG and biotinylated DNA (b), and covalently linked antibody-DNA conjugates (c). These reagents are associated with different approaches to IPCR. The assembly of the compounds in (b) could, for example, be achieved either by several subsequent incubation steps, which is functional but time- and work-intensive, or by self-assembly. The covalent conjugates (c) are well suited for multiplex-IPCR, but their synthesis is more complicated.

The capability of antigen detection systems could be considerably enhanced and potentially broadened by coupling to PCR. Following these ideas, researchers have developed an antigen detection system, termed immuno-PCR, in which a specific antibody-DNA conjugate is used to detect antigens. Immuno-PCR uses the specificity of antigen-antibody reaction and the extremely high sensitivity of PCR amplification to detect antigens, especially for the detection of extremely trace amount of antigens.

In Immuno-PCR, the polymerase chain reaction (PCR) is used to amplify a segment of marker DNA that has been attached specifically to antigen-antibody complexes. Because of the enormous amplification capability and specificity of PCR, immuno-PCR allows considerable enhancement in detection sensitivity of a specific antigen over conventional antigen detection systems, such as ELISA and radioimmunoassays. A variety of superior characteristics and the versatility of immuno-PCR, including high but controllable sensitivity, simplicity, and easy contamination control, offer great promise for its application in various aspects of biological and medical sciences, as well as clinical diagnostics and forensic medicine.

There are three principal steps in the immune-PCR test: ① antigen-antibody reaction, ② binding antigen-antibody complex with (chimeric) linker molecules, and ③ PCR amplification of the chimeric reporter DNA in the antigen-antibody-DNA conjugate (usually a plasmid DNA).

In immuno-PCR, a linker molecule with bispecific binding affinity for DNA and antibodies is used to attach a DNA molecule (marker) specifically to an antigen-antibody complex, resulting in the formation of a specific antigen-antibody-DNA conjugate. The attached marker DNA can be amplified by PCR with the appropriate primers. The presence of specific PCR products demonstrates that marker DNA molecules are attached specifically to antigen-antibody complexes, which indicates the presence of antigen.

The key step of this technique is the preparation of (chimeric) linker molecules. In immuno-PCR, (chimeric) linker molecule plays a role as a bridge. It should possess two binding sites, one is responsible for binding an antibody in the antigen-antibody complex, another is responsible for binding the plasmid DNA. *e.g.*, a (strept)avidin (STR)-protein A chimera has been designed to be used as a linker. The chimera has two independent specific binding abilities; one is to biotin, derived from the STR moiety, and the other is to the Fc portion of an immunoglobulin G (IgG) molecule, derived from the protein A moiety. This bifunctional specificity both for biotin and antibody allows the specific conjugation of any biotinylated DNA molecule to antigen-antibody complexes.

The advantages of immuno-PCR are:

(1) High specificity. Because immuno-PCR is based on the specific reaction of antigen and corresponding antibody, no specificity would be lost.

(2) High sensitivity. Sensibility dramatically improved in comparison to classical ELISA. Given the amazing ability of PCR amplification, the sensitivity of current antigen detection systems can be enhanced by at least a few orders of magnitude simply by the introduction of PCR, *e.g.*, immuno-PCR is 10^5 times more sensitive than ELISA. In principle, the extremely high sensitivity of immuno-PCR should enable this technology to be applied to the detection of single antigen molecules; no method is currently available for this.

(3) Possibility to quantify.

(4) Compatible with biological matrices.

(5) Being simple to operate. It is much easier to amplify a plasmid DNA than a target gene via PCR amplification, even an ordinary laboratory will fill the bill（符合要求）.

(6) Reduced volumes and quantities.

(7) Immuno-PCR can be used for the same applications as classical ELISA — infectious proteins (*e.g.*, prion), toxins (*e.g.*, bacterial toxins), hormones, pesticides, viruses and other antigens.

The controllable sensitivity and the simple procedure of immuno-PCR should allow the development of fully automated assay systems without loss in sensitivity, with a great potential promise for applications in clinical diagnostics.

Applications of PCR Techniques（PCR 技术的应用）

PCR allows isolation of DNA fragments from genomic DNA by selective amplification of a specific region of DNA. Other applications of PCR include DNA sequencing to determine unknown PCR-amplified sequences in which one of the amplification primers may be used in Sanger sequencing, isolation of a DNA sequence to expedite recombinant DNA technologies involving the insertion of a DNA sequence into a plasmid, phage, or cosmid (depending on size) or the genetic material of another

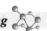

organism. Bacterial colonies (such as *E. coli*) can be rapidly screened by PCR for correct DNA vector constructs. This technique may also be used to determine evolutionary relationships among organisms when certain molecular clocks are used (*i.e.*, the 16S rRNA and recA genes of microorganisms).

Because PCR amplifies the regions of DNA that it targets, it can be used to analyze extremely small amounts of sample. This is often critical for forensic analysis, when only a trace amount of DNA is available as evidence. PCR may also be used in the analysis of ancient DNA that is tens of thousands of years old. These PCR-based techniques have been successfully used on animals, such as a forty-thousand-year-old mammoth (猛犸象), and also on human DNA, in applications ranging from the analysis of Egyptian mummies (木乃伊) to the identification of a Russian tsar (沙皇) and the body of English king Richard Ⅲ.

Quantitative PCR methods allow the estimation of the amount of a given sequence present in a sample — a technique often applied to quantitatively determine levels of gene expression. The mathematical foundations for the reliable quantification of the PCR and RT-qPCR facilitate the implementation of accurate fitting (拟合) procedures of experimental data in research, medical, diagnostic and infectious disease applications.

Research applications

PCR has been applied to many areas of research in molecular genetics:

➢ PCR allows rapid production of short pieces of DNA, even when not more than the sequence of the two primers is known. This ability of PCR augments many methods, such as generating **hybridization probes** for Southern or Northern blot hybridization. PCR supplies these techniques with large amounts of pure DNA, sometimes as a single strand, enabling analysis even from very small amounts of starting material.

➢ The task of **DNA sequencing** can also be assisted by PCR. Known segments of DNA can easily be produced from a patient with a genetic disease mutation. Modifications to the amplification technique can extract segments from a completely unknown genome, or can generate just a single strand of an area of interest.

➢ PCR has numerous applications to the more traditional process of **DNA cloning**, which requires larger amounts of DNA — representing a specific DNA region — for insertion into a vector from a larger genome, which may be only available in small quantities. Using a single set of "vector primers", it can also analyze or extract fragments that have already been inserted into vectors. Some alterations to the PCR protocol can **generate mutations** (general or site-directed) of an inserted fragment.

➢ **Sequence-tagged site** is a process where PCR is used as an indicator that a particular segment of a genome is present in a particular clone. The Human Genome Project found this application vital to mapping the cosmid clones they were sequencing, and to coordinating the results from different laboratories.

➢ An application of PCR is the phylogenic analysis of DNA from **ancient sources**, such as that found in the recovered bones of Neanderthals (尼安德特人), from frozen tissues of mammoths, or from the brain of Egyptian mummies. In some cases, the highly degraded DNA from these sources might be reassembled during the early stages of amplification.

➢ A common application of PCR is the study of patterns of **gene expression**. Tissues (or even individual cells) can be analyzed at different stages to see which genes have become active, or which have been switched off. This application can also use quantitative PCR to quantitate the actual levels of expression.

➤ The ability of PCR to simultaneously amplify several loci from individual sperm has greatly enhanced the more traditional task of **genetic mapping** by studying chromosomal crossovers after meiosis. Rare crossover events between very close loci have been directly observed by analyzing thousands of individual sperms. Similarly, unusual deletions, insertions, translocations, or inversions can be analyzed, all without having to wait (or pay) for the long and laborious processes of fertilization, embryogenesis, *etc*.

➤ **Site-directed mutagenesis:** PCR can be used to create mutant genes with mutations chosen by scientists at will. These mutations can be chosen in order to understand how proteins accomplish their functions, and to change or improve protein function.

Medical and diagnostic applications

PCR has been applied to a large number of medical procedures:

➤ Prospective parents can be tested for being genetic carriers, or their children might be tested for actually being affected by a disease. DNA samples for prenatal testing can be obtained by amniocentesis （羊膜穿刺术）, chorionic villus sampling （绒毛膜绒毛取样检查）, or even by the analysis of rare fetal cells circulating in the mother's bloodstream. PCR analysis is also essential to preimplantation genetic diagnosis （胚胎植入前遗传学诊断）, where individual cells of a developing embryo are tested for mutations.

➤ PCR can also be used as part of a sensitive test for **tissue typing** （组织分型，组织配型）, vital to organ transplantation. As of 2008, there is even a proposal to replace the traditional antibody-based tests for blood type with PCR-based tests.

➤ PCR is being used to characterize mutations associated with carcinogenesis. Many forms of cancer involve alterations to **oncogenes**. PCR is very useful under such circumstances since it allows for the isolation and amplification of tumor suppressors. PCR permits early diagnosis of malignant diseases such as leukemia and lymphomas, which is currently the highest-developed in cancer research and is already being used routinely. PCR assays can be performed directly on genomic DNA samples to detect translocation-specific malignant cells at a sensitivity that is at least 10 000 fold higher than that of other methods. By using PCR-based tests to study these mutations, therapy regimens can sometimes be individually customized to a patient. Quantitative PCR for example, can be used to quantify and analyze single cells, as well as recognize DNA, mRNA and protein confirmations and combinations.

Infectious disease applications

PCR is being used to detect and characterize microbial pathogens. PCR allows for rapid and highly specific diagnosis of infectious diseases, including those caused by bacteria or viruses. PCR also permits identification of non-cultivatable or slow-growing microorganisms such as mycobacteria （分枝杆菌）, anaerobic bacteria, or viruses from tissue culture assays and animal models. The basis for PCR diagnostic applications in microbiology is the detection of infectious agents and the discrimination of non-pathogenic from pathogenic strains by virtue of （因为） specific genes.

Characterization and detection of infectious disease organisms have been revolutionized by PCR in the following ways:

➤ Viral DNA can be detected by PCR. The primers used must be specific to the targeted sequences in the DNA of a virus, and PCR can be used for diagnostic analyses or DNA sequencing of the viral genome. The high sensitivity of PCR permits virus detection soon after infection and even before the onset of disease. Such early detection may give physicians a significant lead time（提前期）in treatment. The amount of virus ("viral load") in a patient can also be quantified by PCR-based DNA quantitation techniques. The **human immunodeficiency virus** (or **HIV**), is a difficult target to find and eradicate. The earliest tests for infection relied on the presence of antibodies to the virus circulating in the bloodstream. However, antibodies don't appear until many weeks after infection, maternal antibodies mask the infection of a newborn, and therapeutic agents to fight the infection don't affect the antibodies. PCR tests have been developed that can detect as little as one viral genome among the DNA of over 50 000 host cells. Infections can be detected earlier, donated blood can be screened directly for the virus, newborns can be immediately tested for infection, and the effects of antiviral treatments can be quantified.

➤ A variant of PCR (RT-PCR) is used for detecting viral RNA rather than DNA. In this test the enzyme reverse transcriptase is used to generate a DNA sequence that matches the viral RNA; this DNA is then amplified as per（按照，依据）the usual PCR method. RT-PCR is widely used to detect the SARS-CoV-2 viral genome.

➤ Some disease organisms, such as that for **tuberculosis**（肺结核，结核病）, are difficult to sample from patients and slow to be grown in the laboratory. PCR-based tests have allowed the detection of small numbers of disease organisms (both live or dead), in convenient samples（便利抽样样本）. Detailed genetic analysis can also be used to detect antibiotic resistance, allowing immediate and effective therapy. The effects of therapy can also be immediately evaluated.

➤ The spread of a **disease organism**（致病有机体，病原体）through populations of domestic or wild animals can be monitored by PCR testing. In many cases, the appearance of new virulent sub-types（子型）can be detected and monitored. The sub-types of an organism that were responsible for earlier epidemics can also be determined by PCR analysis.

➤ Diseases such as pertussis（百日咳）(or whooping cough) are caused by the bacteria *Bordetella pertussis*（百日咳博代氏杆菌）. This bacteria is marked by a serious acute respiratory infection that affects various animals and humans and has led to the deaths of many young children. The pertussis toxin is a protein exotoxin that binds to cell receptors by two dimers and reacts with different cell types such as T lymphocytes which play a role in cell immunity. PCR is an important testing tool that can detect sequences within the gene for the pertussis toxin. Because PCR has a high sensitivity for the toxin and a rapid turnaround time（周转时间）, it is very efficient for diagnosing pertussis when compared to culture.

Forensic applications

PCR may also be used for **genetic fingerprinting**（指纹分析）— a forensic technique used to identify a person or organism by comparing experimental DNAs through different PCR-based methods.

➤ In its most discriminating form, genetic fingerprinting can uniquely discriminate any one person from the entire population of the world. Minute samples of DNA can be isolated from a crime scene, and compared to that from suspects, or from a DNA database of earlier evidence or convicts. Simpler versions of these tests are often used to rapidly rule out suspects during a criminal investigation. Evidence from decades-old crimes can be tested, confirming or exonerating（使免罪，宣判……无罪，证明……的清白）the people originally convicted. PCR is a very powerful and significant analytical tool to use for forensic DNA typing because researchers only need a very small amount of the target DNA to be used for analysis. For example, a single human hair with an attached hair follicle has enough DNA to conduct the analysis. Similarly, a few sperm, skin samples from under the fingernails, or a small amount of blood can provide enough DNA for conclusive analysis.

➢ Some PCR fingerprint methods have high discriminative power and can be used to identify genetic relationships between individuals, such as parent-child or between siblings, and are used in **paternity testing** (亲子鉴定) (Fig. 2-36). Less discriminating forms of DNA fingerprinting can help with DNA paternity testing, where an individual is matched with their close relatives. DNA from unidentified human remains can be tested, and compared with that from possible parents, siblings, or children. Similar testing can be used to confirm the biological parents of an adopted (or kidnapped) child. The actual biological father of a newborn can also be confirmed (or ruled out).

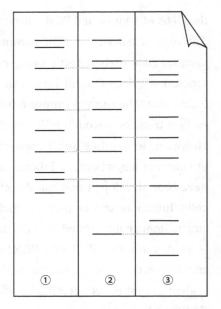

Fig. 2-36 Electrophoresis of PCR-amplified DNA fragments. ① Father. ② Child. ③ Mother. The child has inherited some, but not all of the fingerprints of each of its parents, giving it a new, unique fingerprint.

➢ The PCR AMGX/AMGY design has been shown to not only facilitate in amplifying DNA sequences from a very minuscule amount of genome. However it can also be used for real-time sex determination from forensic bone samples. This provides a powerful and effective way to determine gender in forensic cases and ancient specimens.

Application in agriculture (农业中的应用)

The agricultural biotechnology industry applies PCR technology at numerous steps throughout product development. The major uses of PCR technology during product development include gene discovery and cloning, vector construction, transformant (转化体, 转化株, 转化子) identification, screening and characterization, and seed quality control. Commodity and food companies, as well as third-party diagnostic testing companies, rely on technology to verify the presence or absence of **genetically modified** (GM, 基因改进的, 转基因的) material in a product or to quantify the amount of GM material present in a product. Quantitative PCR technology also has been used to estimate GM copy number and zygosity (接合性, 组织配型, 合子型) in seeds and plants.

The grain handling and grain processing industry uses PCR to certify (证明, 保证) compliance with (符合, 遵守) contracts between buyer and seller. PCR testing is used for 4 specific purposes in the grain handling industry:

PCR testing for unapproved events. — In countries that have a defined approval process for GM crops, an event may be approved for use in the country of production but not yet approved for use in an importing country. In these instances, the importing country often requires that the grain shipment be tested for the presence of specific GM events to ensure that the grain shipment does not contain these unapproved events. Such testing often relies on qualitative PCR because the detection of these events, in most cases, is at a zero-tolerance threshold.

PCR testing for GM content. — Most countries that have adopted mandatory labeling rules for food or feed (饲料) have set tolerances for the adventitious (偶然的, 偶发的) presence of GM material in

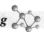

grain products or the final foods based on a percent GM (weight-to-weight) content. In these countries, food and feed manufacturers and retailers often choose to acquire grain and grain products below the defined regulatory threshold to avoid labeling their products. In this case, the grain must come from a non-GM identity preservation program and be certified to contain GM grains at a level below the threshold specified in the contract. To meet this need for testing, several laboratories currently are adopting quantitative PCR for percent GM determinations.

PCR testing for non-GM labeling. — In some cases, food manufacturers and retailers wish to use positive labeling for their non-GM products. These companies hope to gain market share among consumers who wish to avoid GM products. In most cases, the use of positive labeling requires that the grain and grain products originate from a non-GM identity preservation program and test negative or at least below a certain threshold for GM DNA. Qualitative PCR testing is most often used to certify compliance with a non-GM contract.

PCR testing for the presence of a high-value commodity. — In certain cases, it is desirable to show that a commodity is made up of a specific crop commodity [*e.g.*, low phytate (植酸，肌醇六磷酸) maize, soybean with altered oil profile]. PCR could be used for this purpose by testing for the GM trait that conveys (传达) the characteristic, although the grain may also be tested by quantifying the improved quality of the commodity.

2.3.2　DNA sequencing（DNA 的序列测定）

DNA sequencing is the process of determining the precise order of nucleotides within a DNA molecule. It includes any method or technology that is used to determine the order of the four bases — adenine, guanine, cytosine, and thymine — in a strand of DNA. The advent of rapid DNA sequencing methods has greatly accelerated biological and medical research and discovery.

Knowledge of DNA sequences has become indispensable (必不可少的) for basic biological research, and in numerous applied fields such as diagnostic, biotechnology, forensic biology (法医生物学), virology and biological systematics (系统分类学). The rapid speed of sequencing attained with modern DNA sequencing technology has been instrumental in the sequencing of complete DNA sequences, or genomes (基因组，染色体组) of numerous types and species of life, including the human genome and other complete DNA sequences of many animal, plant, and microbial species.

The first DNA sequences were obtained in the early 1970s by academic researchers (学术研究人员) using laborious (费劲的) methods based on two-dimensional chromatography. Following the development of fluorescence-based sequencing methods with automated analysis, DNA sequencing has become easier and orders of magnitude (数量级) faster.

Use of sequencing

DNA sequencing may be used to determine the sequence of individual genes, larger genetic regions (*i.e.,* clusters of genes or operons), full chromosomes or entire genomes. Sequencing provides the order of individual nucleotides (单个核苷酸的顺序) in DNA or RNA (commonly represented as A, C, G, T, and U) isolated from cells of animals, plants, bacteria, archaea, or virtually any other source of genetic information. This is useful for:

- Molecular biology — studying the genome itself, how proteins are made, what proteins are made, identifying new genes and associations with diseases and phenotypes (表型，表现型，显型), and identifying potential drug targets.

- Evolutionary biology (进化生物学) — studying how different organisms are related and how they evolved.

- Metagenomics (宏基因组学，微生物环境基因组学，元基因组学) — identifying species present in a body of water, sewage (污水，下水道，污物), dirt, debris (碎片，碎屑) filtered from the air, or swab (棉签拭子) samples of organisms. Helpful in ecology, epidemiology (流行病学，传染病学), microbiome (微生物组) research, and other fields.

History

RNA sequencing was one of the earliest forms of nucleotide sequencing. The major landmark of RNA sequencing is the sequence of the first complete gene and the complete genome of Bacteriophage MS2, identified and published by Walter Fiers and his coworkers at the University of Ghent (Ghent, Belgium), in 1972 and 1976.

The first method for determining DNA sequences involved a location-specific primer extension strategy established by Ray Wu at Cornell University in 1970. DNA polymerase catalysis and specific nucleotide labeling, both of which figure prominently in current sequencing schemes, were used to sequence the cohesive ends of lambda phage DNA. Between 1970 and 1973, Wu, R Padmanabhan and colleagues demonstrated that this method can be employed to determine any DNA sequence using synthetic location-specific primers. Frederick Sanger then adopted this primer-extension strategy to develop more rapid DNA sequencing methods at the MRC Centre (医学研究委员会中心), Cambridge, UK and published a method for "DNA sequencing with chain-terminating inhibitors" in 1977. Walter Gilbert and Allan Maxam at Harvard also developed sequencing methods, including one for "DNA sequencing by chemical degradation". In 1973, Gilbert and Maxam reported the sequence of 24 need space base-pairs method known as **wandering-spot analysis** (漫游斑分析法) (Fig.2-37). Advancements in sequencing were aided by the concurrent (同时发生的) development of recombinant DNA technology, allowing DNA samples to be isolated from sources other than viruses.

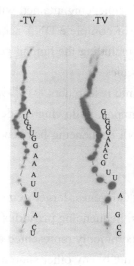

Fig. 2-37　Wandering-spot analysis of 3′-terminal-labeled plus and minus strands of dsRNA segment IV. Partial alkaline digest of the RNA was fractionated by two-dimensional polyacrylamide gel electrophoresis with 10% polyacrylamide gel (pH 3.5) as the first dimension (from left to right) and 20% polyacrylamide–7 M urea gel as the second dimension (from bottom to top).

The first full DNA genome to be sequenced was that of bacteriophage φX174 in 1977. Medical Research Council scientists deciphered the complete DNA sequence of the Epstein-Barr virus in 1984, finding it to be 170 thousand base-pairs long.

A non-radioactive method for transferring the DNA molecules of sequencing reaction mixtures onto an immobilizing matrix during electrophoresis was developed by Pohl and co-workers in the early 1980′s. Followed by the commercialization of the DNA sequencer "Direct-Blotting-Electrophoresis-System GATC 1500" by GATC Biotech, which was intensively used in the framework of the EU genome-sequencing program, the complete DNA sequence of the yeast *Saccharomyces cerevisiae* (酿酒酵母) chromosome Ⅱ. Leroy E. Hood′s laboratory at the California Institute of Technology announced the first semi-automated DNA sequencing machine in 1986. This was followed by Applied Biosystems′ marketing of the first fully automated sequencing machine, the **ABI 370**, in 1987 and by **Dupont′s Genesis 2000** which used a novel fluorescent labeling technique enabling all four dideoxynucleotides to be identified in a single lane. By 1990, the U.S. National Institutes of Health (NIH) had begun large-scale sequencing trials on *Mycoplasma capricolum* (山羊支原体), *Escherichia coli*, *Caenorhabditis elegans* (秀丽隐杆线虫), and *Saccharomyces cerevisiae* for US $0.75 per base. Meanwhile, sequencing of human cDNA sequences called expressed sequence tags (表达序列标签) began in Craig Venter′s lab, an attempt to capture the coding fraction of the human genome. In 1995, Venter, Hamilton Smith, and colleagues at The Institute for Genomic Research (TIGR，美国基因组研究所) published the first complete genome of a free-living organism (独立生存的生物), the bacterium *Haemophilus influenzae* (流感嗜血杆菌). The circular chromosome contains 1 830 137 bases and its publication in the journal *Science* marked the first published use of whole-genome shotgun sequencing, eliminating the need for initial mapping efforts. By 2001, shotgun sequencing methods had been used to produce a draft sequence of the human genome.

Several new methods for DNA sequencing were developed in the mid to late 1990s. These techniques comprise the first of the "next-generation" sequencing methods. On October 26, 1990, Roger Tsien, Pepi Ross, Margaret Fahnestock and Allan J Johnston filed a patent describing stepwise ("base-by-base") sequencing with removable 3′ blockers on DNA arrays (blots and single DNA molecules). In 1996, Pål Nyrén and his student Mostafa Ronaghi at the Royal Institute of Technology in Stockholm (斯德哥尔摩) published their method of pyrosequencing (焦磷酸测序，焦磷酸微测序). On April 1, 1997, Pascal Mayer and Laurent Farinelli submitted patents to the World Intellectual Property Organization (世界知识产权组织) describing **DNA colony sequencing** (DNA 集落测序). The DNA sample preparation and random surface-PCR arraying methods described in this patent, coupled to Roger Tsien *et al.*′s "base-by-base" sequencing method is now implemented in Illumina′s Hi-Seq genome sequencers. Lynx Therapeutics published and marketed "**Massively parallel signature sequencing**" (大规模平行签名测序技术), or **MPSS**, in 2000. This method incorporated a parallelized, adapter/ligation-mediated, bead-based sequencing technology and served as the first commercially available "next-generation" sequencing method, though no DNA sequencers were sold to independent laboratories. In 2004, 454 Life Sciences marketed a parallelized version of pyrosequencing. The first version of their machine reduced sequencing costs 6-fold compared to automated Sanger sequencing, and was the second of the new generation of sequencing technologies, after **MPSS**.

The large quantities of data produced by DNA sequencing have also required development of new methods and programs for sequence analysis. Phil Green and Brent Ewing of the University of Washington described their phred quality score (弗瑞德质量评分) (Fig. 2-38) for sequencer data analysis in 1998.

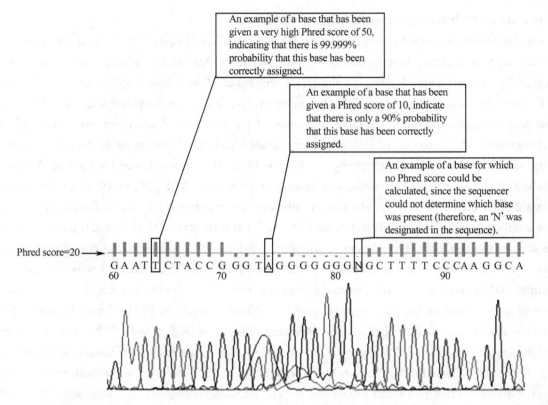

Fig. 2-38 An example of a DNA sequence tracing and the Phred score (grey bars) corresponding to each colored peak. The colored peaks on the trace correspond to each DNA letter. For example 'T's bases are represented in red, and this sequence has four 'T' bases on a row, as viewed by the four red peaks in the sequence. The aqua（浅绿色，浅绿色的）horizontal line placed across the grey bars represents a Phred score of 20 which is considered an acceptable level of accuracy. A Phred score of 20 corresponds to a 99% accuracy in the base call. Therefore, bars above this line indicate base calls that have a higher than 99% probability of being correct. Those below have less than a 99% probability of being correct.

Basic methods

2.3.2.1 *Sanger sequencing/Chain-termination methods*（Sanger 双脱氧链终止法）

Sanger sequencing is a method of **DNA sequencing** based on the selective incorporation of chain-terminating dideoxynucleotides by DNA polymerase during *in vitro* DNA replication. Developed by Frederick Sanger and colleagues in 1977, the chain-termination method soon became the method of choice, owing to its relative ease and reliability. It was the most widely used sequencing method for approximately 25 years. The Sanger method was the method used in the first generation of DNA sequencers, and in mass（规模化）production form, is the technology that produced the first human genome in 2001, ushering in the age of genomics, thanks to great advances made in the technique, such as fluorescent labeling, capillary electrophoresis, and general automation（通用自动化），which allowed much more efficient sequencing and lower costs.

More recently, Sanger sequencing has been supplanted by "Next-Gen" sequencing methods (radically different approaches), especially for large-scale, automated genome analyses (The latter had brought the cost per genome down from $100 million in 2001 to $10 000 in 2011). However, the Sanger method remains in wide use, for smaller-scale projects, validation of Next-Gen results and for obtaining especially long contiguous DNA sequence reads (＞500 nucleotides).

Method

The classical chain-termination method requires a single-stranded DNA template, a DNA primer, a DNA polymerase, normal deoxynucleotide triphosphates (dNTPs), and modified di-deoxynucleotide triphosphates (ddNTPs), the latter of which lack the 3′-OH group to which the next dNTP of the growing DNA chain is added (*i.e.*, the formation of a phosphodiester bond between two nucleotides). Hence the incorporation of a modified ddNTP terminates DNA strand elongation. Without the 3′-OH, no more nucleotides can be added, and DNA polymerase falls off. The resulting newly synthesized DNA chains will be a mixture of lengths, depending on how long the chain was when a ddNTP was randomly incorporated. The ddNTPs may be radioactively or fluorescently labeled for detection in automated sequencing machines.

The DNA sample is divided into four separate sequencing reactions, containing all four of the standard deoxynucleotides (dATP, dGTP, dCTP and dTTP) and the DNA polymerase. To each reaction is added only one of the four dideoxynucleotides (ddATP, ddGTP, ddCTP, or ddTTP), while three other nucleotides are ordinary ones. Putting it in a more sensible (合理的) order, four separate reactions are needed in this process to test all four ddNTPs. Following rounds of template DNA extension from the bound primer, the resulting DNA fragments are heat denatured and separated by size using gel electrophoresis. This is frequently performed using a denaturing polyacrylamide-urea gel with each of the four reactions run in one of four individual lanes (lanes A, T, G, C). The DNA bands may then be visualized by autoradiography or UV light and the DNA sequence can be directly read off the X-ray film or gel image (Figure 2-40). The dark bands correspond to DNA fragments of different lengths. A dark band in a lane indicates a DNA fragment that is the result of chain termination after incorporation of a dideoxynucleotide (ddATP, ddGTP, ddCTP, or ddTTP). The relative positions of the different bands among the four lanes, from bottom to top, are then used to read the DNA sequence.

Technical variations of chain-termination sequencing include tagging (尾随，连接，给……贴标签) with nucleotides containing radioactive phosphorus for radiolabeling, or using a primer labeled at the 5' end with a fluorescent dye. Dye-primer sequencing facilitates reading in an optical system for faster and more economical analysis and automation. The later development by Leroy Hood and coworkers of fluorescently labeled ddNTPs and primers set the stage (做好准备) for automated, high-throughput DNA sequencing.

Chain-termination methods have greatly simplified DNA sequencing. For example, chain-termination-based kits are commercially available that contain the reagents needed for sequencing, pre-aliquoted and ready to use. Limitations include non-specific binding of the primer to the DNA, affecting accurate read-out of the DNA sequence, and DNA secondary structures affecting the fidelity of the sequence.

Manual DNA sequencing example:

- First, anneal the primer to the DNA template (must be single stranded):
- Then split the sample into four aliquots including the following nucleotides:

  "G" tube: All four dNTPs, one of which is radiolabeled, plus ddGTP (low concentration)

  "A" tube: All four dNTPs, one of which is radiolabeled, plus ddATP

  "T" tube: All four dNTPs, one of which is radiolabeled, plus ddTTP

  "C" tube: All four dNTPs, one of which is radiolabeled, plus ddCTP

- When a DNA polymerase (*e.g.*, Klenow fragment) is added to the tubes, the synthetic reaction proceeds until, by chance, a dideoxynucleotide is incorporated instead of a deoxynucleotide. This is a "chain termination" event, because there is a 3′ H instead of a 3′ OH group. Since the synthesized DNA is labeled (classically with ^{35}S-dATP), the products can be detected and distinguished from the template.

Note that the higher the concentration of the ddNTP in the reaction, the shorter the products will be, hence, you will get sequences CLOSER to your primer. With lower concentrations of ddNTP, chain termination will be less likely, and you will get longer products (sequences further AWAY from the primer). If, for example, we were to look only at the "G" reaction, there would be a mixture of the following products of synthesis:

Each newly synthesized strand at some point had a ddGTP incorporated instead of dGTP, Chain termination then occurred (no more polymerization). Because ddGTP incorporation is random, all possible lengths of DNA that end in G are produced.

These products are denatured into single stranded DNA molecules and run on a polyacrylamide/urea gel. (Polyacrylamide gels, unlike agarose, allow resolution of DNA molecules that differ in size by only one nucleotide.) The gel is dried onto chromatography paper and exposed to X-ray film. Since the template strand is not radioactively labeled, it does not generate a band on the X-ray film. Only the labeled top strands (Fig. 2-39) generate bands, which would look like this:

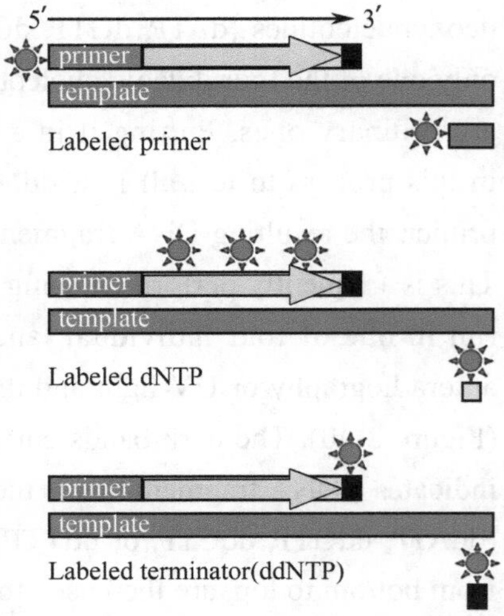

As you can see (Fig. 2-40) from this one reaction (the "G" reaction) the chain termination events produce individual bands on a gel. The chain terminations closest to the primer generate the smallest DNA molecules (which migrate further down the gel), and chain terminations further from the primer generate larger DNA molecules (which are slower on the gel and therefore remain nearer to the top).

Fig. 2-39 DNA fragments are labeled with a radioactive or fluorescent tag on the primer in the new DNA strand with a labeled dNTP, or with a labeled ddNTP.

When similar chain termination reactions are run for each nucleotide, the four reactions can be run next to each other, and the sequence of the DNA can be read off of the "ladder" of bands, 5′ to 3′ sequence being read from bottom to top:

The resolution of the gel electrophoresis is very important in DNA sequencing. Molecule that is n bases in length must be separable from molecule that is (n+1) bases in length (respectively). To accomplish this:

● Polyacrylamide, not agarose, is used

● The gels must be quite large so that the molecules migrate further and are better resolved

● Samples are denatured before they are loaded, and the gels must contain a high concentration of urea (7 to 8 molar) to prevent folding of the molecules and formation of secondary structures by hydrogen bonding that would alter the mobility of the molecule

● The gels are run at higher temperature (about 50℃), also to prevent H bond formation

2.3.2.2 Maxam-Gilbert sequencing （Maxam-Gilbert 化学降解法）

Maxam-Gilbert sequencing is a method of DNA sequencing developed by Allan Maxam and Walter Gilbert in 1976-1977. This method is based on nucleobase-specific partial chemical modification of DNA

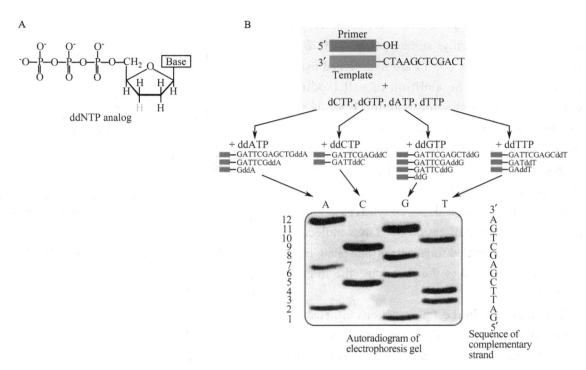

Fig. 2-40   Illustration of classical chain-termination method. A. ddNTP analog. B. Procedures of Sanger sequencing method. Line up all four reactions, and you can "read" the sequence ladder 5′ to 3′ as GATTCGA ... *etc.* in this example.

and subsequent cleavage of the DNA backbone at sites adjacent to the modified nucleotides.

Maxam-Gilbert sequencing was the first widely adopted method for DNA sequencing, and, along with the Sanger dideoxy method, represents the first generation of DNA sequencing methods. Maxam-Gilbert sequencing is no longer in widespread use, having been supplanted by next-generation sequencing methods.

History

Allan Maxam and Walter Gilbert published a DNA sequencing method in 1977 based on chemical modification of DNA and subsequent cleavage at specific bases. Although Maxam and Gilbert published their chemical sequencing method two years after Frederick Sanger and Alan Coulson published their work on plus-minus sequencing, Maxam-Gilbert sequencing rapidly became more popular, since purified samples of double-stranded DNA could be used directly, while the initial Sanger method required that each read start be cloned for production of single-stranded DNA. However, with the improvement of the chain-termination method, Maxam-Gilbert sequencing has fallen out of favor due to its technical complexity prohibiting its use in standard molecular biology kits, extensive use of hazardous chemicals, and difficulties with scale-up.

An automated Maxam-Gilbert sequencing protocol was developed in 1994.

Procedure

Maxam-Gilbert sequencing requires radioactive labeling at one 5′ end of the DNA fragment to be sequenced (typically by a kinase reaction using gamma-^{32}P ATP) and purification of the DNA. Chemical treatment generates breaks at a small proportion of one or two of the four nucleotide bases in each of four reactions (G, A+G, C, C+T). For example, the purines (A+G) are depurinated (脱嘌呤) using formic acid (甲酸),

the guanines (and to some extent the adenines) are methylated by dimethyl sulfate（硫酸二甲酯）, and the pyrimidines (C+T) are hydrolyzed using hydrazine（肼）. The addition of salt (sodium chloride) to the hydrazine reaction inhibits the reaction of thymine for the C-only reaction（胞嘧啶特异性反应）. The modified DNAs may then be cleaved by hot piperidine（哌啶, 氮己烷, 六氢吡啶）at the position of the modified base. The concentration of the modifying chemicals is controlled to introduce on average one modification per DNA molecule. Thus a series of labeled fragments is generated, from the radiolabeled end to the first "cut" site in each molecule.

The fragments in the four reactions are electrophoresed side by side in denaturing acrylamide gels for size separation. To visualize the fragments, the gel is exposed to X-ray film for autoradiography, yielding a series of dark bands each showing the location of identical radiolabeled DNA molecules. From presence and absence of certain fragments the sequence may be inferred (Fig. 2-41).

Basic steps：

(1) Labeling one of the terminals of the DNA fragment which is to be sequenced（typically using radioactive isotope ^{32}P）;

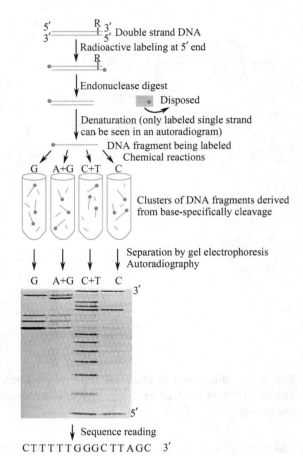

Fig. 2-41 Principles of Maxam–Gilbert sequencing reaction. Cleaving the same tagged segment of DNA at different points yields tagged fragments of different sizes. The fragments may then be separated by gel electrophoresis.

(2) Chemically modifying on special bases (respectively and) separately in every independent chemical reaction among the parallel ones;

(3) Cleaving DNA fragments chemically at the positions of the modified bases;

(4) Size separating the resulting DNA fragment mixtures in a denaturing acrylamide gel;

(5) Directly reading the nucleotide sequence of the DNA fragment according to the dark bands pattern revealed on the autoradiogram.

Chemical reagents commonly used in Maxam-Gilbert sequencing are listed in Table 2-3.

Table 2-3 Chemical reagents commonly used in Maxam–Gilbert sequencing

Base system	Modifying chemicals	Chemical reactions	Breaking point
G	Dimethyl sulphate（硫酸二甲酯）	Methylation	G
A + G	Piperidine formate（哌啶甲酸）	Depurination	G and A
C + T	Hydrazine	Pyrimidine ring opening	C and T
C	Hydrazine + NaCl (1.5 M)	Cytosine ring opening	C
A > C	90℃, NaOH (1.2 M)	Cleavage reaction	A and C

2.3.2.3 *Several approaches to DNA sequencing technology* （DNA 测序技术的若干进展）

1. PCR sequencing approach（PCR 测序）

Polymerase Chain Reaction (PCR)-sequencing

PCR was a major breakthrough for molecular marker research in that for the first time, any genomic region could be amplified and analyzed in many individuals without the requirement for cloning and isolating large amounts of ultra-pure genomic DNA. PCR sequencing involves determination of the nucleotide sequence within a DNA fragment amplified by the PCR, using primers specific for a particular genomic site. The method that has been most commonly used to determine nucleotide sequences is based on the termination of *in vitro* DNA replication. The procedure is initiated by annealing a primer to the amplified DNA fragment, followed by dividing the mixture into four subsamples. Subsequently, DNA is replicated *in vitro* by adding the four deoxynucleotides (adenine, cytosine, guanine, thymidine; dA, dC, dG and dT), a single dideoxynucleotide (ddA, ddC, ddG or ddT) and the enzyme DNA polymerase to each reaction. Sequence extension occurs as long as deoxynucleotides are incorporated in the newly synthesized DNA strand. However, when a dideoxynucleotide is incorporated, DNA replication is terminated. Because each reaction contains many DNA molecules and incorporation of dideoxynucleotides occurs at random, each of the four subsamples（子样品）contains fragments of varying length terminated at any occurrence of the particular dideoxy base used in the subsample. Finally, the fragments in each of the four subsamples are separated by gel electrophoresis.

Strengths

Because all possible sequence differences within the amplified fragment can be resolved（解析）between individuals, PCR sequencing provides the ultimate measurement of genetic variation. Universal primer pairs to target specific sequences in a wide range of species are available for the chloroplast（叶绿体），mitochondrial and ribosomal genomes. Other advantages of PCR sequencing include its high reproducibility and the fact that sequences of known identity are studied, increasing the chance of detecting truly homologous differences. Due to the amplification of fragments by PCR only low quantities of template DNA are required. Moreover, most of the technical procedures are amenable（经得起的，可用某种方式处理的）to automation. Much of this process is now automated.

Weaknesses

Disadvantages include low genome coverage and low levels of variation below the species level. In the event that primers for a genomic region of interest are unavailable, high development costs are involved. If sequences are visualized by polyacrylamide gel electrophoresis and autoradiography, analytical procedures are laborious（费力的）and technically demanding. Fluorescent detection systems and reliable analytical software to score base pairs using automated sequencers are now widely applied. This requires considerable investments for equipment or substantial costs in the case of outsourcing（外购）. Because sequencing is costly and time-consuming, most studies have focused on only one or a few loci（位点，基因座）. This restricts genome coverage and together with the fact that different genes may evolve at different rates, the extent to which the estimated gene diversity reflects overall genetic diversity is yet to be determined.

Applications

Because generally insufficient nucleotide variation is detected below the species level, PCR sequencing is most useful to address questions of interspecific and intergeneric relationships. Until recently, chloroplast DNA and nuclear ribosomal DNA have provided the major datasets (数据集) for phylogenetic (系统发育) inference (推理) because of the ease of obtaining data due to high copy number. Recently, single- to low-copy nuclear DNA markers have been developed as powerful new tools for phylogenetic analyses.

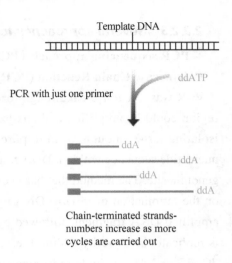

2. Thermal cycle sequencing (热循环测序法)

Thermal cycle sequencing offers an alternative to the traditional methodology.

The discovery of thermostable DNA polymerases, which led to the development of, has also resulted in new methodologies for chain termination sequencing. In particular, the innovation called thermal cycle sequencing has two advantages over traditional chain termination sequencing. First, it uses double-stranded rather than single-stranded DNA as the starting material. Second, very little template DNA is needed (nanogram amounts), so the DNA does not have to be cloned before being sequenced.

Thermal cycle sequencing is carried out in a similar way to PCR but just one primer is used and each reaction mixture includes one of the ddNTPs. Because there is only one primer, only one of the strands of the starting molecule is copied, and the product accumulates in a linear fashion, not exponentially as is the case in a real PCR. The presence of the ddNTP in the reaction mixture causes chain termination, as in the standard methodology, and the family of resulting strands can be analyzed and the sequence read in the normal manner by polyacrylamide gel electrophoresis.

2.3.2.4 *Automated DNA sequencing* (DNA 自动测序)

Most DNA sequencing is now automated. The Sanger method chain termination reactions are still used, but pouring, running and reading polyacrylamide gels have been replaced by automated methods.

Dye-terminator sequencing

Dye-terminator sequencing utilizes labeling of the chain terminator ddNTPs, which permits sequencing in a single reaction, rather than four reactions as in the classical chain-termination method. Instead of labeling the products of all 4 sequencing reactions with the same radioactive deoxynucleotide, each of the four dideoxynucleotides is labeled with a different fluorescent dye (Fig. 2-42). When excited with a laser, the 4 different kinds of products emit light at different wavelengths, hence are detected and the fluorescence intensity translated into a data "peak". Thus all four chain termination reactions can be performed in the same tube, and run on a single lane on a gel. A machine scans the lane with a laser. The wavelength of fluorescence from the label conjugated (结合) to the ddNTPs can be interpreted by the machine as an indication of which reaction (ddG, ddA, ddT, or ddC) a particular DNA band came from. Owing to its greater expediency (方便) and speed, dye-terminator sequencing is now the mainstay (最基本组成部分) in automated sequencing.

Its limitations include dye effects due to differences in the incorporation of the dye-labeled chain terminators into the DNA fragment, resulting in unequal (不均衡) peak heights and shapes in the electronic DNA sequence trace chromatogram after capillary electrophoresis. This problem has been addressed with the use of modified DNA polymerase enzyme systems and dyes that minimize incorporation variability, as well as methods for eliminating "dye blobs" (染料团，大量未掺入的染料

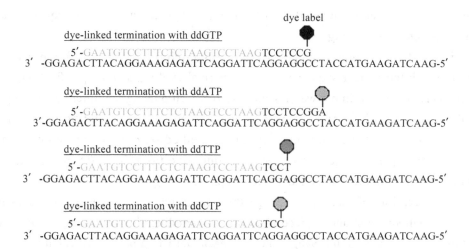

Fig. 2-42 Illustration of dye-terminator sequencing for automated DNA sequencing. Each of the four fluorescent dyes is used to label its respective dideoxynucleotide — G, A, T or C.

终止子）. The dye-terminator sequencing method, along with automated high-throughput DNA sequence analyzers, is now being used for the vast majority of sequencing projects.

Automation and sample preparation

Automated DNA-sequencing instruments (DNA sequencers) can sequence up to 384 DNA samples in a single batch (run) in up to 24 runs a day. DNA sequencers carry out capillary electrophoresis for size separation, detection and recording of dye fluorescence, and data output as fluorescent peak trace chromatograms (Fig. 2-43). Sequencing reactions by thermocycling, cleanup and re-suspension in a buffer solution before loading onto the sequencer are performed separately. A number of commercial and non-commercial software packages can trim（修剪，整理）low-quality DNA traces automatically. These programs score the quality of each peak and remove low-quality base peaks (generally located at the ends of the sequence). The accuracy of such algorithms（算法，演算法，运算法则）is below visual

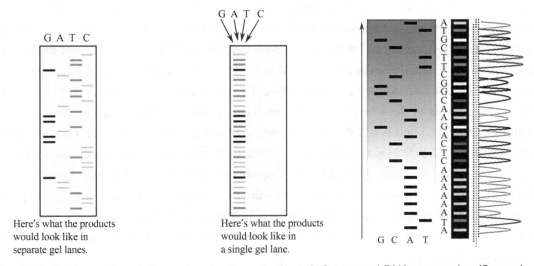

Fig. 2-43 A. Comparison between band patterns in the gels for manual DNA sequencing (Sanger) and automated DNA sequencing. B. An example of the results of automated chain-termination DNA sequencing. Sequence ladder by radioactive sequencing (left) compared to fluorescent peaks (right).

examination by a human operator, but sufficient for automated processing of large sequence data sets.

Microfluidic Sanger sequencing

Microfluidic（微流控）Sanger sequencing is a lab-on-a-chip（芯片实验室）application for DNA sequencing, in which the Sanger sequencing steps (thermal cycling, sample purification, and capillary electrophoresis) are integrated into a wafer-scale（晶圆级）chip using nanoliter-scale sample volumes. This technology generates long and accurate sequence reads, while obviating（避免）many of the significant shortcomings of the conventional Sanger method (*e.g.*, high consumption of expensive reagents, reliance on expensive equipment, personnel-intensive（人才密集型）manipulations, *etc.*) by integrating and automating the Sanger sequencing steps.

In its modern inception（开始，开端）, high-throughput genome sequencing involves fragmenting the genome into small single-stranded pieces, followed by amplification of the fragments by Polymerase Chain Reaction (PCR). Adopting the Sanger method, each DNA fragment is irreversibly terminated with the incorporation of a fluorescently labeled dideoxy chain-terminating nucleotide, thereby producing a DNA "ladder" of fragments that each differ in length by one base and bear a base-specific fluorescent label at the terminal base. Amplified base ladders are then separated by Capillary Array Electrophoresis (CAE) with automated, *in situ* "finish-line" detection of the fluorescently labeled ssDNA fragments, which provides an ordered sequence of the fragments. These sequence reads are then computer assembled into overlapping or contiguous（连续的，邻近的，相连的）sequences (termed "contigs") which resemble the full genomic sequence once fully assembled.

Sanger methods achieve read lengths of approximately 800 bp (typically 500~600 bp with non-enriched DNA). The longer read lengths in Sanger methods display significant advantages over other sequencing methods, especially in terms of sequencing repetitive（多次重复的）regions of the genome. A challenge of short-read sequence（短读序列）data is particularly an issue in sequencing new genomes (*de novo*) and in sequencing highly rearranged genome segments, typically those seen of cancer genomes or in regions of chromosomes that exhibit structural variation.

Device design

The sequencing chip has a four-layer construction, consisting of three 100-mm-diameter glass wafers (on which device elements are microfabricated) and a polydimethylsiloxane (PDMS, 聚二甲基硅氧烷) membrane. Reaction chambers and capillary electrophoresis channels are etched between the top two glass wafers, which are thermally bonded（热粘合热合）. Three-dimensional channel interconnections and microvalves（微型阀）are formed by the PDMS and bottom manifold（多管式，歧管式）glass wafer.

The device consists of three functional units, each corresponding to the Sanger sequencing steps. The **Thermal Cycling** (TC) unit is a 250-nanoliter reaction chamber with an integrated resistive temperature detector（集成电阻温度检测器）, microvalves, and a surface heater. Movement of reagent between the top all-glass layer and the lower glass-PDMS layer occurs through 500-μm-diameter via-holes（通路孔，辅助孔）. After thermal-cycling, the reaction mixture undergoes purification in the capture/purification chamber, and then is injected into the capillary electrophoresis (CE) chamber. The CE unit consists of a 30-cm capillary which is folded into a compact switchback（曲折的）pattern via 65-μm-wide turns.

Sequencing chemistry

- **Thermal cycling**

In the TC reaction chamber, dye-terminator sequencing reagent, template DNA, and primers are loaded into the TC chamber and thermal-cycled for 35 cycles (at 95℃ for 12 seconds and at 60℃ for 55 seconds).

- **Purification**

The charged reaction mixture (containing extension fragments, template DNA, and excess sequencing reagent) is conducted (引导) through a capture/purification chamber at 30℃ via a 33-Volts/cm electric field applied between capture outlet and inlet ports (接口，端口). The capture gel through which the sample is driven, consists of 40 μM of oligonucleotide (complementary to the primers) covalently bound to a polyacrylamide matrix. Extension fragments are immobilized by the gel matrix, and excess primer, template, free nucleotides, and salts are eluted through the capture waste port. The capture gel is heated to 67~75℃ to release extension fragments.

- **Capillary electrophoresis**

Extension fragments are injected into the CE chamber where they are electrophoresed through a 125~167-V/cm field.

Platforms

The Apollo 100 platform (Microchip Biotechnologies Inc., Dublin, CA)

Comparisons to other sequencing techniques

The ultimate goal of high-throughput sequencing is to develop systems that are low-cost, and extremely efficient at obtaining extended (longer) read lengths. Longer read lengths of each single electrophoretic separation, substantially reduces the cost associated with *de novo* DNA sequencing and the number of templates needed to sequence DNA contigs at a given redundancy. Microfluidics may allow for faster, cheaper and easier sequence assembly (Table 2-4).

Table 2-4 Performance values for genome sequencing technologies including Sanger methods and next-generation methods.

Technology	Number of Lanes	Injection Volume (nL)	Analysis Time	Average Read Length	Throughput (including analysis)	Gel Pouring	Lane Tracking
Slab Gel	96	500~1000	6~8 hours	700 bp	67.2 kb/hr	Yes	Yes
Capillary Array Electrophoresis	96	1~5	1~3 hours	700 bp	166 kb/hr	No	No
Microchip	96	0.1~0.5	6~30 minutes	430 bp	660 kb/hr	No	No
454/Roche FLX		<0.001	4 hours	200~300 bp	20~30 Mb/hr	No	
Illumina/Solexa			2~3 days	30~100 bp	20 Mb/hr	No	
ABI/SOLiD			8 days	35 bp	5~15 Mb/hr	No	

Data is from 2008 and has since changed drastically.

Applications of microfluidic sequencing technologies

Other useful applications of DNA sequencing include single nucleotide polymorphism (SNP) detection, single-strand conformation polymorphism (SSCP) heteroduplex analysis (异源双链分析), and short tandem repeat (STR，短串联重复) analysis. Resolving DNA fragments according to differences in size and/or conformation is the most critical step in studying these features of the genome.

2.3.3 Construction of gene library（基因文库的构建）

A gene library is a random collection of cloned DNA fragments in a number of vectors that ideally includes all the genetic information of that species.

In molecular biology, a **library** is a collection of DNA fragments that are stored and propagated（传播，繁殖）in a population of microorganisms through the process of molecular cloning. There are different types of DNA libraries, including cDNA libraries (formed from reverse-transcribed RNA), genomic libraries (formed from genomic DNA) and randomized mutant libraries (formed by *de novo* gene synthesis where alternative nucleotides or codons are incorporated). DNA library technology is a mainstay（支柱，中流砥柱，主要的依靠）of current molecular biology, genetic engineering, and protein engineering, and the applications of these libraries depend on the source of the original DNA fragments. There are differences in the cloning vectors and techniques used in library preparation, but in general each DNA fragment is uniquely inserted into a cloning vector and the pool of recombinant DNA molecules is then transferred into a population of bacteria (a Bacterial Artificial Chromosome or BAC library) or yeast such that each organism contains on average one construct（构建物，构成物）(vector + insert) — the nucleotide sequences of interest are preserved as inserts to a plasmid or the genome of a bacteriophage that has been used to infect bacterial cells. As the population of organisms is grown in culture, the DNA molecules contained within them are copied and propagated (thus, "cloned").

The term "library" can refer to a population of organisms, each of which carries a DNA molecule inserted into a cloning vector, or alternatively to the collection of all of the cloned vector molecules.

By using recombinant DNA technology, the total DNA of some organism would be cut into small pieces by some specific restriction endonucleases, and then those pieces would be randomly inserted into some plasmids or other vectors, and then the latter in turn would be transferred into some appropriate host cells. Through cell proliferation, asexual reproduction system (clones) of the various pieces would be constructed and formed. When there are more than enough clones so as to include all the genes present in an organism, this batch of cloning overall is called the biological gene library. The sum of DNA fragments inserted in those vector molecules represents the whole genome sequence or the whole mRNA sequence of an organism, so the gene library can be categorized into genome libraries and cDNA libraries. This definition also applies to mitochondrial DNA and chloroplast DNA, which are called the mitochondrial or chloroplast gene libraries of an organism, respectively.

In order to store the gene library effectively, bacteria are propagated on solid medium to increase the number of bacteria that contain those specific DNA fragments. By means of molecular hybridization, bacteria (or bacteriophages) with DNA fragments containing the desired genes can be screened out. These bacteria (or phages) are then propagated to a large amount, from which the DNA fragments of the desired genes can be isolated. The establishment and use of a gene library is an effective method to isolate the genes of higher eukaryotes.

Bacteriophage lambda is one of the most commonly used cloning vectors adopted to build the gene pool, with a theoretical capacity of 23 kb to insert exogenous DNA fragments, whereas the actual capacity is 15~20 kb fragments. The size limit of foreign genes that a vector can hold or the total number of elements that the vector can hold without requiring real location is called **vector capacity**.

In 1978 Collins and Hohn *et al.* developed the cosmid plasmid, a special type of plasmid vector containing the *cos* sequence of lambda DNA and plasmid replicons, with a capacity of 31~45 kb, which is suitable for use as a gene library vector. In addition, the YAC plasmid of the yeast system has a capacity of millions of base pairs.

An ideal gene library should meet the following requirements:

(1) The library should include all DNA sequences of that certain organism, which can represent the whole genome sequences or mRNA sequences, thus the construction needs to be randomized.

(2) The size of the library should be moderate, which should be within the order of magnitude to facilitate the screening and cloning. Therefore, lambda vectors and cosmids are the most used vectors with the capacity to insert large fragments, rather than the plasmid vectors with only a capacity to clone small fragments.

(3) The number of recombinants is high in the library.

(4) The library should be built to make it easy to reserve and amplify, proper vectors should therefore be chosen for this purpose.

2.3.3.1   *Genomic libraries*（基因组文库）

A **genomic library** is a collection of the total genomic DNA from a single organism, *i.e.*, a set of clones that together represents the entire genome of a given organism. It can be a population of host bacteria, each of which carries a DNA molecule that was inserted into a cloning vector, such that the collection of cloned DNA molecules represents the entire genome of the source organism; or the collection of all of the identical vector molecules, each carrying a piece of the chromosomal DNA of the organism, prior to the insertion of these molecules into the host cells.

The number of clones that constitute a genomic library depends on (1) the size of the genome in question and (2) the insert size tolerated by the particular cloning vector system. For most practical purposes, the tissue source of the genomic DNA is unimportant because each cell of the body contains virtually identical DNA (with some exceptions).

In order to construct a genomic library, the organism's DNA is extracted from cells and then digested with a restriction enzyme to cut the DNA into fragments of a specific size. The fragments are then inserted into the vector using DNA ligase. Next, the vector DNA can be taken up by a host organism — commonly a population of *Escherichia coli* or yeast — with each cell containing only one vector molecule. Using a host cell to carry the vector allows for easy amplification and retrieval of specific clones from the library for analysis.

There are several kinds of vectors available with various insert capacities. Generally, libraries made from organisms with larger genomes require vectors featuring larger inserts, thereby fewer vector molecules are needed to make the library. Researchers can choose a vector also considering the ideal insert size to find a desired number of clones necessary for full genome coverage.

History

The first DNA-based genome ever fully sequenced was achieved by two-time Nobel Prize winner, Frederick Sanger, in 1977. Sanger and his team of scientists created a library of the bacteriophage, phi X 174, for use in DNA sequencing. The importance of this success contributed to the ever-increasing demand for sequencing genomes to research gene therapy. Teams are now able to catalog（把……编目，分类）polymorphisms in genomes and investigate those candidate genes contributing to maladies such as Parkinson's disease, Alzheimer's disease, multiple sclerosis（多发性硬化）, rheumatoid arthritis, and Type 1 diabetes. These are due to the advance of genome-wide association studies（全基因组关

联研究) from the ability to create and sequence genomic libraries. Prior (在前，居先), linkage and candidate-gene studies were some of the only approaches.

Genomic library construction

Construction of a genomic library involves creating many recombinant DNA molecules. An organism's genomic DNA is extracted and then digested with a restriction enzyme. For organisms with very small genomes (~10 kb), the digested fragments can be separated by gel electrophoresis. The separated fragments can then be excised and cloned into the vector separately. However, when a large genome is digested with a restriction enzyme, there are far too many fragments to excise individually. The entire set of fragments must be cloned together with the vector, and separation of clones can occur after. In either case, the fragments are ligated into a vector that has been digested with the same restriction enzyme. The vector containing the inserted fragments of genomic DNA can then be introduced into a host organism (Fig. 2-44).

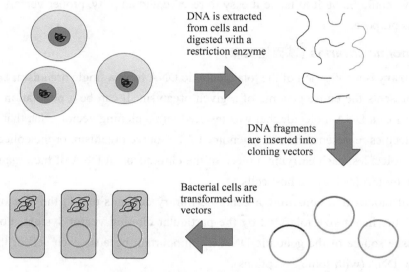

Fig. 2-44   Genomic Library Construction.

Below are the steps for creating a genomic library from a large genome.

(1) Extract and purify DNA.

(2) Digest the DNA with a restriction nuclease to produce a large number of different DNA fragments but all with identical cohesive ends. This creates fragments that are similar in size, each containing one or more genes or **a part of a gene***.

(3) Insert the fragments of DNA into suitable vectors that were cut with the same restriction enzyme. Use the enzyme DNA ligase to seal (密封，封闭) the DNA fragments into the linearized plasmid vector molecules or into a suitable virus vector. This creates a large pool of recombinant molecules.

(4) These recombinant molecules are taken up by a host bacterium or yeast by transformation, transduction or electroporation, creating a DNA library. This library would contain all of the nuclear DNA sequences of the source organism and could be searched for any particular gene of interest from the source organism.

Each clone in the library is called a **genomic DNA clone**.

*Not every genomic DNA clone would contain a complete gene since in many cases the restriction enzyme will have cut at least once within the gene. Thus some clones will contain only **a part of a gene**.

Below is a diagram of the above outlined steps.

1. Vector selection （选择载体）

A. Types of vectors

Genome size varies among different organisms and the cloning vector must be selected accordingly. For a large genome, a vector with a large capacity should be chosen so that a relatively small number of clones are sufficient for coverage of the entire genome. However, it is often more difficult to characterize an insert contained in a higher capacity vector.

Table 2-5 is a list of several kinds of vectors commonly used for genomic libraries and the insert size that each generally holds.

Table 2-5   Commonly used vectors

Vector type	Insert size (thousands of bases)
Plasmids	up to 15 kb
Lambda phage (λ phage) （λ 噬菌体载体）	15~30 kb
Cosmids （柯斯质粒，黏粒载体）	31~45 kb
Bacteriophage P1	70~100 kb
P1 artificial chromosomes (PACs, P1 噬菌体衍生的人工染色体)	100~300 kb
Bacterial artificial chromosomes (BACs)	120~350 kb
Yeast artificial chromosomes (YACs)	100~2 000 kb

Plasmid

Plasmid is an autonomously replicating circular extra-chromosomal DNA. It is a double stranded DNA molecule commonly used for molecular cloning. Plasmids are generally 2 to 4 kilobase-pairs (kb) in length and are capable of carrying inserts up to 15 kb. Plasmids contain an origin of replication allowing them to replicate inside a bacterium independently of the host chromosome. Plasmids commonly carry a gene for antibiotic resistance that allows for the selection of bacterial cells containing the plasmid. Many plasmids also carry a reporter gene that allows researchers to distinguish clones containing an insert from those that do not.

Plasmids are the standard cloning vectors and the most commonly used. Most general plasmids may be used to clone DNA inserts of up to 15 kb in size. One of the earliest commonly used cloning vectors is the pBR322 plasmid. Other cloning vectors include the pUC series of plasmids, and a large number of different cloning plasmid vectors are available. Many plasmids have high copy numbers, for example, pUC19 has a copy number of 500~700 copies per cell, and this high copy numbers is useful as it produces greater yield of recombinant plasmid for subsequent manipulation. However low-copy-number plasmids may be preferably used in certain circumstances, for example, when the protein from the cloned gene is toxic to the cells.

Some plasmids contain an M13 bacteriophage origin of replication and may be used to generate single-stranded DNA. These are called phagemid （噬菌粒）, and examples are the pBluescript series of cloning vectors.

Bacteriophage

The bacteriophages used for cloning are the phage λ and M13 phage. There is an upper limit on the amount of DNA that can be packed into a phage (a maximum of 53 kb), therefore to allow foreign DNA to be inserted into phage DNA, some phage cloning vectors need to have some non-essential genes deleted, for example the genes for lysogeny（溶原现象，溶原性）in phage λ. There is also a lower size limit for DNA that can be packed into a phage, and vector DNA that is too small cannot be properly packaged into the phage. This property can be used for selection — vector without insert may be too small, therefore only vectors with insert may be selected for propagation.

Phage lambda (λ) & Bacteriophage Lambda Vectors（λ 噬菌体载体）**.** Phage λ is a double-stranded DNA virus that infects *E. coli*. The λ chromosome is 48.5 kb long and can carry inserts up to 25 kb. The insert DNA is replicated with the viral DNA; thus, together they are packaged into viral particles. These particles are very efficient at infection and multiplication leading to a higher production of the recombinant λ chromosomes. However, due to the smaller insert size, libraries made with λ phage may require many clones for full genome coverage. There are two kinds of λ phage vectors — **insertion vector** and **replacement vector.**

a. **Insertion vector**（插入型载体）— DNA is inserted into a specific site. Insertion vectors contain a unique cleavage site, say a multiple cloning site whereby foreign DNA ranging in size from 5 to 11 kb may be inserted. A recombinant phage can be identified by insertional inactivation. An insertion vector does not lose any gene of the vector, so the molecular weight of the recombinant vector is larger than the original vector. If the length of the recombinant vector exceeds 5% of that of the wild type λDNA, the packaging efficiency of the recombinant phage would be much lower than that of the original phage. Therefore, the vector capacity is small, and the insert size is mostly within 9 kb.

b. **Replacement vector**（置换型载体）— foreign DNA replaces a piece of DNA. In replacement vectors, the cleavage sites flank a region containing genes not essential for the lytic cycle, and this region may be deleted and replaced by the desired foreign DNA fragment in the cloning process. This non-essential viral sequence is called the "stuffer fragment", the foreign DNA fragment "DNA insert".

Two cleavage sites corresponding to two specific endonucleases are engineered flanking the stuffer fragment, one on each end. After endonuclease cleavage, a bacteriophage λ cloning/expression vector is separated into three DNA fragments — the central nonessential region of phage λ, the left arm and the right arm. Upon removal of the stuffer fragment, a DNA insert is attached in between the two "arms" of phage λ to generate a recombinant phage λ vector whose non-essential sequence is replaced by foreign DNA. While those inserts replace non-essential viral sequences in the λ chromosome, the genes required for formation of viral particles and infection remain intact. The packaging capacity is 38~53 kb. In practice, exogenous DNA fragments of 8~25 kb can be incorporated in this way.

Cosmids

Cosmids are plasmids that incorporate a segment of bacteriophage λ DNA that has the **cohesive end site** (*cos*) which contains elements required for packaging DNA into λ particles.

The *cos* sequence allows the cosmid to be packaged into bacteriophage λ particles. Bacteriophage λ particles — containing a linearized cosmid — are introduced into the host cell by transduction. Once inside the host, the cosmids circularize with the aid of the host's DNA ligase and then function as plasmids.

Cosmid have been developed in the late 1970s and have been improved significantly since. They are predominantly plasmids with a bacterial *ori*V, an antibiotic selection marker and a cloning site, but they carry one, or more recently two *cos* sites derived from bacteriophage lambda. Depending on the particular

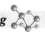

aim of the experiment, broad host range cosmids, shuttle cosmids or "mammalian" cosmids (linked to SV40 *ori*V and mammalian selection markers) are available. The loading capacity of cosmids varies depending on the size of the vector itself but usually lies around 40~45 kb. The cloning procedure involves the generation of two vector arms which are then joined to the foreign DNA (Fig. 2-45). Selection against wildtype cosmid DNA is simply done via size exclusion! Remember however that cosmids always form colonies and not plaques! Also clone density is much lower with around 10^5~10^6 cfu per μg of ligated DNA.

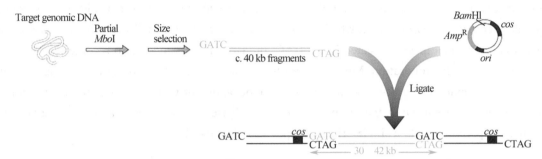

Fig. 2-45   Ligation to cleaved cosmid vector molecules can produce vector-target concatemers（多联体，串联体），resulting in a large exogenous DNA fragment flanked by *cos* sequences.

After the construction of recombinant lambda or cosmid libraries the total DNA is transfered into an appropriate *E. coli* host via a technique called ***in vitro* packaging**. The necessary packaging extracts are derived from *E. coli* cI857 lysogens（溶原性细菌株，溶素原）[red⁻ gam⁻ Sam and Dam (head assembly) and Eam (tail assembly) respectively]. These extracts will recognize and package the recombinant molecules *in vitro*, generating either mature phage particles (lambda-based vectors) or recombinant plasmids contained in phage shells (cosmids). These differences are reflected in the different infection frequencies seen in favor of lambda-replacement vectors. This compensates for their slightly lower loading capacity. Phage library are also stored and screened easier than cosmid (colonies!) libraries.

The *cos* sequences are usually inserted into a small plasmid vector to construct cosmid vectors.

It is normally used to clone large DNA fragments between 28 to 45 kb. Such a large foreign DNA fragments can be cloned using such vectors in an ***in vitro* packaging** reaction because the total size of the cosmid vector is usually only about 8.

Bacteriophage P1 vectors

Bacteriophage P1 vectors can hold inserts 70~100 kb in size. They begin as linear DNA molecules packaged into bacteriophage P1 particles. These particles are injected into an *E. coli* strain expressing *Cre* recombinase（Cre 重组酶）. The linear P1 vector becomes circularized by recombination（重组）between two *loxP* sites in the vector. P1 vectors generally contain a gene for antibiotic resistance and a positive selection marker to distinguish clones containing an insert from those that do not. P1 vectors also contain a P1 plasmid replicon（复制子），which ensures only one copy of the vector is present in a cell. However, there is a second P1 replicon called the **P1 lytic replicon** that is controlled by an inducible promoter. This promoter allows the amplification of more than one copy of the vector per cell prior to DNA extraction.

P1 artificial chromosomes

P1 artificial chromosomes (PACs) is based on the P1 phage. The PAC have features of both P1 vectors and Bacterial Artificial Chromosomes (BACs). Similar to P1 vectors, **PACs** contain a plasmid and a lytic replicon. Unlike P1 vectors, they do not need to be packaged into bacteriophage particles for transduction. Instead they are introduced into *E. coli* as circular DNA molecules through electroporation （电穿孔）just as BACs are. Also similar to BACs, these are relatively harder to prepare due to a single origin of replication.

Bacterial artificial chromosomes

Bacterial artificial chromosomes (BACs) are circular DNA molecules, usually about 7 kb in length, that are capable of holding inserts up to 350 kb in size. BACs are based on F plasmid — they contain a replicon derived from *E. coli* F factor, which ensures they are maintained in *E. coli* with a copy number of only 1 per cell. Once an insert is ligated into a BAC, the BAC is introduced into recombination deficient strains of *E. coli* by electroporation. Most BAC vectors contain a gene for antibiotic resistance and also a positive selection marker. Fig. 2-46 depicts a BAC vector being cut with a restriction enzyme, followed by the insertion of foreign DNA that is re-annealed by a ligase. Overall, this is a very stable vector, but may be hard to prepare due to a single origin of replication just like PACs.

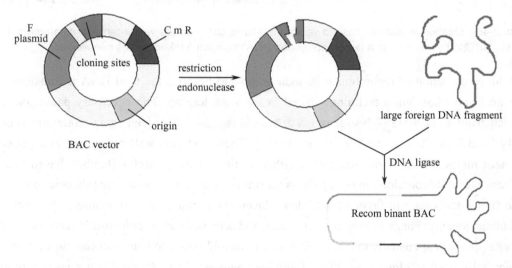

Fig. 2-46　BAC vector

Yeast artificial chromosomes

Yeast artificial chromosomes (YACs) are linear DNA molecules containing the necessary features of an authentic yeast chromosome, including telomeres （端粒，染色体终端）, a centromere （着丝粒，中心粒）, and an origin of replication. Large inserts of DNA can be ligated into the middle of the YAC so that there is an "arm" of the YAC on either side of the insert. The recombinant YAC is introduced into yeast by transformation; selectable markers present in the YAC allow for the identification of successful transformants （转化子）. YACs can hold inserts up to 3 000 kb, but most YAC libraries contain inserts 250~400 kb in size. Theoretically there is no upper limit on the size of insert a YAC can hold. It is the quality in the preparation of DNA used for inserts that determines the size limit. The most challenging aspect of using YAC is the fact they are prone to rearrangement.

Human artificial chromosome

Human artificial chromosome may be potentially useful as gene transfer vectors for gene delivery into human cells, and a tool for expression studies and determining human chromosome function. It can carry very large DNA fragment (there is no upper limit on size for practical purposes), therefore it does not have the problem of limited cloning capacity of other vectors, and it also avoids possible insertional mutagenesis caused by integration into host chromosomes by viral vector.

Animal and plant viral vectors

Viruses that infect plant and animal cells have also been manipulated to introduce foreign genes into plant and animal cells. The natural ability of viruses to adsorb to cells, introduce their DNA and replicate have made them ideal vehicles to transfer foreign DNA into eukaryotic cells in culture. A vector based on Simian virus 40 (SV40) was used in first cloning experiment involving mammalian cells. A number of vectors based on other type of viruses like Adenoviruses and Papilloma virus（乳头瘤病毒）have been used to clone genes in mammals. At present, retroviral vectors are popular for cloning genes in mammalian cells. In case of plants like Cauliflower mosaic virus（花椰菜花叶病毒）, Tobacco mosaic virus and Gemini viruses（双粒病毒）have been used with limited success.

B. How to select a vector

Vector selection requires one to ensure the library made is representative of the entire genome. Any insert of the genome derived from a restriction enzyme should have an equal chance of being in the library compared to any other insert. Furthermore, recombinant molecules should contain large enough inserts, ensuring that the library size is able to be handled conveniently. This is particularly determined by the amount of clones needed to have in a library. The amount of clones to get a sampling of all the genes is determined by the size of the organism's genome as well as the average insert size. This is represented by the formula (also known as the Carbon and Clarke formula):

$$N = ln (1-P) / ln (1-f)$$

where, N is the necessary number of recombinants

P is the desired probability that any fragment in the genome will occur at least once in the library created

f is the fractional proportion of the genome in a single recombinant

f can be further shown to be: $f = i/g$

where,

i is the insert size

g is the genome size

Thus, increasing the insert size (by choice of vector) would allow for fewer clones needed to represent a genome. The proportion of the insert size versus the genome size represents the proportion of the respective genome in a single clone. Here is the equation with all parts considered:

$$N = ln (1-P) / ln (1- i/g)$$

2. Target DNA preparation（外源 DNA 制备）

The genomic DNA to be cloned has to be cut into restriction fragments within the appropriate size range. For constructing genomic library, large insert DNAs should be prepared, and shear force should not be adopted in this process.

In order to make the size of gene library suitable for screening, partial restriction digestion of chromosome DNA with enzymes such as *Sau*3AI or *Mbo*I, which recognize 4 base pair sequences, are mostly used; followed by size fractionation, dephosphorylation [using calf-intestine phosphatase （磷酸酶）], or filling in receded 3′ end of DNA fragments with the Klenow fragment, in order to avoid chromosome scrambling（致乱，加扰）, *i.e.*, the ligation of physically unlinked fragments —

connection of the newly formed fragments of the genome in a non-adjacent way. The length of the extracted genomic DNA fragments is about 20~50 kb in general. Agarose gel electrophoresis or density gradient centrifugation was used to separate DNA fragments in this size range.

3. Ligation and *in vitro* Packaging（连接及包装）

Ligation

Once the DNA to be cloned exists as a defined fragment (called the **target** or **insert**), it can be joined to the vector by the process called **ligation**. The tool used for this process is DNA ligase, an enzyme that catalyzes the formation of a phosphodiester bond between juxtaposed（并置）5′-phosphate and 3′-hydroxyl termini in duplex DNA. The desired product in a ligation reaction is a functional hybrid molecule that consists exclusively of the vector plus the insert. However, a number of other events can occur in a ligation reaction, including circularization of the target fragment, ligation of vector without the addition of an insert, ligation of a target molecule to another target molecule, and any number of other possible combinations.

Two vector types are used in recombinant DNA research: circular molecules such as plasmids and cosmids, and linear cloning vectors such as those derived from the bacteriophage λ. In either case, for joining to a target DNA fragment, a vector is first cut with a restriction enzyme that produces compatible ends with those of the target. Circular vectors, therefore, are converted to a linear form prior to ligation to target. The insert fragment is then ligated to the prepared vector to create a recombinant molecule capable of replication once introduced into a host cell.

Dugaiczyk *et al.* (1975) identified the two factors that play the biggest role in determining the outcome of any particular ligation. First, the readiness with which two DNA molecules join is dependent on the concentration of their ends — the higher the concentration of compatible ends (those capable of being joined), the greater the likelihood that two termini will meet and be ligated. This parameter is designated by the term i and is defined as the *total* concentration of complementary ends in the ligation reaction. Second, the amount of circularization occurring within a ligation reaction is dependent on the parameter j, the concentration of same-molecule ends in close enough proximity to each other that they could potentially and effectively interact. For any DNA fragment, j is a constant value dependent on the fragment's length, not on its concentration in the ligation reaction.

For a linear fragment of duplex DNA with self-complementary, cohesive ends (such as those produced by *Eco*RI), i is given by the formula

$$i = 2N_0M \times 10^{-3} \text{ ends/ml}$$

where N_0 is Avogadro's number (6.023×10^{23}) and M is the molar concentration of the DNA.

Some DNA fragments to be used for cloning are generated by a double digest, say by using both *Eco*RI and *Hind*III in the same restriction reaction. In such a case, one end of the fragment will be cohesive with other *Eco*RI-generated termini while the other end of the DNA fragment will be cohesive with other *Hind*III-generated termini. For such DNA fragments with ends that are not self-complementary, the concentration of each end is given by

$$i = N_0M \times 10^{-3} \text{ ends/ml}$$

A value for j, the concentration of one end of a molecule in the immediate vicinity of its other end, can be calculated using the equation

$$j = \left(\frac{3}{2\pi ld} \right)^{3/2} \text{ ends/ml}$$

where l is the length of the DNA fragment, b is the minimal length of DNA that can bend around to form a circle, and π is the ratio of the circumference of a circle to its diameter.

λ DNA is 48 502 bp in length. When l and b are assigned values of 13.2×10^{-4} cm and 7.7×10^{-6} cm for λ DNA in ligation buffer, respectively, the j value for λ (j_λ) is calculated to be 3.22×10^{11} ends/ml.

The j value for any DNA molecule can be calculated in relation to j_λ using the equation

$$j = j_\lambda \left(\frac{\mathrm{MW}_\lambda}{\mathrm{MW}} \right)^{1.5} \text{ ends/ml}$$

where j_λ is equal to 3.22×10^{11} ends/ml and MW represents molecular weight.

Under circumstances in which j is equal to i ($j = i$, or $j/i = 1$), the end of any particular DNA molecule is just as likely to join with another molecule as it is to interact with its own opposite end. If j is greater than i ($j > i$), intramolecular ligation events predominate and circles are the primary product. If i is greater than j ($i > j$), intermolecular ligation events are favored and hybrid linear structures predominate.

Ligation of restriction endonuclease-generated DNA fragments（限制性酶切片段的连接）

① ***Ligation of compatible cohesive ends***（匹配黏端连接）. After digestion with nucleases, same or different, the compatible cohesive ends can be generated and ligated by DNA ligase.

② ***Ligation of blunt ends***（平末端连接）. Blunt ends can be directly ligated by ligase, but the ligation efficiency of blunt ends is lower than that of cohesive ends.

③ ***Ligation of incompatible cohesive ends***（不匹配黏端连接）. A couple of methods can be used to blunt cohesive ends and then ligate. One is to use DNA polymerase I Klenow fragment to fill-in 3′ end or use the enzyme S1 nuclease to remove the 5′ overhang and then ligate the cohesive ends. Whereas Klenow fragment can also be used to fill-in part of the 3′ recessed ends to generate the compatible cohesive ends and then ligate. *Pfu* DNA polymerase can be used to remove 3′ overhangs (polishing) or to fill-in 5′ overhangs with greater efficiencies than either Klenow polymerase or T4 DNA polymerase.

Ligation using plasmid vectors

Ligation using a plasmid vector requires that two types of events occur. First, a linear hybrid molecule must be formed by ligation of one end of the target fragment to one complementary end of the linearized plasmid. Second, the other end of the target fragment must be ligated to the other end of the vector to create a circular recombinant plasmid. The circularization event is essential since only circular molecules transform *E. coli* efficiently. Ligation conditions must be chosen, therefore, that favor intermolecular ligation events followed by intramolecular ones.

It was suggested by Maniatis *et al.* (1982) that optimal results will be achieved with plasmid vectors when i is greater than j by two- to threefold. Such a ratio will favor intermolecular ligation but will still allow for circularization of the recombinant molecule. Furthermore, Maniatis *et al.* recommend that the concentration of the termini of the insert (i_{insert}) be approximately twice the concentration of the termini of the linearized plasmid vector ($i_{\text{insert}} = 2i_{\text{vector}}$).

Ligation using λ-derived vectors

The vectors derived from phage λ carry a cloning site within the linear genome. Cleavage at the cloning site by a restriction enzyme produces two fragments, each having a λ cohesive end sequence (*cos*) at one end and a restriction enzyme-generated site at the other. Successful ligation of target with λ vector actually requires three primary events.

① Joining of the target segment to one of the two λ fragments.

② Ligation of the other λ fragment to the other end of the target fragment to create a full-length λ genome equivalent.

③ Joining of the *cos* ends between other full-length λ molecules to create a **concatemer**（串联体）, a long DNA molecule in which a number of λ genomes are joined in a series, end-to-end. Only from a concatemeric structure can individual λ genomes be efficiently packaged into a protein coat allowing for subsequent infection and propagation.

In ligation of a fragment to the arms of a λ vector, both ends of the fragment will be compatible with the cloning site of either λ arm, but each arm has only one compatible end with the insert. The ligation is mainly affected by two factors: the molar ratio between an insert fragment and the two arms of a λ vector, and the concentration of each DNA molecule. In experiments, the concentration of phage vector is usually 0.5~1.0 μg/ml. For the most efficient ligation, the reaction should contain equimolar amounts of the restriction enzyme-generated ends of each of the three fragments, the λ left arm, the insert, and the λ right arm. However, since there are two fragments of λ and one insert fragment per recombinant genome, when preparing the ligation reaction, the molar ratio of annealed arms to insert should be 2 : 1 so that the three molecules have a ratio of 2 : 1 : 2 (left arm : insert : right arm). Furthermore, since ligation of insert DNA into a bacteriophage λ-derived cloning vector requires the formation of linear concatemers of the form λ left arm : insert : λ right arm : λ left arm : insert : λ right arm : λ left arm : insert : λ right arm, *etc.* — linear ligation products need to predominate, for this reaction to be favored, i needs to be much higher than j ($i \gg j$). The concentration of ends (i) and the molecule's length (j) must be manipulated such that j is less than i, thereby favoring the production of linear hybrid molecules over circular ones.

The reaction volume should be as small as possible, and the ligating reaction should be carried out at 16°C for 4~6 h. For other details of ligation reaction, see **2.4.2 DNA ligase** for reference.

Packaging

Packaging of recombinant λ genomes

Following ligation of an insert fragment to the arms of a λ vector and concatemerization of recombinant λ genomes, the DNA must be packaged into phage protein head and tail structures, rendering them fully capable of infecting sensitive *E. coli* cells. This is accomplished by adding ligated recombinant λ DNA to a prepared extract containing the enzymatic and structural proteins necessary for complete assembly of mature virus particles. The packaging mixture is then plated with host cells that allow the formation of plaques on an agar plate. Plaques can then be analyzed for the presence of the desired clones. The measurement of the effectiveness of these reactions is called the **packaging efficiency** and can be expressed as the number of plaques (PFUs) generated from a given number of phage genomes or as the number of plaques per microgram of phage DNA.

Packaging extracts purchased commercially can have packaging efficiencies for wild-type concatemeric λ DNA of between 1×10^7 and 2×10^9 pfu/μg DNA.

The Mechanism of Viral DNA Packaging

Common development pathways exist in large double-stranded (ds)DNA viruses including the tailed bacteriophages and the eukaryotic herpes-, pox-, and adenoviruses, despite their obvious differences. Infection of the host cell ultimately leads to the synthesis of capsid proteins that are assembled into "procapsid" structures. Concurrently, viral DNA is replicated producing numerous copies of the viral

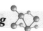

genome. Many double-stranded DNA viruses have replication and recombination pathways that produce concatemers composed of multiple genomes linked in a head-to-tail fashion (immature DNA) by rolling circle replication of the viral genome and recombination of monomeric DNA. Such a linear DNA concatemer is often the preferred viral DNA substrate for the packaging process. The assembly of an infectious virus requires that a single genome be "packaged" into the restricted confines of preformed empty shells, called procapsids or proheads. This extraordinary process represents the intersection (交点) of the capsid and DNA synthetic pathways, and is an essential step in virus assembly.

The details of DNA packaging vary with each virus; however, the similarities are striking and indicate a common strategy. Even the prokaryotic RNA packaging system shows functional similarity to the eukaryotic reoviruses (呼肠孤病毒). Indeed, a general packaging mechanism may be universal and traverse the prokaryotic-eukaryotic boundary.

For viruses such as phage λ that have unique (non-permuted) chromosomes, the assembly of an infectious virus requires that specific chromosome ends must be generated by recognition and cleavage of specific DNA sites from the concatemer by viral packaging proteins. The cutting of concatemeric DNA occurs during DNA packaging — individual genomes is generated by the introduction of nicks, staggered by 12 bp, into the concatemeric DNA, and concurrently packaged into an empty procapsid.

Cohesive ends (*cos*)

Phage λ chromosomes are 48 502 bp long linear duplex, with complementary, 12-base-long single-stranded extensions at the 5' ends of the strands. These extensions, called cohesive ends, or *cos*, is the junction between individual genomes in concatemeric λ DNA and is the site where terminase assembles to initiate the packaging process, enabling the chromosome to cyclize in an infected cell, hence is required for efficient packaging of a λ chromosome. Late during infection, an individual genome is excised by terminase from the concatemer and concomitantly the "matured" DNA is translocated into the capsid.

cos is composed of three subsites: *cosN*, *cosB*, and *cosQ* (Fig. 2-47A). These *cos* subsites, which are located in a ~200-bp segment, orchestrate the recognition, processing, and packaging of λDNA (Fig. 2-47).

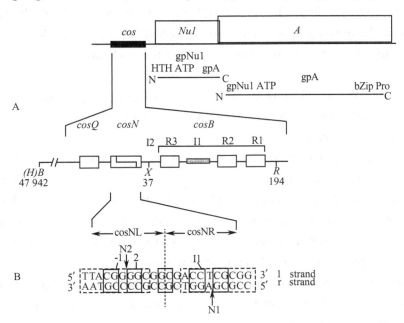

Fig. 2-47 Structure of λ *cos*.

cosN and *cosB* are critical to the assembly of a terminase packaging complex at *cos* and the initiation of genome packaging.

cosN. The site at which terminase introduces staggered nicks is *cosN*. Defined functionally as the terminase nicking site, *cosN* is located between two other sites, *cosQ* and *cosB*, and is to the left of *cosB*. *cosN* contains a 22 bp long segment with 10 bp exhibiting 2-fold rotational symmetry (Fig. 2-47B). The top strand nick position (N2) is in *cosNL*, the left *cosN* half-site, and the bottom strand nick position (N1) is in *cosNR*, the right *cosN* half-site. *cosN*'s 2-fold rotational symmetry suggests that a symmetrically disposed (安排) dimer of gpA subunits whose dyad structure matches the 2-fold rotational symmetry of *cosN* is responsible for symmetric duplex nicking activity at *cosN*, which introduce site-specific nicks into the duplex 12 bases apart (the *cos* cleavage reaction).

cosB. In addition to *cosN*, the adjacent site *cosB* is required for cutting at *cosN* to initiate DNA packaging. *cosB* is defined functionally as a terminase binding site, and has been shown to stimulate the efficiency and accuracy of the *cos* cleavage reaction — nicking of *cosN*, and to be essential for a post-cleavage step required for initiation of DNA packaging. Within *cosB* there are three distinct gpNul binding sites: R1, R2, and R3, located in a segment extending from λ bp 53~166. Terminase binding to the R sites is mediated by a helix-turn-helix DNA binding motif at the amino terminus of gpNul (amino acid residues 5~24). Between R3 and R2 is I1, a binding site for **integration host factor (IHF)**, the *E. coli* site-specific DNA binding and bending protein. The sharp bend imposed by IHF at I1 is proposed to facilitate cooperative interactions between terminase protomers (原体) anchored at the R2 and R3 sites. Between *cosN* and *cosB* is a segment of unknown function called I2.

cosQ. Whereas terminase requires *cosB* of λ for initiation of packaging, the *cosQ* subsite is required and plays an important role in the DNA packaging termination. However, a downstream *cos* consisting of *cosQ* and *cosN* is inadequate to support efficient packaging termination — the sequences within *cosB* function with *cosQ* and *cosN* to promote packaging termination and processivity. *cosQ* acts in presenting a gpA subunit to the bottom strand of *cosN* by forming a bend in the region of DNA between *cosQ* and *cosN*, forming a loop for *cosQ* and *cosN* to be aligned in the same orientation. A second version of the model proposes that *cosQ* is needed for a pause in the packaging process to recruit the second of two gpA subunits from solution to the *cosN* site for the nicking of the bottom strand of DNA.

The key components of the packaging machine are the packaging enzyme (terminase, motor) and the portal protein that forms the unique DNA entrance vertex (顶点) of prohead.

Portal protein & portal vertex

As late DNA replication produces concatemers, the procapsid components assemble an icosahedron (二十面体) that is generally formed of many copies of a major capsid protein. Of the 12 fivefold (五重的) vertexes of the icosahedron, one is the unique portal vertex, which is occupied by a dodecameric (十二聚体的) portal protein ring. The portal protein gpB is the product of the *B* gene of λ, which assembles into a gear-, or a doughnut-shaped structure, situated at a unique vertex of an empty procapsid shell — the head shell precursor, with 12 portal protein monomers arranged radially, creating a central channel through which DNA enters and exits the shell during packaging and injection, respectively. The portal also serves as an initiator for assembly of the major capsid protein and the scaffolding protein(s) into an icosahedral lattice, also the site of tail attachment.

Terminase（末端酶）

Terminase enzymes are a central component of the DNA packaging motors in both prokaryotic and eukaryotic dsDNA viruses, and are responsible for the ATP-dependent insertion of viral DNA into an empty procapsid, a process called **DNA packaging**.

The tailed phages and herpesviruses produce a multifunctional DNA packaging enzyme that contains the endonuclease activity that cuts concatemers at specific sites to generate virion chromosomes, which is coordinated with packaging of the DNA into an empty protein shell. All of the characterized terminase enzymes are composed of a large subunit (49~72 kDa) , which provides the packaging activities of the enzyme, and a small subunit (18~21 kDa) that is responsible for specific recognition of viral DNA. The functional holoenzyme is hetero-oligomer of these subunits.

In the case of bacteriophage λ, the functional terminase holoenzyme is composed of a heteromultimer of gpA (73.3 kDa, 641 amino acid residues) and gpNul (20.4 kDa) subunits, the products of the lambda *A* and *Nul* genes, respectively, isolated as a heterotrimeric holoenzyme complex of $gpA_1 \cdot gpNul_2$ protomers. Purified, recombinant λ terminase also forms a homogeneous, heterotrimeric structure, consisting of one gpA molecule associated with two gpNu1 molecules (114.2 kDa).

The larger gpA subunit possesses all of the catalytic activities required for DNA maturation and packaging. These include site specific endonuclease (*cos*-cleavage) and strand separation (helicase，解旋酶) activities required to excise an individual genome from the concatemer (DNA maturation activity), DNA translocase (packaging) activity and ATPase activity that powers DNA packaging.

The small gpNul subunit that is required for specific recognition of viral DNA, contains a DNA-binding motif that targets the enzyme to a cleavage site on the concatemer, binds *cosB* to anchor gpA during *cosN* cutting.

Lambda terminase holoenzyme is a complex biological machine that contains a nuclease catalytic site, a strand-separation "helicase" catalytic site, a DNA translocation catalytic site and four ATPase sites (two in gpA and one in each of the gpNu1 dimer subunits). Each of these catalytic sites must be regulated both spatially and temporally（时空，空间和时间）to ensure site-specific assembly of the DNA maturation machinery, appropriate maturation of the genome end, binding to the procapsid and activation of DNA translocation motor. Complex allosteric interactions between all of the catalytic sites have been demonstrated which likely reflects the regulated activation and deactivation of the sites.

Model for the packaging motor

It has long been presumed that a dimer of gpA is required to nick the duplex at the *cosN* site to prepare viral DNA for packaging. Conversely, it has been suggested that a gpA hexamer is the relevant species in the packaging motor.

Nasib K. Maluf *et al.* further show that λ terminase adopts a heterogeneous mixture of higher-order structures. Terminase holoenzyme adopts at least two distinct hetero-oligomeric species, a heterotrimer and a 13.3 S hetero-oligomer, with an average molecular mass of 528 ($\pm$ 34) kDa. Both the heterotrimer and the higher-order species possess similar site-specific *cos* cleavage (endonuclease) activity, as well as DNA packaging activities (in the presence of IHF). The heterotrimer is dependent upon *Escherichia coli* IHF for these activities.

A simpler model would envision a single, stable hetero-oligomer that was involved in all aspects of terminase function. Such kind of model was proposed for the terminase packaging motor (Fig. 2-48).

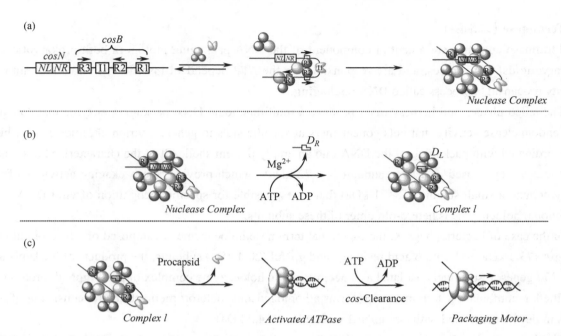

Fig. 2-48   Model for DNA packaging in bacteriophage. (a) Assembly of an activated nuclease complex (step 1). The *cos* sequence is shown at top left, with the R-elements, the I1 element and *cosN* shown; the *cosNL* and *cosNR* half-sites are indicated as *NL* and *NR*, respectively. A terminase heterotrimer is composed of a gpNu1 dimer (blue spheres) and one gpA subunit (red sphere). The packaging motor is assembled from five heterotrimers. A core interaction in motor assembly and stability is binding of a gpNu1 dimer at the R3 and R2 elements, supported by duplex bending by IHF (cyan lobes). Additional bending and/or wrapping involves multiple interactions between the pentamer ring and all of *cosB*. The nature of these interactions is at present speculative. (b) Maturation of the genome end (step 2). Duplex nicking and strand separation, catalyzed by gpA subunits in the ring, require Mg^{2+} and ATP. This reaction ejects the D_R fragment from the complex and yields complex I. (c) Assembly of the packaging motor (step 3). gpA subunits in the ring bind to the portal vertex (purple ring) of an empty procapsid. This completes the packaging motor and activates the packaging ATPase. *cos* clearance requires that IHF dissociate from I1, and that gpNu1 switch from a specific to a non-specific DNA binding mode.

Step 1: assembly of an activated nuclease complex. Packaging of viral DNA initiates with the assembly or specific binding of the terminase subunits at a packaging initiation site on the viral DNA concatemer — *cos*, concatemeric λ DNA is recognized, bound by terminase at *cosB*. Specific recognition of viral DNA and assembly of the packaging machinery is mediated by the small subunit of terminase, gpNu1, which specifically recognizes the three R-elements (R3, R2 and R1) found within the *cosB* subsite and binds to them, and introduces staggered nicks at an adjacent site, a subsite of *cos*, *cosN*, to generate the cohesive ends found on virion DNA. A critical interaction is simultaneous binding of R3 and R2 elements in *cosB* by the two gpNu1 subunits in a terminase heterotrimer, which is promoted by IHF-induced bending at the I1 site. This represents an initial interaction that is mediated by the two gpNu1 subunits in a terminase hetero-trimer. IHF binding and bending are required to facilitate the assembly of additional heterotrimers onto *cos* DNA, thus forming the active packaging complex. Additional heterotrimers then are recruited to *cos* that form a pentameric terminase ring (the 13.3 S species), which encircles DNA within the central channel, and that further bends and/or wraps the duplex.

Step 2: maturation of the genome end. Once assembled, and in the presence of $Mg^{2+}\cdot ATP$, a nuclease activity centered in the large subunit cuts the duplex, thus forming a mature genome end in preparation for DNA packaging. The so-called "helicase" activity of gpA then separates the nicked, annealed strands, ejecting the D_R DNA fragment from the complex. The gpA subunits within the terminase ring catalyze both duplex nicking and strand separation reactions; the intact ring remains bound to the mature genome end (D_L), which represents the exceptionally stable complex I packaging intermediate.

Step 3: assembly of the packaging motor. The terminase-viral DNA complex next docks on the portal vertex of a procapsid. During prohead assembly, a majority of the gpB is processed to gpB* by removal of the N-terminal 20 amino acids. The C-terminus of the large terminase subunit, gpA, interacts with the portal proteins in an empty procapsid during DNA packaging, assembling a motor complex containing five large terminase subunits that leads to DNA packaging. This interaction completes the packaging motor, which activates the packaging ATPase site(s) in gpA that fuels the machine to translocate the DNA into the procapsid (or prohead). This is followed by "***cos*-clearance**" — the transition from the site-specifically bound complex I to the mobile packaging motor, *cos* clearance requires un-wrapping of the duplex, which involves dissociation of IHF and that gpNu1 transitions from a site-specific DNA binding protein bound at *cosB*, to an actively translocating non-specific DNA binding protein. gpNu1 remains part of the translocating packaging complex. ATP affects specific DNA binding by gpNu1, thus modulating a molecular switch that facilitates *cos* clearance and the transition to an active packaging complex. DNA remains encircled by the terminase ring, facilitating processive translocation of the DNA into the capsid (Fig. 2-49). The nuclease activity of the enzyme is presumed to be simultaneously inactivated to prevent

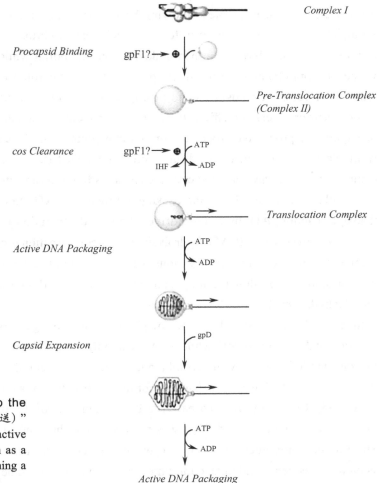

Fig. 2-49   Translocation of DNA into the Procapsid (原壳体). "Propagation（传送）" steps require *cos*-clearance, followed by active DNA packaging. The procapsid is shown as a large cyan (青色，蓝绿色) sphere containing a portal (门的，入口) complex (purple oval).

duplex nicking during packaging.

The interaction between complex I and the portal triggers two critical events. (i) Terminase switches from a *cos*-specific single-stranded DNA binding protein to a mobile complex that binds tightly, but non-specifically to duplex DNA; and (ii) the packaging activity of the enzyme is activated, which translocates DNA into the capsid.

The pentameric motor processively translocates DNA into the capsid until the head shell is full with one viral genome and the next *cos* sequence (the end of the genome) is encountered.

In many viruses, DNA packaging triggers procapsid expansion. Shell expansion occurs early during DNA packaging. For example, in phage l , a pausing of DNA translocation occurs when about 30% of the DNA has been packaged.

The rate of DNA packaging does decrease as packaging proceeds. The translocating motor ultimately fills the capsid with DNA, packaging a single viral genome condensed to near liquid crystalline density. This represents an energetically demanding process, and the DNA packaging motor is among the most powerful biological motors thus far characterized. The portal vertex has a role in sensing the amount of DNA that has been packaged, by sensing (1) the packaging density, (2) the rate of DNA translocation, or (3) the energy required to continue packaging. After the interior of the shell is filled with DNA ("headful" packaging), the endonuclease cuts the DNA, completing DNA packaging. Upon packaging a complete genome, terminase again cuts the duplex, which separates the DNA-filled capsid from the terminase·concatemer complex, allowing head-finishing proteins to assemble on the portal, sealing the portal, and constructing a platform for tail attachment. Addition of a viral tail completes the assembly of an infectious virus. Terminase then undocks from the portal while remaining bound to the concatemer, poised to capture another prohead and package the next chromosome on the concatemer. The terminase concatemer complex binds a second procapsid to initiate a second round of DNA packaging. All these events occur precisely and efficiently in about 5 min during the late phase of phage life cycle. Thus, DNA packaging is a processive process, with multiple genomes in the concatemer packaged per DNA binding event. There is a universal "head-full" component. That is, the nuclease activity of the terminase large subunit is in some way activated once the capsid is filled to capacity.

ATP plays multiple roles in the packaging process — ATP modulates the rate and fidelity of the *cos*-cleavage reaction, ATP hydrolysis drives the strand separation reaction and DNA packaging is fueled by the hydrolysis of ATP. ATP hydrolysis-driven conformational changes in the packaging motor (large terminase) power DNA motion. Various parts of the motor subunit, such as the ATPase, arginine finger, transmission (传动) domain, hinge, and DNA groove, work in concert to translocate about 2 bp of DNA per ATP hydrolyzed.

In general, the expected number of plaques for λ phage should be about 1.8×10^8 pfu/μg upon infection of *Escherichia coli*, while λDNA can only form $10^4 \sim 10^6$ pfu/μg. Therefore, in order to improve the transduction efficiency of recombinant phage, it is essential to effectively package the recombinant phage *in vitro*, which is in turn essential for the construction of a complete gene library.

In 1985, Rosenberg prepared bacterial lysate using *E. coli* C strain. When DNA was added to lysate, *cos* sites were identified and DNA was packaged into the head of phages, forming transfecting phages. Any polycos monomer 25 kb in size or smaller could be used, so long as it contains a packaging recognition sequence and ligated multimers allow the *cos* sites to be spaced 38~51 kb apart. Since polycos packaging is efficient, this may represent an excellent method to introduce large plasmids or phagemids, which are difficult to transfer by standard methods, into *E. coli* cells. This vector system is intrinsically versatile and should help circumvent many cloning limitations.

Many companies currently sell kits that can be used directly to construct genomic libraries.

Vectors such as λZAP® and ZAP Express® are available for constructing small-insert libraries. PWE15 and SuperCos 1 are cosmid vectors for generating cosmid libraries, with a cloning capacity of 30~42 kb. The use of these kits will greatly simplify the construction of genomic libraries.

λZAP®. The Bluescript SK (−) phagemid sequences in lambda ZAP — pBluescript® SK (−) — were positioned between the two partial origin domains so that the excision of the plasmid DNA from the lambda ZAP vector would generate a complete pBluescript SK (−) phagemid, including an intact, reconstituted f1 origin of replication. The excision process eliminates the need to subclone DNA inserts from the lambda phage into a plasmid by restriction digestion and ligation. Entire DNA inserts within the lambda ZAP vector can be recovered within the Bluescript SK (−) phagemid, positioned within the pBluescript polylinker in a manner suitable for further analysis. The ability to rapidly and efficiently convert lambda phage clones to phagemids reduces time for analysis of cloned genes. The vector also has an insert capacity of up to 10 kb without exceeding the packaging limit, which is 105% of wild type lambda phage (51 kb). This large capacity, in addition to the choice of cloning sites and *in vivo* excision process, makes the lambda ZAP vector attractive for the construction of genomic libraries. It can also be used efficiently as a cDNA expression vector.

ZAP Express®. The ZAP Express vector allows both eukaryotic and prokaryotic expression, while also increasing both cloning capacity and the number of unique lambda cloning sites. The ZAP Express vector has 12 unique cloning sites which will accommodate DNA inserts from 0 to 12 kb in length. Inserts cloned into the ZAP Express vector can be excised out of the phage in the form of the kanamycin-resistant pBK-CMV phagemid vector by the same excision mechanism found in the lambda ZAP vectors. Clones in the ZAP Express vector can be screened with either DNA probes or antibody probes, and *in vivo* rapid excision of the pBK-CMV phagemid vector allows insert characterization in a plasmid system.

pWE15. pWE15 is a cosmid cloning vector for construction of DNA libraries, Amp^r, which allows for the insertion of DNA fragments of 20~40 kb. It is a cosmid vector for rapid genomic walking, restriction mapping and gene transfer, with selectable markers in either *Escherichia coli* or mammalian cell lines.

SuperCos 1. SuperCos 1 is a novel, 7.9-kb cosmid vector that contains bacteriophage promoter sequences flanking a unique cloning site. This structure allows rapid synthesis of "walking" probes specific for the extreme ends of insert DNA. The SuperCos 1 vector is also engineered to contain genes for the amplification and expression of cosmid clones in eukaryotic cells. In addition, most genomic inserts can be excised as a single large restriction fragment using the *Not*I restriction site that flanks the SuperCos 1 polylinker.

The above gene libraries which have been ligated and packaged under appropriate reaction conditions should be stored at 4°C. Generally, the constructed gene libraries were used directly for screening the target genes without further amplification.

4. Library Titer Determination

Library with a viral vector. After a genomic library is constructed with a viral vector, such as lambda phage, the titer of the library can be determined. Calculating the titer allows researchers to approximate how many infectious viral particles were successfully created in the library. To do this, dilutions of the library are used to transfect cultures of *E. coli* of known concentrations. The cultures are then plated on agar plates and incubated overnight. The number of viral plaques is counted and can be used to calculate the total number of infectious viral particles in the library. Most viral vectors also carry a marker that allows clones containing an insert to be distinguished from those that do not have an insert. This allows researchers to also determine the percentage of infectious viral particles actually carrying a fragment of the library.

Library with a non-viral vector. A similar method can be used to titer genomic libraries made with non-viral vectors, such as plasmids and BACs. A test ligation of the library can be used to transform *E. coli*. The transformation mixture is then spread on agar plates and incubated overnight. The titer of the transformation is determined by counting the number of colonies present on the plates. These vectors generally have a selectable marker allowing the differentiation of clones containing an insert from those that do not. By doing this test, researchers can also determine the efficiency of the ligation and make adjustments as needed to ensure they get the desired number of clones for the library.

5. Screening DNA libraries

In order to isolate clones that contain regions of interest from a library, the library must first be screened. One method of screening is hybridization. Each transformed host cell of a library will contain only one vector with one insert of DNA. The whole library can be plated onto a filter（滤膜）over media. The filter and colonies are prepared for hybridization and then labeled with a probe. The target DNA, insert of interest, can be identified by detection such as autoradiography due to the hybridization with the probe (Fig. 2-50).

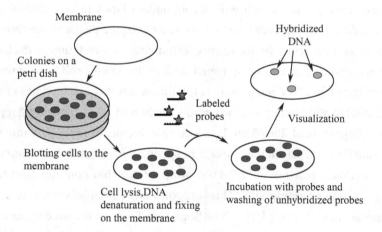

Fig. 2-50　Colony Blot Hybridization.

Genomic libraries are screened by hybridization with a DNA probe that is complementary to part of the nucleotide sequence of the desired gene. The probe may be a DNA restriction fragment or perhaps part of a cDNA clone. Another approach is possible if some of the protein sequence for the desired gene is known. Using the genetic code, one can then deduce the DNA sequence of this part of the gene and synthesize an oligonucleotide with this sequence to act as the DNA probe.

When using a plasmid vector, a typical procedure for screening would be to take agar plates bearing bacterial colonies that make up the genomic library and overlay each plate with a nitrocellulose

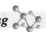

membrane. This is peeled off and is a **replica** of the plate in that some of the colonies will have adhered to it and in the same pattern as the colonies on the plate. This filter is often called a "**colony lift**"（菌落转印）. It is treated with alkali to lyse the bacterial cells and denature the DNA and then hybridized with a radiolabeled DNA probe. After washing away the unreacted probe, autoradiography of the filter shows which colonies have hybridized with the probe and thus contain the desired sequences. These are then recovered from the agar plate.

When a bacteriophage is used as the cloning vector, the gene library is screened as an array of plaques in a bacterial lawn（菌苔）. A hybridization screening method is used similar to that described for plasmid screening above; in this case the replica filter is called a "**plaque lift**"（噬菌斑转印）.

For cDNA libraries, screening can similarly be carried out by hybridization. In addition, it is possible to make the cDNA library using a vector that will actually transcribe the inserted cDNA and then translate the resulting mRNA to form protein corresponding to the cloned gene. A library made with such an **expression vector** is an **expression cDNA library**. It can be screened using a labeled antibody that recognizes the specific protein and hence identifies those bacteria which contain the desired gene and are synthesizing the protein. Not just antibody but any ligand that binds to the target protein can be used as a probe. For example, labeled hormone may be used to identify clones synthesizing hormone receptor proteins.

Another method of screening is with polymerase chain reaction (PCR). Some libraries are stored as pools of clones and screening by PCR is an efficient way to identify pools containing specific clones.

Applications

After a library is created, the genome of an organism can be sequenced to elucidate how genes affect an organism or to compare similar organisms at the genome level. The aforementioned genome-wide association studies can identify candidate genes stemming from（出自，来源于，发生于）many functional traits. Genes can be isolated through genomic libraries and used on human cell lines or animal models to further research. Furthermore, creating high-fidelity clones with accurate genome representation and no stability issues would contribute（做出贡献）well as intermediates for shotgun sequencing or the study of complete genes in functional analysis.

Genomic libraries are commonly used for sequencing applications. They have played an important role in the whole genome sequencing of several organisms, including the human genome and several model organisms. Genomic libraries are also utilized in comparison studies between differing species. Applications of genomic libraries include:

- Determining the complete genome sequence of a given organism
- Serving as a source of genomic sequence for generation of transgenic animals through genetic engineering
- Study of the function of regulatory sequences *in vitro*
- Study of genetic mutations in cancer tissues

Hierarchical sequencing（等级排序）

One major use of genomic libraries is hierarchical shotgun sequencing, which is also called top-down, map-based or clone-by-clone sequencing. This strategy was developed in the 1980s for sequencing whole genomes before high throughput techniques for sequencing were available. Individual clones from genomic libraries can be sheared into smaller fragments, usually 500 bp to 1 000 bp, which are more manageable for sequencing. Once a clone from a genomic library is sequenced, the sequence can be used to screen the library for other clones containing inserts which overlap with the sequenced clone. Any new overlapping clones can then be sequenced forming a contig（片段重叠群）. This technique, called **chromosome walking,** can be exploited to sequence entire chromosomes.

Whole genome shotgun sequencing is another method of genome sequencing that does not require a library of high-capacity vectors. Rather, it uses computer algorithms to assemble short sequence reads to cover the entire genome. Genomic libraries are often used in combination with whole genome shotgun sequencing for this reason. A high resolution map can be created by sequencing both ends of inserts from several clones in a genomic library. This map provides sequences of known distances apart, which can be used to help with the assembly of sequence reads acquired through shotgun sequencing (Fig. 2-51). The

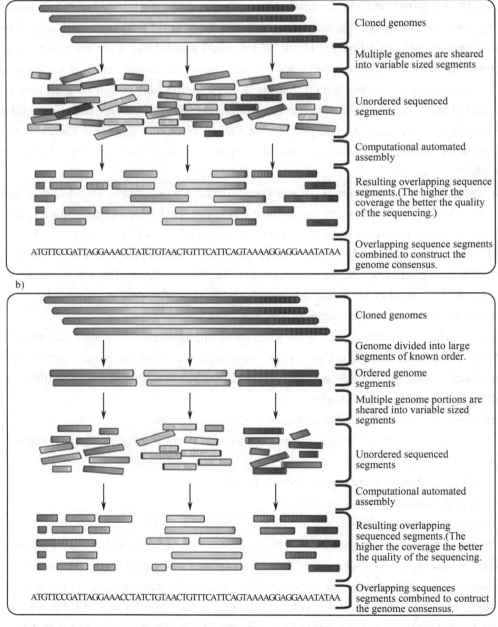

Fig. 2-51   Whole genome shotgun sequencing versus Hierarchical shotgun sequencing.

human genome sequence, which was declared complete in 2003, was assembled using both a BAC library and shotgun sequencing.

Genome-wide association studies

Genome-wide association studies（全基因组关联研究）are general applications to find specific gene targets and polymorphisms within the human race. In fact, the International HapMap project（人类基因组单体型图计划）was created through a partnership of scientists and agencies from several countries to catalog and utilize this data. The goal of this project is to compare genetic sequences of different individuals to elucidate similarities and differences within chromosomal regions. Scientists from all of the participating nations are cataloging these attributes with data from populations of African, Asian, and European ancestry（血统）. Such genome-wide assessments may lead to further diagnostic and drug therapies while also helping future teams focus on orchestrating（精心安排）therapeutics with genetic features in mind. These concepts are already being exploited in genetic engineering. For example, a research team has actually constructed a PAC shuttle vector that creates a library representing two-fold coverage of the human genome. This could serve as an incredible（难以置信的，惊人的）resource to identify genes, or sets of genes, causing disease. Moreover, these studies can serve as a powerful way to investigate transcriptional regulation as it has been seen in the study of baculoviruses（杆状病毒）. Overall, advances in genome library construction and DNA sequencing have allowed for efficient discovery of different molecular targets. Assimilation（同化，吸收）of these features through such efficient methods can hasten the employment of novel drug candidates.

2.3.3.2 cDNA libraries（cDNA 文库）

A **cDNA library** is a combination of cloned cDNA (complementary DNA) fragments inserted into a collection of host cells, which together constitute some portion of the transcriptome（转录物组）of the organism. A cDNA library represents a sample of the mRNA purified from a particular source (either a collection of cells, a particular tissue, or an entire organism), which has been converted back to a DNA template by the use of the enzyme reverse transcriptase. cDNA is produced from fully transcribed mRNA found in the nucleus and therefore contains only the expressed genes of an organism. Similarly, tissue-specific cDNA libraries can be produced. It thus represents the genes that were being actively transcribed in that particular source under the physiological, developmental, or environmental conditions that existed when the mRNA was purified.

cDNA libraries are useful in reverse genetics（反向遗传学，逆遗传学）, but they only represent a very small (less than 1%) portion of the overall genome in a given organism. In eukaryotic cells the mature mRNA is already spliced, hence the cDNA produced lacks introns and can be readily expressed in a bacterial cell. While information in cDNA libraries is a powerful and useful tool since gene products are easily identified, the libraries lack information about enhancers, introns, and other regulatory elements found in a genomic DNA library.

cDNA libraries can be generated using techniques that promote "full-length" clones or under conditions that generate shorter fragments used for the identification of "expressed sequence tags".

cDNA Library Construction

cDNA is created from a mature mRNA from a eukaryotic cell with the use of an enzyme known as reverse transcriptase. In eukaryotes, a polyA tail (consisting of a long sequence of adenine nucleotides) distinguishes mRNA from tRNA and rRNA and can therefore be used as a primer site for reverse transcription (Fig. 2-52). This has the problem that not all transcripts, such as those for the histone（组蛋白）, encode a polyA tail.

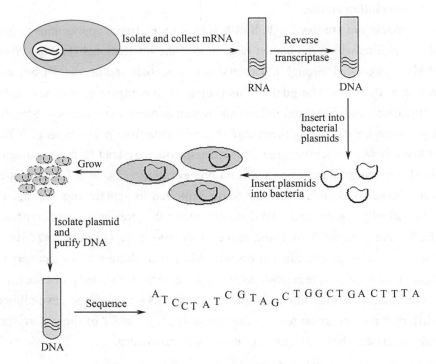

Fig. 2-52　Formation of a cDNA library.

mRNA extraction

Firstly, the mRNA is obtained and purified from the rest of the RNAs. Several methods exist for purifying RNA such as trizol extraction（trizol 抽提试剂盒）and column purification. Column purification is done by using oligomeric dT nucleotide coated resins where only the mRNA having the polyA tail will bind. The rest of the RNAs are washed out. The mRNA is eluted by using eluting buffer and some heat to separate the mRNA strands from oligo-dT.

The organs with highly abundant mRNA are commonly chosen as the source material for extracting the desired mRNA. Hence the content of target mRNA should be determined in various candidate organs or body fluids before its extraction. While for those cases with only lowly abundant mRNA available, methods such as agarose gel electrophoresis and sucrose gradient centrifugation are used to enrich the Target sequence. In those processers, care should be taken on the RNase activity and measures should be taken to inhibit it.

cDNA construction

Minus strand DNA synthesis（cDNA 第一链的合成）: Once mRNA is purified, *oligo-dT* (a short sequence of deoxy-thymine nucleotides) is tagged as a complementary primer which binds to the polyA tail providing a free 3′-OH end that can be extended by reverse transcriptase to create the complementary DNA strand. Adding random primer mixture facilitates cloning the sequence near 5′ end in an exceptionally long mRNA. Reverse transcriptase derived from Avian myelogenous leukemia virus（AMV, 禽髓系白血病病毒）and that derived from MORONI mouse leukemia virus（M-MLV, 莫洛尼鼠白血病病毒）are the two majorly used enzymes in this process.

Plus strand DNA synthesis（cDNA 第二链的合成）: Now, the mRNA is removed by using an RNase enzyme leaving a single stranded cDNA (sscDNA). This sscDNA is converted into a double stranded DNA with the help of DNA polymerase. However, for DNA polymerase to synthesize a complementary strand a free 3′-OH end is needed. This is provided by the sscDNA itself by generating a *hairpin loop*（发夹环）at the 3′ end by coiling on itself. The polymerase extends the 3′-OH end and later the loop at 3′ end is opened by the scissoring action of S_1 *nuclease*. This approach is seldom used nowadays.

Alternatively, Ribonuclease H (RNase H) can be used to cleave the 3′-O-P bond of RNA in a DNA/RNA duplex substrate to produce 3′-hydroxyl and 5′-phosphate terminated products. And the fragments generated from enzyme treatment of RNase H, still attached on the minus strand DNA, can serve as the primers for synthesizing newly formed plus strand DNA, with the help of ligase to ligate the newly elongated "Okazaki fragments" to form the whole length plus strand DNA hence the whole length double strand cDNA. Since the purification step could be omitted after the minus strand DNA synthesis, a one tube reverse transcription characterize this RNase H method.

Another approach is tailing an oligodeoxynucleotide **adaptor** [*i.e.*, poly(dC)] on the free 3′-OH end and/or 5′-OH end of minus strand DNA by terminal transferase, followed by synthesizing plus strand DNA with a primer complementary to the adaptor sequence [in this case poly(dG)]. A whole length cloning of a cDNA is possible with this approach. A special restriction site designed within the primer would facilitate cloning manipulation.

Restriction endonucleases and DNA ligase are then used to clone the sequences into bacterial plasmids. The cloned bacteria are then selected, commonly through the use of antibiotic selection. Once selected, stocks（品系，原种，群体）of the bacteria are created which can later be grown and sequenced to compile the cDNA library.

Phage vectors λgt10, λgt11 and λZAP are vectors frequently used in cDNA cloning.

Applications of cDNA libraries

cDNA libraries are commonly used when reproducing（复制，再造）eukaryotic genomes, as the amount of information is reduced to remove the large numbers of non-coding regions from the library. cDNA libraries are used to express eukaryotic genes in prokaryotes. Prokaryotes do not have introns in their DNA and therefore do not possess any enzymes that can cut them out during transcription process. cDNA does not have introns and therefore can be expressed in prokaryotic cells. cDNA libraries are most useful in reverse genetics（反向遗传学，逆遗传学）where the additional genomic information is of less use. Additionally, cDNA libraries are frequently used in functional cloning to identify genes based on the encoded protein's function. When studying eukaryotic DNA, expression libraries are constructed using complementary DNA (cDNA) to help ensure the insert is truly a gene. Applications of cDNA libraries include:

- Discovery of novel genes
- Cloning of full-length cDNA molecules for *in vitro* study of gene function
- Study of the repertoire of mRNAs expressed in different cells or tissues
- Study of alternative splicing in different cells or tissues

cDNA Library vs. Genomic DNA Library

cDNA library lacks the non-coding and regulatory elements found in genomic DNA. Genomic DNA libraries provide more detailed information about the organism, but are more resource-intensive（资源密集型的，大量占用资源的）to generate and maintain.

Cloning of cDNA

cDNA molecules can be cloned by using restriction site **adapters**. **Adapters** are short, double stranded pieces of DNA (**oligodeoxyribonucleotide**) about 8 to 12 nucleotide pairs long that include a restriction endonuclease cleavage site, *e.g.*, *Bam*HI. Both the cDNA and the **adapter** have blunt ends which can be ligated together using a high concentration of T4 DNA ligase. Then sticky ends are produced in the cDNA molecule by cleaving the cDNA ends (which now have **adapters** with an incorporated site) with the appropriate endonuclease. A cloning vector (plasmid) is then also cleaved with the appropriate endonuclease. Following "sticky end" ligation of the insert into the vector the resulting recombinant DNA molecule is transferred into *E. coli* host cell for cloning.

Lambda vectors used for making cDNA libraries do not require a large insert capacity (most cDNAs are <5 kb long). Design of insertion vectors often involves modification of the λ genome to permit insertional cloning into the cI gene.

Methods of cDNA cloning（cDNA 的克隆）

Incorporating cDNA into the vector.

The next challenge is to incorporate this collection of cDNAs into a vector so that it can be manipulated. One of the most convenient ways of doing this is to attempt to manipulate the cDNAs so that each one has a unique restriction site at those ends. To do this, the cDNAs are frequently methylated with a specific methyl transferase that incorporates a methyl group into a particular restriction site to protect them from the restriction enzyme that will be used later. Any 3' or 5' extensions must be then either eliminated by exonuclease treatment or filled in with polymerase. This produces a "blunt ended" molecule in which the 3' and 5' bases are in "register". It is then possible to ligate a synthetic oligonucleotide to the ends of this cDNA. Blunt end ligation is generally a low efficiency process; but, by using a high concentration of these synthetic oligonucleotides, it is possible to drive the reaction to near completion. These synthetic oligonucleotides can either be "**linkers**" (which are synthesized to have one blunt end and one end that have an "overhang" (*i.e.*, region of single stranded DNA) that is complementary to that produced by restriction enzymes or they can be "**adapters**" (which are a double-stranded DNA molecule that can be treated with an endonuclease to produce the appropriate overhang).

The value of producing an overhang is that it will facilitate the introduction of the cDNA into a vector. The vector can also be prepared by treating it with the same endonuclease, or an endonuclease that produces the same restriction site, to produce a single-stranded region that is complementary to the single-stranded region in the cDNA. Mixing the cDNA of interest with the vector in the presence of ligase allows incorporation of the cDNA into the vector. One of the experimental difficulties in doing this is that the vector itself will have a high tendency to re-ligate to form a vector without any cDNA insert. This is frequently minimized by treating the vector with phosphatase to remove the terminal phosphates. These phosphates are required for ligase to act, so this strategy prevents this unwanted side reaction.

① *Adaptor cloning*（接头克隆）

Two artificially synthesized adaptors each carrying one designed restriction site are introduced at both the 5' and 3' ends of the targeted cDNA respectively. After enzymatic cleavage with appropriate endonucleases, the adaptor-ligated cDNA can be cloned into the vector directionally.

② *Linker cloning*（引物 - 接头克隆）

Linkers with one end blunt and another sticky are adopted. After ligated to dscDNA with their blunt ends, the resulting linker-cDNA can be incorporated into an appropriate vector without enzymatic cleavage by endonucleases.

③ *Cloning cDNA via homopolymer tailing* (同聚尾克隆)

Double strand cDNA may be cloned by tailing a DNA or RNA with a homopolymer. This method is known as "homopolymer tailing".

With the homopolymer tailing method, using the terminal transferase, single strands are formed at the 3′ end of the HLZ DNA (a cDNA coding for human lysozyme) by the addition of nucleotides (preferably dGTP) at their "blunt" or "staggered" ends. In a separate reaction, the bacterial plasmid is linearized with a restriction endonuclease (when cloning HLZ cDNA the vector pUC9 was preferred) and given complementary tails (preferably dCTP) in order to obtain complementary single strands at the 3′ ends. In the next step, the homopolymer-extended double strand cDNA is mixed with the correspondingly complementarily-tailed vector in order to link it under suitable conditions. After recombination has occurred, CaCl$_2$-treated *E. coli* cells are transformed with this mixture and spread on selective plates. The clones containing HLZ cDNA may be identified by various known methods (*e.g.*, the colony hybridization technique). After the identification of corresponding clones, the plasmid DNA of each clone was extracted and the insertion was sequenced using the Maxam and Gilbert method or the Sanger method. Determination of the DNA sequence from the cDNA insertion from positive clones makes it possible to infer the amino acid sequence of the potential protein.

The main drawback of this method is that only plasmids can be used as vectors, hence it is difficult to preserve and screen such libraries. The reactions between plasmid and cDNA are uncontrollable. Since there is an extra homopolymeric tail on the synthesized cDNA, it is difficult to do further research such as expression. As a result, this method is seldom used nowadays.

④ *Okayama-Berg method* (*Okayama-Berg* 载体克隆)

The method of Okayama and Berg provided a major improvement in the quality of cDNA libraries. They employed a plasmid primer for first strand synthesis and used RNase H and DNA Pol I mediated nick translation to produce the cDNA second strand. Their procedure requires restriction endonuclease digestion of the mRNA:cDNA duplex, followed by the addition of a complementary linker piece to prime the second strand repair reaction. The Okayama and Berg procedure preferentially selects for long cDNAs (*i.e.*, the full- or nearly full length cDNA can be cloned), apparently due to preferential tailing of such templates. The resulting cDNA is then ligated to a vector, and a successful transformant is selected out using immunoscreening. Their procedure provides for moderately complex libraries with good representation of long cDNAs. However, their method is significantly more involved (复杂的) and demanding (苛刻的，要求高的) than most other procedures for generating cDNA libraries. It has already become the basis of many cDNA cloning approaches presently used.

Gubler and Hoffman adapted the second strand synthesis method of Okayama and Berg into their oligo dT primed procedure. Many different procedures now exist employing RNase H and DNA Pol I mediated second strand cDNA synthesis. These procedures vary in how the cDNA is inserted into the vector and which vector is chosen. For most oligonucleotide primed procedures, linkers or adaptors are added prior to cloning into an appropriately cut vector (either plasmid or phage). These procedures require restriction endonuclease treatment of the duplex cDNA prior to cloning and so run the risk of cleavage of the cDNA itself. Furthermore, these procedures suffer from a considerable number of null-insert clones. To decrease this background, size fractionation via chromatography must be done to remove free adaptors, oligonucleotides and the shorter cDNAs. Plasmid primed methods lead to very few null-insert clones, and hence avoid the need for fractionation.

Spickofsky and Margolskee describe modifications of the vectors and methods of Okayama and Berg which leads to a cDNA library construction procedure of increased efficiency (*i.e.*, higher complexity libraries). This new method also simplifies the cloning procedure, omitting the need for a separate linker piece. The procedure uses an asymmetrically tailed linker-primer plasmid: one end of the linker-primer has a 3′ terminal deoxythymidylate (脱氧胸苷酸) extension (the primer end), the other end has a 3′ terminal deoxycytidylate (脱氧胞苷酸) extension (the linker end). The linker end of the plasmid contains a 3′ phosphate group which blocks further 3′ extension at that end. The linker-primer plasmid can be used to prime first strand cDNA synthesis, and then as a bridge to initiate second strand cDNA synthesis. Libraries made by the linker-primer method are equivalent in final form to those made by the procedure of Okayama and Berg. However, the number of steps involved in library preparation is decreased and significantly greater numbers of independent transformants are generated by this method: typically 9×10^8 colonies per microgram of linker-primer DNA were obtained. This method should be useful for cases in which only small quantities of mRNA are available or cDNAs corresponding to extremely rare mRNAs are sought. These libraries are more convenient to prepare than phage based libraries, and yield 50-fold more clones per microgram of starting mRNA than do phage based methods.

⑤ *Single-stranded vector cloning* (单链载体克隆)

The method of hybrid and deletion is mainly applied to screen and identify cDNA clones encoding any subunits of multimeric protein. Based on this method, a specific group of mRNAs from all the subunits of the multi-function protein hybridize with cDNA library constructed with single-stranded cloning vector. If the mRNA that encodes one of subunits of this protein forms the hybrid molecule of DNA:RNA, the corresponding construction of mRNA deletion will be generated, which, as a result, is unable to translate to a functional protein. In case of a lack of the appropriate immunological reagents or nucleic acid probes, this method can be applied to screen cDNA clones encoding constitutive polypeptide subunits.

⑥ *MRNA:cDNA cloning* (*mRNA-cDNA* 克隆)

After first strand DNA is synthesized, the resulting mRNA-cDNA hybrid is arranged to be tagged with dA, then the newly formed hybrid is annealed to a plasmid tagging with dT at both the 5′ and 3′ ends. The polyA tail of cDNA forms hydrogen bond with plasmid dT, and polyA at 3′ end of mRNA forms hydrogen bond with dT at the end of plasmid. Then the recombinant (mRNA:cDNA hybrid-incorporated) vector is used directly to transform *E. coli*, and inside the host cell the mRNA on the hybrid will be decomposed and new strand DNA (second strand) will be complemented on the remaining single stranded DNA (first strand).

Amplification of a bacteriophage λ library (λ 噬菌体文库的扩增)

This protocol may be used for genomic DNA or cDNA libraries. A freshly packaged and titered library is adsorbed to log phase plating bacteria. The mixture is then plated at high density and allowed to grow until the plaques are just subconfluent. The phage are eluted from the plate by overnight incubation with phage buffer and the library is titered and stored.

Expression cDNA library（表达型 cDNA 文库）

Cloning vector

A **cloning vector** is a small piece of DNA, taken from a virus, a plasmid, or the cell of a higher organism, that can be stably maintained in an organism, and into which a foreign DNA fragment can be inserted for cloning purposes. The vector therefore contains features that allow for the convenient insertion or removal of DNA fragment in or out of the vector, for example by treating the vector and the foreign DNA with a restriction enzyme that creates the same overhang, then ligating the fragments together. After a DNA fragment has been cloned into a cloning vector, it may be further subcloned into another vector designed for more specific use.

There are many types of cloning vectors, but the most commonly used ones are genetically engineered plasmids. Cloning is generally first performed using *Escherichia coli*, and cloning vectors in *E. coli* include plasmids, bacteriophages (such as phage λ), cosmids, and bacterial artificial chromosomes (BACs). Some DNA however cannot be stably maintained in *E. coli*, for example very large DNA fragment, and other organisms such as yeast may be used. Cloning vectors in yeast include yeast artificial chromosomes (YACs).

Features of a cloning vector

All commonly used cloning vectors in molecular biology have key features necessary for their function such as a suitable cloning site and selectable marker. Others may have additional features specific to their use. For reason of ease and convenience, cloning is often performed using *E. coli*. Thus, the cloning vectors used often have elements necessary for their propagation and maintenance in *E. coli* such as a functional origin of replication (*ori*). The ColE1 origin of replication is found in many plasmids. Some vectors also include elements that allow them to be maintained in another organism in addition to *E. coli*, and these vectors are called **shuttle vector**.

Cloning site

All cloning vectors have features that allow a gene to be conveniently inserted into the vector or removed from it. This may be a **multiple cloning site (MCS)** which contains many unique restriction sites. The restriction sites in the MCS are first cleaved by restriction enzymes, and a PCR-amplified target gene, also digested with the same enzymes, is then ligated into the vectors using DNA ligase. The target DNA sequence can be inserted into the vector in a specific direction if so desired. The restriction sites may be further used for sub-cloning into another vector if necessary.

Other cloning vectors may use topoisomerase（拓扑异构酶）instead of ligase and cloning may be done more rapidly without the need for restriction digest of the vector or insert. In this **TOPO cloning** method a linearized vector is activated by attaching topoisomerase I to its ends, and this "TOPO-activated" vector may then accept a PCR product by ligating both the 5′ ends of the PCR product, releasing the topoisomerase and forming a circular vector in the process.

As illustrated in the Fig. 2-53, the "A" overhang on the blue PCR product insert comes from using *Taq* polymerase for the amplification step since *Taq* polymerase leaves a single deoxyadenosine (A) at the 3′ ends of PCR products. The complimentary "T" in the pair comes from a topoisomerase I-linearized backbone. DNA topoisomerase I (depicted as a green cloud) functions both as a restriction endonuclease and as a ligase by cleaving and rejoining supercoiled DNA ends to facilitate replication.

The TOPO technique specifically uses Vaccinia virus-isolated topoisomerase I as this enzyme recognizes the DNA sequence 5′- (C/T)CCTT-3′ and digests double stranded DNA at this sequence. The

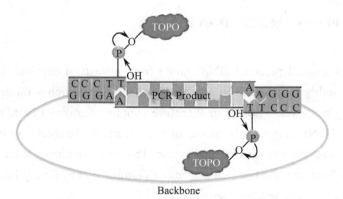

Fig. 2-53   Schematic diagram of TOPO cloning.

energy from this breakage is stored as a covalent bond between the cleaved 3′ DNA strand and a tyrosyl residue of topoisomerase I. If a 5′ hydroxyl group from a different DNA strand comes along, it can attack this covalent bond thus joining the two DNA strands and releasing topoisomerase.

Another method of cloning without the use of DNA digest and ligase is by DNA recombination, for example as used in the Gateway cloning system (通路克隆系统). The gene, once cloned into the cloning vector (called entry clone in this method), may be conveniently introduced into a variety of expression vectors by recombination.

Selectable marker

A selectable marker is carried by the vector to allow the selection of positively transformed cells. Antibiotic resistance is often used as marker, an example is the β-lactamase (β- 内酰胺酶) gene which confers resistance to the penicillin group of β-lactam (β- 内酰胺类) antibiotics like ampicillin (氨苄青霉素). Some vectors contain two selectable markers, for example the plasmid pACYC177 has both ampicillin and kanamycin (卡那霉素) resistance genes. Shuttle vector which is designed to be maintained in two different organisms may also require two selectable markers, although some selectable markers such as resistance to zeocin (吉欧霉素，腐草霉素 D1) and hygromycin B (潮霉素 B) are effective in different cell types. Auxotrophic (营养缺陷型的) selection markers that allow an auxotrophic organism to grow in minimal growth medium may also be used; examples of these are *LEU2* and *URA3* which are used with their corresponding auxotrophic strains of yeast.

Another kind of selectable marker allows for the positive selection of plasmid with cloned gene. This may involve the use of a gene lethal to the host cells, such as barnase (芽孢杆菌 RNA 酶), Ccda, and the parD/parE toxins. This typically works by disrupting or removing the lethal gene during the cloning process, and unsuccessful clones where the lethal gene still remains intact would kill the host cells, therefore only successful clones are selected.

Reporter gene

Reporter genes are used in some cloning vectors to facilitate the screening of successful clones by using features of these genes that allow successful clone to be easily identified. Such features present in cloning vectors may be the *lacZα* fragment for α complementation in **blue-white selection**, and/or marker gene or reporter genes in frame with and flanking the MCS to facilitate the production of fusion proteins. Examples of fusion partners that may be used for screening are the green fluorescent protein (GFP) and luciferase (荧光素酶).

Elements for expression

A cloning vector need not contain suitable elements for the expression of a cloned target gene, many however do, and may then work as an **expression vector**. The target DNA may be inserted into a site that is under the control of a particular promoter necessary for the expression of the target gene in the chosen host. Where the promoter is present, the expression of the gene is preferably tightly controlled and inducible so that proteins are only produced when required. Some commonly used promoters are the T7 and *lac* promoters. The presence of a promoter is necessary when screening techniques such as blue-white selection are used.

Cloning vectors without promoter and **ribosomal binding site** (RBS) for the cloned DNA sequence are sometimes used, for example when cloning genes whose products are toxic to *E. coli* cells. Promoter and RBS for the cloned DNA sequence are also unnecessary when first making a genomic or cDNA library of clones since the cloned genes are normally subcloned into a more appropriate expression vector if their expression is required.

Types of cloning vectors

A large number of cloning vectors are available, and choosing the vector may depend on a number of factors, such as the size of the insert, copy number and cloning method. Large insert may not be stably maintained in a general cloning vector, especially for those with a high copy number, therefore cloning large fragments may require more specialized cloning vector.

The pUC plasmid has a high copy number, contains a multiple cloning site, a gene for ampicillin antibiotic selection, and can be used for blue-white screen.

For more details, see section **2.3.3.1** and section **2.5**.

Screening: example of the blue/white screen

Many general purpose vectors such as pUC19 (Fig. 2-54) usually include a system for detecting the presence of a cloned DNA fragment, based on the loss of an easily scored phenotype. The most widely used is the gene coding for *E. coli* β-galactosidase, whose activity can easily be detected by the ability of the enzyme it encodes to hydrolyze the soluble, colorless substrate X-gal (5-bromo-4-chloro-3-indolyl-beta-d-galactoside) into an insoluble, blue product (5,5′-dibromo-4,4′-dichloro indigo). Cloning a fragment of DNA within the vector-based *lacZα* sequence of the β-galactosidase prevents the production of an active enzyme. If X-gal is included in the selective agar plates, transformant colonies are generally blue in the case

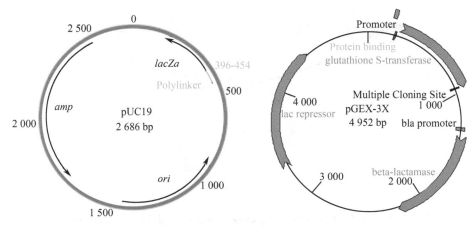

Fig. 2-54   Vector maps of cloning vector pUC19 and expression vector pGEX-3X.

of a vector with no inserted DNA and white in the case of a vector containing a fragment of cloned DNA.

Expression vector（表达型载体）

An **expression vector**, otherwise known as an **expression construct**, is usually a plasmid or virus designed for protein expression in cells. The vector is used to introduce a specific gene into a target cell, and can commandeer（征用，强占）the cell's mechanism for protein synthesis to produce the protein encoded by the gene. The plasmid is engineered to contain regulatory sequences that act as enhancer and promoter regions and lead to efficient transcription of the gene carried on the expression vector. The goal of a well-designed expression vector is the production of significant amount of stable messenger RNA, and therefore proteins. Expression vectors are basic tools for biotechnology and the production of proteins, for example insulin which is used for medical treatments of diabetes.

Elements of expression vectors（表达载体上的元件）

An expression vector has features that any vector may have, such as an **origin of replication**, a **selectable marker**, and a suitable site for the insertion of a gene such as the **multiple cloning site**. The cloned gene may be transferred from a specialized **cloning vector** to an **expression vector**, although it is possible to clone directly into an expression vector. The cloning process is normally performed in *Escherichia coli*, and vectors used for protein expression in organisms other than *E. coli* may have, in addition to a suitable origin of replication for its propagation in *E. coli*, elements that allow them to be maintained in another organism — **shuttle vectors**.

Elements for expression

An expression vector must have elements necessary for protein expression (Fig. 2-55). These may include a strong promoter, the correct translation initiation sequence such as a **ribosomal binding site** and **start codon**, a strong **termination codon**, and a **transcription termination sequence**. There are differences in the machinery for protein synthesis between prokaryotes and eukaryotes, therefore the

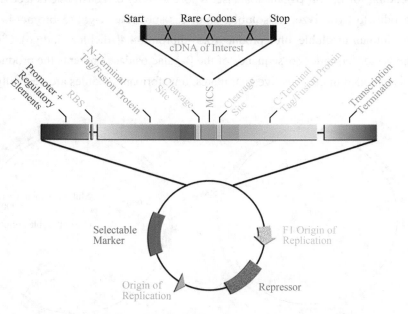

Fig. 2-55 Vector map of an expression vector. Highlighting the elements responsible for expression.

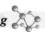

expression vectors must have the **elements for expression** that is appropriate for the chosen host. For example, prokaryotes expression vectors would have a **Shine-Dalgarno sequence**（SD 序列）at its **translation initiation site** for the binding of ribosomes, while eukaryotes expression vectors would contain the Kozak consensus sequence（科扎克共有序列）.

The promoter initiates the transcription and is therefore the point of control for the expression of the cloned gene. The promoters used in expression vector are normally inducible, meaning that protein synthesis is only initiated when required by the introduction of an inducer such as IPTG（异丙基 -β-D-1-硫代半乳糖苷）. Protein expression however may also be constitutive (*i.e.,* protein is constantly expressed) in some expression vectors. Low level of constitutive protein synthesis may occur even in expression vectors with tightly controlled promoters.

Protein tags

After the expression of the gene product, it is usually necessary to purify the expressed protein; however, separating the protein of interest from the great majority of proteins of the host cell can be a protracted process. To make this purification process easier, a purification tag may be added to the cloned gene. This tag could be **histidine (His) tag**, other marker peptides, or a **fusion partners** such as **glutathione S-transferase**（谷胱甘肽 S- 转移酶）or **maltose-binding protein**（麦芽糖结合蛋白）. Some of these fusion partners may also help to increase the solubility of some expressed proteins. Other fusion proteins such as **green fluorescent protein** may act as a **reporter gene** for the identification of successfully cloned genes.

Others

The expression vector is transformed or transfected into the host cell for protein synthesis. Some expression vectors may have elements for transformation or the insertion of DNA into the host chromosome, for example the *vir* genes for plant transformation, and integrase（整合酶）sites for chromosomal insertion.

Some vectors may include targeting sequence that may target the expressed protein to a specific location such as the **periplasmic space**（细胞周质间隙）of bacteria.

Applications

Laboratory use

Expression vector in an expression host is now the usual method used in laboratories to produce proteins for research. Most proteins are produced in *E. coli*, but for glycosylated proteins and those with disulfide bonds, yeast, baculovirus and mammalian systems may be used.

Production of peptide and protein pharmaceuticals

Most protein pharmaceuticals are now produced through recombinant DNA technology using expression vectors. These peptide and protein pharmaceuticals may be hormones, vaccines, antibiotics, antibodies, and enzymes. The first human recombinant protein used for disease management was insulin and it was introduced in 1982. Biotechnology allows these peptide and protein pharmaceuticals, some of which were previously rare or difficult to obtain, to be produced in large amount. It also reduces the risks of contaminants such as host viruses, toxins and prions（朊病毒）. For example, growth hormone extracted from pituitary glands harvested from human cadavers had caused Creutzfeldt-Jakob disease（克雅氏病）in patients receiving treatment for dwarfism（侏儒症）due to prion contamination, and viral contaminants in clotting factor Ⅷ isolated from human blood had resulted in the transmission of viral diseases such as hepatitis and AIDS. Such risk is reduced or removed completely when these proteins are produced in non-human cell-lines.

Transgenic plant and animals

In recent years, expression vectors have been used to introduce specific genes into plants and animals to produce transgenic organisms, for example in agriculture it is used to produce transgenic plants. Expression vectors have been used to introduce a vitamin A precursor, β-carotene（β-胡萝卜素）, into rice plants. This product is called **golden rice**. This process has also been used to introduce a gene into plants that produces an insecticide（杀虫剂）, called *Bacillus thuringiensis* **toxin**（苏云金杆菌毒素）or **Bt toxin** which reduces the need for farmers to apply insecticides since it is produced by the modified organism. In addition, expression vectors are used to extend the ripeness of tomatoes by altering the plant so that it produces less of the chemical that causes the tomatoes to rot. There has been controversy over using expression vectors to modify crops due to the fact that there might be unknown health risks, possibilities of companies patenting certain genetically modified food crops, and ethical concerns. Nevertheless, this technique is still being used and heavily researched.

Transgenic animals have also been produced to study animal biochemical processes and human diseases, or used to produce pharmaceuticals and other proteins. They may also be engineered to have advantageous or useful traits. **Green fluorescent protein** is sometimes used as tags which results in an animal that can fluoresce, and this has been exploited commercially to produce the fluorescent GloFish（荧光热带鱼）.

Gene therapy

Gene therapy is a promising treatment for a number of diseases where a "normal" gene carried by the vector is inserted into the genome, to replace an "abnormal" gene or supplement the expression of particular gene. Viral vectors are generally used but other nonviral methods of delivery are being developed. The treatment is still a risky option due to the viral vector used which can cause ill-effects, for example giving rise to（使发生，引起）insertional mutation that can result in cancer. However, there have been promising results.

cDNA non-expression library（非表达型 cDNA 文库）

Non-expression library：

In non-expression library, a target gene would not be expressed as a protein. However, every fragment is part of the screen, the screen is hybridization-based, *e.g.*, target gene can be screened by hybridization with nucleotide probe.

Non-expression library is suitable for the separation research of target gene which can be screened by hybridization with a nucleotide probe.

2.4 Tool enzyme commonly used in gene engineering（基因工程常用的工具酶）

In the research on genetic engineering, the most important tools are the enzymes that play a key role in various enzymatic reactions, such as nucleic acid restriction endonucleases, exonucleases, DNA ligases, reverse transcriptases, *etc*.

2.4.1 Restriction endonuclease（核酸限制性内切酶）

A **restriction enzyme** (or **restriction endonuclease**) is an enzyme that cleaves DNA into fragments at or near specific recognition nucleotide sequences known as **restriction sites**. Restriction enzymes are commonly classified into five types, which differ in their structure and whether they cut their DNA substrate at their recognition site, or if the recognition and cleavage sites are separate from one another. To cut DNA, all restriction enzymes make two incisions, once through each **sugar-phosphate backbone** (*i.e.,* each strand) of the DNA double helix.

These enzymes are found in bacteria and archaea and provide a defense mechanism against invading viruses. Inside a prokaryote, the restriction enzymes selectively cut up **foreign** DNA in a process called **restriction digestion**; meanwhile host DNA is protected by a modification enzyme (a methyltransferase) that modifies the prokaryotic DNA and blocks cleavage. Together, these two processes form the **restriction modification system**.

Over 3 600 restriction endonucleases are known, which represent over 250 different DNA specificities, and over 3 000 of them have been studied in detail, and more than 800 of these are available commercially. These enzymes are routinely used for DNA modification in laboratories, and are a vital tool in **molecular cloning**.

History

The term restriction enzyme originated from the studies of phage λ and the phenomenon of host-controlled restriction and modification of such bacterial phage or bacteriophage. The phenomenon was first identified in work done in the laboratories of Salvador Luria, Jean Weigle and Giuseppe Bertani in early 1950s. It was found that a bacteriophage λ that can grow well in one strain of *Escherichia coli*, for example *E. coli* C, when grown in another strain, for example *E. coli* K, its yields can drop significantly, by as much as 3~5 orders of magnitude. The host cell, in this example *E. coli* K, is known as the restricting host, and appears to have the ability to reduce the biological activity of the phage λ. If a phage becomes established in one strain, the ability of that phage to grow also become restricted in other strains. In the 1960s, it was shown in work done in the laboratories of Werner Arber and Matthew Meselson that the restriction is caused by an enzymatic cleavage of the phage DNA, and the enzyme involved was therefore termed a restriction enzyme.

The restriction enzymes studied by Arber and Meselson were type I restriction enzymes that cleave DNA randomly away from the recognition site. In 1970, Hamilton O. Smith, Thomas Kelly and Kent Wilcox isolated and characterized the first type II restriction enzyme, *Hind* II, from the bacterium *Haemophilus influenzae*. Restriction enzymes of this type are more useful for laboratory work as they cleave DNA at the site of their recognition sequence. Later, Daniel Nathans and Kathleen Danna showed that cleavage of simian virus 40 （SV40，猿猴空泡病毒 40）DNA by restriction enzymes yields specific fragments that can be separated using polyacrylamide gel electrophoresis, thus showing that restriction enzymes can also be used for mapping of the DNA. For their work in the discovery and characterization of restriction enzymes, the 1978 Nobel Prize for Physiology or Medicine was awarded to Werner Arber, Daniel Nathans, and Hamilton O. Smith. Their discovery of restriction enzymes allows DNA to be manipulated, leading to the development of recombinant DNA technology that has many applications, for example, the large scale production of human insulin for diabetics using *E. coli* bacteria.

Origins

Restriction enzymes likely evolved from a common ancestor and became widespread via **horizontal gene transfer**. In addition, there is mounting （逐渐增加的）evidence that restriction endonucleases evolved as a selfish（利己的）genetic element.

Recognition site

$$
\begin{array}{l}
5'\cdots GAT \mid ATC\cdots3' \\
3'\cdots CTA \mid TAG\cdots5'
\end{array}
$$

A palindromic（回文结构的，旋转对称的）recognition site reads the same on the reverse strand as it does on the forward strand when both are read in the same orientation.

Restriction enzymes recognize a specific sequence of nucleotides and produce a double-stranded cut in the DNA. The recognition sequences can also be classified by the number or bases in its recognition site, usually between 4 and 8 bases, and the number of bases in the sequence will determine how often the site will appear by chance in any given genome, *e.g.*, a 4-base pair sequence would theoretically occur once every 4^4 or 256 bp, 6 bases, 4^6 or 4 096 bp, and 8 bases would be 4^8 or 65 536 bp. Many of them are palindromic, meaning the base sequence reads the same backwards and forwards. In theory, there are two types of palindromic sequences that can be possible in DNA. The *mirror-like* palindrome is similar to those found in ordinary text, in which a sequence reads the same forwards and backwards on a single strand of DNA strand, as in GTAATG. The *inverted repeat* palindrome is also a sequence that reads the same forwards and backwards, but the forwards and backwards sequences are found in complementary DNA strands (*i.e.*, of double-stranded DNA), as in GTATAC (GTATAC being complementary to CATATG). Inverted repeat palindromes are more common and have greater biological importance than mirror-like palindromes.

*Eco*RI digestion produces "sticky" ends,

$$
\begin{array}{l}
G \mid AATTC \\
CTTAA \mid G
\end{array}
$$

whereas *Sma*I restriction enzyme cleavage produces "blunt" ends:

$$
\begin{array}{l}
CCC \mid GGG \\
GGG \mid CCC
\end{array}
$$

Recognition sequences in DNA differ for each restriction enzyme, producing differences in the length, sequence and strand orientation (5′ end or the 3′ end) of a sticky-end "overhang"（突出端，单链突出端）of an enzyme restriction.

Different restriction enzymes that recognize the same sequence are known as **neoschizomers**（异裂酶）. These often cleave in different locales（场所）of the sequence. Different enzymes that recognize and cleave in the same location are known as **isoschizomers**（同裂酶）.

Restriction enzyme digestion

Restriction enzymes recognize specific nucleotide sequences (**recognition sequences**) in double-stranded DNA, that are usually four, five or six nucleotides long, and then cut both strands of the DNA at specific locations. There are basically three ways in which the DNA can be cut; a staggered cut to leave a **5′ overhang** (*i.e.*, a short single-stranded region of DNA is left that has a 5′ end and overhangs the end of the double-stranded DNA), a staggered cut to leave a **3′ overhang**, or a cut in the same place on both strands to leave a **blunt end** (Fig. 2-56). For enzymes that cut in the staggered manner, the single-stranded tails are called **cohesive ends** because they allow any two DNA fragments produced by the same restriction enzyme to form complementary base pairs (Fig. 2-56). The cut ends can then be joined together (**ligated**) by an enzyme called **DNA ligase**. The new DNA molecule that has been made by joining the DNA fragments is called a **recombinant DNA molecule** (Fig. 2-11B). Blunt-ended DNA molecules can also be joined together by DNA ligase but the reaction is far less favorable.

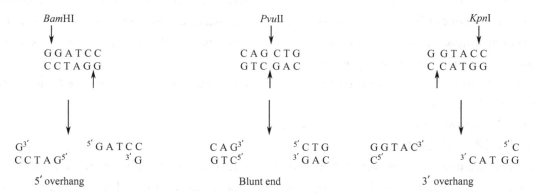

Fig. 2-56   The three types of cleavage by commonly used restriction enzymes.

Principles of nomenclature (命名原则)

Restriction endonucleases are generally named according to the bacterium from which they were isolated. Each enzyme is named after the bacterium from which it was isolated using a naming system based on bacterial **genus**, **species** and **strain**.

The first three letters of the enzyme name are the first letter of the genus name (属名) and the first two letters of the species name (种名). Additional letters or numbers indicate the strain of bacteria or specific enzyme from this organism — since each bacterium may contain several different restriction enzymes, a Roman numeral is also used to identify each enzyme. For example, the name of the *Eco*RI restriction enzyme was derived as shown in (Table 2-6).

Table 2-6   Derivation of the *Eco*RI name

Abbreviation	Meaning	Description
E	*Escherichia*	genus
co	*coli*	specific epithet （绰号，诨名）
R	RY13	strain
I	First identified	order of identification in the bacterium

Types

Naturally occurring restriction endonucleases are categorized into four groups (Types Ⅰ, Ⅱ, Ⅲ, and Ⅳ) based on their composition and enzyme cofactor requirements, the nature of their target sequence, and the position of their DNA cleavage site relative to the target sequence. DNA sequence analyses of restriction enzymes however show great variations, indicating that there are more than four types. All types of enzymes recognize specific short DNA sequences and carry out the endonucleolytic cleavage of DNA to give specific fragments with terminal 5′-phosphates. They differ in their recognition sequence, subunit composition, cleavage position, and cofactor requirements, as summarized below:

- Type Ⅰ enzymes (EC 3.1.21.3) cleave at sites remote from a recognition site; require both ATP and S-adenosyl-L-methionine to function; multifunctional protein with both restriction digestion and methylase (EC 2.1.1.72) activities.

- Type II enzymes (EC 3.1.21.4) cleave within or at short specific distances from a recognition site; most require magnesium; single function (restriction digestion) enzymes independent of methylase.

- Type III enzymes (EC 3.1.21.5) cleave at sites a short distance from a recognition site; require ATP (but do not hydrolyze it); S-adenosyl-L-methionine stimulates reaction but is not required; exist as part of a complex with a modification methylase (EC 2.1.1.72).

- Type IV enzymes target modified DNA, *e.g.*, methylated, hydroxymethylated and glucosyl-hydroxymethylated DNA.

- Type V enzymes utilize guide RNAs (gRNAs).

Type I （I型限制性内切酶）

Type I restriction enzymes were the first to be identified and were first identified in two different strains (K-12 and B) of *E. coli*. These enzymes cut at a site that differs, and is a random distance (at least 1 000 bp) away, from their recognition site. Cleavage at these random sites follows a process of DNA translocation, which shows that these enzymes are also molecular motors （分子马达，分子发动机）. The recognition site is asymmetrical and is composed of two specific portions — one containing 3~4 nucleotides, and another containing 4~5 nucleotides — separated by a non-specific spacer of about 6~8 nucleotides. These enzymes are multifunctional and are capable of both restriction digestion and modification activities, depending upon the methylation status of the target DNA. The cofactors S-Adenosyl methionine (AdoMet), hydrolyzed adenosine triphosphate (ATP), and magnesium (Mg^{2+}) ions, are required for their full activity. Type I restriction enzymes possess three subunits called *Hsd*R, *Hsd*M, and *Hsd*S; *Hsd*R is required for restriction; *Hsd*M is necessary for adding methyl groups to host DNA (methyltransferase activity) and *Hsd*S is important for specificity of the recognition (DNA-binding) site in addition to both restriction digestion (DNA cleavage) and modification (DNA methyltransferase) activity.

Type II （II型限制性内切酶）

Typical type II restriction enzymes differ from type I restriction enzymes in several ways. They are homodimers, with recognition sites usually undivided, palindromic and 4~8 nucleotides in length. They recognize and cleave DNA at the same site, and they do not use ATP or AdoMet for their activity — they usually require only Mg^{2+} as a cofactor (Fig. 2-57). These enzymes cleave the phosphodiester bond of double helix DNA. It can either cleave at the center of both strands to yield a blunt end, or at a staggered position leaving overhangs called sticky ends. These are the most commonly available and used restriction enzymes. In the 1990s and early 2000s, new enzymes from this family were discovered that did not follow all the classical criteria of this enzyme class, and new subfamily nomenclature was developed to divide this large family into subcategories based on deviations from typical characteristics of type II enzymes. These subgroups are defined using a letter suffix.

Type IIB restriction enzymes (*e.g.*, *Bcg*I and *Bpl*I) are multimers, containing more than one subunit. They cleave DNA on both sides of their recognition to cut out the recognition site. They require both AdoMet and Mg^{2+} cofactors. Type IIE restriction endonucleases (*e.g.*, *Nae*I) cleave DNA following interaction with two copies of their recognition sequence. One recognition site acts as the target for cleavage, while the other acts as an allosteric effector that speeds up or improves the efficiency of enzyme

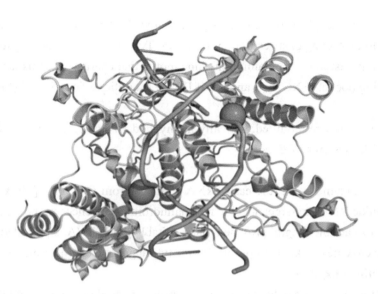

Fig. 2-57   Type II site-specific deoxyribonuclease. Structure of the homodimeric restriction enzyme *Eco*RI (cyan and green cartoon diagram) bound to double stranded DNA (brown tubes). Two catalytic magnesium ions (one from each monomer) are shown as magenta spheres and are adjacent to the cleaved sites in the DNA made by the enzyme (depicted as gaps in the DNA backbone).

cleavage. Similar to type II E enzymes, type II F restriction endonucleases (*e.g.*, *Ngo*MIV) interact with two copies of their recognition sequence but cleave both sequences at the same time. Type II G restriction endonucleases (*e.g.*, RM.*Eco*57I) do have a single subunit, like classical Type II restriction enzymes, but require the cofactor AdoMet to be active. Type II M restriction endonucleases, such as *Dpn*I, are able to recognize and cut methylated DNA. Type II S restriction endonucleases (*e.g.*, *Fok*I) cleave DNA at a defined distance from their non-palindromic asymmetric recognition sites, this characteristic is widely used to perform *in-vitro* cloning techniques such as Golden Gate cloning. These enzymes may function as dimers. Similarly, Type II T restriction enzymes (*e.g.*, *Bpu*10I and *Bsl*I) are composed of two different subunits. Some recognize palindromic sequences while others have asymmetric recognition sites.

Type III（III型限制性内切酶）

Type III restriction enzymes (*e.g.*, *Eco*P15) recognize two separate non-palindromic sequences that are inversely oriented. They cut DNA about 20~30 base pairs after the recognition site. These enzymes contain more than one subunit and require AdoMet and ATP cofactors for their roles in DNA methylation and restriction digestion, respectively. They are components of prokaryotic DNA restriction-modification mechanisms that protect the organism against invading foreign DNA. Type III enzymes are hetero-oligomeric, multifunctional proteins composed of two subunits, Res and Mod. The Mod subunit recognizes the DNA sequence specific for the system and is a modification methyltransferase; as such, it is functionally equivalent to the M and S subunits of type I restriction endonuclease. Res is required for restriction digestion, although it has no enzymatic activity on its own. Type III enzymes recognize short 5~6 bp-long asymmetric DNA sequences and cleave 25~27 bp downstream to leave short, single-stranded 5′ protrusions（突出，突出物）. They require the presence of two inversely oriented unmethylated recognition sites for restriction digestion to occur. These enzymes methylate only one strand of the DNA, at the N-6 position of adenosyl residues, so newly replicated DNA will have only one strand methylated, which is sufficient to protect against restriction digestion. Type Ⅲ enzymes belong to the beta-subfamily of N6 adenine methyltransferases, containing the nine motifs that characterize this family, including motif I, the AdoMet binding pocket (FXGXG), and motif IV, the catalytic region [S/D/N (PP) Y/F].

Type IV

Type IV enzymes recognize modified, typically methylated DNA and are exemplified (例证，例示) by the McrBC and Mrr systems of *E. coli*.

Type V

Type V restriction enzymes (*e.g.*, the cas9-gRNA complex from CRISPRs [成簇规则间隙短回文重复序列）] utilize guide RNAs to target specific non-palindromic sequences found on invading organisms. They can cut DNA of variable length, provided that a suitable guide RNA is provided. The flexibility and ease of use of these enzymes make them promising for future genetic engineering applications.

Artificial restriction enzymes

Artificial restriction enzymes can be generated by fusing a natural or engineered DNA-binding domain to a nuclease domain (often the cleavage domain of the type Ⅱ S restriction enzyme *Fok*I). Such artificial restriction enzymes can target large DNA sites (up to 36 bp) and can be engineered to bind to desired DNA sequences. Zinc finger nucleases (锌指核酸酶) are the most commonly used artificial restriction enzymes and are generally used in genetic engineering applications, but can also be used for more standard gene cloning applications. Other artificial restriction enzymes are based on the DNA binding domain of TAL effectors (转录激活子样效应器).

In 2013, a new technology CRISPR-Cas9, based on a prokaryotic viral defense system, was engineered for editing the genome, and it was quickly adopted in laboratories.

In 2017, a group from University of Illinois reported using an Argonaute protein (阿尔古蛋白) taken from *Pyrococcus furiosus* (强烈火球菌) (PfAgo) along with guide DNA to edit DNA *in vitro* as artificial restriction enzymes.

Artificial ribonucleases that act as restriction enzymes for RNA have also been developed. A PNA-based system, called a PNAzyme, has a Cu(Ⅱ)-2,9-dimethylphenanthroline group that mimics ribonucleases for specific RNA sequence and cleaves at a non-base-paired region (RNA bulge) of the targeted RNA formed when the enzyme binds the RNA. This enzyme shows selectivity by cleaving only at one site that either does not have a mismatch or is kinetically preferred out of two possible cleavage sites.

Examples

Examples of restriction enzymes are listed in Table 2-7.

Table 2-7　Commonly used restriction enzymes and their Recognition Sequence

Enzyme	Source	Recognition Sequence	Cut
*Eco*RI	*Escherichia coli*	5′GAATTC 3′CTTAAG	5′---G　　　AATTC---3′ 3′---CTTAA　　　G---5′
*Eco*R Ⅱ	*Escherichia coli*	5′CCWGG 3′GGWCC	5′---　　　CCWGG---3′ 3′---GGWCC　　　---5′
*Bam*HI	*Bacillus amyloliquefaciens*	5′GGATCC 3′CCTAGG	5′---G　　　GATCC---3′ 3′---CCTAG　　　G---5′

continued

Enzyme	Source	Recognition Sequence	Cut
*Hind*III	*Haemophilus influenzae*	5′AAGCTT 3′TTCGAA	5′---A AGCTT---3′ 3′---TTCGA A---5′
*Taq*I	*Thermus aquaticus*	5′TCGA 3′AGCT	5′---T CGA---3′ 3′---AGC T---5′
*Not*I	*Nocardia otitidis*	5′GCGGCCGC 3′CGCCGGCG	5′---GC GGCCGC---3′ 3′---CGCCGG CG---5′
*Hin*FI:"Hin"FI	*Haemophilus influenzae*	5′GANTC 3′CTNAG	5′---G ANTC---3′ 3′---CTNA G---5′
*Sau*3AI	*Staphylococcus aureus*	5′GATC 3′CTAG	5′--- GATC---3′ 3′---CTAG ---5′
*Pvu*II *	*Proteus vulgaris*	5′CAGCTG 3′GTCGAC	5′---CAG CTG---3′ 3′---GTC GAC---5′
Sma I *	*Serratia marcescens*	5′CCCGGG 3′GGGCCC	5′---CCC GGG---3′ 3′---GGG CCC---5′
*Hae*III *	*Haemophilus aegyptius*	5′GGCC 3′CCGG	5′---GG CC---3′ 3′---CC GG---5′
*Hga*I	*Haemophilus gallinarum*	5′GACGC 3′CTGCG	5′---NN NN---3′ 3′---NN NN---5′
*Alu*I*	*Arthrobacter luteus*	5′AGCT 3′TCGA	5′---AG CT---3′ 3′---TC GA---5′
*Eco*RV*	*Escherichia coli*	5′GATATC 3′CTATAG	5′---GAT ATC---3′ 3′---CTA TAG---5′
*Eco*P15I	*Escherichia coli*	5′CAGCAGN$_{25}$NN 3′GTCGTCN$_{25}$NN	5′---CAGCAGN$_{25}$ NN---3′ 3′---GTCGTCN$_{25}$NN ---5′
*Kpn*I	*Klebsiella pneumoniae*	5′GGTACC 3′CCATGG	5′---GGTAC C---3′ 3′---C CATGG---5′
*Pst*I	*Providencia stuartii*	5′CTGCAG 3′GACGTC	5′---CTGCA G---3′ 3′---G ACGTC---5′
*Sac*I	*Streptomyces achromogenes*	5′GAGCTC 3′CTCGAG	5′---GAGCT C---3′ 3′---C TCGAG---5′
*Sal*I	*Streptomyces albus*	5′GTCGAC 3′CAGCTG	5′---G TCGAC---3′ 3′---CAGCT G---5′
*Sca*I*	*Streptomyces caespitosus*	5′AGTACT 3′TCATGA	5′---AGT ACT---3′ 3′---TCA TGA---5′
*Spe*I	*Sphaerotilus natans*	5′ACTAGT 3′TGATCA	5′---A CTAGT---3′ 3′---TGATC A---5′
*Sph*I	*Streptomyces phaeochromogenes*	5′GCATGC 3′CGTACG	5′---GCATG C---3′ 3′---C GTACG---5′
*Stu*I*	*Streptomyces tubercidicus*	5′AGGCCT 3′TCCGGA	5′---AGG CCT---3′ 3′---TCC GGA---5′
*Xba*I	*Xanthomonas badrii*	5′TCTAGA 3′AGATCT	5′---T CTAGA---3′ 3′---AGATC T---5′

Applications

Isolated restriction enzymes are used to manipulate DNA for different scientific applications.

They are used to assist the insertion of genes into vectors (*e.g.*, plasmid vectors) during gene cloning and protein production experiments. For optimal use, plasmids that are commonly used for gene cloning are modified to include a short *polylinker* (多接头多位点人工接头) sequence (called the **multiple cloning site**, or **MCS**) rich in restriction enzyme recognition sequences. This allows flexibility when inserting gene fragments into the vector; restriction sites contained naturally within genes influence the choice of endonuclease for digesting the DNA, since it is necessary to avoid undesigned restriction digestion taking place within the **gene of interest** while intentionally digesting the **DNA to be inserted** at its terminal restriction endonuclease recognition sites. To clone a gene fragment into a vector, both the **DNA vector** and the **gene insert** are typically cut with the same restriction enzymes, and then glued together with the assistance of an enzyme known as a **DNA ligase**.

Restriction enzymes can also be used to distinguish gene alleles by specifically recognizing single base changes in DNA known as **single nucleotide polymorphisms (SNPs)**. This is however only possible if a SNP alters the restriction site present in the allele. In this method, the restriction enzyme can be used to genotype (确定基因型) a DNA sample without the need for expensive gene sequencing. The sample is first digested with the restriction enzyme to generate DNA fragments, and then the different sized fragments are separated by gel electrophoresis. In general, alleles with correct restriction sites will generate two visible bands of DNA on the gel, and those with altered restriction sites will not be cut and will generate only a single band. A DNA map by restriction digest (**restriction mapping**, 限制性酶切作图) that can give the relative positions of the genes and a specific pattern of bands after gel electrophoresis due to the different lengths of DNA generated by restriction digest reveals the sample subject's genotype.

In a similar manner, restriction enzymes are used to digest genomic DNA for gene analysis by Southern blot. This technique allows researchers to identify how many copies [or paralogues (旁系同源)] of a gene are present in the genome of one individual, or how many gene mutations (polymorphisms) have occurred within a population. The latter example is called **restriction fragment length polymorphism (RFLP)**.

Artificial restriction enzymes created by linking the *FokI* DNA cleavage domain with an array (大批, 一系列) of DNA binding proteins or zinc finger arrays, denoted by **zinc finger nucleases (ZFN)**, are a powerful tool for host genome editing (宿主基因组编辑) due to their enhanced sequence specificity. ZFN work in pairs, their dimerization being mediated *in-situ* through the *FokI* domain. Each zinc finger array (ZFA) is capable of recognizing 9~12 base-pairs, making for 18~24 for the pair. A 5~7 bp spacer (间隔区, 间隔子) between the cleavage sites further enhances the specificity of ZFN, making them a safe and more precise tool that can be applied in humans. A recent Phase I clinical trial of ZFN for the targeted abolition (废除) of the CCR5 co-receptor for HIV-1 has been undertaken.

Others have proposed using the bacteria restriction-modification system (R-M system) as a model for devising human anti-viral gene or genomic vaccines and therapies since the R-M system serves an innate defense role in bacteria by restricting tropism (生物向性反应) by bacteriophages. There is research on REases and ZFN that can cleave the DNA of various human viruses, including HSV-2 (单纯疱疹病毒2型), high-risk HPVs (人乳头状瘤病毒) and HIV-1, with the ultimate goal of inducing target mutagenesis（突变，诱变）and aberrations（畸变，失常）of human-infecting viruses. Interestingly, the human genome already contains remnants（残迹）of retroviral genomes that have been inactivated and harnessed（驾驭，利用，维护）for self-gain（自增益）. Indeed, the mechanisms for silencing active L1 genomic retroelements（逆转录因子，逆转录元件）by the **three prime repair exonuclease 1 (TREX1)** and **excision repair cross complementing 1（ERCC，切除修复交叉互补基因）** appear to mimic the action of R-M systems in bacteria, and the non-homologous end-joining（NHEJ，非同源性末端接合，非同源末端连接）that follows the use of ZFN without a repair template.

Isoschizomers（同裂酶）

Restriction enzymes from different organisms may recognize the same DNA sequence. If the enzymes recognize the same site (and cleave at the same position), they are labeled **isoschizomers**. For example, *Sph*I (CGTAC/G) and *Bbu*I (CGTAC/G) are isoschizomers of each other. The first enzyme discovered which recognizes a given sequence is known as the prototype; all subsequently identified enzymes that recognize that sequence (and cleave at the same position) are isoschizomers. Isoschizomers are isolated from different strains of bacteria and therefore may require different reaction conditions.

In some cases, only one out of a pair of isoschizomers can recognize both the methylated as well as unmethylated forms of restriction sites. In contrast, the other restriction enzyme can recognize only the unmethylated form of the restriction site. This property of some isoschizomers allows identification of methylation state of the restriction site while isolating it from a bacterial strain. For example, the restriction enzymes *Hpa*II and *Msp*I are isoschizomers, as they both recognize the sequence 5′-CCGG-3′ when it is unmethylated. But when the second C of the sequence is methylated, only *Msp*I can recognize it while *Hpa*II cannot.

Isocaudamers（同尾酶）

Isocaudamers are pairs of restriction enzymes that have slightly different recognition sequences but upon cleavage generate compatible cohesive ends with identical termini (overhang). For example the enzymes *Mbo*I and *Bam*HI are isocaudamers:

e.g.,   *Group 1*

*Mbo*I	*Bam*HI	*Sau*3AI
N↓GATCN	G↓GATCC	N↓GATCN
NCTAG↑N	CCTAG↑G	NCTAG↑N

Group 2

*Sal*I	*Xho*I
G↓TCGAC	C↓TCGAG
CAGCT↑G	GAGCT↑C

N represents any of the four nucleotides. Independently of which nucleotide is present when cleaving with *Mbo*I, after cleavage with either enzyme, all termini have the central tetranucleotide -GATC. This allows fragments generated with one enzyme to anneal with fragments generated with the other enzyme.

Neoschizomer（异裂酶）

Neoschizomers are restriction enzymes that recognize the same nucleotide sequence as their prototype but cleave at a different site. In some special applications this is a very helpful feature. Neoschizomers are a specific subset of isoschizomer.

For example: Prototype *Mae*II A^CGT produces DNA fragments with a 2-base 5′ extension.

Neoschizomer *Tai*I ACGT^ produces DNA fragments with a 4-base 3' extension.

Tai I
Recognition sequence

$$
\begin{array}{c}
\text{A C G T} \\
\text{T G C A}
\end{array}
\longrightarrow
\begin{array}{cc}
\text{xxxACGT} & \text{xxx} \\
\text{xxx} & \text{TGCAxxx}
\end{array}
$$

Mae II
Recognition sequence

$$
\begin{array}{c}
\text{A C G T} \\
\text{T G C A}
\end{array}
\longrightarrow
\begin{array}{cc}
\text{xxxA} & \text{CGTxxx} \\
\text{xxxTGC} & \text{Axxx}
\end{array}
$$

Recognition sequences and products of neoschizomers

Prototype *Apa*I GGGCC^C produces DNA fragments with a 4-base 3' extension. Neoschizomer *Bsp*120I G^GGCCC produces DNA fragments with a 4-base 5' extension.

*Sma*I (CCC/GGG) and *Xma*I (C/CCGGG) are neoschizomers of each other.

There are also other pairs of neoschizomers.

Factors affecting the action of restriction endonucleases （影响限制性内切酶活性的因素）

Concentration of DNA. Attention should be paid to removing proteins, residual organic solvents and salts in DNA samples. Samples can be treated with the corresponding RNase to remove RNAs.

The DNA conformation. Linear DNA strands are more readily cleaved by restriction endonuclease enzymes than superhelical DNAs. The efficiencies of certain restriction endonuclease enzymes to different restriction sites are not the same, which may be due to the difference in nucleotide composition between their flanking sequences.

Degree of DNA methylation. The endonuclease activity can be significantly inhibited by certain methylated nucleotides in the recognition sequence. The plasmid DNA isolated from *Escherichia coli* was in most cases mixed with two residual methylases: a) *dam* methylase, which catalyzes methylation of the adenine residue in a GATC sequence; b) *dem* methylase, which catalyzes the methylation of cytosine residue in a CCA/TGG sequence. Therefore plasmid DNA isolated from *E. coli* can only be partially cleaved by the restriction endonuclease enzymes. For this reason, some methylase (−) *Escherichia coli* strains are adopted to prepare plasmid DNAs for gene cloning. Whereas under certain conditions, the feature that restriction endonucleases can not cleave restriction sites with methylated nucleotides can be used as a way to achieve experimental purposes. If the restriction endonuclease recognition site is adjacent to a methylated sequence, the endonuclease activity at the recognition site will be inhibited, thus changing the sequence specificity of the endonuclease enzyme. In addition, when the DNA ends are modified with synthetic adapters, the internal restriction sites must be protected by methylation before the adapters are digested.

The temperature. Temperature is one of the important factors affecting the rate of enzymatic reaction. Different restriction endonuclease enzymes have different optimum temperature, most of which is 37℃. But some restriction endonuclease enzymes have lower optimum temperatures, such as 25℃ for *Sma*I, 30℃ for *Apa*I; Some restriction endonuclease enzymes require higher temperatures, such as 45℃ for *Mae*I and 50℃ for *Bcl*I.

Buffer. The buffer for restriction endonuclease contains magnesium chloride, sodium chloride or potassium chloride, Tris-HCl, β-mercaptoethanol or dithiothreitol and bovine serum albumin, among which the divalent cation (such as Mg^{2+}) is an absolutely necessary condition for the restriction endonuclease activity. If the reaction concentration is not appropriate, not only will the endonuclease activity decrease, the recognition sequence specificity will also change. For most restriction endonuclease enzymes, the optimum pH is 7.4. At present, many manufacturers provide MULTI-CORE™ buffer packs, suitable for a variety of endonuclease digestion reactions.

2.4.2 DNA ligase (DNA 连接酶)

In molecular biology, **DNA ligase** is a specific type of enzyme, a ligase (EC 6.5.1.1), that facilitates the joining of DNA strands together by catalyzing the formation of a phosphodiester bond. It plays a role in repairing single-strand breaks in duplex DNA in living organisms, but some forms (such as DNA ligase IV) may specifically repair double-strand breaks (*i.e.,* a break in both complementary strands of DNA). Single-strand breaks are repaired by DNA ligase using the complementary strand of the double helix as a template, with DNA ligase creating the final phosphodiester bond to fully repair the DNA (Fig. 2-58).

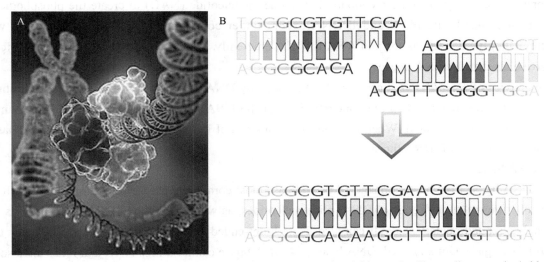

Fig. 2-58   A. DNA ligase repairing chromosomal damage; B. A pictorial example of how a ligase works (with sticky ends).

The ends created by a single enzyme are complementary, and can hydrogen bond over the short region of the overhang. However the weak hydrogen bonds between the bases are not sufficient to keep the DNA together, unless covalent bonds are regenerated in the phosphosugar backbone.

The lines above and below the sequence represent the phosphate-sugar backbone, which still contains a nick at the site where the two fragments came together. A few phosphodiester bond can be made by the enzyme DNA ligase (the same enzyme used in DNA replication), in an ATP dependent reaction. A single intact DNA molecule has now been regenerated. If this new arrangement for the fragments or they are from different sources, this is now a recombinant DNA molecule.

DNA ligase is used in both DNA repair and DNA replication (see *Mammalian ligases*). In addition, DNA ligase has extensive use in molecular biology laboratories for recombinant DNA experiments. Purified DNA ligase is used in gene cloning to join DNA molecules together to form recombinant DNA.

Ligase will also work with blunt ends, although higher enzyme concentrations and different reaction conditions are required.

Ligase mechanism

The mechanism of DNA ligase is to form two covalent phosphodiester bonds between 3′ hydroxyl ends of one nucleotide ("acceptor"), with the 5′ phosphate end of another ("donor"). Two ATP molecules are consumed for each phosphodiester bond formed. AMP is required for the ligase reaction, which proceeds in four steps:

(1) Reorganization of activity sites such as nicks in DNA segments or Okazaki fragments, *etc*.

(2) Adenylation (addition of AMP) of a lysine residue in the active center of the enzyme, pyrophosphate is released.

(3) Transfer of the AMP to the 5′ phosphate of the so-called donor, formation of a pyrophosphate bond.

(4) Formation of a phosphodiester bond between the 5′ phosphate of the donor and the 3′ hydroxyl of the acceptor.

Types of ligases

E. coli DNA ligase

The *E. coli* DNA ligase is encoded by the *lig* gene. DNA ligase in *E. coli*, as well as most prokaryotes, uses energy gained by cleaving nicotinamide adenine dinucleotide (NAD) to create the phosphodiester bond. It does not ligate blunt-ended DNA except under conditions of molecular crowding with polyethylene glycol, and cannot join RNA to DNA efficiently. *E. coli* DNA ligase is more specific for cohesive ends than T4 DNA ligase.

The activity of *E. coli* DNA ligase can be enhanced by DNA polymerase at the right concentrations. Enhancement only works when the concentrations of the DNA polymerase I are much lower than the DNA fragments to be ligated. When the concentrations of Pol I DNA polymerases are higher, it has an adverse effect on *E. coli* DNA ligase.

T4 DNA ligase

The DNA ligase from bacteriophage T4 is the ligase most-commonly used in laboratory research. It can ligate cohesive or "sticky" ends of DNA, oligonucleotides, as well as RNA and RNA-DNA hybrids, but not single-stranded nucleic acids. It can also ligate blunt-ended DNA with much greater efficiency than *E. coli* DNA ligase. Unlike *E. coli* DNA ligase, T4 DNA ligase cannot utilize NAD and it has an absolute requirement for ATP as a cofactor. Some engineering has been done to improve the *in vitro* activity of T4 DNA ligase; one successful approach, for example, tested T4 DNA ligase fused to several alternative DNA binding proteins and found that the constructs with either p50 or NF-κB as fusion partners were over 160% more active in blunt-end ligations for cloning purposes than wild type T4 DNA ligase. A typical reaction for inserting a fragment into a plasmid vector would use about 0.01 (sticky ends) to 1 (blunt ends) units of ligase. The optimal incubation temperature for T4 DNA ligase is 16℃.

Mammalian ligases

In mammals, there are four specific types of ligase:

• DNA ligase I: ligates the nascent DNA of the lagging strand after the Ribonuclease H has removed the RNA primer from the Okazaki fragments.

• DNA ligase III: complexes with DNA repair protein XRCC1 to aid in sealing DNA during the process of nucleotide excision repair and recombinant fragments. Of the all known mammalian DNA ligases, only Lig III has been found to be present in mitochondria.

• DNA ligase IV: complexes with XRCC4. It catalyzes the final step in the non-homologous end joining DNA double-strand break repair pathway. It is also required for V (D)J recombination, the process that generates diversity in immunoglobulin and T-cell receptor loci during immune system development.

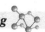

DNA ligase from eukaryotes and some microbes uses adenosine triphosphate (ATP) rather than NAD.

Thermostable ligases

Ligases from various thermophilic bacteria have been cloned and sequenced, and are available commercially for use in **ligase amplification reactions** because of their thermostable properties. For instance, Ampligase DNA Ligase is stable and active at much higher temperatures than conventional DNA ligases. Its half-life is 48 hours at 65℃ and greater than 1 hour at 95℃. Ampligase DNA Ligase has been shown to be active for at least 500 thermal cycles (94℃/80℃) or 16 hours of cycling. This exceptional thermostability permits extremely high hybridization stringency and ligation specificity.

Measurement of ligase activity

There are at least three different units used to measure the activity of DNA ligase:

● **Weiss unit** — the amount of ligase that catalyzes the exchange of 1 nmole of ^{32}P from inorganic pyrophosphate to ATP in 20 minutes at 37℃. This is the one most commonly used

● **Modrich-Lehman unit** — this is rarely used, and one unit is defined as the amount of enzyme required to convert 100 nmoles of $d(A-T)_n$ to an exonuclease-III resistant form in 30 minutes under standard conditions

● Many commercial suppliers of ligases use an arbitrary unit based on the ability of ligase to ligate cohesive ends. These units are often more subjective than quantitative and lack precision

Applications in molecular biology research

DNA ligases have become indispensable tools in modern molecular biology research for generating recombinant DNA sequences. For example, DNA ligases are used with restriction enzymes to insert DNA fragments, often genes, into plasmids.

Controlling the optimal temperature is a vital aspect of performing efficient recombination experiments involving the ligation of cohesive-ended fragments. Most experiments use T4 DNA ligase (isolated from bacteriophage T4), which is most active at 37℃. However, for optimal ligation efficiency with cohesive-ended fragments ("sticky ends"), the optimal enzyme temperature needs to be balanced with the melting temperature T_m of the sticky ends being ligated, the homologous pairing of the sticky ends will not be stable because the high temperature disrupts hydrogen bonding. A ligation reaction is most efficient when the sticky ends are already stably annealed, and disruption of the annealing ends would therefore result in low ligation efficiency. The shorter the overhang, the lower the T_m.

Since blunt-ended DNA fragments have no cohesive ends to anneal, the melting temperature is not a factor to consider within the normal temperature range of the ligation reaction. However, the higher the temperature, the lower the chance that the ends to be joined will be aligned (匹配，使成一对) to allow for ligation (molecules move around the solution more at higher temperatures). The limiting factor in blunt end ligation is not the activity of the ligase but rather the number of alignments between DNA fragment ends that occur. The most efficient ligation temperature for blunt-ended DNA would therefore be the temperature at which the greatest number of alignments can occur. The majority of blunt-ended ligations are carried out at 14~25℃ overnight. The absence of stably annealed ends also means that the ligation efficiency is lowered, requiring a higher ligase concentration to be used.

History

The first DNA ligase was purified and characterized in 1967. The common commercially available DNA ligases were originally discovered in bacteriophage T4, *E. coli* and other bacteria.

2.4.3   Polymerases (聚合酶)

2.4.3.1   *Escherichia coli DNA polymerase I* (大肠埃希菌 *DNA* 聚合酶 *I*)

The *E. coli* **DNA polymerase I** (or **Pol I**) is an enzyme that participates in the process of DNA replication. Discovered by Arthur Kornberg in 1956, it was the first known DNA polymerase (and, indeed, the first known of any kind of polymerase). It was initially characterized in *E. coli* and is ubiquitous in prokaryotes. In *E. coli* and many other bacteria, the gene that encodes Pol I is known as ***polA***. The *E. coli* form of the enzyme is composed of 928 amino acids, a single chain protein with a molecular weight of 109 000, and is an example of a processive (前进的，进行的，向前的) enzyme — it can sequentially catalyze multiple polymerizations.

E. coli **DNA Polymerase I is a DNA-dependent DNA polymerase that possesses both 3′→5′ and 5′→3′ exonuclease activities.** It requires magnesium as a cofactor. Each of its three enzymatic activities is encapsulated into distinct domains of the holoenzyme, such that proteolytic deletions can be generated that lack one or more of the activities. The so-called Klenow fragment is one such molecule that is widely used in recombinant DNA work.

DNA Polymerase I

Pol I possesses four enzymatic activities:

(1) A 5′→3′ (forward) DNA-Dependent DNA polymerase activity, requiring a 3′ primer site and a template strand.

(2) A 3′→5′ (reverse) exonuclease activity that mediates proofreading.

(3) A 5′→3′ (forward) exonuclease activity mediating nick translation during DNA repair.

(4) A 5′→3′ (forward) RNA-Dependent DNA polymerase activity. Pol I operates on RNA templates with considerably lower efficiency (0.1%~0.4%) than it does DNA templates, and this activity is probably of only limited biological significance.

In the replication process, RNase H removes the RNA primer (created by Primase) from the lagging strand and then Polymerase I fills in the necessary nucleotides between the Okazaki fragments in a 5′→3′ direction, proofreading for mistakes as it goes. It is a template-dependent enzyme — it only adds nucleotides that correctly base pair with an existing DNA strand acting as a template. DNA ligase then joins the various fragments together into a continuous strand of DNA.

Despite its early characterization, it quickly became apparent that Polymerase I was not the enzyme responsible for most DNA synthesis — DNA replication in *E. coli* proceeds at approximately 1 000 nucleotides/second, while the rate of base pair synthesis by Polymerase I averages only between 10 and 20 nucleotides/second. Moreover, its cellular abundance of approximately 400 molecules per cell did not correlate with the fact that there are typically only two replication forks in *E. coli*. Moreover, it is insufficiently processive to copy an entire genome, as it falls off after incorporating only 25~50 nucleotides. Its role in replication was proven when, in 1969, John Cairns isolated a viable Polymerase I mutant that lacked the polymerase activity. Cairns′ lab assistant, Paula De Lucia, created thousands of cell free extracts from *E. coli* colonies and assayed them for DNA-polymerase activity. The 3 478th clone contained the polA mutant, which was named by Cairns to credit (归功于，赞颂) "Paula" [De Lucia]. It was not until the discovery of DNA polymerase Ⅲ that the main replicative DNA polymerase was finally identified.

The physiological role of Pol I

Is DNA polymerase I the major replicative polymerase of *E. coli*? For more than 10 years, this was thought to be the case; however, there were some problems:

➢ Pol I is not processive enough [~ 200 NT on a gapped（有缺口的）DNA template].

➢ Pol I turnover number is too low (only ~ 600 nt/min/mol; or 10 nt/sec). The replication fork in *E. coli* moves at roughly 1 000 nt/sec. at 37℃. (Based on 4.7×10^6 bp, and a known chromosomal replication time of ~40 min.)

The most important challenge arrived with the isolation of *E. coli* mutants severely deficient in Pol I (in 1969). Since then, several mutants have been isolated (the original was called polA). All viable（能生存的）polA mutants make some residual amount of enzyme, and all have $5' \rightarrow 3'$ exonuclease activity. The original polA mutants grow at a normal rate, but are very susceptible to UV irradiation and other agents that damage DNA. This indicates a role for Pol I in DNA repair (more later).

But it also turns out that Pol I is essential for chromosomal replication — it plays an important role in primer removal and joining of nascent DNA fragments (Okazaki fragment processing; more later). This is why all viable polA mutants have at least some function, and more precisely why all have $5' \rightarrow 3'$ exonuclease activity. Both of these processes (repair and primer removal) require $5' \rightarrow 3'$ exonuclease activity.

Therefore, Pol I is an essential enzyme, even if not the major replicative polymerase. Pol I mutations that destroy polymerase activity are not lethal. (Presumably another pol can substitute.) But Pol I mutations that destroy $5' \rightarrow 3'$ exonuclease activity are lethal.

Research applications

DNA polymerase I can be used in:

(1) Nick translation of DNA（DNA 缺口平移）

Nick translation is a tagging technique in molecular biology in which DNA Polymerase I is used to replace some of the nucleotides of a DNA sequence with their labeled analogues, creating a tagged DNA sequence which can be used as a probe in Fluorescent *in situ* hybridization or blotting techniques.

This process is called nick translation because the DNA to be processed is treated with DNase to produce single-stranded "nicks"（缺口）. This is followed by replacement in nicked sites by DNA polymerase I, which elongates the 3' hydroxyl terminus, removing nucleotides by $5' \rightarrow 3'$ exonuclease activity, and replacing them with dNTPs (Fig. 2-59). To radioactively label a DNA fragment for use as a probe in blotting procedures, one of the incorporated nucleotides provided in the reaction is radiolabeled in the alpha phosphate position. Similarly, a fluorophore（荧光团）can be attached instead for fluorescent labeling, or an

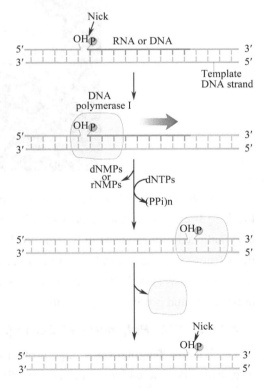

Fig. 2-59   Nick translation of DNA.

antigen for immunodetection. When DNA polymerase I eventually detaches（脱落）from the DNA, it leaves another nick in the phosphate backbone. The nick has "translated（转移）" some distance depending on the processivity of the polymerase. This nick could be sealed by DNA ligase, or its 3′ hydroxyl group could serve as the template for further DNA polymerase I activity. Proprietary（专有的）enzyme mixes are available commercially to perform all steps in the procedure in a single incubation.

(2) 3′-protruding end labeling of DNA（3′黏端的末端标记）

DNA polymerase I was used frequently in the early days of recombinant DNA technology for radiolabeling DNA and synthesizing cDNA. However, other enzymes have proven to be more effective for these purposes, including a proteolytic fragment of DNA polymerase I called Klenow fragment and T4 DNA polymerase. The holoenzyme DNA polymerase I is no longer frequently used.

In 1984, Yousaf S.I., *et al* published their findings about 3′-end labeling of DNA: Blunt and 3′-protruding ends were labeled more efficiently with [alpha-^{32}P] ddATP using than were the 5′-ends with [gamma-^{32}P] ATP using by standard methods. This improvement in efficiency of labeling DNA and the simplicity of the method allows 3′-end labeling of DNA to become a realistic alternative to 5′-end labeling.

For radiolabeling DNA, 2 steps are involved:

First, the overhanging 3′ terminus is cleaved by the 3′→5′ exonuclease activity of **Pol I** and leave 3′ recessed terminus; then the polymerase activity of **Pol I** will reconcile with the 3′→5′ exonuclease activity of **Pol I,** hence there is an equilibrium between 3′ exonuclease degradation and 3′ dNTP incorporation, provided that a high concentration of dNTPs are present. If dNTPs are labeled, then the resulting products are 3′ labeled DNA.

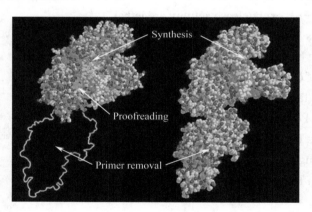

DNA polymerase I obtained from *E. coli* is used extensively for molecular biology research. However, the 5′→3′ exonuclease activity makes it unsuitable for many applications. Fortunately this undesirable enzymatic activity can be simply removed from the holoenzyme（全酶）to leave a useful molecule called the Klenow fragment, widely used in molecular biology. Exposure of DNA polymerase I to the protease subtilisin（枯草杆菌蛋白酶）cleaves the molecule into a smaller fragment, which retains only the DNA polymerase and proofreading activities.

2.4.3.2 *DNA Polymerase I, Large (Klenow) Fragment*（大肠埃希菌 DNA 聚合酶 I 大片段）

The **Klenow fragment** is a large protein fragment produced when DNA polymerase I from *E. coli* is enzymatically cleaved by the protease subtilisin. First reported in 1970, it retains the 5′→3′ polymerase activity and the 3′→5′ exonuclease activity for removal of precoding（预编码）nucleotides and proofreading, but loses its $5'\rightarrow 3'$ exonuclease activity.

The other smaller fragment formed when DNA polymerase I from *E. coli* is cleaved by subtilisin retains the $5'\rightarrow 3'$ exonuclease activity but does not have the other two activities exhibited by the Klenow fragment (*i.e.*, $5'\rightarrow 3'$ polymerase activity, and $3'\rightarrow 5'$ exonuclease activity).

Research

Because the $5'\rightarrow 3'$ exonuclease activity of DNA polymerase I from *E. coli* makes it inapplicable to many applications, the Klenow fragment, which lacks this activity, can be very useful in research. The Klenow fragment is extremely useful for research-based tasks such as:

➢ Synthesis of double-stranded DNA from single-stranded templates.
➢ Filling in receded 3′ ends of DNA fragments to make 5′ overhang blunt.
➢ Digesting away protruding 3′ overhangs.
➢ Preparation of radioactive DNA probes.

The Klenow fragment was also the original enzyme used for greatly amplifying segments of DNA in the polymerase chain reaction (PCR) process, before being replaced by thermostable enzymes such as *Taq* polymerase.

The exo-Klenow fragment

Just as the $5'\rightarrow 3'$ exonuclease activity of DNA polymerase I from *E. coli* can be undesirable, the $3'\rightarrow 5'$ exonuclease activity of Klenow fragment can also be undesirable for certain applications. This problem can be overcome by introducing mutations in the gene that encodes Klenow. This results in forms of the enzyme being expressed that retain $5'\rightarrow 3'$ polymerase activity, but lack any exonuclease activity ($5'\rightarrow 3'$ or $3'\rightarrow 5'$). This form of the enzyme is called the **exo-Klenow fragment**.

The exo-Klenow fragment is used in some fluorescent labeling reactions for microarray（微阵列，微阵列芯片）, and also in dA and dT tailing, an important step in the process of ligating DNA adapters to DNA fragments, frequently used in preparing DNA libraries for Next-Gen sequencing.

The Klenow fragment of DNA polymerase I

Pol I actually appears to be three enzymes in one polypeptide (**polymerase,** $3'\rightarrow 5'$ exonuclease, $5'\rightarrow 3'$ exonuclease). Interestingly, mild digestion of Pol I with protease (trypsin, subtilisin) cleaves the 109 kDa protein into two active fragments: a large C-terminal (Klenow) fragment (76 kDa) containing the **polymerase** and $3'\rightarrow 5'$ exonuclease, and a small fragment that contains the $5'\rightarrow 3'$ exonuclease activity.

The separation of Pol I has practical consequences, because the **Klenow fragment** (KF) is a very valuable enzyme in the laboratory. It can be used for cDNA synthesis, flush-ending restriction fragments with 5′-overhangs, and labeling DNA (random primer method, *etc.*).

It is also important to note that, when mixed together, the large and small subunits of Pol I can carry out nick translation. Besides being interesting from an evolutionary point of view, this observation illustrates an important concept: exonuclease activities are not always an intrinsic part of a polymerase. In some cases, exonucleases functionally associate with the polymerase.

The structure of DNA polymerase I

As we have seen, the $5'\rightarrow 3'$ exonuclease and polymerase activities act coordinately in nick translation, even though they use different termini. It is easy to visualize how this might occur — different termini are bound by different active sites on the enzyme, with the $5'\rightarrow 3'$ exonuclease domain ahead of the Klenow fragment (KF).

Insight into this and other important questions has come from analysis of the crystal structures of KF and other polymerases. High-resolution analysis of the crystal structure of KF (residues 324~928) shows that the polymerase domain resembles a right hand gripping a double helix, with a separate juxtaposed（并列的）exonuclease domain (Fig. 2-60).

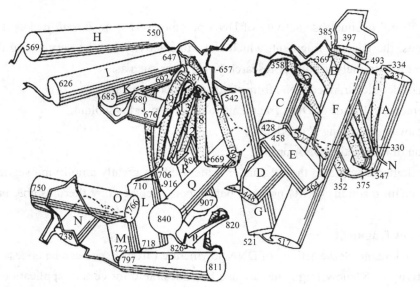

Fig. 2-60 Schematic drawing of the course of the polypeptide in the Klenow fragment. Regions in β-sheet structure are represented by arrows numbered from the fragment N-terminus and those in α-helix are represented by tubes lettered from the N-terminus. The break indicated between helices I and H is at the position of a partially disordered 50 residues (not included). The division between large and small domains is the loop between helices F and G.

The 3′→5′ exonuclease domain

As noted above, KF can be divided into two domains. The 3′→5′ exonuclease domain is the smaller of the two (amino acids 324~517). It is composed of 4 antiparallel β sheets surrounded by α helices. This domain contains a dNMP binding site, which corresponds to the exonuclease active site. The 3′-OH can hydrogen bond with threonine 358 (ddNMPs can't do this, which explains why ddNTPs bind poorly and are not efficiently removed by the exonuclease). Also, there is no apparent hydrogen bonding between the dNMP purine and pyrimidine bases and the protein; this is expected because all four dNMPs must fit into this site. Mutants in the dNMP binding site lack exonuclease activity but retain polymerase activity. This confirms that the primer terminus can be bound by two different sites in the Klenow fragment: the exonuclease active site and the polymerase active site (formerly called the primer terminus site).

The polymerase domain

The polymerase domain is the larger of the two, and binds both template primers and dNTPs. When separately expressed, it has polymerase but not exonuclease activity. In addition, mutations in amino acids that contribute to the polymerase catalytic site affect polymerase activity but not exonuclease activity.

The polymerase domain encompasses amino acids 521~928. It is mainly helical, and its most distinctive feature is a deep cleft ("palm") that is large enough to accommodate B-form duplex DNA (20~25 Å wide and 25~35 Å deep). The cleft is located between helices I and O. A six-stranded β sheet forms the bottom of the cleft, and α helices form the sides. One side is longer than the other and could curl over like "fingers", the opposite side resembles a "thumb". Positive charge is distributed in the cleft, which facilitates interaction with the negatively charged DNA backbone. As the DNA passes through the crevice (palm) , it enters from the direction of the exonuclease domain and is bent by as much as 45° .

Structural contributions to processivity

The thumb domain has been implicated in processivity (*i.e.,* the ability of the enzyme to remain associated with the template-primer over many catalytic cycles). At the tip of the thumb, a disordered "flap" of about 50 amino acids that can close over the helix is apparent. (The flap is between helices H and I). Closure of the flap apparently slows the rate of DNA dissociation and contributes to processivity. In support of this idea, deletion of the tip of the KF thumb reduces processivity by about a factor of four（四倍）. Thus the flap is sometimes called the "processivity domain".

Structural contributions to catalysis (nucleotidyl transfer) and fidelity — a stepwise mechanism of DNA synthesis

The active site residues lie in palm domain. The primer terminus is believed to interact with tyrosine 776 (Y776). In addition, two essential aspartate residues, D705 and D882, also lie at the base of the palm. As we shall see later, it is these acidic residues that bind the Mg^{2+} ions that are essential for catalysis. The second substrate, dNTP, is bound by a pocket in the fingers domain. Interestingly, there are no hydrogen bonds formed between the enzyme and the new base pair formed by the template and the incoming nucleotide. This is useful, because there are four different types of nucleotides that must enter the dNTP site.

The fidelity of a polymerase, its ability to discriminate between correct and incorrect dNTPs, is obviously critical. As we have just learned, however, discrimination is not based on interactions with individual bases. Instead, the correct addition (and error discrimination) depends on relative nucleotide affinity and ultimately is based on shape. Consider:

➤ Since there are no base-specific interactions between the enzyme and dNTP, all four have an equal opportunity to enter the dNTP site.

➤ However, those that can form a Watson-Crick base pair have a higher affinity for the template base than those that do not. Hence they are more likely to be incorporated.

➤ A correct Watson-Crick base pair has the correct shape (steric complementarity) , and "fits" better than a mispair.

To see this more clearly, we can break the polymerase reaction down into a series of steps, some of which are associated with changes in the shape of the enzyme. The multistep process provides several opportunities to discriminate between correct and incorrect nucleotides.

➤ The initial step involves binding the template-primer (to form a binary complex). This results in a conformational change in which the thumb closes down around the DNA.

➤ Binding of the correct dNTP forms a productive polymerizing complex (a ternary complex). This favors the correct nucleotide by a factor of 10^2 to 10^3.

➤ Once a dNTP is bound, another conformational change occurs in which the fingers rotate toward the palm. This moves the correct dNTP closer to the active site and into position for catalysis. This strongly favors a correct Watson-Crick base pair, as only these have the correct fit. This has the effect of increasing polymerase fidelity to about 10^4 to 10^5. The closing of the fingers may be the rate limiting step.

➤ After polymerization the fingers open again to release pyrophosphate and permit entry of another

Fundamentals, Approaches and Breakthroughs in R & D Genetically Engineered Biotherapeutics

dNTP. The template-primer translocates（易位）and rotates relative to the enzyme so that the new primer terminus is in the primer-binding site.

Adding an incorrect base greatly decreases the rate of polymerization, primarily because the primer terminus is efficiently bound to the primer binding site only when it is properly base paired. This gives the $3'{\rightarrow}5'$ exonuclease activity a chance to act on the primer terminus. This editing function further increases fidelity by a factor of about 10^2.

Structural data indicate that the $3'{\rightarrow}5'$ exonuclease and polymerase activities reside on separate domains of KF, and are about 30 Å apart. Yet both the polymerase active site and the exonuclease active site compete for the same primer terminus. So DNA binding must differ in the polymerase and exonuclease reactions.

A hypothesis to explain this suggests that mispairing stimulates exonuclease activity by leading to partial melting of duplex DNA (~3 bp or so). DNA bending would further help to destabilize the helix and help shift the equilibrium toward ssDNA in a mispaired duplex. Melting seems to be important, because while the palm cleft can accommodate a duplex, the crevice leading to the exonuclease site isn't big enough and can only accept ssDNA. Conversely, proper base pairing favors interaction between the primer terminus and the polymerase active site.

2.4.3.3　T4 DNA polymerase（T4 DNA 聚合酶）

T4 is a bacteriophage of *E. coli*. The activities of T4 DNA polymerase are very similar to Klenow fragment of DNA polymerase I — it functions as a $5'{\rightarrow}3'$ DNA polymerase and a $3'{\rightarrow}5'$ exonuclease, but does not have $5'{\rightarrow}3'$ exonuclease activity.

In general, T4 DNA polymerase is used for the same types of reactions as Klenow fragment, particularly in blunting the ends of DNA with 5' or 3' overhangs. There are, however, two differences between the two enzymes that have practical signficance:

The $3'{\rightarrow}5'$ exonuclease activity of T4 DNA polymerase is roughly 200 times that of Klenow fragment, making it preferred by many investigators for blunting DNAs with 3' overhangs. While Klenow fragment will displace downstream oligonucleotides as it polymerizes, T4 DNA polymerase will not. This attribute makes T4 DNA polymerase the more efficient choice for certain types of oligonucleotide mutagenesis reactions.

The bacteriophage T4 DNA polymerase was also initially used in PCR. It has a higher fidelity of replication than the Klenow fragment, but is also destroyed by heat.

Description

T4 DNA Polymerase catalyzes the $5'{\rightarrow}3'$ synthesis of DNA from a primed single-stranded DNA template. Although possessing a potent $3'{\rightarrow}5'$ proofreading exonuclease, T4 DNA Polymerase contains no $5'{\rightarrow}3'$ exonuclease activity.

T4 DNA Polymerase can be used to fill 5' protruding ends with labeled or unlabeled dNTPs or for the generation of blunt ends from DNA molecules with 3' overhangs.

Features

High Fidelity: T4 DNA Polymerase is the enzyme of choice for applications where misincorporation is a concern.

Flexible: T4 DNA Polymerase may be used in a variety of molecular applications. Active in many Promega 1 × restriction enzyme buffers.

240

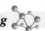

May Be Heat-Inactivated: T4 DNA Polymerase is inactivated by heating at 75℃ for 10 minutes.

Provided with 10 × Reaction Buffer: 250 mM Tris-acetate (pH 7.7), 1 M potassium acetate and 10 mM DTT.

Applications

Flush（齐平）5′ protruding ends with labeled or unlabeled dNTPs.

Blunt 3′ overhangs.

In vitro mutagenesis.

2.4.3.4　T7 DNA polymerase（T7 DNA 聚合酶）

The T7 DNA polymerase of the T7 bacteriophage is a DNA-dependent DNA polymerase responsible for the fast rate of T7 phage DNA replication *in vivo*. The polymerase consists of a 1 : 1 complex of the viral T7 gene 5 protein (80 kDa) and the *E. coli* thioredoxin（硫氧还蛋白）(12 kDa).

It lacks a 5′→3′ exonuclease domain, but the 3′→5′ exonuclease activities are approximately 1 000-fold greater than that of Klenow fragment. The exonuclease activity appears to be responsible for the high fidelity of this enzyme and prevents strand displacement（移位，转位，置换）synthesis.

This polymerase is unique due to its considerable processivity, or ability to stay on DNA for a greater than average number of base pairs. This makes it particularly useful for recombinant protein expression systems; Using the T7 promoter and T7 polymerase strongly drive the inserted gene of interest without inducing host protein overexpression. It is also suitable for site-directed mutagenesis, but is not recommended for DNA sequencing applications.

Applications

Labeling 3′-termini of DNA fragments with protruding 5′ ends (Fill-In Reaction).

Labeling the 3′-termini of blunt-ended DNA fragments or the termini of DNA fragments with protruding 3′-termini (Exchange Reaction).

Site-directed mutagenesis.

Not suitable for DNA sequencing due to high exogenous levels of exonuclease activities.

Another Pol I family enzyme — T7 DNA polymerase

T7 is an *E. coli* bacteriophage that encodes its own DNA polymerase. Phage T7 polymerase is a small, single polypeptide enzyme (gp5, ~80 kDa) that contains a highly active 3′→5′ exonuclease activity in addition to a 5′→3′ polymerase activity. It is the enzyme responsible for replicating the ~35 kbp dsDNA phage genome.

A 5′→3′ exonuclease activity is encoded by another phage gene. Its product (gp6) can associate with T7 pol during replication. The gp6 protein shows strong homology to the 5′→3′ exonuclease domain of Pol I. So T7 is an example of a divided Pol I type enzyme; it has separate polypeptides which provide the Klenow (5′→3′ polymerase and 3′→5′ exonuclease) and 5′→3′ exonuclease activities.

T7 pol is structurally homologous to the KF of Pol I and like Pol I, it is not a very processive polymerase. However, a high degree of processivity is required to rapidly duplicate the relatively large phage genome. How is this achieved?

The answer to this question is quite surprising. In the cell, T7 pol exists in a tight 1 : 1 complex with thioredoxin (12 kDa). Thioredoxin is a cellular protein that normally functions as a redox coenzyme for ribonucleotide（核糖核苷酸）reductase, an enzyme system that synthesizes deoxyribonucleotides（脱氧核苷酸）from ribonucleotide diphosphates.

In the T7 system, thioredoxin is recruited as a processivity factor. In a complex with T7 pol, thioredoxin clamps pol to the template primer, resulting in a 50-fold increase in activity and about a 1 000-fold increase in processivity. It does this without binding DNA, and without the help of other accessory factors. How this unique association of cellular and viral proteins came to be is not clear, but we now know how it works.

Recently, the structure of T7 pol complexed with a template primer, dNTP, and *E. coli* thioredoxin was solved. As expected, the enzyme is quite similar to Pol I in structure, while some important information regarding dNTP binding and polymerase translocation was obtained from this study. Most interestingly, it was found that thioredoxin associates with a flexible loop extending from the thumb region (the processivity domain) of the polymerase. This suggested that the thumb and thioredoxin could swing across the DNA binding groove to encircle the template primer — essentially forming a lid over the active site that functions like a clamp. So the thioredoxin clamp converts a Pol I-like enzyme into a highly processive, replicative polymerase.

Further support for this mechanism has come from genetic and biochemical studies in which the thumb region of T7 pol was grafted onto the tip of KF. These studies showed that the T7 thumb could confer a thioredoxin-dependent increase in KF processivity.

The T7 pol-thioredoxin (gp5-trx) complex is highly active and processive and today is widely used for the Sanger sequencing reaction (in preference to Klenow). A modified form of the enzyme, minus the $3' \rightarrow 5'$ exonuclease domain, is marketed commercially (as "Sequenase"). T7 polymerase has several advantages over the Klenow fragment for DNA sequencing:

➢ Its high processivity allows it to read through secondary structure(s) in the template better than Klenow.

➢ It better tolerates nucleoside analogues (dITP vs. dGTP) that can improve electrophoretic resolution in sequencing gels.

2.4.3.5 *Sequenase*（测序酶）

Sequenase DNA Polymerase is derived from Bacteriophage T7 DNA polymerase which has been chemically or genetically modified to eliminate its $3' \rightarrow 5'$ exonuclease activity, and became the first easy-to-use DNA sequencing products.

Sequenase is the modified form of T7 DNA polymerase developed by the United States Biochemical Corporation, which has more than 99% of its 3' to 5' exonuclease activity excised. While Sequenase Version 2 has its whole $3' \rightarrow 5'$ exonuclease activity excised, hence an ideal enzyme for sequencing long DNA fragments using dideoxy chain termination approach.

The modified version of the T7 DNA polymerase is the sequencing enzyme most commonly used, T7 gene 5 encodes a protein with a molecular weight of 80 kDa, which consists of two independent domain structures, with one of the structural domains highly homologous to the DNA binding domain and polymerization domain of *E. coli* DNA polymerase I. This binding and polymerization domain occupies the sequence of the protein close to the C-terminal, while the N-terminal is responsible for its strong $3' \rightarrow 5'$ exonuclease activity. When T7 DNA polymerase is incubated with oxygen, a reducing agent and low concentration of ferric ion for several days, the exonuclease activity of the enzyme would be inactivated, while the polymerase activity of the protein would not be significantly changed. So the modified version of T7 gene 5 protein-thioredoxin complex (namely Sequenase) exhibits an extremely high processivity, and has become an ideal enzyme for sequencing long DNA fragments in dideoxy chain termination reaction. Currently, the enzyme has been produced and commercialized by United States Biochemical Co. with a registered trademark of sequenase®.

Sequenase™ Version 2.0 DNA Polymerase is a re-modified form of T7 DNA polymerase. It has virtually no $3' \rightarrow 5'$ exonuclease activity, which is more favorable for DNA sequencing.

Sequenase Version 2.0 is highly processive, incorporates nucleotide analogs (dITP, thio-dNTPs, dideoxy-NTPs, *etc.*), is not impeded by secondary structures, and can carry out strand displacement synthesis. It is an excellent enzyme for dideoxy-sequencing, and is useful in other applications, especially where the absence of associated exonuclease activity is desirable.

Sequenase Version 2.0 has two subunits, one is the *E. coli* protein thioredoxin (MW 12 000) and the other is a genetically engineered version of bacteriophage T7 gene 5 protein (MW 76 000). The genetic changes in this subunit (a deletion of 28 amino acids accomplished by *in vitro* mutagenesis) eliminate all measurable exonuclease activity without changing the DNA polymerase activity.

Bacteriophage T7 DNA polymerase — sequenase

An ideal DNA polymerase for chain-terminating DNA sequencing should possess the following features: (1) incorporate dideoxy and other modified nucleotides at an efficiency similar to that of the cognate deoxynucleotides; (2) high processivity; (3) high fidelity in the absence of proofreading/exonuclease activity; and (4) production of clear and uniform signals for detection. The DNA polymerase encoded by bacteriophage T7 is naturally endowed with or can be engineered to have all these characteristics. The chemically or genetically modified enzyme (Sequenase) expedited significantly the development of DNA sequencing technology.

DNA polymerases catalyze the synthesis of DNA, a pivot（关键的）process in both living organisms and in biotechnology. Family A DNA polymerases including *Escherichia coli* DNA polymerase I, *Taq* DNA polymerase, and T7 DNA polymerase have served as prototypes for biochemical and structural studies on DNA polymerases and have been widely used as molecular reagents.

A DNA polymerase activity from bacteriophage T7 was first observed in an *E. coli* mutant deficient in DNA polymerase I infected with bacteriophage T7. The initial characterization of T7 DNA polymerase was intriguing. Although the gene responsible for the polymerase activity was mapped to gene 5, gene 5 protein (gp5) itself had what appeared to be no DNA polymerase activity but only ssDNA exonuclease activity. Apparently a host component was required to reconstitute the full DNA polymerase. This host factor turned out to be a small redox protein-*E. coli* thioredoxin. The redox capacity of thioredoxin, however, is not required for stimulation of the DNA polymerase activity. Instead thioredoxin plays a structural role in stabilizing the binding of gene 5 protein to a primer-template and increases the processivity of the polymerase more than 100-fold, representing a unique function of this universal protein. Thioredoxin binds to a 71-residue loop of T7 gene 5 protein, which is not present in other Pol I -type polymerases, resulting in a stable 1 : 1 complex ($K_D = 5$ nM).

Another intriguing finding during the initial characterization of T7 DNA polymerase is on its exonuclease activity. T7 DNA polymerase lacks the $5' \rightarrow 3'$ exonuclease activity found in *E. coli* DNA polymerase I but does possess a strong $3' \rightarrow 5'$ single and double stranded DNA exonuclease activity. The double stranded DNA exonuclease activity requires the presence of thioredoxin. Interestingly, various protein purification procedures, depending on the presence or absence of EDTA in the buffer, can generate T7 DNA polymerases that differ significantly in their exonuclease activity, resulting in two forms of DNA polymerase. By comparison of the two forms of polymerase and careful tracking of the purification procedures, it was revealed that the exonuclease activity of T7 DNA polymerase could be specifically inactivated in an oxidation reaction by oxygen, a reducing agent and ferrous ion. The easily modifiable exonuclease and extraordinary processivity of T7 DNA polymerase kindled the emergence of a powerful tool in the DNA sequencing era.

Sequenase era

Invented by Sanger *et al.* (1977), the method of chain-terminating sequencing initiated a revolution toward the genome-sequencing era. However, the enzymes initially used for chain-terminating sequencing, the Klenow fragment of *E. coli* DNA polymerase I and avian myeloblastosis virus (AMV, 禽成髓细胞瘤病毒) reverse transcriptase, had low processivity (~15 nt for Klenow fragment and 200 for AMV reverse transcriptase, the latter has a relatively higher processivity but its rate of DNA synthesis is only several nucleotides per second). Processivity describes the number of nucleotides continuously incorporated by a DNA polymerase using the same primer-template without dissociation. Thus if the DNA polymerase used for chain-terminating sequencing is non-processive, artifactual bands will arise at positions corresponding to the nucleotide at which the polymerase dissociated. Frequent dissociation will create a strong background that obscures the true DNA sequence. Although the issue can be partially improved by long time incubation with a high concentration of substrates that may "chase" those artifactual bands up to higher molecular weight. The procedure is not an ideal solution since reinitiation of primer elongation at dissociation sites (usually regions of compact secondary structure or hairpins) is inefficient and may result in the incorporation of incorrect nucleotides. Although T7 DNA polymerase itself has a processivity of only a few nucleotides, the association with *E. coli* thioredoxin dramatically increases its processivity. Consequently, with T7 DNA polymerase termination of a sequencing reaction will occur only at positions where a chain-termination agent (such as a dideoxynucleotide) is incorporated, yielding a long DNA sequence.

A more severe problem with DNA polymerase used prior to T7 DNA polymerase is the discrimination against dideoxynucleotides, the chain-terminating nucleotides used in Sanger sequencing. Most of the known DNA polymerase strongly discriminate against ddNTP. For example, T4 DNA polymerase, *E. coli* DNA polymerase I, *Taq* DNA polymerase, and Vent DNA polymerase incorporate a dideoxynucleoside monophosphate (ddNMP) at least 1 000 times slower than the corresponding deoxynucleoside monophosphate (dNMP). To use these polymerases in DNA sequencing a high radio of ddNTP to dNTP must be used for efficient chain termination. Even though the overall incorporation of ddNMP can be improved in such an uneconomic way, wide variation in the intensity of adjacent fragments still occurs because the extent of discrimination varies with different DNA sequences and structures. T7 DNA polymerase, however, is at the other end of the spectrum, discriminating against ddNTP only several fold. Thus a much lower concentration of ddNTP can be used with T7 DNA polymerase and the uniformity of DNA bands on the gel is much higher. The discrimination was further lowered by replacing magnesium with manganese in the sequencing reaction. With Mn^{2+} in an isocitrate buffer, T7 DNA polymerase incorporates dNMP and ddNMP at same rate, resulting in uniform terminations of sequencing reactions.

With the naturally endowed high processivity and the lack of discrimination against ddNTP, the only hindrance for T7 DNA polymerase as a DNA sequencing enzyme is its robust $3' \rightarrow 5'$ exonuclease activity. Exonuclease activity increases the fidelity of DNA synthesis by excising newly synthesized bases incorrectly base-paired to the template. For applications like PCR it is often a desired feature. While for DNA sequencing such activity is detrimental since when the dNTP concentration falls, the rate of exonuclease activity increases close to that of polymerase activity, resulting in no net DNA synthesis or degradation of DNA. The associated exonuclease activity will also cause DNA polymerase to idle at regions with secondary structures in the template, producing variability in the intensity of signals. The iron-catalyzed oxidation mentioned above can produce modified T7 DNA polymerase with greatly reduced exonuclease activity, and this chemically modified enzyme was the basis for sequenase and the first easy-to-use DNA sequencing kits commercialized by United States Biochemical Co. However, the residual exonuclease activity can still result in some loss of labeled DNA bands upon prolonged incubation. Tabor and Richardson carried out an extensive chemical and mutagenesis screen for selective elimination of the exonuclease activity of T7 DNA polymerase. The rapid screening of a large number of mutants was based on the observation that exonuclease minus mutants of T7 DNA polymerase can synthesize through a specific hairpin region in the DNA template. As a result many mutants deficient in exonuclease activity were revealed and among them a mutant lacking 28 amino acids in the N-terminal exonuclease domain had no detectable exonuclease activity, while its polymerase activity is significantly higher than that of the wild type protein. This mutant was the basis of version 2 of Sequenase. Sequenase pioneered development of thermostable enzymes and facilitated the automation of high-throughput sequencing.

Degradation of a DNA fragment can occur via a nucleophilic attack on the 3'-terminal internucleotide linkage by H_2O or pyrophosphate (PPi). The $3' \rightarrow 5'$ exonuclease catalyzes the former reaction, generating dNMP or ddNMP. The latter reaction is called pyrophosphorolysis（焦 磷 酸 解）. As the reversal of polymerization, pyrophosphorolysis generates dNTP or ddNTP, sometimes resulting in "holes": the disappearance of ddNMP labeled DNA fragments on the gel. By adding pyrophosphatase to the reaction to cleave PPi the pyrophosphorolysis can be eliminated. The combination of modified T7 DNA polymerase, manganese ion, and pyrophosphatase can generate accurate and uniform bands on a DNA sequencing gel to the extent that, the DNA sequence can be directly determined by the relative intensity of each band if different amount of the four ddNTPs are added at certain ratio.

Themostability is a highly desired feature for DNA polymerase. A thermostable enzyme like *Taq* DNA polymerase is superior for cycle sequencing, in which multiple rounds of DNA synthesis are carried out from the same template, with the newly synthesized DNA strand released after each cycle by heat denaturation. The heat stable DNA polymerase survives the denaturation step and is available for the next cycle of polymerization. Cycle sequencing allows much less DNA template and polymerase to be used in a sequencing reaction. In cycle sequencing, low processivity is an advantage because a polymerase with low processivity cycles rapidly, decreasing the chance of strong specific stops. However, the strong discrimination against ddNTP (at least 100-fold, often 10 000-fold) by most thermostable DNA polymerase was a significant obstacle for their use in cycle sequencing. Although the use of manganese ion can decrease the discrimination, manganese has several disadvantages compared with magnesium such as narrow working concentration, precipitation, and less activity of DNA polymerase than that supported by magnesium ion.

Studies on T7 DNA polymerase led to one of the most elegant demonstrations of enzyme engineering and turned *Taq* DNA polymerase into "Thermo sequenase". To pursue the molecular mechanism underlying the discrepancy in discrimination against ddNTP among family A DNA polymerases, Tabor and Richardson swapped (交换) the five most conserved regions in the crevice (裂缝，裂隙) responsible for binding DNA and NTPs between T7 DNA polymerase and *E. coli* DNA polymerase I, based on the 3D structure of *E. coli* DNA polymerase I. By an SDS-DNA activity assay, the "Helix O" from *E. coli* DNA polymerase I was observed to confer strong discrimination against ddNTP to T7 DNA polymerase. Further mutagenesis in this region revealed that the tyrosine-526 in T7 DNA polymerase or the homologous position phenylalanine-762 in *E. coli* DNA polymerase I was the single determinant for discrimination against ddNTP. When the corresponding residue, F667 in *Taq* DNA polymerase was replaced with tyrosine, the modified *Taq* DNA polymerase F667Y actually preferred ddNTP 2-fold over dNTP, comparing to the 6 000-fold discrimination against ddNTP by the wild-type enzyme. *Taq* DNA polymerase F667Y, with its naturally endowed superior thermostability and engineered elimination of discrimination against ddNTP, was the basis for "Thermo sequenase" , an enzyme that greatly expedited the Human Genome Project.

2.4.3.6 *Reverse transcriptase* (逆转录酶)

A **Reverse transcriptase (RT)** is an enzyme used to generate complementary DNA (cDNA) from an RNA template, a process termed *reverse transcription*. It is mainly associated with retroviruses. However it should be noted that non-retroviruses also use RT (for example, the hepatitis B virus, a member of the Hepadnaviridae (肝脱氧核糖核酸病毒科，嗜肝病毒种), which are dsDNA-RT viruses, while retroviruses are ssRNA viruses). RT inhibitors are widely used as antiretroviral drugs. RT activities are also associated with the replication of chromosome ends [telomerase (端粒酶)] and some mobile genetic elements [retrotransposons (反转录转座子)].

Retroviral RT has three sequential biochemical activities:

(a) RNA-dependent DNA polymerase activity

(b) Ribonuclease H (核糖核酸酶 H)

(c) DNA-dependent DNA polymerase activity

These activities are used by the retrovirus to convert single-stranded genomic RNA into double-stranded cDNA which can integrate into the host genome, potentially generating a long-term infection that can be very difficult to eradicate. The same sequence of reactions (一系列的反应) is widely used in the laboratory to convert RNA to DNA for use in molecular cloning, RNA sequencing, polymerase chain reaction (PCR), or genome analysis.

Well studied reverse transcriptases include:

● HIV-1 reverse transcriptase from human immunodeficiency virus type 1 (PDB 1HMV) has two subunits, which have respective molecular weights of 66 and 51 kilodaltons.

● M-MLV reverse transcriptase from the Moloney murine leukemia virus [M-MLV，莫洛尼 (氏) 鼠白血病病毒] is a single 75 kDa monomer.

● AMV reverse transcriptase from the avian myeloblastosis virus (禽成髓细胞性白血病病毒) like HIV also has two subunits, a 63 kDa subunit and a 95 kDa subunit.

● Telomerase reverse transcriptase (端粒酶逆转录酶) that maintains the telomeres (端粒) of eukaryotic chromosomes.

Function in viruses

The enzymes are encoded and used by reverse-transcribing viruses, which use the enzyme during the process of replication. Reverse-transcribing RNA viruses, such as retroviruses, use the enzyme to reverse-transcribe their RNA genomes into DNA, which is then integrated into the host genome and replicated along with it. Reverse-transcribing DNA viruses, such as the hepadnaviruses（嗜肝 DNA 病毒）, can allow RNA to serve as a template in assembling, and making DNA strands. HIV infects humans with the use of this enzyme. Without reverse transcriptase, the viral genome would not be able to incorporate into the host cell, resulting in failure to replicate.

Process of reverse transcription

Reverse transcriptase creates single-stranded DNA from an RNA template.

In virus species with reverse transcriptase lacking DNA-dependent DNA polymerase activity, creation of double-stranded DNA can possibly be done by host-encoded DNA polymerase δ, mistaking the viral DNA-RNA for a primer and synthesizing a double-stranded DNA by a similar mechanism as in **primer removal**, where the newly synthesized DNA displaces the original RNA template.

The process of reverse transcription is extremely error-prone and it is during this step that mutations may occur. Such mutations may cause **drug resistance**.

Retroviral reverse transcription

Retroviruses, also referred to as class VI ssRNA-RT viruses, are RNA reverse transcribing viruses with a DNA intermediate. Their genomes consist of two molecules of positive-sense（正义链，正链）single stranded RNA with a 5′ cap and 3′ polyadenylated tail. Examples of retroviruses include the human immunodeficiency virus (HIV) and the human T-lymphotropic virus (HTLV，人体 T 细胞白血病病毒). Creation of double-stranded DNA occurs in the cytosol（细胞溶质）as a series of these steps:

(1) A specific cellular tRNA acts as a primer and hybridizes to a complementary part of the virus genome called the **primer binding site** or **PBS.**

(2) Complementary DNA then binds to the U5 (non-coding region) and R region (a direct repeat found at both ends of the RNA molecule) of the viral RNA.

(3) A domain on the reverse transcriptase enzyme called RNase H degrades the 5′ end of the RNA which removes the U5 and R region.

(4) The primer then 'jumps' to the 3′ end of the viral genome and the newly synthesized DNA strands hybridizes to the complementary R region on the RNA.

(5) The first strand of complementary DNA (cDNA) is extended and the majority of viral RNA is degraded by RNase H.

(6) Once the strand is completed, second strand synthesis is initiated from the viral RNA.

(7) There is then another 'jump' where the PBS from the second strand hybridizes with the complementary PBS on the first strand.

(8) Both strands are extended further and can be incorporated into the hosts genome by the enzyme integrase.

Creation of double-stranded DNA also involves **strand transfer**, in which there is a translocation of short DNA product from initial RNA dependent DNA synthesis to acceptor template regions at the other end of the genome, which are later reached and processed by the reverse transcriptase for its DNA-dependent DNA activity.

Retroviral RNA is arranged in 5′ terminus to 3′ terminus. The site where the primer is annealed to viral RNA is called the **primer-binding site (PBS).** The RNA 5′ end to the PBS site is called **U5**, and the RNA 3′ end to the PBS is called the **leader**. The tRNA primer is unwound between 14 and 22 nucleotides and forms a base-paired duplex with the viral RNA at PBS. The fact that the PBS is located near the 5′ terminus of viral RNA is unusual because reverse transcriptase synthesize DNA from 3′ end of the primer in the 5′ to 3′ direction (with respect to the RNA template). Therefore, the primer and reverse transcriptase must be relocated to 3′ end of viral RNA. In order to accomplish this reposition (复位), multiple steps and various enzymes including DNA polymerase, ribonuclease H (RNase H) and polynucleotide unwinding are needed.

The HIV reverse transcriptase also has ribonuclease activity that degrades the viral RNA during the synthesis of cDNA, as well as DNA-dependent DNA polymerase activity that copies the *sense* cDNA strand into an *antisense* DNA to form a double-stranded viral DNA intermediate (vDNA).

In eukaryotes

Self-replicating stretches of eukaryotic genomes known as retrotransposons (逆转录转座子) utilize reverse transcriptase to move from one position in the genome to another via an RNA intermediate. They are found abundantly in the genomes of plants and animals. Telomerase is another reverse transcriptase found in many eukaryotes, including humans, which carries its own RNA template; this RNA is used as a template for DNA replication.

In prokaryotes

Initial reports of reverse transcriptase in prokaryotes came as far back as 1971. These have since been broadly described as part of bacterial **Retron（反转录子）msr RNAs**, distinct sequences which code for reverse transcriptase, and are used in the synthesis of msDNA（多拷贝单链 DNA）. In order to initiate synthesis of DNA, a primer is needed. In bacteria, the primer is synthesized during replication.

Evolutionary role

Valerian Dolja of Oregon State argues that viruses due to their diversity have played an evolutionary role in the development of cellular life, with reverse transcriptase playing a central role.

Structure

Reverse transcriptase enzymes include an RNA-dependent DNA polymerase and a DNA-dependent DNA polymerase, which work together to perform transcription. In addition to the transcription function, retroviral reverse transcriptases have a domain belonging to the RNase H family which is vital to their replication.

Replication fidelity

There are three different replication systems during the life cycle of a retrovirus. First of all, the reverse transcriptase synthesizes viral DNA from viral RNA, and then from newly made complementary DNA strand. The second replication process occurs when host cellular DNA polymerase replicates the integrated viral DNA. Lastly, RNA polymerase II transcribes the proviral DNA into RNA which will be packed into virions. Therefore, mutation can occur during one or all of these replication steps.

Reverse transcriptase has a high error rate when transcribing RNA into DNA since, unlike most other DNA polymerases, it has no proofreading ability. This high error rate allows mutations to accumulate at an accelerated rate relative to proofread forms of replication. The commercially available reverse transcriptases produced by Promega are quoted by their manuals as having error rates in the range of 1 in 17 000 bases for AMV and 1 in 30 000 bases for M-MLV.

Other than creating single nucleotide polymorphisms, reverse transcriptases have also been shown to be involved in processes such as **transcript fusions**, **exon shuffling** (外显子改组) and creating artificial antisense transcripts. It has been speculated that this **template switching** (模板转换) activity of Reverse Transcriptase, which can be demonstrated completely *in vivo*, may have been one of the causes for finding several thousand unannotated (未注释的) transcripts in the genomes of model organisms.

Applications

Antiviral drugs

As HIV uses reverse transcriptase to copy its genetic material and generate new viruses (part of a retrovirus proliferation circle), specific drugs have been designed to disrupt the process and thereby suppress its growth. Collectively, these drugs are known as reverse transcriptase inhibitors and include the nucleoside and nucleotide analogues zidovudine (齐多夫定) (trade name Retrovir), lamivudine (拉米夫定) (Epivir) and tenofovir (替诺福韦) (Viread), as well as non-nucleoside inhibitors, such as nevirapine (奈韦拉平) (Viramune).

Molecular biology

Reverse transcriptase is commonly used in research to apply the polymerase chain reaction technique to RNA in a technique called reverse transcription polymerase chain reaction (RT-PCR). The classical PCR technique can be applied only to DNA strands, but, with the help of reverse transcriptase, RNA can be transcribed into DNA, thus making PCR analysis of RNA molecules possible. Reverse transcriptase is also used to create cDNA libraries from mRNA. The commercial availability of reverse transcriptase greatly improved knowledge in the area of molecular biology, as, along with other enzymes, it allowed scientists to clone, sequence, and characterize RNA.

Reverse transcriptase has also been employed in insulin production. By inserting eukaryotic mRNA for insulin production along with reverse transcriptase into bacteria, the mRNA could be inserted into the prokaryote's genome. Large amounts of insulin can then be created, sidestepping (回避, 横跨一步 躲避) the need to harvest pig pancreas and other such traditional sources. Directly inserting eukaryotic DNA into bacteria would not work because it carries introns, so would not translate successfully using the bacterial ribosomes. Processing in the eukaryotic cell during mRNA production removes these introns to provide a suitable template. Reverse transcriptase converted this edited RNA back into DNA so it could be incorporated in the genome.

2.4.3.7   *Taq DNA polymerase* (*Taq DNA* 聚合酶)

Another Pol I family enzyme — *Thermus aquaticus* DNA polymerase

Structurally, *Taq* polymerase (Fig. 2-61) shows considerable homology to Pol I and T7 polymerases in the cleft (palm) region and its $5' \rightarrow 3'$ exonuclease domain also resembles that of Pol I. However, the $3' \rightarrow 5'$ exonuclease domain, while present, is dramatically altered and non-functional.

The error-prone nature of *Taq* polymerase can sometimes cause problems in PCR. For this reason, several other heat stable DNA polymerases which have proofreading activities are commercially marketed. Two examples are *Pwo* polymerase from *Pyrococcus woesei* (乌兹炽热球菌, 伍斯氏火球 菌, 沃斯氏热球菌) and *Pfu* polymerase from *P. furiosus* (both are thermophilic archaebacteria).

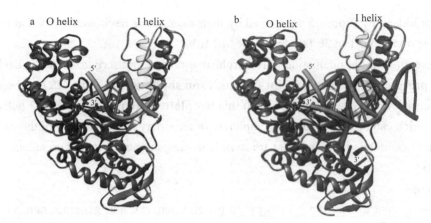

Fig. 2-61   The interaction of duplex DNA with *Taq* polymerase. a. Duplex portion of DNA on a ribbon representation of the KF portion of *Taq* polymerase. The O helix is in green, the I helix in yellow and the catalytically essential carboxylates, Asp610[705], Asp785[882] and Glu786[883], are shown near the 3′ terminus. The template strand is orange and the primer strand is red. b. Superposition of DNAs bound in editing and in polymerizing modes. To orient the two DNAs, the polymerase domains of the KF and *Taq* polymerase complexes were superimposed and the DNA from the editing complex added to the *Taq* polymerase — DNA complex. Particularly striking（惊人的，显著的）is the difference in the positions of the primer backbones relative to the loop at the tip of the I helix. The template strand of editing-complex DNA is in cyan and its primer strand is in blue.

For other details of this enzyme, see **2.3.1.2** for reference.

2.4.3.8   *Terminal deoxynucleotidyl transferase*（末端脱氧核苷酸转移酶）

Terminal deoxynucleotidyl transferase (TdT), also known as **DNA nucleotidylexotransferase (**DNTT**)** or **terminal transferase**, is a specialized DNA polymerase expressed in immature, pre-B, pre-T lymphoid cells, and acute lymphoblastic leukemia（急性淋巴细胞白血病）/lymphoma cells. TdT adds N-nucleotides to the V, D, and J exons（variable, diversity, and joining exons）during antibody gene recombination, enabling the phenomenon of junctional diversity. In humans, terminal transferase is encoded by the *DNTT* gene.

TdT is absent in fetal liver HSCs（hepatic stellate cells，肝星状细胞），significantly impairing junctional diversity in B-cells during the fetal period.

Function

TdT catalyzes the addition of nucleotides to the 3′ terminus of a DNA molecule. Unlike most DNA polymerases, it does not require a template. The preferred substrate of this enzyme is a 3′-overhang, but it can also add nucleotides to blunt or recessed（凹陷的）3′ ends. Cobalt is a necessary cofactor, however the enzyme catalyzes reaction upon Mg and Mn administration *in vitro*.

Uses

Terminal transferase has applications in molecular biology. It can be used in RACE（末端快速扩增法）to add nucleotides that can then be used as a template for a primer in subsequent PCR. It can also be used to add nucleotides labeled with radioactive isotopes, for example in the **TUNEL** assay (**T**erminal deoxynucleotidyl transferase d**U**TP **n**ick **e**nd **l**abeling) for the demonstration of apoptosis (which is marked, in part, by fragmented DNA). Also used in the immunofluorescence assay for the diagnosis of acute lymphoblastic leukemia（急性成淋巴细胞性白血病）.

In immunohistochemistry, antibodies to TdT can be used to demonstrate the presence of immature T and B cells and multipotent hematopoietic stem cells, which possess the antigen, while mature lymphoid cells are always TdT-negative. While TdT-positive cells are found in small numbers in healthy lymph nodes and tonsils（扁桃体，扁桃腺）, the malignant cells of acute lymphoblastic leukemia are also TdT-positive, and the antibody can, therefore, be used as part of a panel（一组实验对象）to diagnose this disease and to distinguish it from, for example, small cell tumors of childhood.

2.4.4 DNA/RNA modifying enzymes（核酸修饰酶）

2.4.4.1 *Alkaline phosphatase* (BAP, 碱性磷酸酶)

Alkaline phosphatase (ALP, ALKP, ALPase, Alk Phos) (EC 3.1.3.1) is a hydrolase enzyme responsible for removing phosphate groups from many types of molecules, including nucleotides, proteins, and alkaloids（生物碱）. The process of removing the phosphate group is called **dephosphorylation**（脱磷酸作用）. As the name suggests, alkaline phosphatases are most effective in an alkaline environment. The optimal pH for the activity of the *E. coli* enzyme is 8.0 while the bovine enzyme optimum pH is slightly higher at 8.5. It is sometimes used synonymously（同义）as **basic phosphatase**.

Use in research

Typical use in the lab for alkaline phosphatases includes removing phosphate monoester to prevent self-ligation.

Alkaline phosphatase has become a useful tool in molecular biology laboratories, since DNA normally possesses phosphate groups on the 5′ end. Removing these phosphates prevents the DNA from ligating (the 5′ end attaching to the 3′ end), thereby keeping DNA molecules linear until the next step of the process for which they are being prepared; also, removal of the phosphate groups allows radiolabeling (replacement by radioactive phosphate groups) in order to measure the presence of the labeled DNA through further steps in the process or experiment. For these purposes, the alkaline phosphatase from shrimp is the most useful, as it is the easiest to inactivate once it has done its job.

Another important use of alkaline phosphatase is as a label for enzyme immunoassays.

Undifferentiated pluripotent stem cells have elevated levels of alkaline phosphatase on their cell membrane, therefore alkaline phosphatase staining is used to detect these cells and to test pluripotency [*i.e.*, embryonic（胚胎的）stem cells or embryonal（胚胎型）carcinoma cells].

Common alkaline phosphatases used in research includes:

➢ Shrimp（虾）alkaline phosphatase (SAP), from a species of Arctic shrimp (*Pandalus borealis*，北极虾). This phosphatase is easily inactivated by heat, a useful feature in some applications.

➢ Calf-intestinal alkaline phosphatase (CIP).

➢ Placental alkaline phosphatase (PLAP) and its C terminally truncated version that lacks the last 24 amino acids (constituting the domain that targets for GPI membrane anchoring) — the secreted alkaline phosphatase (SEAP).

➢ Bacterial alkaline phosphatase (BAP), from *Escherichia coli* C4 cells.

Inhibitors

All mammalian alkaline phosphatase isoenzymes except placental (PALP and SEAP) are inhibited by homoarginine（高精氨酸）, and, in similar manner, all except the intestinal and placental ones are blocked by levamisole（左旋咪唑）. Heating for ~2 hours at 65℃ inactivated most isoenzymes except Placental isoforms (PALP and SEAP). Phosphate is another inhibitor which competitively inhibits alkaline phosphatase.

2.4.4.2 *T4 polynucleotide kinase*（T4 多核苷酸激酶）

Polynucleotide kinase (or PNK) is a T7 bacteriophage/T4 bacteriophage enzyme that catalyzes the transfer of a gamma phosphate from ATP to the free hydroxyl end of the 5′ DNA or RNA.

2.4.5 Other enzyme tools （其他工具酶）

2.4.5.1 *BAL 31 nuclease*（Bal.31 核酸酶）

BAL 31 Nuclease, a product secreted by the marine bacterium *Alteromonas espejiana*（艾氏交替单胞菌）BAL 31 (*A. espejiana* BAL 31), is an endonuclease specific for single-stranded DNA (activity I).

It also has exonuclease activity (activity II), and degrades double-stranded DNA from both the 3′- and 5′- ends when single-stranded DNA are not present. The final products are 5′-P mononucleotides.

There are two kinds of this enzyme, [F] type and [S] type. The [F] type has a relatively high activity II, and the [S] type has a relatively low activity II compared with their activities I. Although the types differ in their relative activity, there are no differences in the reaction conditions. TaKaRa has been selling BAL 31 Nuclease that consists mainly of the [F] type.

Applications

Deletion from both ends of DNA fragments. Suitable to delete 100~1 000 bases.

2.4.5.2 *S1 nuclease*（S1 核酸酶）

Aspergillus（曲霉菌）**nuclease S1** is an endonuclease enzyme derived from *Aspergillus oryzae*（米曲霉）that splits single-stranded DNA (ssDNA) and RNA into oligo- or mononucleotides. It is an extracellular, single-strand-specific, sugar non-specific, fungal nuclease with 3′-mononucleotidase activity. It acts as phosphoesterases cleaving the P—O 3′ bond and producing 5′-mononucleotides as end products.

This enzyme catalyzes the following chemical reaction—

Endonucleolytic cleavage to 5′-phosphomononucleotide and 5′-phosphooligonucleotide end-products

S1 nuclease is an endonuclease that is active against single-stranded DNA and RNA molecules, and is more active on single-stranded nucleic acids with preference for ssDNA over RNA and 3′-AMP. It is five times more active on DNA than RNA. Its reaction products are oligonucleotides or single nucleotides with 5′ phosphoryl groups. Although its primary substrate is single-stranded, it can also occasionally introduce single-stranded breaks in double-stranded DNA or RNA, or DNA-RNA hybrids. The enzyme hydrolyzes single stranded region in duplex DNA such as loops or gaps.

Nomenclature

Alternative names include EC 3.1.30.1, endonuclease S1 (Aspergillus), single-stranded-nucleate endonuclease, deoxyribonuclease S1, nuclease S1, *Neurospora crassa*（粗糙脉孢菌，红面包菌）single-strand specific endonuclease, S1 nuclease, single-strand endodeoxyribonuclease, single-stranded DNA specific endonuclease, single-strand-specific endodeoxyribonuclease, single strand-specific DNase and *Aspergillus oryzae* S1 nuclease.

Properties

Aspergillus nuclease S1 is a monomeric protein of a molecular weight of 38 kilodalton. It requires Zn^{2+} as a cofactor and is relatively stable against denaturing agents like urea, SDS, or formaldehyde.

The optimum pH for its activity lies between 4~4.3. Aspergillus nuclease S1 is known to be inhibited somewhat by 50 μM ATP and nearly completely by 1 mM ATP. Phosphate ion and 5′-AMP are also reported to be two independent inhibitors.

Uses

Aspergillus nuclease S1 is used in the laboratory as a reagent in nuclease（核酸酶）protection assays. In molecular biology, it is used in removing single stranded tails from DNA molecules to create blunt ended molecules and opening hairpin loops generated during synthesis of double stranded cDNA. It is also used as an analytical tool for determination of the secondary structure of nucleic acids.

2.4.5.3   *Mung bean nuclease*（绿豆核酸酶）

Mung bean nuclease (Nuclease MB) is a nuclease derived from sprouts of the mung bean (*Vigna radiata,* 绿豆) that removes nucleotides in a step-wise manner from single-stranded DNA molecules (ssDNA) and is used in biotechnological applications to remove such ssDNA from a mixture also containing double-stranded DNA (dsDNA). This enzyme is useful for transcript mapping, removal of single-stranded regions in DNA hybrids or single-stranded overhangs produced by restriction enzymes, *etc.* It has an activity similar to Nuclease S1 (both are EC 3.1.30.1), but it has higher specificity for single-stranded molecules.

The enzyme degrades single-stranded DNA or RNA to nucleoside 5′-monophosphates, but does not digest double-stranded DNA, double-stranded RNA, or DNA/RNA hybrids. Mung Bean Nuclease catalyzes the specific degradation of single-stranded DNA or RNA, and produces mono- and oligonucleotides carrying a 5′-P terminus. Mung bean nuclease has a stringent single-stranded specificity for DNA or RNA.

Physicochemical properties

Mung bean nuclease has an estimated molecular weight of 39 kDa by SDS-PAGE. It is a glycoprotein, 29% of this mass is sugars. As of April 2019, the specific gene encoding for this protein is unknown, and all production relies on a purification process on bean sprouts from 1980. It is believed to possess 3 pairs of disulfide bonds and one exposed cysteine residue.

Mung bean nuclease activity requires Zn^{2+}. The addition of EDTA or SDS causes irreversible inactivation. Mung bean nuclease is not active at pH below 4.6, nor at low salt concentration.

Description

Nuclease MB is a specific DNA and RNA exo-endonuclease which will degrade single-stranded extensions from the ends of DNA and RNA molecules, leaving blunt, ligatable ends. Its higher single-strand specificity makes it the enzyme of choice for most applications requiring a single-strand-specific nuclease. More than 1 000- fold amount of enzyme can degrade oligomer into all mononucleotides.

Its ability to recognize double-stranded nucleic acids depends on the base sequence. An excess of the enzyme is required to degrade double-stranded DNA or RNA and DNA-RNA hybrids, and in this case, AT-rich regions are selectively degraded.

This enzyme tends to cleave and work well at A↓pN, T↓pN sites, and especially A↓pN sites which are 100% degraded. However, it is difficult to degrade C↓pC, C↓pG sites. Unlike S1 Nuclease, Mung Bean Nuclease will not cleave the intact strand of nicked duplex DNA.

Unit Definition

One unit of Mung Bean Nuclease converts 1 μg of heat-denatured calf thymus DNA into an acid-soluble form in 1 minute at 37℃ under standard assay conditions.

Applications in biotechnology and biochemical research

➢ Removal of hairpin loops during cDNA synthesis.

➢ High-resolution mapping of the termini and exon structures of RNA transcripts (commonly termed Berk-Sharp or S1 Mapping) using either internal-labeled or end-labeled probes.

➢ Restriction-site modification or removal by digestion of single-stranded protruding ends.

➢ Cleavage of single-basepair mismatches, as a replacement for CEL 1 Nuclease in TILLING.

➢ Unidirectional deletion of large DNA (in combination with Exonuclease III) to generate ordered deletions for sequencing.

➢ Removal of 3′ and 5′ extensions from DNA or RNA termini.

➢ Transcriptional mapping.

➢ Cleavage of hairpin loops.

➢ Excision of gene coding sequences from genomic DNA.

2.4.5.4 *Ribonuclease*（*RNase,* 核糖核酸酶）

Ribonuclease (commonly abbreviated **RNase**) is a type of nuclease that catalyzes the degradation of RNA into smaller components. Ribonucleases can be divided into endoribonucleases and exoribonucleases, and comprise several sub-classes within the EC 2.7 (for the phosphorolytic enzymes) and 3.1 (for the hydrolytic enzymes) classes of enzymes.

All organisms studied contain many RNases of many different classes, showing that RNA degradation is a very ancient and important process. As well as cleaning of cellular RNA that is no longer required, RNases play key roles in the maturation of all RNA molecules, both messenger RNAs that carry genetic material for making proteins, and non-coding RNAs that function in varied cellular processes. In addition, active RNA degradation systems are a first defense against RNA viruses, and provide the underlying machinery for more advanced cellular immune strategies such as RNAi.

Some cells also secrete copious quantities of non-specific RNases such as A and T1. RNases are, therefore, extremely common, resulting in very short lifespans for any RNA that is not in a protected environment. It is worth noting that all intracellular RNAs are protected from RNase activity by a number of strategies including 5′ end capping, 3′ end polyadenylation, and folding within an RNA protein complex (ribonucleoprotein particle or RNP).

Another mechanism of protection is **ribonuclease inhibitor (RI)**, which comprises a relatively large fraction of cellular protein (~ 0.1%) in some cell types, and which binds to certain ribonucleases with the highest affinity of any protein-protein interaction; the dissociation constant for the RI-RNase A complex is ~20 fM under physiological conditions. RI is used in most laboratories that study RNA to protect their samples against degradation from environmental RNases.

Similar to restriction enzymes, which cleave highly specific sequences of double-stranded DNA, a variety of endoribonucleases that recognize and cleave specific sequences of single-stranded RNA have been recently classified.

RNases play a critical role in many biological processes, including angiogenesis（血管生成）and self-incompatibility（自交不亲和性）in flowering plants（有花植物，显花植物）(angiosperms，被子植物). Also, RNases in prokaryotic toxin-antitoxin systems are proposed to function as plasmid stability loci, and as stress-response elements when present on the chromosome.

Major types of endoribonucleases

➢ **RNase A**（EC 3.1.27.5）is an RNase that is commonly used in research. RNase A (*e.g.*, bovine pancreatic ribonuclease A: PDB 2AAS) is one of the hardiest enzymes in common laboratory usage; one method of isolating it is to boil a crude cellular extract until all enzymes other than RNase A are denatured. It is specific for single-stranded RNAs. It cleaves the 3′-end of unpaired C and U residues, ultimately forming a 3′-phosphorylated product via a 2′,3′-cyclic monophosphate intermediate. It does not require any cofactors for its activity.

➢ **RNase H** (EC 3.1.26.4) is a ribonuclease that cleaves the RNA in a DNA/RNA duplex to produce ssDNA. RNase H is a non-specific endonuclease and catalyzes the cleavage of RNA via a hydrolytic mechanism, aided by an enzyme-bound divalent metal ion. RNase H leaves a 5′-phosphorylated product.

➢ **RNase III** (EC 3.1.26.3) is a type of ribonuclease that cleaves rRNA (16S rRNA and 23S rRNA) from transcribed polycistronic RNA operon in prokaryotes. It also digests double strands RNA (dsRNA) — Dicer family of RNase, cutting pre-miRNA (60~70 bp long) at a specific site and transforming it in miRNA (22~30 bp), which is actively involved in the regulation of transcription and mRNA life-time.

➢ **RNase L** (EC 3.1.26.-) is an endoribonuclease that functions in the interferon (IFN) antiviral response. In INF treated and virus infected cells, RNase L probably mediates its antiviral effects through a combination of direct cleavage of single-stranded viral RNAs, inhibition of protein synthesis through the degradation of rRNA, induction of apoptosis, and induction of other antiviral genes. Activation of RNase L could lead to elimination of virus infected cells under some circumstances due to cytochrome C release from mitochondria and caspase-dependent apoptosis.

➢ **RNase P** (EC 3.1.26.5) is a type of ribonuclease that is unique in that it is a ribozyme — a ribonucleic acid that acts as a catalyst in the same way as an enzyme. Its function is to cleave off an extra, or precursor, sequence on tRNA molecules. RNase P is one of two known multiple turnover ribozymes in nature (the other being the ribosome). A form of RNase P that is a protein and does not contain RNA has recently been discovered.

➢ **RNase PhyM** is a type of endoribonuclease that is sequence specific for single-stranded RNAs. It cleaves 3′-end of unpaired A and U residues.

➢ **Ribonuclease T$_1$** [EC 3.1.27.3, *guanyloribonuclease, Aspergillus oryzae ribonuclease, RNase N1, RNase N2, ribonuclease N3, ribonuclease U1, ribonuclease F1, ribonuclease Ch, ribonuclease PP1, ribonuclease SA, RNase F1, ribonuclease C2, binase, RNase Sa, guanyl-specific RNase, RNase G, RNase T$_1$, ribonuclease guaninenucleotido-2′-transferase (cyclizing), ribonuclease N3, ribonuclease N1*] is a fungal endonuclease that is sequence specific for and cleaves single-stranded RNA after unpaired guanine (G) residues, *i.e.*, on their 3′ end; the most commonly studied form of this enzyme is the version found in the mold *Aspergillus oryzae* （米曲霉）. Owing to its specificity for guanine, RNase T$_1$ is often used to digest denatured RNA prior to sequencing. Similar to other ribonucleases such as barnase （芽孢杆菌 RNA 酶） and RNase A, ribonuclease T$_1$ has been popular for folding studies. Structurally, ribonuclease T$_1$ is a small α+β protein (104 amino acids) with a four-stranded, antiparallel beta sheet covering a long alpha helix (almost five turns). RNase T$_1$ has two disulfide bonds, Cys2-Cys10 and Cys6-Cys103, of which the latter contributes more to its folding stability; complete reduction of both disulfides usually unfolds the protein, although its folding can be rescued with high salt concentrations. RNase T$_1$ also has four prolines, two of which (Pro39 and Pro55) have *cis* isomers of their X-Pro peptide bonds. Nonnative isomers of these prolines can retard conformational folding dramatically, folding on a characteristic time scale of 7 000 seconds (almost two hours) at 10℃ and pH 5.

➤ **Ribonuclease T2, or RNase T2** (EC 3.1.27.1) is an enzyme that in humans is encoded by the *RNASET2* gene. It is a type of endoribonuclease, which is sequence specific for single-stranded RNAs. It cleaves 3′-end of all 4 residues, but preferentially 3′-end of As. This ribonuclease gene is a novel member of the Rh/T2/S-glycoprotein class of extracellular ribonucleases.

➤ **Ribonuclease U2** [EC 3.1.27.4, *purine specific endoribonuclease, ribonuclease U3, RNase U3, RNase U2, purine-specific ribonuclease, purine-specific RNase, Pleospora RNase, Trichoderma koningi RNase III, ribonuclease (purine)*] is an enzyme **which** is sequence specific for single-stranded RNAs. It cleaves 3′-end of unpaired A residues. This enzyme catalyzes the following chemical reaction—

Two-stage endonucleolytic cleavage to nucleoside 3′-phosphates and 3′-phosphooligonucleotides ending in Ap or Gp with 2′,3′-cyclic phosphate intermediates

➤ **Ribonuclease V** (EC 3.1.27.8, *endoribonuclease V*) is an enzyme specific for polyadenine and polyuridine RNA. This enzyme catalyzes the hydrolysis of poly(A), forming oligoribonucleotides and ultimately 3′-AMP. This enzyme also hydrolyzes poly(U).

Major types of exoribonucleases

➤ **Polynucleotide Phosphorylase (PNPase，多核苷酸磷酸化酶)** (EC 2.7.7.8) functions as an exonuclease as well as a nucleotidyltransferase（核苷酸基转移酶）. It is a bifunctional enzyme with a phosphorolytic 3′ to 5′ exoribonuclease activity and a 3′-terminal oligonucleotide polymerase activity. It also synthesizes long, highly heteropolymeric tails *in vivo*. It is involved in mRNA processing and degradation in bacteria, plants, and in humans. In humans, the enzyme is encoded by the *PNPT1* gene. In its active form, the protein forms a ring structure consisting of three PNPase molecules. Each PNPase molecule consists of two RNase PH domains, an S1 RNA binding domain and a K-homology domain. The protein is present in bacteria and in the chloroplasts and mitochondria of some eukaryotic cells.

➤ **RNase PH** (EC 2.7.7.56) is a tRNA nucleotidyltransferase, present in archaea and bacteria, that is involved in tRNA processing. Contrary to hydrolytic enzymes, it is a phosphorolytic enzyme. RNase PH functions as an exonuclease as well as a nucleotidyltransferase. The active structure of the proteins is a homohexameric complex, consisting of three ribonuclease (RNase) PH dimers.

➤ **RNase R**, or Ribonuclease R, is a 3′→5′ exoribonuclease, which belongs to the RNase II superfamily, a group of enzymes that hydrolyze RNA in the 3′→5′ direction. RNase R has been shown to be involved in selective mRNA degradation, particularly of non stop mRNAs in bacteria. RNase R ensures translation accuracy, correct rRNA maturation and elimination of abnormal rRNAs, and is employed by the *trans*-translation system to break down damaged mRNAs. In *Escherichia coli*, RNase R is a 92 kD protein, with the characteristic capacity to degrade structured RNA substrates without displaying sequence specificity. Therefore, RNase R acts over a range of substrates, such as, ribosomal, transfer, messenger and small non-coding RNAs. RNase R is associated with ribonucleoprotein complex that contains tmRNA and SmpB, and is involved in the development of tmRNA under cold-shock. RNase R is also associated with ribosomes and participates in ribosomal RNA quality control processes. RNase R has an *in vitro* affinity for rRNA. In several rRNA quality control pathways, RNase R behaves as a mainfactor by enhancing the removal of faulty rRNA molecules. This protein is also critical for handling rRNA precursors and for observing the ribosome integrity. RNase R has two cold shock domains, an RNase catalytic domain, an S1 domain and a basic domain. RNase R is more active and more effective in breaking down RNAs than the other bacterial exoribonucleases, such as RNase II. It can, unlike RNase II, degrade RNA with secondary structures without help of accessory factors. Besides the substrate RNAs that construct double-stranded RNA with 3′ overhangs shorter than seven nucleotides, RNase R can degrade all linear RNAs. For the methodical digestion of eukaryotic linear RNAs, RNase R is a good 3′ to 5′ exoribonuclease but there are infrequent cases of RNase R resistance.

➤ **RNase D** (EC 3.1.13.5) is one of the seven exoribonucleases identified in *E. coli*. It is a 3′→5′ exoribonuclease which has been shown to be involved in the 3′ processing of various stable RNA molecules, including pre-tRNA.

➤ **Ribonuclease T** (*RNase T, exonuclease T, exo T*), a member of the larger DEDD family of exoribonucleases, is the major contributor for the 3′→5′ maturation of many stable RNAs — it is a ribonuclease enzyme involved in the maturation of transfer RNA and ribosomal RNA (*i.e.*, 5S and 23S rRNA domains) in bacteria as well as in DNA repair pathways — it can play a role in DNA repair by cleaving the 3′ end of bulge DNA. It is a member of the DnaQ family of exonucleases and non-processively acts on the 3′ end of single-stranded nucleic acids. RNase T catalyzes the removal of nucleotides from the 3′ end of both RNA and DNA. It is inhibited by both double stranded DNA and RNA, as well as cytosine residues on the 3′ end of RNA. Two cytosines at the 3′ end of RNA appear to remove the activity of RNase T entirely. This cytosine effect, however, is observed less with ssDNA. This lack of sequence specificity in ssDNA, combined with its ability to act on ssDNA close to a duplex region, has led to its use in creating blunt ends for DNA cloning. Structurally, RNase T exists as an anti-parallel dimer and requires a divalent cation to function. In *E. coli*, RNase T is encoded by the rnt gene.

➤ **Exoribonuclease I** (核糖核酸外切酶 I) (EC 3.1.11.1) degrades single-stranded RNA from 5′→3′, exists only in eukaryotes. **5′-3′ exoribonuclease 1** (Xrn1) is a protein that in humans is encoded by the XRN1 gene. Xrn1 hydrolyses RNA in the 5′ to 3′ direction. As a member of the 5′→3′ exonuclease family, the encoded protein may be involved in replication-dependent histone mRNA degradation, and interacts directly with the enhancer of mRNA-decapping protein 4. In addition to mRNA metabolism, a similar protein in yeast has been implicated in a variety of nuclear and cytoplasmic functions, including transcription, translation, homologous recombination, meiosis, telomere maintenance, and microtubule assembly. Mutations in this gene are associated with osteosarcoma, suggesting that the encoded protein may also play a role in bone formation. Alternative splicing results in multiple transcript variants.

➤ **Exoribonuclease II** [EC 3.1.13.1, *ribonuclease II, ribonuclease Q, BN ribonuclease, Escherichia coli exo-RNase II, RNase II, exoribonuclease (misleading), 5′-exoribonuclease*] is an enzyme, a close homolog of Exoribonuclease I. This enzyme catalyzes the exonucleolytic cleavage in the 3′→5′ direction to yield nucleoside 5′-phosphates with preference for single-stranded RNA.

RNase specificity

Although, usually most of exo- and endoribonucleases are not sequence specific, recently CRISPR-Cas system natively recognizing and cutting DNA was engineered to cleave ssRNA in sequence specific manner.

RNase contamination during RNA extraction

The extraction of RNA in molecular biology experiments is greatly complicated by the presence of ubiquitous and hardy ribonucleases that degrade RNA samples. Certain RNases can be extremely hardy and inactivating them is difficult compared to neutralizing DNases. In addition to the cellular RNases that are released, there are several RNases that are present in the environment. RNases have evolved to have many extracellular functions in various organisms. For example, RNase 7, a member of the RNase A superfamily, is secreted by human skin and serves as a potent antipathogen defence. In these secreted RNases, the enzymatic RNase activity may not even be necessary for its new, exapted（扩展适应，伸延 适应）function. For example, immune RNases act by destabilizing the cell membranes of bacteria.

2.4.5.5 Deoxyribonuclease I（DNase I, 脱氧核糖核酸酶 I）

Deoxyribonuclease I (usually called **DNase I**), is an endonuclease coded by the human gene **DNASE1**. DNase I is a nuclease that cleaves DNA preferentially at phosphodiester linkages adjacent to a pyrimidine nucleotide, yielding 5′-phosphate-terminated polynucleotides with a free hydroxyl group on position 3′, on average producing tetranucleotides. It acts on single-stranded DNA, double-stranded DNA, and chromatin（染色质）. In addition to its role as a waste-management endonuclease, it has been suggested to be one of the deoxyribonucleases responsible for DNA fragmentation during apoptosis.

DNase I binds to the cytoskeletal protein actin（肌动蛋白）. It binds actin monomers with very high (sub-nanomolar) affinity and actin polymers with lower affinity. The function of this interaction is unclear. However, since actin-bound DNase I is enzymatically inactive, the DNase-actin complex might be a storage form of DNase I that prevents damage of the genetic information.

This gene encodes a member of the DNase family. This protein is stored in the zymogen（酶原）granules of the nuclear envelope and functions by cleaving DNA in an endonucleolytic manner. At least six autosomal（常染色体的）codominant（共显性的，等显性的）alleles have been characterized, DNASE1*1 through DNASE1*6, and the sequence of DNASE1*2 represented in this record. Mutations in this gene, as well as factor inactivating its enzyme product, have been associated with systemic lupus erythematosus (SLE，系统性红斑狼疮), an autoimmune disease. A recombinant form of this protein is used to treat one of the symptoms of cystic fibrosis（囊胞性纤维症）by hydrolyzing the extracellular DNA in sputum（痰，唾液）and reducing its viscosity. Alternate transcriptional splice variants of this gene have been observed but have not been thoroughly characterized.

In genomics

In genomics, DNase I hypersensitive sites are thought to be characterized by open, accessible chromatin; therefore, a DNase I sensitivity assay is a widely used methodology in genomics for identifying which regions of the genome are likely to contain active genes.

DNase I Sequence Specificity

It has been recently reported that DNase I shows some levels of sequence specificity that may depend on experimental conditions.

2.4.5.6 Exonuclease（核酸外切酶）

Exonucleases are enzymes that work by cleaving nucleotides one at a time from the end (exo) of a polynucleotide chain. A hydrolyzing reaction that breaks phosphodiester bonds at either the 3′ or the 5′ end occurs. Its close relative is the endonuclease, which cleaves phosphodiester bonds in the middle (endo) of a polynucleotide chain. Eukaryotes and prokaryotes have three types of exonucleases involved in the normal turnover of mRNA: 5′ to 3′ exonuclease, which is a dependent decapping protein, 3′ to 5′

exonuclease, an independent protein, and poly(A)-specific 3′ to 5′ exonuclease.

In both archaebacteria（古细菌）and eukaryotes（真核生物）, one of the main routes of RNA degradation is performed by the multi-protein exosome（外来体）complex, which consists largely of 3′ to 5′ exoribonucleases.

Significance to polymerase

RNA polymerase II is known to be in effect during transcriptional termination; it works with a 5′ exonuclease (human gene Xrn2) to degrade the newly formed transcript downstream, leaving the polyadenylation site and simultaneously shooting the polymerase. This process involves the exonuclease's catching up to the pol II and terminating the transcription.

Pol I then synthesizes DNA nucleotides in place of the RNA primer it had just removed. DNA polymerase I also has 3′ to 5′ and 5′ to 3′ exonuclease activity, which is used in editing and proofreading DNA for errors. The 3′ to 5′ only remove one mononucleotide at once, and the 5′ to 3′ activity can remove mononucleotides or up to 10 nucleotides at once.

E. coli types

In 1971, Lehman IR discovered exonuclease I in *E. coli*. Since that time, there have been numerous discoveries including: **exonuclease II**, **III**, **IV**, **V**, **VI**, **VII**, and **VIII**. Each type of exonuclease has a specific type of function or requirement.

Exonuclease I breaks apart single-stranded DNA in a 3′→5′ direction, releasing deoxyribonucleoside 5′-monophosphates one after another. It does not cleave DNA strands without **terminal 3′-OH groups** because they are blocked by phosphoryl or acetyl groups.

Exonuclease II is associated with DNA polymerase I, which contains a 5′ exonuclease that clips off（削去）the RNA primer contained immediately upstream from the site of DNA synthesis in a 5′→3′ manner.

Exonuclease III has four catalytic activities:
> 3′ to 5′ exodeoxyribonuclease activity, which is specific for double-stranded DNA
> RNase activity
> 3′ phosphatase activity（磷酸酶活性）
> AP endonuclease activity (later found to be called endonuclease II).

Exonuclease IV adds a water molecule, so it can break the bond of an oligonucleotide to nucleoside 5′ monophosphate. This exonuclease requires Mg^{2+} in order to function and works at higher temperatures than exonuclease I.

Exonuclease V is a 3′ to 5′ hydrolyzing enzyme that catalyzes linear double-stranded DNA and single-stranded DNA, which requires Ca^{2+}. This enzyme is extremely important in the process of homologous recombination（同源重组）.

Exonuclease VIII is 5′ to 3′ dimeric protein that does not require ATP or any gaps or nicks in the strand, but requires a **free 5′ OH group** to carry out its function.

Discoveries in humans

The 3′ to 5′ human type endonuclease is known to be essential for the proper processing of histone pre-mRNA（组蛋白信使核糖核酸前体）, in which U7 snRNP directs the single cleavage process. Following the removal of the downstream cleavage product (DCP) Xrn1 continues to further breakdown the product until it is completely degraded. This allows the nucleotides to be recycled. Xrn1 is linked to a co-transcriptional cleavage (CoTC) activity that acts as a precursor to developing a free 5′ unprotected end, so the exonuclease can remove and degrade the downstream cleavage product (DCP). This initiates transcriptional termination because one does not want DNA or RNA strands building up in their bodies.

Discoveries in yeast

CCR4-NOT is a general transcription regulatory complex in budding yeast that is found to be associated with mRNA metabolism, transcription initiation, and mRNA degradation. CCR4 has been found to contain RNA and single-stranded DNA 3′ to 5′ exonuclease activities. Another component associated with the CCR4-NOT is CAF1 protein, which has been found to contain 3′ to 5′ or 5′ to 3′ exonuclease domains in the mouse and *Caenorhabditis elegans*（秀丽隐杆线虫）. This protein has not been found in yeast, which suggests that it is likely to have an abnormal exonuclease domain like the one seen in a metazoan（后生动物，多细胞动物）. Yeast contains two exonucleases, Rat1 and Xrn1. The Rat1 works just like the human type (Xrn2) and Xrn1 function in the cytoplasm in the 5′ to 3′ direction to degrade RNAs (pre-5.8S and 25S rRNAs) in the absence of Rat1.

2.5　Brief introduction on the major systems and vectors for gene expression（基因表达的主要体系及载体简介）

Since the very first exogenous gene had been successfully expressed in *Escherichia coli* by Cohen *et al.* in 1973, great progress has been made in genetic engineering, especially in several major prokaryotic and eukaryotic expression systems and even in whole organism (like plants or animals) expression systems (*i.e.*, transgenic plants and transgenic animals).

All expression systems have some advantages as well as some disadvantages that should be considered in selecting which one to use. Choosing the best one requires evaluating the options — from yield to glycosylation, to proper folding to economics of scale-up.

Expression systems

Different organisms may be used to express a target protein, the expression vector used therefore will have elements specific to a particular organism. The most commonly used organism for protein expression is the bacterium *Escherichia coli*. However not all proteins can be successfully expressed in *E. coli*, and other systems may therefore be used.

2.5.1　Prokaryotic expression system（原核表达体系）

The main characteristics of prokaryotic cell structure include: absence of a distinct membrane-bounded nucleus and membrane-bounded organelles; Prokaryotic cells divide by binay fission, in which the DNA replicates and then the cell divides in two. That is all — no mitosis, no spindle, no nothing!

Proteobacteria（变形菌门）, Firmicutes（厚壁菌门）and Actinobacteria（放线菌门）are prokaryotes. In recent years, prokaryotes, especially *Escherichia coli*, have played an important role in the development of genetic engineering. Other expression systems such as *Bacillus* and *Streptomyces*（链霉菌属）have also developed greatly.

2.5.1.1　Escherichia coli (molecular biology)（大肠埃希菌）

The expression host of choice for the expression of many proteins is *Escherichia coli*, as the production of heterologous protein in *E. coli* is relatively simple and convenient, as well as being rapid and cheap. A large number of *E. coli* expression plasmids are also available, suitable for a wide variety of needs.

Escherichia coli (/ˌɛʃɨˈrɪkiəˈkoʊlaɪ/; commonly abbreviated ***E. coli***) is a gamma proteobacterium（γ-变形菌纲）commonly found in the lower intestine of warm-blooded animals.

E. coli is one of the most widely used expression hosts, and heterologous DNA is normally introduced in a plasmid expression vector. The techniques for overexpression in *E. coli* are well developed and work by increasing the number of copies of the gene or increasing the binding of transcription factors to the promoter region so as to facilitate transcription.

For example a DNA sequence for a protein of interest could be cloned or subcloned into a high copy-number plasmid containing the *lac* promoter, which is then transformed into the bacterium *Escherichia coli*. Addition of IPTG (a lactose analog) activates the *lac* promoter and causes the bacteria to express the protein of interest.

Diversity of *Escherichia coli*

Escherichia coli is one of the most diverse bacterial species with only 20% of the genes in a typical *E. coli* genome shared among all strains.

History

In 1885, Theodor Escherich, a German-Austrian pediatrician（儿科医师），first discovered this organism in the feces of healthy individuals and called it *Bacterium coli commune* due to the fact it is found in the colon. Early classifications of Prokaryotes placed these in a handful of genera based on their shape and motility (at that time Ernst Haeckel's classification of Bacteria in the kingdom Monera（原核生物界）was in place（得其所，在应有的位置上）).

Following a revision of *Bacterium* it was reclassified as *Bacillus coli* by Migula in 1895 and later reclassified in the newly created genus *Escherichia* as *Escherichia coli*.

Due to its ease of culture and fast doubling it was used in the early microbiology experiments, however bacteria were considered primitive（原始的，简单的）and pre-cellular（前细胞的）and received little attention before 1944, when Avery, Macleod and McCarty demonstrated that DNA was the genetic material using *Salmonella typhimurium*（鼠伤寒杆菌，鼠伤寒沙门菌），following which *Escherichia coli* was used for linkage mapping studies.

Strains

Four of the many *E. coli* strains (K-12, B, C, and W) are thought of as model organism strains. These are classified in Risk Group 1（第一级危险群）in biosafety guidelines.

Therapeutic use & Role in biotechnology

Nonpathogenic *E. coli* strain Nissle 1917 (EcN) (Mutaflor) and *E. coli* O83:K24:H31 (Colinfant) are used as probiotic（益生菌）agents in medicine, mainly for the treatment of various gastrointestinal diseases, including inflammatory bowel disease. It is thought that the EcN strain might impede the growth of opportunistic pathogens（机会致病菌），including *Salmonella*（沙门菌）and other coliform（大肠埃希菌的）enteropathogens, through the production of microcin（微菌素）proteins the production of siderophores（铁载体，含铁细胞）.

Because of its long history of laboratory culture and ease of manipulation, *E. coli* also plays an important role in modern biological engineering and industrial microbiology. The work of Stanley Norman Cohen and Herbert Boyer in *E. coli*, using plasmids and restriction enzymes to create recombinant DNA, became a foundation of biotechnology. Considered a very versatile host for the production of heterologous （不同的，异种的）proteins, researchers can introduce genes into the microbes using plasmids, allowing for the mass production of proteins in industrial fermentation processes. Genetic systems have also been developed which allow the production of recombinant proteins using *E. coli*. One of the first useful applications of recombinant DNA technology was the manipulation of *E. coli* to produce human insulin. Modified *E. coli* have been used in vaccine development, bioremediation （生物修复，生物降解，生物除污）, and production of immobilized enzymes.

The *E. coli* K-12 strains and their derivatives (DH1, DH5α, MG1655, RV308 and W3110) are the strains most widely used by the biotechnology industry.

Model organism

E. coli is frequently used as a model organism in microbiology studies. Cultivated strains (*e.g.*, *E. coli* K12) are well-adapted to the laboratory environment, and, unlike wild type strains, have lost their ability to thrive in the intestine. Many lab strains lose their ability to form biofilms （生物膜，菌膜）. These features protect wild-type strains from antibodies and other chemical attacks, but require a large expenditure of energy and material resources.

In 1946, Joshua Lederberg and Edward Tatum first described the phenomenon known as bacterial conjugation （细菌接合）using *E. coli* as a model bacterium, and it remains a primary model to study conjugation. *E. coli* was an integral part of the first experiments to understand phage genetics, and early researchers, such as Seymour Benzer, used *E. coli* and phage T4 to understand the topography （拓扑图）of gene structure. Prior to Benzer's research, it was not known whether the gene was a linear structure, or if it had a branching pattern.

E. coli was one of the first organisms to have its genome sequenced; the complete genome of *E. coli* K-12 was published by *Science* in 1997.

(1) Specific properties of *Escherichia coli* expression system（大肠埃希菌体系的特点）

Due to the low cost and speed with which it can be grown and modified in laboratory settings, *E. coli* is a popular expression platform for the production of recombinant proteins used in therapeutics. One advantage to using *E. coli* over another expression platform is that *E. coli* naturally does not export many proteins into the periplasm, making it easier to recover a protein of interest without cross-contamination.

➢ Molecular genetic studies have already been conducted very thoroughly in *E. coli* expression systems.

➢ As *E. coli* is a strain with high reproductivity, it is suitable for large scale culture.

➢ Exogenous genes can be expressed in *E. coli* at high levels.

➢ The downstream technology is mature enough for *E. coli* to be controlled easily.

The disadvantages （缺点）：

➢ *E. coli*'s application is restricted due to its lacking of post-translational modification system.

➢ *E. coli* contains endotoxin and pyrogen, which can hardly be gotten rid off.

➢ Newly formed heterologous proteins can not fold properly in *E. coli*, and it is difficult to renature them.

➢ In most of the cases, a heterologous protein would form inclusion bodyies, which are tedious to extract.

(2) The main factors affecting expression of eukaryotic gene in *E. coli*（影响真核基因在大肠埃希菌表达的主要因素）

① A prokaryotic vector can not distinguish an eukaryotic intron from exons, hence it is cDNA rather than chromosome fragments that was usually adopted as the coding gene, and the signal peptide sequence of the eukaryotic protein should be deleted.

② It is necessary to choose an expression vector with an appropriate strong promoter.

③ The mRNA acquired through transcription should possess effective ribosome binding sites.

④ When PCR primers should be designed, or genes should be synthesized, *E. coli* biased coden should be chosen.

⑤ Expression products should be somewhat stable.

⑥ An appropriate *E. coli* host strain should be chosen.

⑦ The culturing condition of the engineered bacterium should be optimized.

(3) Construction of *Escherichia coli* expression vector（大肠埃希菌表达载体的构建）

In order for eukaryotic genes to be normally transcribed and translated into corresponding proteins in *Escherichia coli*, effective expression vectors need to be constructed. Typical *Escherichia coli* expression vectors are mainly composed of promoters, operons, multiple cloning sites, transcription and translation signals, origins of replication and screening marker genes.

I. Promoter 启动子

Promoter is a *cis*-acting element instrumental in turning on gene expression, which can be specifically recognized and bound by RNA polymerase and acts as the transcription initiation site. Promoters are generally divided into two categories: one type of promoter can be recognized directly by RNA polymerase, while the other requires the presence of protein cofactors when binding to RNA polymerase.

A promoter consists of a core promoter and an upstream promoter elements, and in those two regions there are some special sequences that can be recognized by an RNA polymerase — universal sequences（通用序列）or consensus sequences（共有序列）. In prokaryotes, there is a consensus sequence, TATAAT, called **Pribnow box**, localized at −10 upstream of the transcription initiation site, and another consensus sequence, TTGACA, at −35. The two sets of sequences are usually separated by 16~18 bp. Alteration of the consensus sequence may cause functional disruption. A few prokaryotes lack either or both of these consensus sequences. In this case, RNA polymerases are often unable to recognize those sequences independently, and protein cofactors are needed to facilitate in recognizing adjacent sequences to compensate for the deficiency of promoters.

The promoters used in *E. coli* expression vectors are usually based on the promoter of the ***lac* operon**（乳糖操纵子）or the T7 promoter, and they are normally regulated by the *lac* operator. The promoters may also be hybrids of different promoters, for example, the *tac* promoter is a hybrid of *trp* and *lac* promoters. Note that most commonly used *lac* or *lac*-derived promoters are based on the ***lac*UV5** mutant which is insensitive to **catabolite repression**（分解代谢产物阻遏）. This mutant allows for expression of protein under the control of the *lac* promoter even when the growth medium contains glucose; whereas if wild-type *lac* promoter is used, glucose would inhibit protein expression. Nevertheless, presence of glucose may still be used to reduce background expression through residual inhibition（后效抑制）in some systems.

Commonly used promoters in *E. coli* expression vectors are as follows:

A. *lac* promoter (P*lac*) & *lac*UV5 promoter (P*lac*~UV5~) 〔lac 启动子和 lacUV5 启动子〕

The *lac* promoter is a medium-strength promoter derived from the lactose operon in *Escherichia coli*. The latter consists of a promoter capable of attracting RNA polymerase, an operator gene, a binding site for catabolite gene activating protein (CAP) and part of the β-galactosidase structural genes (*LacZ*).

The *Escherichia coli* LacUV5 promoter is a mutant derivative of the *lac* promoter, which has two base substitution mutations (G→A, T→A) in its Pribnow box, and its sequence is ATAAT (**P*lac*** : TAT**G**T**T** → **P*lac*~UV5~** : AT**A**A**T**). The *lac*UV5 promoter is insensitive to catabolite repression, and transcription can proceed effectively even when CAP and cAMP are deficient. The *lac*UV5 promoter with deletion of the CAP site used to be the promoter chosen for construction of expression vectors.

Either the *lac* promoter or the *lac*UV5 promoter is usually tailed with the gene fragment encoding β-galactosidase (*lacZ*), and when a foreign DNA is inserted into this region, it is expressed as a fusion protein. For the plasmids containing the *lac* promoter, the formation of functional β-galactosidase can cleave X-gal, resulting in blue colonies on the plate containing IPTG and X-gal.

B. Bacteriophage lambda promoters P~L~ and P~R~ (Phage λ left arm promoter λP~L~ & phage λ right arm promoter λP~R~)

λP~L~ and λP~R~ are the transcriptional control regions of the left and right arms of early promoter region of bacteriophage λ development, including promoter sequences that attract RNA polymerase and operon sequences that attract repressor protein *c*I, which are negatively regulated by *c*I proteins.

λP~L~ is a temperature-sensitive promoter with high RNA transcription promotion efficiency and is strictly regulated by repressor proteins. As a prokaryotic promoter, it is widely used to construct vectors such as pKC30 and pCP series. A series of expression vectors that direct high-level overproduction of gene products in *Escherichia coli* have been constructed. All contain strong bacteriophage lambda promoters, P~L~ and P~R~, arranged in tandem to further enhance transcription level.

C. *trp* promoter (P*trp*)

P*trp* was derived from the regulatory region of the *trp* operon in *Escherichia coli*. A complete regulatory region includes promoter, operon, leading sequence and attenuator.

P~trp~ possesses the consensus -10 and -35 regions of sigma(70)-dependent promoters, while the -10 region is within the operon ($-21 \sim +1$), therefore the binding of the repressor to the operon O~trp~ completely excludes RNA polymerase binding.

P~trp~ is turned off (repressed) in tryptophan-rich culture medium, and as the tryptophan level decreases to a value low enough for derepression to occur, the initiation of transcription begins with the binding of RNA polymerase to the P~trp~. P~trp~ is a strong promoter, its initiation effect is stronger than P~lac~, whereas its regulatory effect is inferior to that of P~lac~. Examples of plasmid vectors containing P~trp~ are pWT121, *etc*.

D. *tac* promoter

tac promoter is a hybrid *trp-lac* promoter, derived by fusing the -35 region of P~trp~ and the -10 region of P~lac~. By site-directed mutagenesis, the distance between the -35 and -10 regions was constructed to be 17 bp. P~tac~ can be inhibited by the repressor *lac*I and induced by IPTG. This promoter has a typical TTGACA (-35)··· (N)~17~···TATAAT (-10) promoter sequence. *tac* promoter, which combine the advantages of both parental promoters, exhibited extremely higher transcriptional activity — several to tens of times stronger than P~trp~ or P~lac~, and is one of the most commonly used transcriptional regulation system. The plasmid vectors with *tac* promoter(s) are pDR540, pKK177-3, and pGEX series, *etc*. The *tac* promoter can be negatively regulated by the regulatory gene of the *lac* operon, *lac*I.

E. T7 promoter (P_{T7})

T7 promoter is derived from the promoter for late gene transcription of T7 bacteriophage, which has a conserved sequence of 23 bp ($-17 \sim +6$), namely P_{T7}. This promoter could not be recognized by *Escherichia coli* RNA polymerase, but could only be recognized by T7 RNA polymerase and initiates transcription.

P_{T7} demonstrated high transcriptional activity and specificity. The activity of T7 polymerase was 6 times higher than that of *Escherichia coli* polymerase. Examples of plasmid vectors with T7 promoter(s) are pET series.

II. Transcription Terminator in Prokaryotes 转录终止子

In genetics, a transcription terminator is a section of nucleic acid sequence that marks the end of a gene or operon in genomic DNA during transcription. This sequence mediates transcriptional termination by providing signals in the newly synthesized transcript RNA that trigger processes which release the transcript RNA from the transcriptional complex. These processes include the direct interaction of the mRNA secondary structure with the complex and/or the indirect activities of recruited termination factors. Release of the transcriptional complex frees RNA polymerase and related transcriptional machinery to begin transcription of new mRNAs.

Two classes of transcription terminators, Rho-dependent and Rho-independent, have been identified throughout prokaryotic genomes. These widely distributed sequences are responsible for triggering the end of transcription upon normal completion of gene or operon transcription, mediating early termination of transcripts as a means of regulation such as that observed in transcriptional attenuation and ensuring the termination of runaway (失控的) transcriptional complexes that manage to escape earlier terminators by chance which prevents unnecessary energy expenditure for the cell.

Rho-dependent terminators

Rho-dependent transcription terminators (Fig. 2-62) reguire a protein called Rho factor, which exhibits RNA helicase (解旋酶) activity, to disrupt the mRNA-DNA-RNA polymerase transcriptional complex. Rho-dependent terminators are found in bacteria and phage. The Rho-dependent terminator occurs downstream of translational stop codons and consists of an unstructured, cytosine-rich sequence on the mRNA known as a **Rho utilization site (*rut*)** for which a consensus sequence has not been identified, and a downstream **transcription stop point (*tsp*)**. The ***rut*** serves as a mRNA loading site and as an activator for Rho activation enables Rho to efficiently hydrolyze ATP and translocate down the mRNA while it maintains contact with the ***rut*** site. Rho is able to catch up with the RNA polymerase, which is stalled (暂缓，停顿) at the downstream ***tsp*** sites. Contact between Rho and the RNA polymerase complex stimulates dissociation of the transcriptional complex through a mechanism involving allosteric effects of Rho on RNA polymerase.

Rho-independent terminators

Intrinsic transcription terminators or Rho-independent terminators (Fig. 2-62) are strong terminators, which are characterized by inverted repeats (palindromic sequence) rich in GC before the transcription termination point to form a self-annealing hairpin structure (Fig. 2-63) on the elongating transcript, which results in the disruption of the **mRNA-DNA-RNA polymerase ternary complex**. The terminator sequence in DNA contains a 7~20 base pair GC-rich region of dyad symmetry followed by a short

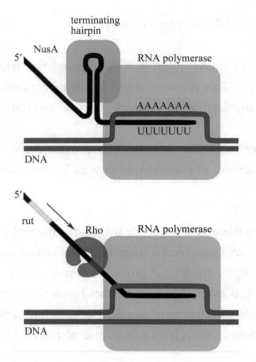

Fig. 2-62 Simplified schematics of the mechanisms of prokaryotic transcriptional termination in vector version. Rho-independent termination, a terminating hairpin forms on the nascent mRNA interacting with the NusA protein to stimulate release of the transcript from the RNA polymerase complex(top). In Rho-dependent termination, the Rho protein binds at the upstream *rut* site, translocates down the mRNA, and interacts with the RNA polymerase complex to stimulate release of the transcript(bottom).

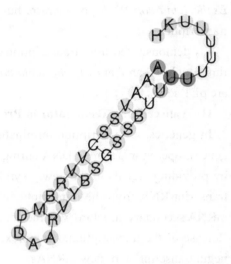

Fig. 2-63 A predicted conserved secondary structure and sequence conservation annotation for 90 bacterial Rho-independent termination elements.

poly-T tractor "T stretch" which is transcribed to form the terminating hairpin and a 7~9 nucleotide "U tract" respectively. The mechanism of termination is hypothesized to occur through a combination of direct promotion of dissociation through allosteric effects of hairpin binding interactions with the RNA polymerase and "competitive kinetics". The hairpin formation causes RNA polymerase stalling and destabilization, leading to a greater likelihood that dissociation of the complex will occur at that location due to an increased time spent paused at that site and reduced stability of the complex. Additionally, the elongation protein factor NusA interacts with the RNA polymerase and the hairpin structure to stimulate transcriptional termination.

There is no transcriptional terminator sequence at the 3′ end of the cDNA reverse transcribed from a eukaryotic mRNA. Therefore, when eukaryotic genes are to be expressed in *Escherichia coli*, especially when a strong promoter is adopted, a strong transcriptional terminator should be placed downstream of eukaryotic genes. The closer the distance between the exogenous gene and the transcriptional terminator, the higher the expression level.

III. Ribosome binding site (RBS) (核糖体结合位点)

A. The initiation codon and the Shine-dalgarno Sequence (起始密码子，SD 序列)

A Ribosome Binding Site (RBS) is an RNA sequence found at the 5′ end of mRNA to which ribosomes can bind and initiate translation. Translation initiation in bacteria almost always requires both the initiation codon (ATG), and the Shine-Dalgarno sequence — the purine-rich DNA sequence preceding the initiation codon in mRNA. SD sequence can complement and bind with the 3′ end of 16S rRNA, the pyrimidine-rich sequence in the small subunit of the ribosome.

The 30S ribosomal subunit initiates protein synthesis by binding mRNA and initiator tRNA. During translation initiation, the 30S ribosomal subunits first recognize and bind to the ribosomal binding site. By base-pairing of the ORF-preceding SD sequence with the 3′-tail of the 16S ribosomal RNA (rRNA) of the 30S subunit, the mRNA-30S ribosomal subunit complex is formed thus facilitate placement of the mRNA open-reading frame (ORF). The SD sequence base pairs in a Watson-Crick fashion with the complementary anti-SD sequence (aSD) at the 3′ end of the 16S RNA, which directly positions the start codon to the P-site of the 30S subunit and stimulates translation initiation. Prior to and after initiation, the SD-duplex causes strong anchoring of 5′ end of mRNA onto the 30S subunit.

B. Nature, Length and Distance to Start Codon of SD Sequence

Since base-pairing of SD-aSD may limit the movement of mRNA along the ribosome, the nature, the length of the SD motif, and distance of SD to start codon are key factors in translation initiation. The nature and length determine the stability and hybridization of the SD-aSD interaction.

The generic SD motif is AGGAG (G), although it may vary in length from about 3~9 nucleotides (*e.g.*, UAAGGAGGU). In the dynamic cellular environment, SD can base pair either fully or partially to its complement, resulting in variations of SD motifs. Different SD sequences had different effects on gene expression.

The length of the SD motif also affects the rate of translation. Varying the length of the *E. coli* SD sequence from five to eight bases results in a fourfold increase in gene expression level. However, a longer SD motif increases SD-aSD interactions and inhibits translation from progressing into elongation phase.

Most of the genes in *Escherichia coli* had AUG as the initiation coden (about 90%), and a few were GUG. Therefore, the first amino acid of almost all proteins expressed in bacteria is formylmethionine, and part of the protein′s formylmethionine is removed in the peptide synthesis process.

The spacing between the SD sequence and the initiation codon varies considerably in natural messages, with the average being 7 nucleotides. SD motif is usually found 3~13 nucleotides (nt) upstream of translation initiation codon. within the ribosome binding site (RBS).

(4) Major categories of *E. coli* plasmid vector (大肠埃希菌质粒载体的主要类型)

I. pSC101 plasmid vector

pSC101

pSC101 is a DNA plasmid that is used as a cloning vector in genetic cloning experiments. The plasmid is a natural plasmid from *Salmonella panama* (巴拿马沙门菌).

pSC101 is a low copy number stringent plasmids, whose replication is subject to stringent control, as an overall result of a complex set of interactions, each of which contributes to the final efficiency of replication of the plasmid. pSC101 is an iteron (重复子) plasmid, with a molecular weight of 5.8×10^6 U.

History

In the early 1970s, Herbert Boyer and Stanley Norman Cohen produced pSC101, the first plasmid vector for cloning purposes. Soon after successfully cloning two pSC101 plasmids together to create one large plasmid, they published the results describing the experiment, in 1973. Then they demonstrated that a gene from a frog could be transferred into bacterial cells and then expressed by the bacterial cells (well adapted to *E. coli*). In 1980, pSC101 became the first patented commercial DNA cloning vector when patents were awarded to Boyer and Cohen. The "SC" stands for Stanley Cohen. Although the original pSC101 only contained tetracycline resistance and a restriction site for *Eco*RI, the commercially available pSC101 gained restriction sites for several enzymes, including *Hin*dIII, in addition to the *Eco*RI site.

II. ColE1 plasmid vector

ColE1

ColE1 is a plasmid found in bacteria, with a molecular weight of 4.2×10^6 U. ColE1 is a multicopy plasmid, whose replication is subject to relaxed control.

The name **ColE1** derives from the fact that it carries a gene for colicin（大肠埃希菌素）(a type of bacteriocin（细菌素）produced by and toxic to some strains of *Escherichia coli*) E1 (the *cea* gene). It also codes for immunity from this product with the *imm* gene. In addition, the plasmid has a series of **mobility** (*mob*) genes. Its size and the presence of a single *Eco*RI recognition site caused it to be considered as a vector candidate.

Replication

ColE1 replication begins at the origin. 555 bp upstream from this point, RNA polymerase initiates transcription of RNA II which acts as a pre-primer and begins the synthesis of the leader strand. The transcript folds into a secondary structure which stabilizes the interaction between the nascent RNA and the origin's DNA. This hybrid is attacked by RNase H, which cleaves the RNA strand, exposing a 3′ hydroxyl group. This allows the extension of the leading strand by DNA Polymerase I. Lagging strand synthesis is later initiated by a primase encoded by the host cell. Replication is carried out entirely by host proteins (RNA polymerase, DNA polymerase I and RNase H) so that inhibition of translation will stop the growth of the cells, but not the replication of ColE1. Since the translation of Rop protein will also be inhibited, a higher than normal copy number will result in these cells.

Copy number control

RNA I is a counter-transcript to a section of RNA II and so binds to its 5′ end. This alters the folding of RNA II so that the DNA-RNA hybrid is not stabilized and cleavage does not occur. This ensures that at high copy numbers, replication is slowed down due to increased RNA I concentration. Rop is a secondary replication repressor, it stabilizes the RNA I-RNA II hybrid. Rop may be especially important at preventing runaway replication at slow growth rates (Fig. 2-64).

ColE1 has a relatively high copy number of 10~15 or even more.

III. pBR322 plasmid vector

pBR322

pBR322 is an artificially constructed plasmid and was one of the first widely used *E. coli* cloning vectors. Created in 1977 in the laboratory of Herbert Boyer at the University of California, San Francisco, it was named after the postdoctoral researchers who constructed it. The p stands for "plasmid," and BR for "Bolivar" and "Rodriguez."

pBR322 has the following advantages: a. Low molecular weight; b. High copy number; c. Dozens of types of sole restriction sites for various restriction enzymes to cleave and insert exogenous genes without affecting plasmid replication.

pBR322 is 4361 base pairs in length and has two antibiotic resistance genes — the gene *bla* encoding

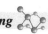

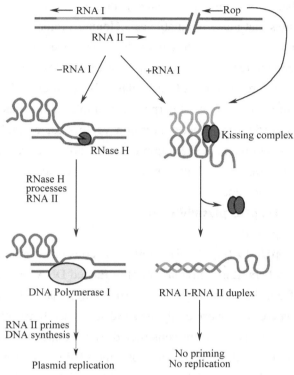

Fig. 2-64   ColE1 replication control. The copy number of plasmids with the *ori* of ColE1 is regulated by two RNA transcripts, RNA II and RNA I. RNA II is needed for the initiation of replication, whereas RNA I acts as its repressor. The nascent RNA II, whose transcription is initiated 555 bp upstream of the replication origin, forms a hybrid with the template DNA near the *ori*. RNase H cleaves the RNA strand and exposes a 3′ hydroxyl group. The processed RNA II can then serve as a primer for DNA synthesis by DNA Polymerase I. The primer formation is inhibited by RNA I, a shorter transcript which is complementary to the 5′ end of RNA II. When RNA I is present, it forms a hybrid with RNA II. This alters the folding of RNA II so that the DNA-RNA hybrid is not stabilized and cleavage does not occur. The binding of RNA I to RNA II is enhanced by the rop protein.

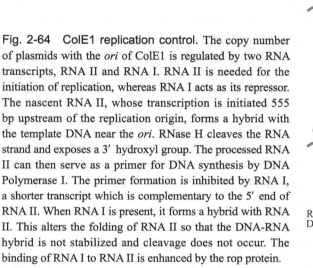

the ampicillin resistance (Amp^R) protein, and the gene *tetA* encoding the tetracycline resistance (Tet^R) protein (Fig. 2-23). It contains the origin of replication of pMB1, and the *rop* gene, which encodes a restrictor of plasmid copy number. The plasmid has unique restriction sites for more than forty restriction enzymes. Eleven of these forty sites lie within the *Tet*^{r} gene. There are two sites for restriction enzymes *Hin*dIII and *Cla*I within the promoter of the *Tet*^{r} gene. There are six key restriction sites inside the *Amp*^{r} gene.

The circular sequence is numbered such that 0 is the middle of the unique *Eco*RI site and the count increases through the *Tet*^{r} gene. The *Amp*^{r} gene is penicillin beta-lactamase. Promoters P1 and P3 are for the beta-lactamase gene. P3 is the natural promoter, and P1 is artificially created by the ligation of two different DNA fragments to create pBR322. P2 is in the same region as P1, but it is on the opposite strand and initiates transcription in the direction of the tetracycline resistance gene.

Background

Early cloning experiments may be conducted using natural plasmids such the ColE1 and pSC101. Each of these plasmids may have its advantages and disadvantages. For example, the ColE1 plasmid and its derivatives have the advantage of higher copy number and allow for chloramphenicol amplification of plasmid to produce a high yield of plasmid, however screening for immunity to colicin E1 is not technically simple. The plasmid pSC101, a natural plasmid from *Salmonella panama*, confers tetracycline resistance which allows for simpler screening process with antibiotic selection, but it is a low copy number plasmid which does not give a high yield of plasmid. Another plasmid, RSF2124, which is a derivative of ColE1, confers ampicillin resistance but is larger.

Many other plasmids were artificially constructed to create one that would be ideal for cloning purpose, and pBR322 was found to be most versatile by many and was therefore the one most popularly used. It has two antibiotic resistance genes, as selectable markers, and a number of convenient unique restriction sites that made it suitable as a cloning vector. The plasmid was constructed with genetic material from 3 main sources — the tetracycline resistance gene of pSC101, the ampicillin resistance gene of RSF2124, and the replication elements of pMB1, a close relative of the ColE1 plasmid.

A large number of other plasmids based on pBR322 have since been constructed specifically designed for a wide variety of purposes. Examples include the pUC series of plasmids, pBR324, pBR325, pBR327, pAT153, *etc*. Most expression vectors for extrachromosomal protein expression and shuttle vectors contain the pBR322 origin of replication, and fragments of pBR322 are very popular in the construction of intraspecies shuttle or binary vectors and vectors for targeted integration and excision of DNA from chromosome.

IV. pUC plasmid vector

pUC19

pUC19 (Fig. 2-54) is one of a series of plasmid cloning vectors created by Joachim Messing and co-workers. It is a circular double stranded DNA and has 2686 base pairs. The designation "pUC" is derived from the classical "p" prefix (denoting "plasmid") and the abbreviation for the University of California, where early work on the plasmid series had been conducted.

pUC series were constructed by introducing *lacZ* gene, which contains a multiple cloning site at its 5′-terminal, to the original plasmid pBR322, hence acquiring a new plasmid vector series with a feature of bifunctional detection of both antibiotic resistance and blue-white screen. pUC19 is one of the most widely used vector molecules as the recombinants（重组子）, or the cells into which foreign DNA has been introduced, can be easily distinguished from the non-recombinants based on color differences of colonies on growth media. pUC18 is similar to pUC19, but the MCS region is reversed.

Components

a. Notably, it has a *lacZα* gene of *E. coli* which encodes the first 59 residues of β-galactosidase *lacZ*, the α-peptide.

b. The promoter region of the *lac* operon of *E. coli*.

c. The *ori* site, or origin of replication, is derived from the plasmid pMB1.

d. The multiple cloning site (MCS) region is split into codons 6~7 of the *lacZ* gene, providing for many restriction endonucleases restriction sites. The recognition sites for *Hind*III, *Sph*I, *Pst*I, *Sal*I, *Xba*I, *Bam*HI, *Sma*I, *Kpn*I, *Sac*I and *Eco*RI restriction enzymes have been derived from the vector M13mp19.

e. In addition to β-galactosidase, pUC19 also encodes for an ampicillin resistance gene (*amp^r*), via a β-lactamase enzyme that functions by degrading ampicillin and reducing its toxicity to the host.

Function

This plasmid is introduced into a bacterial cell by a process called "transformation", where it can multiply and express itself. However, due to the presence of MCS and several restriction sites, a foreign piece of DNA of choice can be introduced into it by inserting it into place in MCS region. The cells which have taken up the plasmid can be differentiated from cells that have not taken up the plasmid by growing it on media with ampicillin. Only the cells with the plasmid containing the ampicillin resistance (*amp^r*) gene will survive. Furthermore, the transformed cells containing the plasmid with the gene of interest can be distinguished from cells with the plasmid but without the gene of interest, just by looking at the color of the colony they make on agar media supplemented with IPTG and X-gal. Recombinants are white, whereas non-recombinants are blue.

Mechanism

The *lacZ* fragment, whose synthesis can be induced by IPTG, is capable of intra-allelic complementation（等位基因内互补）with a defective form of β-galactosidase enzyme encoded by host chromosome (mutation lacZDM15 in *E. coli* JM109, DH5α and XL1-Blue strains). In the presence of IPTG in growth medium, bacteria synthesize both fragments of the enzyme. Both the fragments can together hydrolyze X-gal (5-bromo-4-chloro-3-indolyl-beta-D-galactopyranoside) and form blue colonies when grown on media where it is supplemented (Figure 2-24).

Insertion of foreign DNA into the MCS located within the *lacZ* gene causes insertional inactivation of this gene at the N-terminal fragment of β-galactosidase and abolishes intra-allelic complementation. Thus bacteria carrying recombinant plasmids in the MCS cannot hydrolyze X-gal, giving rise to white colonies, which can be distinguished on culture media from non-recombinant cells, which are blue.

Therefore, the media used should contain ampicillin, IPTG, and X-gal.

Use in research

Due to its extensive use as a cloning vector in research and industry, pUC19 is frequently used in research as a model plasmid. For example, biophysical studies on its naturally supercoiled state have determined its radius of gyration（旋转）to be 65.6 nm and its Stokes radius to be 43.6 nm.

Advantages:

a. pUC19 is small but has a high copy number. The high copy number is a result of the lack of the *rop* gene and a single point mutation in the *ori* of pMB1;

b. The recombinants can be easily distinguished based on color differences of colonies in the presence of IPTG and X-gal;

c. pUC19 contains a multiple cloning site region for inserting foreign DNA.

Other examples of *E. coli* expression vectors are the pGEX series of vectors, and the pET series of vectors.

V. Novel plasmid vectors

On the basis of the above important plasmid vectors, many novel plasmid vectors have been developed.

A. Plasmids with their migration ability lost（丧失了迁移功能的质粒）: For example, in plasmid pBR327, the deletion of a 1090 bp DNA fragment resulted in change of plasmid replication and conjugation performance, while the genes encoding ampicillin resistance and tetracycline resistance were still retained.

B. Plasmid vectors constructed to be able to transcribe and clone exogenous genes *in vitro*（能在体外转录克隆基因的质粒载体）: For example, the main difference between pGEM-3Z and pUC plasmid is that pGEM-3Z has two phage promoters T7 and SP6 in the flanking MCS region of *lacZ* gene. Therefore, in the presence of T7 or SP6 RNA polymerase, the cloned exogenous genes can be transcribed into corresponding mRNAs in *vitro*. Nowadays, a large number of novel pUC-based plasmids have been constructed, and promoters for phage RNA polymerase, were inserted adjacent to the multiple cloning sites, *e.g.*, pSP64, pSP65, pGEM3 and pGEM4.

C. Shuttle plasmid（穿梭载体）: A shuttle plasmid is an artificially constructed plasmid vectors with two different sets of replication origin and selectable marker, hence can survive, replicate and propagate in two different host cells/species. Shuttle plasmids can propagate in eukaryotes and prokaryotes (*e.g.*, both

Saccharomyces cerevisiae and *Escherichia coli*) or in different species of bacteria [*e.g.*, both *E. coli* and *Rhodococcus erythropolis* (红串红球菌)]. Therefore, DNA inserted into a shuttle plasmid can be tested or manipulated in two different cell types. The main advantage of these plasmid vectors is they can be manipulated in *E. coli*, then used in a system which is more difficult or slower to manipulate (*e.g.*, yeast). Shuttle plasmids are frequently used to quickly make multiple copies of the gene in *E. coli* (amplification). They can also be used for *in vitro* experiments and modifications (*e.g.*, mutagenesis, PCR).

One of the most common types of shuttle plasmids is the yeast shuttle plasmid. Almost all commonly used *S. cerevisiae* vectors are shuttle plasmids. Yeast shuttle plasmids have components that allow for replication and selection in both *E. coli* cells and yeast cells. The *E. coli* component of a yeast shuttle plasmid includes an origin of replication and a selectable marker, *e.g.*, antibiotic resistance, β-lactamase, β-galactosidase (半乳糖苷酶). The yeast component of a yeast shuttle plasmid includes an autonomously replicating sequence (*ARS*), a yeast centromere (*CEN*, 着丝粒), and a yeast selectable marker [*e.g.*, *URA3*, a gene that encodes an enzyme for uracil (尿嘧啶) synthesis]. Commonly used shuttle plasmids are *E. coli-bacillus subtilis* (枯草芽孢杆菌) (such as pHV14), *E. coli*-yeast (such as pPIC9K), *E. coli*-animal cells (such as pBPV-BV1) shuttle plasmid. They have been playing an important role in genetic engineering research.

D. Fusion expression vectors（融合表达载体）：Besides direct expression of recombinant protein, a recombinant protein can be fused to C-terminal end of a protein or peptide which is highly expressed or easily purified. Fusion expression usually leads to high expression of the exogenous gene. Through designed enzymatic site or chemical reagent breaking site, fusion partner can be easily cut off *in vitro*. Examples of *E. coli* fusion expression vectors are the pGEX series of vectors where glutathione-S-transferase is used as a fusion partner and protein expression is under the control of the *tac* promoter, and the pETGST series of vectors which use a T7 promoter.

E. Secretory expression vector（分泌表达载体）：Some genes coding for signal peptides can be designed and constructed in a secretory expression vector. After expression, the signal peptide would lead the newly formed recombinant protein into periplasm or extracellular medium.

F. Coexpression vector（共表达载体）：Many eukaryotic expression products would form an enzymatic complex. Only in this way, can their activity be exerted. Therefore, a coexpression vector is usually constructed to contain all these relevant genes. Sometimes chaperons are coexpressed to assist target protein folding properly.

a. Co-expression of protein complexes in *E. coli*

Many different techniques are used to co-express proteins in cells. It is possible to simultaneously express two or more different proteins in *E. coli* using different plasmids. However, when 2 or more plasmids are used, each plasmid needs to use a different antibiotic selection as well as a different origin of replication, otherwise the plasmids may not be stably maintained. Many commonly-used plasmids are based on the ColE1 replicon and are therefore incompatible with each other. In order for a ColE1-based plasmid to coexist with another in the same cell, the other would need to be of a different replicon, *e.g.*, a p15A replicon-based plasmid such as the pACYC series of plasmids. Another approach would be to use a single two-cistron (双顺反子) vector or design the coding sequences in tandem as a bi- or poly-cistronic construct.

（a）**Multiple vectors.** In *E. coli*, the easiest approach for co-expressing proteins is to use vectors with

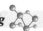

different resistance markers, each vector bearing a single gene. Vectors with the same origin of replication can be used as long as their resistance markers are different. However, plasmids with same origin of replication can 'compete' inside a cell and one of the plasmids might end up being less amplified than the others within the cell (especially in high-density cultures). This can lead to complexes with poor stoichiometry or even missing subunits. In this respect, a theoretically sound and practically proven approach is to use vectors with different origins of replication. More than two vectors can be used, but the question of the correct maintenance of all the plasmids within the cell remains since the amplification of some of them could be down-regulated.

（b）**Single vector, single RNA transcript.**

Another coexpression strategy is to have the various genes cloned on a single vector. This can be achieved by cloning all genes under the control of a single promoter, each gene having its own ribosome-binding site (RBS). This strategy results in a long polycistronic mRNA: its length is restricted by the capabilities of the polymerase used and the intrinsic stability of mRNA. Moreover, the efficiency of ribosome binding to the RBS depends on mRNA structure. Typically, a linker DNA sequence between the end of one gene and the RBS for the next one needs to be introduced. Expression levels and efficiency are sometimes, albeit not always, crucially dependent on the order with which the complex components appear on the common mRNA.

A bicistronic construct has the following advantages over the use of two separate plasmids. First, it is the method of choice in cases where strict control of stoichiometry is necessary to form a functional protein unit. Second, it requires the use of only one antibiotic-resistance marker for plasmid selection.

（c）**Single vector, multiple RNA transcripts.** The use of separate promoters for each gene on a single plasmid results in multiple RNA transcripts, offering an alternative to the method described above in **(b) Single vector, single RNA transcript** section. In this case, the plasmid is larger but the mRNAs are smaller and different promoters can be used. A recent study suggests that a multi-transcript approach appears to give higher yields than a single-transcript polycistronic system. It must be noted that all these techniques (*i.e.,* several vectors, several genes on a single promoter and several promoters on a single plasmid) are compatible and therefore can be combined to increase the number of proteins coexpressed within a single *E. coli* cell.

b. A novel co-expression strategy for *E. coli*

The Strasbourg laboratory has previously developed a co-expression system (Fribourg *et al.*, 2001) based on two vectors [pET15b (Novagen) and pACYC11b, having different resistance markers and compatible origins of replication] that has proved successful in numerous cases. The major limitation of this system was that only two genes could be co-expressed at the same time.

To overcome this limitation, a new set of vectors (pET-MCN; pET multi-cloning and expression) were developed that allows the expression of more than two genes, but is also sufficiently flexible to test the influence of the purification tag without requiring extensive cloning. Initially, all genes of interest are cloned into both vectors; cloning into the pET15b vector results in a His-tagged version of each gene, while cloning into the pACYC11b vector results in an untagged version. Performing all pairwise co-expression experiments, the possible influence of the tag in complex formation can be tested easily. To be able to express more than two genes at a time (one from each vector), both the pET15b and pACYC11b vectors were modified to enable an easy 'cut-and-paste' strategy. In the 'cut' step, a piece of the T7 promoter containing the RBS and the gene of interest (that is already cloned to this vector) is excised (cut). In the 'paste' step, the excised piece is ligated into the T7 promoter of another vector that already contains another gene (paste). This construction leads to a single promoter with two different genes, each one preceded by its own RBS. This mechanism is based on the compatibility of the restriction sites *Spe*I, *Xba*I, *Nhe*I and *Avr*II, which are not affected in each cloning step, and thus this procedure can be repeated as many times as desired, leading to multi-cistronic constructs. Further modifications of the pET15b vector in Strasbourg allowed replacement of its N-terminal His tag by either a C-terminal His tag or an N-terminal fusion protein (thioredoxin, glutathione-S-transferase, maltose-binding protein or NusA) associated or not with an N- or a C-terminal His tag. These different combinations have been made to improve the success rate for expressing poorly soluble proteins as soluble fusion proteins that could then be stabilized by interacting with their natural partner(s). So far, two protease sites have been used: thrombin or TEV. Restriction sites have been introduced to be able to easily replace either the fusion protein or the protease site onto the plasmids and therefore abolish possible solubility problems or degradation through cryptic（隐藏的）protease sites. Altogether, when considering all different fusions, 34 vectors have been generated that are all compatible with the cut-and-paste cloning procedure.

A typical workflow using the pET-MCN system is shown in Fig. 2-65 and is described below. (i) The different constructs generated from the genes of interest are cloned into both the modified pET15b and pACYC11b vectors. Different fusions could be used for constructs that seem to be poorly soluble. (ii) At this stage each possible pair can be tested for interaction by co-expression in *E. coli*. (iii) Constructs coding for interacting protein pairs are transferred onto a single vector following the cut-and-paste procedure described above. (iv) These vectors are used for interaction studies against the initial pool of vectors (looking for trimeric complexes) but also against themselves (looking for tetrameric complexes). If novel interactions are found in this round, new vectors are generated and a new cycle is initiated. Since one cannot exclude the case that soluble complexes will only be obtained upon co-expression of three or four subunits, it might be interesting to generate 'random' bi-cistronic vectors for step (iv) regardless of results in step (ii). Control experiments in Strasbourg showed that in either single expression or two-vector pairwise（成对发生的）expression no decrease in protein yields was observed. Moreover, bicistronic vectors showed identical expression as with two vectors. The presence of the pRare plasmid (encoding several *E. coli* rare tRNAs; Novagen), which can be used when all genes are cloned onto a single plasmid with different antibiotic resistance, sometimes results in an increase in the yield of soluble purified protein. Finally, the three subunit transcription factor NFY was co-expressed, with His-tagged NFYA cloned into modified pET15b and the non-tagged NFYB/ NFYC histone-like pair cloned as a bicistron into modified pACYC11b. Expression tests show proper formation of the ternary NFY. The pET-MCN system has also been tested in other laboratories in Europe. Notably, at EMBL a trimeric complex was expressed as a combination of two vectors, one containing a single gene and the second containing two genes on a single promoter. This complex was expressed, purified and its structure solved. More recently, the genes coding for the three subunits were appended into a single promoter and the complex was expressed and purified as the one expressed from two vectors.

G. Univector plasmid-fusion system（通用载体质粒融合系统）: Univector plasmid-fusion system (UPS) is the central cloning method of a series of new cloning methods that facilitate the rapid and systematic construction of recombinant DNA molecules. The UPS uses Cre-*lox* site-specific recombination to

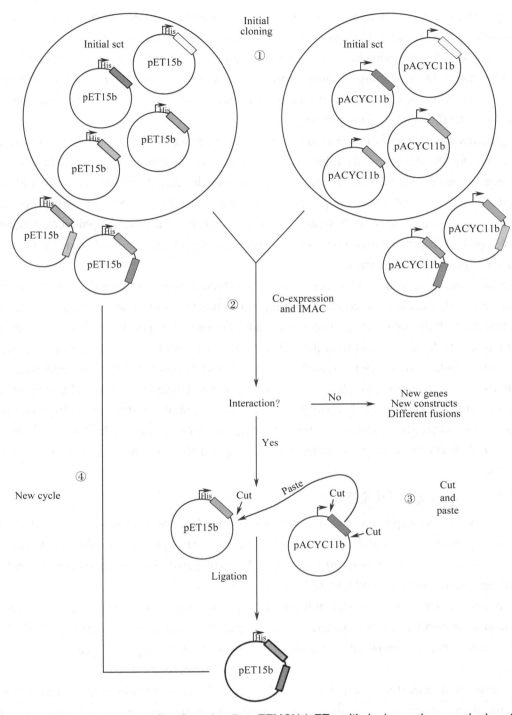

Fig. 2-65   The suggested workflow for using the pETMCN (pET multi-cloning and expression) system.

catalyze plasmid fusion between the univector — a plasmid containing the gene of interest — and host vectors containing regulatory information. Fusion events are genetically selected and place the gene under the control of new regulatory elements. A second UPS-related method allows for the precise transfer of coding sequences only from the univector into a host vector. The UPS eliminates the need for restriction enzymes, DNA ligases and many *in vitro* manipulations required for subcloning, and allows for the rapid construction of multiple constructs for expression in multiple organisms. UPS can also be used to transfer whole libraries into new vectors. Additional adaptations include directional PCR cloning and the generation of 3′ end gene fusions using homologous recombination in *Escherichia coli*. Together, these recombination-based cloning methods constitute a new comprehensive approach for the rapid and efficient generation of recombinant DNA that can be used for parallel processing of large gene sets, a feature that will facilitate future genomic analysis.

Most proteins are expressed in the cytoplasm of *E. coli*, however, not all proteins formed may be soluble in the cytoplasm. Incorrectly folded proteins formed in cytoplasm can form **inclusion body**（包涵体）which will require refolding. Where necessarily, for example when the protein can only fold correctly in an oxidizing environment due to the presence of disulphide bonds, the protein may be targeted to the periplasmic space by the use of an N-terminal signal sequence. Other more sophisticated systems are being developed; such systems may allow for the expression of proteins previously thought impossible in *E. coli*, such as glycosylated proteins.

Escherichia. coli has been used successfully to produce proteins previously thought difficult or impossible in *E. coli*, such as those containing multiple disulfide bonds or those requiring post-translational modification for stability or function. The cellular environment of *E. coli* is normally too reducing for disulphide bonds to form, proteins with disulphide bonds therefore may be secreted to its periplasmic space, however, mutants in which the reduction of both thioredoxins（硫氧还蛋白）and glutathione is impaired also allow disulphide bonded proteins to be produced in the cytoplasm of *E. coli*. It has also been used to produce proteins with various post-translational modifications, including glycoproteins by using the N-linked glycosylation system of *Campylobacter jejuni*（空肠弯曲杆菌）engineered into *E. coli*. Efforts are currently under way to expand this technology to produce complex glycosylations.

2.5.1.2 *Bacillus spp.*（芽孢杆菌）

Bacillus is one of the important industrial microorganisms. It is the main producer of many industrial enzymes, occupies nearly 60% of the enzyme market share. Bacteria in Genus *Bacillus* are Gram-positive organisms. Among them, *Bacillus subtilis* is one of the most popularized microorganisms employed in molecular genetics research, second only to *E. coli.*.

A significant progress also has been achieved in the molecular biology research and expression of heterologous gene cloning of other Bacteria in Genus *Bacillus*, such as *Bacillus brevis*（短芽孢杆菌）（renamed as *Brevibacillus brevis* later), *Bacillus licheniformis*（地衣芽孢杆菌）, *etc*.

1990s

➤ Cultures of *B. subtilis* were popular worldwide before the introduction of antibiotics as an immunostimulatory agent to aid treatment of gastrointestinal and urinary tract diseases. It was used throughout the 1950s as an alternative medicine, which upon digestion has been found to significantly stimulate broad-spectrum immune activity including activation of secretion of specific antibodies IgM, IgG and IgA and release of CpG dinucleotides inducing INF A/Y producing activity of leukocytes and cytokines（细胞因子，细胞激素）important in the development of cytotoxicity towards tumor cells. It was marketed throughout America and Europe from 1946 as an immunostimulatory aid in the treatment of gut and urinary tract diseases such as Rotavirus（轮状病毒）and *Shigella*（志贺氏杆菌）, but declined in popularity after the introduction of cheap consumer（消费类，日需）antibiotics, despite causing fewer allergic reactions and significantly lower toxicity to normal gut flora. It is still widely used in Western Europe and the Middle East as an alternative medicine. The high stability of *B. subtilis* in harsh environmental conditions makes this microorganism a perfect candidate for probiotics（益生菌，微生态制剂）applications either in baked and pasteurized（用巴氏法消毒，用加热杀菌法）foods/beverages or in other galenic forms（药物剂型）like tablets, capsules, and powder.

➤ Wild-type isolates of *B. subtilis* are difficult to work with compared to laboratory strains that have undergone domestication（驯化，驯养）processes of mutagenesis and selection. These strains often have improved capabilities of transformation (uptake and integration of environmental DNA), growth, and loss of abilities needed "in the wild". And, while dozens of different strains fitting this description exist, the strain designated '168' (*B. subtilis* 168) is the most widely used.

➤ A strain of *B. subtilis* formerly known as *Bacillus natto*（纳豆芽孢杆菌）is used in the commercial production of the Japanese food *natto*, as well as the similar Korean food *cheonggukjang*（清国酱）.

2000s

➤ As a model organism, *B. subtilis* is commonly used in laboratory studies directed at discovering the fundamental properties and characteristics of Gram-positive spore-forming bacteria. In particular, the basic principles and mechanisms underlying formation of the durable endospore（内生孢子）have been deduced from studies of spore formation in *B. subtilis*.

➤ Due to its excellent fermentation properties, with high product yields (20 to 25 grams per liter) it is used to produce various enzymes, such as amylase（淀粉酶）and proteases.

➤ Other enzymes produced by *B. subtilis* and *Bacillus licheniformis*（地衣芽孢杆菌）are widely used as additives in laundry detergents.

➤ It is used to produce hyaluronic acid（透明质酸）, which is used in the joint-care sector（关节护理行业）in healthcare and cosmetics.

The extensive knowledge of the molecular biology of *Bacillus subtilis* has led to the development of this bacterium as a host for industrial production of heterologous proteins. At present, some foreign genes have been successfully cloned and expressed in *Bacillus*. *Bacillus* as a gene expression system has the following characteristics ——

Characteristics of the expression system of *Bacillus*（芽孢杆菌的表达体系特点）:

1. Multiple sigma factor: RNA polymerase holoenzyme is composed of 5 subunits ($\alpha_2\beta\beta + \sigma$).

Ten sigma factors have been identified in *Bacillus subtilis*— σA (σ43, σ55), σB (σ37), σC (σ32), σD (σ28), σH (σ30), σL, σE (σ29), σF ($\sigma^{SPDIIAC}$), σG, σK (they sited on different genes, perform different functions, recognize different sequences of −35 and −10 regions and distances in between) — while only two in *E. coli*. Therefore, the genes of most Gram-negative bacteria cannot be directly expressed in *Bacillus* — the promoter and other components need to be replaced.

2. Ribosome binding site (RBS) : the most typical SD sequence of *Bacillus subtilis* is -GGAGG, while that of *E. coli* is -AAGGA.

3. *Escherichia coli* usually secretes proteins between two membranes (plasma membrane and outer membrane), whereas *Bacillus subtilis* has only one membrane and can secrete proteins into the culture medium in large quantities.

According to computer analysis, *Bacillus subtilis* has nearly 300 proteins with N-terminal signaling peptides for transmembrane use. However, the signal peptides used to express and secrete cloned genes mainly come from proteases, amylases and cell wall surface proteins.

Cytosolic Chaperones

Most proteins that are destined for export can only be translocated across the membrane in a more or less unfolded conformation that allows them to pass through the translocation channel of the Sec pathway. To facilitate this, cytosolic factors aid in maintaining these preproteins in a so-called translocation-competent state. Such factors, called chaperones, bind to preproteins and prevent their folding and aggregation. Some of these chaperones are secretion dedicated and assist in protein targeting to the translocase.

Secretion-dedicated chaperones. In *B. subtilis*, the only secretion-specific chaperone thus far identified is the Ffh protein (fifty-four homologue), a GTPase that is homologous to the 54-kDa subunit of the eukaryotic signal recognition Particle (Srp54).

(1) Advantages of Bacillus expression system

This Gram-positive bacterium has the following advantages.

A. *Bacillus subtilis* has no known pathogenic interactions with humans or animals, except for a few species, *i.e.*, *Bacillus anthracis*（炭疽杆菌）and *Bacillus cereus*（蜡样芽孢杆菌）.

B. Transformation can be readily carried out when natural *B. subtilis* competent cell is adopted; the mechanism of transforming exogenous DNA into competent cell also applies to transforming recombinant DNA.

C. An in-depth research has already been conducted on the genetics of *Bacillus subtilis*.

D. It is easy to manipulate *B. subtilis* under lab conditions.

E. Genome sequencing of *B. subtilis* has already been completed.

F. Both plasmids and bacteriophages can be used as cloning vectors. A lot of useful plasmid vectors are now available for *B. subtilis*.

G. Efficient secretory expression capacity — homologous and heterologous proteins can be secreted into culture media with *B. subtilis* serving as the host cell.

Some extracellular proteins (homologous proteins) can be secreted in a large amount. After crossing the plasma membrane, the proteins are either processed or released directly to the culture media rather than aggregate, therefore facilitate the recovery and purification process, *e.g.*, α-amylase, protease, and pesticidal crystal protein（杀虫晶体蛋白）, *etc*.

H. There is no obvious coden preference in *Bacillus*, and the expression products do not form inclusion bodies in general. In a *E.coli* expression system, if there are a large number of consecutive rare codens in an ORF encoding for the exogenous proteins to be recombinantly expressed, the expression level is usually low, or the translation would terminate prematurely. Formation of inclusion body of the target protein product will make the protein insoluble, which in turn will bring a lot of inconvenience to the separation, purification and recovery of the target protein. While *B. subtilis* expression system has no such problems in both aspects.

I. Some ponderable（有重要意义的）signal peptide sequences are available.

J. The fermentation technology is already mature. Good fermentation foundation and production technology made it possible to reach rather high cell density with rather simple culture media.

K. A genetically engineered strain with *B. subtilis* serving as host cell can grow effectively even though only a low-cost approach of strain preservation is used.

L. The cell wall composition of *Bacillus* is simple. Only peptidoglycan and teichoic acid are included. Therefore no endotoxin impurities would be found among the secreted protein products.

M. Prolonged product shelf life.

Hence, *Bacillus* species have been found in many industrial applications, and **Bacillus expression systems** are well developed for scale cultivation.

(2) Shortcomings

Nevertheless, the production of recombinant proteins by *Bacillus subtilis* can be limited by some disadvantages:

A. Industrial strains are difficult to be transformed. Rare strains in Genus *Bacillus* would autonomously enter the competent state, and the duration of cell maintaining competent state is so transient, leading to low molecular cloning efficiency.

B. The efficiency of plasmid transformation is low with the ligation mixture.

C. The secretory expression level is low for most of the heterogenous proteins and there are degradation issues — the high levels of proteases secreted would cause substantial degradation of secreted foreign proteins.

D. There are some restriction-modification systems [RM system] in *Bacillus* strains, hence the recombinant plasmids are usually unstable in such hosts.

E. The lack of understanding about the genetic and physiological processes of fermentation of *B. subtilis*, *e.g.*, the lack of information about its secretion pathway, and the plasmid structure and segregational instability.

Bacillus subtilis（枯草杆菌，枯草芽孢杆菌）

Bacillus subtilis, known also as the *hay bacillus* or *grass bacillus*, is a Gram-positive, catalase-positive bacterium（过氧化氢酶阳性菌）, found in soil and the gastrointestinal tract of ruminants and humans. A member of the genus *Bacillus*（杆菌属，芽孢杆菌属）, *B. subtilis* is rod-shaped, and can form a tough, protective endospore（内生孢子）, allowing it to tolerate extreme environmental conditions of temperature and desiccation（干燥，极端干旱）. *B. subtilis* is heavily flagellated（生有鞭毛的）, which gives it the ability to move quickly in liquids. *B. subtilis* has historically been classified as an obligate aerobe（专性需氧微生物）, though evidence exists that it is a facultative aerobe（兼性需氧微生物）. *B. subtilis* has proven highly amenable（可用某种方式处理的）to genetic manipulation, and is considered the best studied Gram-positive bacterium. *B. subtilis* has become widely adopted as a model organism to study bacterial chromosome replication and cell differentiation (especially of sporulation（孢子形成）, which is a simplified example of cellular differentiation). It is one of the bacterial champions（冠军）in secreted enzyme production and used on an industrial scale by biotechnology companies.

Transcription system

Promoter

The canonical −35 recognition site and −10 Pribnow box of the σA-dependent-promoter in *Bacillus subtilis* are similar to that of *E. coli*, with conservative sequences of TTGACA and TATAAT, respectively. The distance between those regions of promoter is 17~18 bp for the σA-dependent promoter, while those for other RNA polymerase vary, being 15~16 bp, mostly. In general, the promoter becomes weaker when the distance deviates from 17 bp, either longer or shorter.

In *Bacillus subtilis*, many promoters have their regions upstream of the −35 region rich in AT, and the AT rich region is called the transcriptional enhancement region, which is very important for gene transcription.

At least in *Bacillus subtilis*, many promoters contain an important TGTG sequence motif (−16) upstream of the −10 region, and mutations in this region can significantly reduce the promoter strength. Although this −16 region is also found in *E. coli*, such promoters often lack the −35 region which is found in the *Bacillus subtilis*.

In addition, the region between −10 region and −1 region is also usually rich in A, which facilitates the local unwinding of DNA at the beginning of transcription. Studies of many σA-dependent promoters of *Bacillus subtilis* have shown that they carry the canonical −10 and −35 sequences present in *E. coli* promoters.

The above promoters retains a lot of polyA and polyT regions upstream of the −35 region.

So far, promoters of *Bacillus subtilis* have been found in two forms: in the first category are single promoters, most of which are expressed in rapid growth period;

In the second category are compound promoters (the most common example is P43), which include tandem promoters and overlapping promoters. Overlapping promoters have the following characteristics :

(1) Two different types of promoters overlap.

(2) Those two promoters have different transcription initiation sites or the same initiation site.

(3) Some promoters may be regulated by timing sequence. These promoters play an important role in the perception of environmental changes and spore formation of *Bacillus subtilis*.

Terminator

Once the RNA polymerase initiates transcription, it continues to synthesize nucleic acids until it reaches the termination site.

Bacterial DNA has two types of transcription termination sites: ρ-dependent and ρ-independent. In *Bacillus subtilis* gene transcriptional termination, only a few genes have been well studied. Their termination regions are rich in reversed repeats of GC, followed by a series of A (T), *i.e.*, ρ-independent termination of transcription. Some data show that the terminators of *Bacillus subtilis* are similar to that of *E. coli* in structure and sequence, and it is found that the terminating structures of *E. coli* also function in *Bacillus subtilis*.

Currently, the terminators commonly used for exogenous gene expression are rrnT1 and rrnT2 derived from rRNA operon of *E. coli* and Tφ derived from T7 phage DNA.

For some terminators with weak chain-terminating effect a special tandem structure of terminator dimer can be used to enhance their transcriptional terminating effect. Terminators can also be cloned and screened from bacterial or phage genomic DNA by special probe plasmids, as what has been done to promoters.

Translation system

1. Ribosomal binding site (RBS) of *Bacillus subtilis* mRNA, also known as SD sequence. The typical SD sequence of *Bacillus subtilis* is GGAGG, which is different from *E. coli*'s AAGGA.

Generally speaking, the stronger the binding degree between mRNA and ribosome, the higher the efficiency of translation initiation, and the binding degree is mainly determined by the base complementarity of SD sequence and 16S rRNA, among which the four base sequence GGAG is especially important. For most genes, a switch to a C or a T for any of the four bases will cause a dramatic reduction in translation efficiency.

2. The 3′ end of 16S rRNA of ribosomes is involved in mRNA recognition and initial translation, while the 3′ end of 16S rRNA of *Bacillus subtilis* is different from that of *E. coli*. The ribosomes of *Bacillus subtilis* can only recognize homologous mRNAs.

The ribosomes of *E. coli* can support the mRNAs of both Gram-positive and Gram-negative bacteria to direct protein synthesis.

Therefore, as a Gram-negative bacteria *Escherichia coli*, its genes, with some exceptions, generally can not be expressed directly in the Gram-positive bacteria *Bacillus*, while *Bacillus* genes can be expressed in the *Escherichia coli*.

Note: this is because the 30S subunit of ribosome of Gram-positive bacteria lacks S1 protein, which may involve in the ribosome binding. Furthermore, the promoter of Gram-negative bacteria cannot be recognized by *Bacillus subtilis*.

The sequence between the SD sequence and the start codon also affects translation efficiency, with the region rich in A+T usually 15~50 times more efficient than that rich in G+C.

If the base sequence downstream of a SD sequence is AAAA or UUUU, the translation efficiency would be the highest. If it is CCCC and GGGG, the translation efficiency is just 50% and 25% of the maximum, respectively.

The first three bases next to AUG also affect the translation initiation.

For the mRNA encoding beta-galactose in *E. coli*, the best combination of bases at this location is UAU or CUU, and the expression level of the enzyme would be 20 times lower if it was replaced with UUC, UCA, or AGG.

The precise distance between the SD sequence and the initiation codon ensures that after the mRNA attaches to the ribosome, the translation initiation codon AUG will be docked at the P position of the ribosomal complex, which is a prerequisite for translation initiation. In general, the last G of the GGAG G consensus sequence is 7~9 bases away from the start codon. In this interval — one single base less or more — can lead to different levels of reduction of translation initiation efficiency.

In *Bacillus subtilis*, the initiation codon of most genes is AUG, with a few exception of GUG or UUG. Here AUG is still the best choice of initiation codon.

In *E. coli*, the initial tRNA molecule can recognize all AUG, GUG, and UUG, while with different recognition probabilities（概率）.

The base sequence of the first few codons, starting from AUG, is also critical. It should not form a stem-loop structure with the non-coding region of the 5′-end of the mRNA, otherwise the accurate localization（定位）of the mRNA on the ribosome would be seriously interfered.

Secretion pathways

According to the study of proteomics, the protein secretion pathways mainly include (1) Sec secretion pathway and (2) Tat secretion pathway. Other secretion pathways include ABC Transporter（ABC 转运子途径）, which is mainly used to output molecules such as bacteriocin（细菌素）, (3) Com secretion pathway, which is related to the competence formation of *B. subtilis*, and responsible for the binding and ingestion（吸收）of DNA in this process. Through actions of 4 proteins ComGC, ComGE, ComGD and ComGG, the signal peptide of preprotein output via this pathway is cleaved off by type IV signal peptidase (type IV SPase).

Hosts and vectors commonly used in *Bacillus*

Bacillus subtilis has many attractive features to serve as an expression host for foreign protein production. These features include the non-pathogenic nature of *B. subtilis*, well-established safety record, ability to secrete extracellular proteins directly to culture medium, easy genetic manipulation, non-biased codon usage and fast growth rate. However, there are at least two major problems associated with the use of *B. subtilis* as the expression host. These include the presence of high level of extracellular proteases and the formation of inclusion bodies for certain proteins. With the extensive characterization of structural genes encoding proteases and molecular chaperones, protease deficient strains and strains that can constitutively coproduce molecular chaperones at a higher level have been constructed. These strains have been demonstrated to improve both the quality and quantity of the secreted foreign proteins by increasing protein stability, minimizing N-terminal heterogeneity and promoting protein solubility. In combination with appropriate expression vectors, optimized culture media and fermentation technology, staphylokinase（葡激酶）, a promising blood-clot dissolving agent, can be overproduced up to 350 mg/L in high quality. With the characterization of key secretory components involved in different secretory pathways and the availability of sequence information of the entire genome, it is possible to engineer *B. subtilis* to be an idealized expression host using rational approaches.

Besides the expression host, a key component for an expression system is the expression vector. Significant progress has been made in the research on *Bacillus subtilis* plasmid vectors. The plasmid vectors of *Bacillus subtilis* are basically applicable to other bacteria of the genus *Bacillus*.

Now there are six main methods that can be used for heterologous DNA transforming into *B. subtilis*: a. electrotransformation (electroporation); b. competent cell transformation; c. competent cell transformation (Spizizen method); d. protoplast transformation and regeneration (Takashi method); e. protoplast transformation and resuscitation（复苏）; f. bacteriophage mediated transformation.

At present, the commonly used vectors in *Bacillus* mainly include three kinds of plasmids, they are self-replicating plasmids, integrated plasmids and phages. Self-replicating plasmids which have been isolated from *Bacillus* are all cryptic（隐藏的）plasmids without any resistance marker only with a few exceptions (such as pBC16).

The plasmids with resistance markers were mainly from other G$^+$ bacteria, especially from *Staphylococcus aureus*. With the findings that several staphylococcal plasmids can be functional in *B. subtilis*, these plasmids form the basis for the development of various cloning and expression vectors for this microorganism.

Commonly used (drug) selectable markers（抗药性标记）in cloning vectors include: chloramphenicol resistance（抗氯霉素）, erythromycin resistance（抗红霉素）, neomycin resistance（抗新霉素）, spectinomycin resistant（抗壮观霉素）, tetracycline resistance（抗四环素）.

Replicons（复制子）of replicable plasmids can be categorized into Rolling circle Replicon (or Rolling circle Mechanism Replicon, RCM Replicon) and Theta Replicon.

pUB110, pC194 and pE194 (Table 2-8) are typical RCM replicon plasmids, while pAMβ1 is a Theta replicon plasmid.

pBS72, a recently discovered endogenous plasmid of *B. subtilis,* contains a new type of Theta replicator.

With some exceptions, RCM replicon plasmids are usually unstable and can be easily lost when there

Table 2-8   Plasmid vectors commonly used in *Bacillus* expression system.

	pUB110	pE194	pC194
Molecular weight	2.9×10^6 dalton (intact)/4.5 kb	2.4×10^6 dalton/3.7 kb (3728 bp)	1.8×10^6 dalton/2.9 kb
Plasmid copy numbers	30~100/cell 30~50/cell (*Bacillus subtilis*) Plasmid pUB110 regulates its copy number by an antisense RNA that controls the synthesis of the rate limiting RepU protein.	10~25/cell (*Staphylococcus aureas*) 10/cell (37℃) (*Bacillus subtilis*)	Medium 15 1. the medium copy number (20~50 per chromosome) plasmid pC194 2. the low copy number (1~2 per chromosome) plasmid pMTL500Eres [*Bacillus cereus* (蜡样芽孢杆菌)] spores)
Resistance/ Plasmid marker	Neomycin sulfate, neomycin resistance gene, kanamycin (Km)* resistance Neomycin (kanamycin) and phleomycin (腐草霉素) (bleomycin, 博莱霉素)	Erythromycin-resistant Co-resistance to microlide, lincosamide, and streptogramin type B (MLS) antibiotics	Chloramphenicol (氯霉素) resistance, Cmʳ
Common features	Originally isolated from *Staphylococcus aureas* and transferred to *Bacillus subtilis*. pC194, pE194 and pUB110 plasmids replicate like the *E. coli* bacteriophage ϕX174. The replication proceeds **unidirectionally in a counterclockwise direction.** pUB110 replicates asymmetrically like other Gram-positive plasmids, such as pC194 and pE194. pC194, pE194 and pUB110 plasmids replicate by the **rolling circle type mechanism,** they are now collectively known as the **rolling circle (RC) plasmids.** Replication of those plasmids requires a double-stranded origin equivalent to the phage plus origin, a replication protein (Rep), and a single-stranded origin equivalent to the phage minus origin. Rolling circle replication is initiated and terminated at the same site in the plus-origin of replication.		

is no antibiotic resistance gene. Whereas the Theta replicon plasmid is much more stable and is a good candidate for the construction of recombinant expression system.

So far, double-labeled plasmids, *Bacillus-Escherichia coli* shuttle plasmids, expression plasmids, integrating plasmid and probe plasmids have been constructed on the basis of the above plasmids.

Generally speaking, the copy number of most vectors in Gram-positive bacteria is relatively low.

The first generation plasmid vectors include pUB110, pE194 and pC194, *etc*. Vectors developed one after another in recent years (such as pTA1060 and pHP13) have been widely used in shotgun cloning experiments.

pUB110

Plasmid PUB110 and its derivatives have been used widely in *B. subtilis* as cloning and expression vectors, secretion vectors and promoter probe vectors. It has been used as a vector to clone DNA for expression and secretion studies.

The orientation of the inserted gene in pUB110-based vector can greatly affect gene expression.

A majority of plasmids (60%~80%) pUB110 bind to the membrane, which is necessary for pUB110 intiation of replication *in vivo*.

TCAGCAA/AGTCGTT frequently found in or adjacent to the type-II binding area open reading frame α (ORFα) corresponding to 334 amino acids adjacent to the **replication origin** may be essential for the **initiation of replication** of pUB110.

The PepU protein binds to the pUB110 superhelical DNA origin, generating a specific **nick** and a "**functional gap**". DNA helicase and DNA polymerase III account for asymmetric replication. RepU terminates DNA synthesis after a full round of replication.

Since the plasmid copy number for pUB110 (30~100 copies per cell) is much higher than that for PE194 (10 copies per cell), pUB110 and its derivatives have been used extensively for expression studies.

pE194

pE194 is a covalently closed circular DNA. It is a small, multicopy plasmid, which confers resistance to the macrolide-lincosamide-streptogramin B group of antibiotics.

Cop — a protein involved in the copy number control of plasmid pE194, possessing a trimer-like structure.

The region to drive autonomous replication, is contained within the 0.9-kilobase segment. This segment contains *ori*, an incompatibility determinant (*incA*), and specifies（规定）a trans-acting substance, the product of *rep*, which is required for the stable replication of pE194 derivatives. It also contains the target sites for the *rep* and *cop (incA)* products.

Wild-type pE194 cannot replicate above about 43℃.

pE194 appears to **replicate unidirectionally** from an origin located $20.4 \pm 2.7\%$ from the *Hae*III site. The most likely location for the pE194 origin is near 40~50.

The replication origin has been localized to a 199 bp segment between position 1 588 and 1 389 that lies within the coding region of *repF*. This segment also contains the site of action of the *repF* gene product, since it is sufficient for replication when driven in *trans* by the *repF* gene product.

pC194

All pC194-type rolling circle plasmids contain a double (plus) strand origin (*dso*).

The single stranded origin of replication of the pC194 group of plasmids is a critical determinant of the host range of the plasmids.

An antisense RNA IncA regulates the RepH synthesis by a mechanism that seems to involve RNA/RNA interaction in a manner that interferes with translation. IncA may be a micRNA (mRNA-interfering complementary RNA). The consequence of the RNA-RNA interaction would be the formation of a fully base paired sequence at the ribosomal binding site, making this product unavailable for initiation of *rep*H translation.

pC194 is **nicked** at a specific site within the replication region by its replication protein. The **nick site sequence** CTTGATA is found at the **double-stranded origin** (previously called the plus origin) of most of the members of the pC194 group of plasmid.

The plasmid replication origin is localized in a 55 bp region containing the nick site. The pC194 origin sequence (the 55 bp region) contains two palindromes, 14 and 5 bp long, which have the potential to fold into two hairpins, respectively. The latter contains the nick site. Formation of the hairpin may be important for origin activity. The importance of the smaller palindrome was confirmed.

Three features of pC194 replication emerged from these studies.

(1) First, the signal (sequence requirements) for initiation of pC194 replication is apparently more stringent than that for termination. The complete wild-type 55 bp origin was necessary for initiation,

while termination occurred with full efficiency at a shortened 36 bp origin.

(2) Second, both the sequence and the structure of the origin are important for its activity and affect termination. In the wild type origin the nick site is contained within a sequence that can be folded into a hairpin.

(3) Third, successful termination of one replication cycle is not followed by reinitiation of another.

Replication mode, whose replication depends on a plasmid encoded replication initiation protein. pC194 encodes a replication protein which introduces a nick at the plasmid replication origin.

pUB110 & pE194

pE194 and pUB110 are compatible.

pUB110 and PE194 are two commonly used plasmids in *B. subtilis*. Since they can coexist in the same host, these vectors are key components for a binary expression system in *B. subtilis*. One of these plasmids can be applied to direct the expression of the inserted DNA fragment encoding the protein of interest while the other plasmid can coproduce accessory factors such as molecular chaperones and transcription activation factors for enhanced production of foreign proteins.

pUB110 & pC194

A 18-bp consensus sequence appears at the origin of replication (the 5′ end of the **replication region**) of both pUB110 and pC194. In the case of pC194, the 18-bp region includes the site that is nicked by the plasmid replication protein. This nick site is considered to be the site of both initiation and termination of DNA replication.

5′-TTCTTTCTTATCTTG↓ATA

A sequence similar to the consensus sequence of 18 bp also appears at the site of the origin of replication of φX174 which also replicates via a rolling circle mechanism.

In spite of the high degree of homology between pC194 and pUB110 either at the *ori*U DNA sequence or the Rep protein levels, they show a distinct pattern with regard to the amount of single stranded circular DNA that is accumulated during replication. pC194 and pUB110 show the same directionality（方向性）(**counterclockwise**) of replication.

pE194 & pC194

The apparent functional and structural similarities of two sets of inverted complementary repeat sequences in pE194 and pC194 appear to be associated with replication.

pE194 and pC194 plasmids have been enthusiastically adopted by *Bacillus* workers, particularly as potential cloning vehicles in *B. subtilis*. Antibiotic resistance specified by these two plasmids — erythromycin-resistance by pE194 and chloramphenical resistance by pC194 is inducible by the respective antibiotics.

Escherichia coli-bacillus shuttle plasmids, such as plasmid pGK12, plasmid pHV1431, and temperature-sensitive plasmids were also constructed, which would be more conducive to gene manipulation.

pGK12

pGK12 is a small cloning vector composed of fragments derived from pC194, pUB110, pWV01 [a cryptic *Streptococcus cremoris*（乳脂链球菌）Wg2 plasmid] and pE194 *cop-6*, respectively (Fig. 2-66). The recombinant plasmid constructed is a broad-host-range plasmid. Coding for erythromycin (*Em*ʳ) (from pE194 *cop-6*) and chloramphenicol resistance (*Cm*ʳ) (from pC194), it replicates and is expressed in

Bacillus subtilis, Escherichia coli, Streptococcus lactis（乳酸链球菌）and *Lactobacillus paracasei*（副干酪乳杆菌）, and they can be used as a bridge vector (shuttle vector) between these three species.

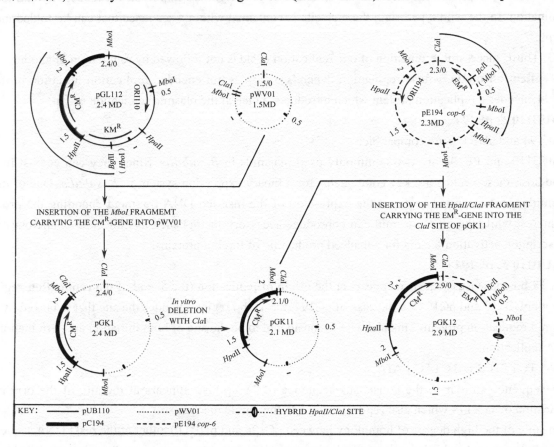

Fig. 2-66 Cloning strategy and restriction maps of plasmids pGL112, pE194 *cop-6*, pGK1, pGK11, and pGK12. The origins of plasmid segments are indicated in the key. For reasons of clarity only those sites relevant for the construction and properties of the recombinant vectors are shown. The concentric arcs span the fragments used for insertion.

This plasmid (pGK12, 2.9 megadaltons) contained a unique *Bcl*I site in the *Em*ʳ gene and unique *Cla*I and *Hpa*II sites outside both resistance genes. It was stably maintained in *B. subtilis* at a copy number of approximately 5. pGK12 also transformed *Escherichia coli* competent cells to *Cm*ʳ and *Em*ʳ. The copy number in *E. coli* was about 60. Moreover, pGK12 transformed protoplasts of *Streptococcus lactis*. In this host both resistance genes are expressed. pGK12 is stably maintained in *S. lactis* at a copy number of 3.

The plasmid pGK12 is an insertion-inactivation vector. The *Bcl* I site is situated in the coding sequence of the *Em*ʳ gene, and insertion of DNA fragments into this site inactivates *Em*ʳ. Therefore, pGK12 can be used to select for recombinant plasmids by insertional inactivation.

pHV1431

Plasmid pHV1431 (10.9 kb, 40 copies, *Cm*ʳ[*Ap*ʳ *Tc*ʳ]) (Fig. 2-67) is a chimeric plasmid derives from plasmid

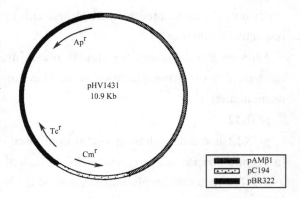

Fig. 2-67 Plasmid of pHV1431.

pBR322, *Staphylococcus aureus* plasmid pC194 and *Enterococcus faecalis*（粪肠球菌）plasmid pAMβ1 and contains a *Hind*III-*Eco*RI insert from pAMβ1, encoding stabilization functions. Plasmid pHV1431 is a shuttle vector that replicates in *E. coli* and *B. subtilis*.

Plasmid pAMβ1 has a **theta mode of replication** that enhances its stability in Gram-positive hosts. Plasmid pHV1431 was considered to be structurally stable because it has a **theta mode of replication** of pAMβ1 and not a rolling circle replication (RCR). In *Bacillus subtilis* many plasmids from *Staphylococcus aureus* replicate via RCR and generate single-stranded (ss) DNA intermediates, which strongly stimulate recombination between homologous sequences. Plasmid pHV1431 was segregationally stable also because of the presence of a fragment of pAMβ1 that codes for a resolvase（游离酶）, thus decreasing the plasmid polymerization.

Bacillus subtilis (pHV1431) cultivated in continuous cultures was maintained **structurally stable but segregationally unstable**.

The frequency of plasmid loss is not zero: 10^{-4} plasmid loss occurs per cell per generation in continuous cultures, and **competition exists between plasmid-carrying and plasmid-free cells that favors plasmid-free cells** because **they grow faster**. Then, at a great generation number, the plasmid was segregationally unstable. **An improvement** in the stability was obtained **through implemention of immobilization systems**. The immobilization involves a compartmentalized type of cell growth that limits the **competition** between plasmid-free and plasmid-harboring cells, and therefore provides a higher plasmid stability (*e.g.*, immobilization of cells in **κ-carrageenan gel beads**). This increased plasmid stability in immobilized cells may have resulted from the mechanical properties of the gel bead system that allow only a limited number of cell divisions to occur in each microcolony before the cells escape from the gel beads. The immobilized cells can be considered to be a reservoir of plasmid-containing cells that are saved from the **competition** with plasmid-free cells. **Immobilization gave rise to higher retention（保存）of plasmid-bearing cells**. Previous studies have shown that **in immobilized systems the copy number of the plasmid remains stable. The plasmid was maintained stable for longer periods**.

Temperature-sensitive (Ts) plasmids

Progress has been made in the study of temperature-sensitive plasmids.

The typical temperature-sensitive plasmid replicon pE194Ts of *Bacillus spp.* was obtained from the plasmid pE194. pE194Ts is a mutant of pE194 (isolated by S. Gruss) which cannot replicate above 37℃. Usually useful mutant strains could be selected above 38℃. Plasmid pE194 is naturally Ts at 51℃, while this mutant derivative was obtained which is Ts at 39 to 42℃. As the growth temperature is increased, the replication rate of the pE194 (Ts) will decrease.

The mutational lesion in pE194Ts may, in fact, affect a *trans*-acting replication effector, *i.e.*, the temperature-sensitive lesion in pE194Ts affects the repF function. The pE194 lesion is in a relatively conserved stretch of the protein sequence. One of the two sequence changes associated with the temperature-sensitive defect is located at position 1431, within the large ORF located between positions 1244 and 1856. This ORF encodes a 25 kDa protein, maybe the *repF* gene product. The other at position 1235.

A thermosensitive (Ts) replicon's subsequent shut-off at elevated temperature would allow selection of low-frequency events like transposition（转座，移位）and recombination in a large cell population. Most of the vectors currently in use carry the temperature-sensitive replicon (pE194Ts) that was originally developed for use in *Bacillus subtilis*.

In order to facilitate genetic analysis, an integrated plasmid vector has also been developed.

The promoters for transcriptional regulation in *Bacillus* include *aprE* (alkaline protease E) promoter, alpha-amylase promoter, *sacB* levansucrase（果聚糖蔗糖酶）promoter and *spac* promoter. *Spac* promoter (P_{spac}) is a fusion promoter of *Bacillus* phage SP01 and *lac* operon sequence.

Brevibacillus brevis

There are some advantages of secretory protein expression: (1) The expression products are soluble and properly folded, hence possessing biological activity. (2) The expression products are segregated from intracellular proteins by the plasma membrane and the cell wall, hence there is no need to tear cells apart, that in turn facilitate the separation and purification, simplify the technology. The existing prokaryotic secretory expression system is unsatisfactory. When exogenous protein is being expressed efficiently in *E. coli*, inclusion bodies would form. The level of secretory expression is low, and usually the product is secreted to periplasmic space rather than extracellularly. Though *Bacillus subtilis* possesses good secretory ability and non-pathogenicity, *Brevibacillus brevis* possesses higher protein secretory capacity and lower extracellular protease activity, hence an ideal host for secretory exogenous protein expression.

Brevibacillus brevis is a new genus that has just emerged from the genus *Bacillus* in recent years. *Bacillus brevis* was originally a subordinate genus of *Bacillus*. While in 1996, Osanu Shida *et al.* found that some species including *Bacillus brevis*, were phylogenetically distinct from other *Bacillus* after gene sequence analysis of their 16S rRNA gene sequences. Thus they proposed reclassification of the *B. brevis* cluster as *Brevibacillus* gen. nov. Hence, the status of *Breviballus* is similar to that of *Bacillus*, with either one being independent Genus, respectively.

The main proteins secreted extracellularly by *Brevibacillus brevis*, are one or two kind high molecular weight cell wall protein(s). The transcription of the genes encoding cell wall proteins are controlled by five tandem promoters (P1 to P5) with high transcriptional activity. Furthermore, P2 and P3, which play a leading role in the process of cell wall protein expression, are regulated by time sequence.

The signal peptide sequences of cell wall proteins possess the typical characteristics of that of common Gram-positive bacteria — they can effectively mediate the secretion of cell wall proteins, hence this kind of promoters and signal peptide coding sequence should be the ideal elements which promote secretory exogenous gene expression in *Brevibacillus brevis*.

Furthermore, disulfide bond oxidoreductase (Dsb) and peptide proline *cis-trans* isomerase (PPIase) were found existing in culture supernatants of *Brevibacillus brevis*. Those enzymes can facilitate proper folding of the peptide chain, forming biologically active nature proteins.

As an expression strain, *Brevibacillus brevis* has several advantages:

1. It hardly secretes protease to the extracellular environment (*Bacillus subtilis* secretes at least 8 different proteases), which is conducive to the stability of the target protein.

2. The cell wall is thinner than that of *Bacillus subtilis*, which is conducive to the secretion of exogenous proteins.

3. There are factors in the fermentation broth that can promote the formation of disulfide bonds in proteins hence promote the folding of exogenous proteins.

In conclusion, with the deepening of research, the secretory mechanism of proteins of *Bacillus subtilis* will be more clearly understood, and many new secretory elements and proteases will be recognized. It is believed that the issues affecting the development of the *Bacillus subtilis* expression system will be well settled in the near future. In addition to the above, there are still other issues about the secretory and expression system of *Bacillus* to be further studied.

First of all, it is necessary to probe into the secretory mechanism and understand the protein transport and folding process thoroughly, especially the speed limiting factors of secretion, which will play an important role in guiding the construction of genetically engineered strains.

Secondly, advanced fermentation technology and optimized protein design should be used to compensate for some defects of the strain itself and increase the yield of the target protein(s).

In addition, the exocrine efficiency of exogenous protein can be improved more significantly by organically combining various ameliorated strategies.

In a word, great progress has been made in the study of secreting and expressing exogenous proteins in *Bacillus* in recent years, and a series of effective exogenous protein expression systems have been established. In particular, the *Bacillus subtilis* and *Brevibacillus brevis* expression systems have been successfully used in the production of some valuable peptides, showing promising application prospects.

In the future, the host/vector expression system of *Bacillus* will continue to be improved and expanded, providing more and more inexpensive and high-quality products for the benefit of mankind.

According to the literature, *Bacillus* has also been applied in the following fields, but these bacteria are not genetically engineered bacteria:

Detergent, food industry, chemical industry, agriculture, environment protection and in medical treatment, such as treating chronic hepatitis, viral disease and AIDS, anti-tumor, antihyperlipidemia (降血脂) and reducing blood alcohol concentration after drinking, and so on.

2.5.1.3   *Streptomyces* (链霉菌)

Streptomyces, one of the important industrial microorganisms, has attracted considerable attention as a highly differentiated prokaryote. *Streptomycetes* exhibit a unique metabolic diversity and enzymatic capabilities. The compounds they produce as secondary metabolites are valuable for industrial and pharmaceutical purposes. It can produce a large number of metabolites, being considered as primary sources of economically important antibiotics. Moreover, their versatile activities of transcription and translation systems may prove of practical use for the expression of heterologous genes, because *E. coli* and *B. subtilis* are relatively fastidious (需复杂营养地) in this respect.

Streptomyces is the largest genus of Actinomycetes (放线菌) and the type genus (模式属) of the family Streptomycetaceae (链霉菌科). The genus *Streptomyces* includes aerobic (需氧的), filamentous bacteria that produce well-developed vegetative hyphae (营养菌丝) with branches. As with the other Actinobacteria, streptomycetes (链霉菌) are Gram-positive bacteria with a high GC content, with an average of 74%. *Streptomyces* currently covers close to 576 species with the number increasing every year. Species nomenclature are usually based on their color of hyphae (菌丝) and spores.

Genomics & Biotechnology

In recent years, with in-depth research of *Streptomyces* species on molecular biology, especially the accomplishment of complete genome sequencing of *S. Coelicolor* (天蓝色链霉菌) strain A3 (2) (2002), and *S. avermitilis* (阿维链霉菌) (2003), *Streptomyces griseus* (灰色链霉菌) (2008) and *Streptomyces scabies* (疮痂病链霉菌) (2009) biotechnology researchers show great interest in *Streptomyces* species and have begun using it as a new system for heterologous expression of proteins. Each of these genomes forms a chromosome with a linear structure, unlike most bacterial genomes, which exist in the form of circular chromosomes. The genomic molecule is about 8 Mb, 1.5 times as large as that of *Escherichia coli*. There are covalently bound proteins at both ends of the chromosome.

Traditionally, *Escherichia coli* was the species of choice to express eukaryotic genes, since it was well understood and easy to work with. Expression of eukaryotic proteins in *E. coli* may be problematic. Sometimes, proteins do not fold properly, which may lead to insolubility, deposition in inclusion bodies, and loss of bioactivity of the product. Though *E. coli* strains have secretion mechanisms, these are of low efficiency and result in secretion into the periplasmic space, whereas secretion by a Gram-positive bacterium such as a *Streptomyces* species results in secretion directly into the extracellular medium. In addition, *Streptomyces* species have more efficient secretion mechanisms than *E. coli*. The properties of the secretion system is an advantage for industrial production of heterologously（异源地）expressed protein because it simplifies subsequent purification steps and may increase yield.

Since the natural habitat of *streptomycetes* is the soil, they need to exploit complex organic material in the soil for nutrient acquisition. Therefore, it is obvious that these soil bacteria can secrete a large variety of hydrolytic enzymes. Several of the enzymes produced by *streptomycetes* are economically valuable, and are widespread used for a variety of applications in medicine, food industries, and textile and leather industries and also in analytical processes. As a consequence, several of these are produced at an industrial scale, where they are secreted into the culture medium at high concentration driven by a potent secretion apparatus. This efficient secretion system can also be applied for the production of heterologous proteins.

These properties among others make *Streptomyces* spp. an attractive alternative to other bacteria such as *E. coli* and *Bacillus subtilis*.

(1) Promoters of *Streptomyces*（链霉菌的启动子）

Different promoters possess different transcription efficiency. The location of the promoter relative to the assayed gene can greatly affect the apparent transcriptional activity.

Common features of *streptomycete* promoter regions

Streptomycete genes have thus far shown a wide diversity in promoter sequences and transcriptional patterns. Studies around early 1980s had indicated that while typical promoters from several other bacterial genera function in *Streptomyces* the converse does not generally occur. Studies of transcription signals in *Streptomyces* have shown that very few nucleotide sequences that serve as promoters in *Streptomyces* can function in *E coli*. The analysis of a variety of *Streptomyces* promoters and the discovery of more than one sigma factor for the RNA polymerase of *S coelicolor* A3(2) have demonstrated the occurrence of multiple classes of promoter sequence in *Streptomyces*. In Strohl's study, of the 87 genes described, 27 of them (ca. 31%) have multiple promoters. Theretofore（在那以前，直到那时）, 13 loci have been shown to contain overlapping, divergent promoters, a structure which has been postulated to be involved in complex regulatory patterns. In some cases, the overlapping divergent promoters are located within, or partially within, the open reading frame of the gene. Some promoter regions are divergent from the same region, but the +1 to ca. −40 regions do not overlap. Some promoters initiate transcription from the middle of multi-gene operons in which other promoters are found upstream of the first gene in the operon, those promoters apparently provide additional transcriptional capabilities to their respective operons. Some promoters lie within open reading frames of *streptomycete* genes.

Thirty-six of 139 *streptomycete* apparent transcription start sites (26%) were located to multiple adjacent (or nearby) nucleotides rather than to a single nucleotide.

At the same time, reports of *E coli* promoters that have activity in *Streptomyces* imply that the same or overlapping sequences are recognized in both genera and that *S. lividans* and *S. coelicolor* may contain an RNA polymerase holoenzyme form which is similar in transcriptional specificity to the major RNA polymerase species in *E. coli*. The data in 1987 (Mark J Buttner *et al.*) strongly support the idea that one type of RNA polymerase holoenzyme in *Streptomyces* recognizes a class of promoters similar to the major consensus promoters of *E. coli*, and that the manner of promoter recognition is similar in both genera. Analyses also showed that some transcription start sites were at the same nucleotide or within 1-2 nucleotides in *S. lividans* and *E. coli*, indicating that the transcription initiation sites for these genes in these two very different organisms were nearly identical.

Streptomycete promoters with sequences similar to *E. coli* Eσ^{70}-like promoters

In Strohl's study, of the 139 apparent *streptomycete* promoter sequences, 29 appear to fall into a group which has been previously described as *streptomycete E. coli* σ^{70}-like promoter sequences. Those promoters have a consensus slightly different from that of *E. coli*.

Hence, the promoters were categorized into two groups, those categorized into Group 1 were based on two criteria:

(i) Their sequences are relatively similar to the consensus sequence for *E. coli* promoters recognized by Eσ^{70} (in which the −35 hexamer is TTGACA and the −10 hexamer is TATAAT);

(ii) The −10 and −35 hexamers of these promoters are 16 to 18 nucleotides apart.

The latter requirement is especially important because >92% of all *E. coli* promoters recognized by Eσ^{70} have spacers between −10 and −35 of 16 to 18 nucleotides (57% of those have spacers of 17 nucleotides), spacer mutations have been shown to yield strong effects on promoter activities, and the RNA polymerase holoenzyme appears to contact only one side of the DNA helix. Mutational studies in 1989 on sigma factors have confirmed the premise that sigma factors generally contact nucleotides in both the −10 and −35 hexamers.

While in Group 2, the conserved sequences of the corresponding −10 and −35 areas are NANNNT and NTGNNN, respectively.

Highly conserved nucleotides of the "−10" and "−35" consensus sequences

Each promoter contains, in front of the transcriptional start points, a region that shows considerable similarity to the "−10" sequence of the consensus prokaryotic promoter. The two most highly conserved nucleotides of the "−10" consensus sequence [*i.e.*, T and A in position 6 and 2, respectively, 3' T (*i.e.*, T in position 6) is considered to be the most strongly conserved nucleotide of the −10 region] are found in 25 out of the 29 (86.21%) within the range of −16 to −5 in Group 1, 73 out of the 110 (66.36%) within the range of −22 to −1 in Group 2. Whereas the two most highly conserved nucleotides (*i.e.*, T and G in position 2 and 3, respectively) are found in sequences corresponding to the consensus "−35" region [29 out of the 29 (100%) within the range of −40 to −27 in Group 1, 63 out of the 110 (57.27%) within the range of −40 to −30 in Group 2], hence can also be recognized in each of the promoters.

Site-specific mutations in the −10 and −35 regions, making an *Streptomycete* promoter identical to the consensus *E. coli* promoter sequence, resulted in higher transcription activities in both *E. coli* and *S. lividans*. These increases in promoter activity, however, were significantly smaller than the increase caused by changing the spacer region from 16 to 17 nucleotides.

Bibb and Jansson's experiments, as a whole suggest a minor role for the interaction of *Streptomycete* RNA polymerases with −35 regions of these particular promoter. Data seem to corroborate the results that certain *actinomycete* promoters may have reduced requirements for upstream sequence (*e.g.*, −35, −10). This phenomenon is more apparent in members of *Streptomycetes* promoters Group 2 than those in Group 1, with the latter sharing similar features with *E. coli*. While there are cases where hexamer sequences such as GGGGGG appear to be important for promoter activity of members of Group 2.

The average distance between the −10 and −35 hexameric regions

The average distance between the −10 and −35 hexameric regions of the promoters in Group 1 is 17.3 nucleotides. This is similar to *E. coli* promoters recognized by $E\sigma^{70}$, in which the optimal spacer distance is 17 ± 1 nucleotides. A spacing (between the "−10" and "−35" regions) which is significantly large or less than the optimal distance (17 bp) suggests that this promoter would function poorly, if at all. Jaurin and Cohen found that addition of 1 nucleotide to the 16 nucleotide spacer region of the *E. coli ampC* promoter increased transcription efficiency 16-fold in *E. coli* and 30-fold in *S. lividans*. Thus, it is apparent that the size of the spacer also is important to the activity in *S. lividans* of $E\sigma^{70}$-like promoters.

The G+C content of DNA isolated from different species vary significantly

In addition to the suboptimal spacing between the presumptive "−10" and "−35" regions, other features may prevent their recognition. For example, Bibb *et al.* noted that the mol% G+C composition of the sequences extending 20 nt either way from the midpoint between the −10 and −35 hexamers (40 nucleotides total), is 43 mol% in *E. coli* promoters, whereas in the *ermE* promoters, the G+C content was found to be 62 to 65 mol%. The apparent *streptomycete* promoter sequences shown in Groups 1 and 2 have an average G+C content of 57 mol% and 62 mol%, respectively.

It is not surprising that the promoters shown in Group 1 would have the lowest G+C content of the different analyses, especially since several of these are functional in *E. coli* (see section on $E\sigma^{70}$-like promoters). Putative promoters from Group 1 (SEP2, SEP3, SEP6, SEP8, pIJ101A-p, pIJ101B-p, and pIJ101-pc, and XP55-p) transcribed in *E. coli*, possessing G+C content of 47.9 mol%.

On the other hand, The promoters shown in Group 2 are, on the average, slightly more G+C-rich than those shown in Group 1. Where tested, these promoters are not typically expressed in *E. coli.*, *i.e.*, the *vph*, *tsr*, *aph*, and *ermE* genes were not expressed from their own promoters in *E. coli*. As would be expected, most of the promoters (*e.g.*, *ermE*-pl, *aph*-p1, *aph*-p2, *tsr*-pl, *tsr*-p2, *vph*-pl, *vph*-p2) of these genes do not have sequences resembling $E\sigma^{70}$-like promoters, so their function in *E. coli* would not be expected.

Recombinant protein production and *streptomycetes*

Heterologous protein secretion in *Streptomyces* spp.

A wide variety of host-vector systems have been developed, many of which are based on plasmid pIJ101, such as pIJ702 and pIJ486M.

Yield vary a lot among *Streptomyces spp.*, while the reason is unknown. While *Streptomycetes* have a high GC (>70%), and as a consequence a high GC codon bias, CDSs (Coding DNA sequence, 编码 DNA 序列) with a lower GC content could nevertheless also efficiently be expressed, and could therefore not account for failure in some cases. This could be further confirmed by the fact that adaptation of the heterologous gene to the host codon usage does not necessarily lead to improved production, although in some cases it did. It is obvious that secretion by *S. lividans* of proteins from prokaryotic origin is in general more successful.

A large number of proteins which are characteristics of prokaryotes have been cloned and expressed in *Streptomyces*, and promoters derived from the genes themselves have been mostly used in the research, indicating that *Streptomyces* can recognize promoters of many heterogenous prokaryotes, while promoters derived from their host — *Streptomyces* promoter, are usually required for eukaryotic gene expression.

The promoters with better gene expression in *Streptomyces* include the erythromycin resistance gene (*ermE*) (红霉素抗性基因) from *Saccharopolyspora erythraea* (糖多孢红霉菌) (formerly *Streptomyces erythreus*), the aminoglycoside phosphotransferase gene (*aph*) (氨基糖苷类磷酸转移酶基因) from *S. fradiae* (弗氏链霉菌), *tipA* promoter, which can be induced by streptomycin, and promoter *gal*-p1 of β-galactosidase gene, casease promoter *melC* and serine protease inhibitor STI-II promoter, *etc*.

Sequences other than just the −10 and −35 regions and other features of the promoter regions

Considering the broad ranges of metabolism that are encompassed (完成) by the promoters described, it is likely that sequences other than just the −10 and −35 regions are important to the regulation of transcription. *e.g.*, DnaA boxes are also parts of the regulatory region, which are located upstream of the promoter of the *Streptomyces dnaA* gene. They were demonstrated to be necessary for efficient binding of the *Streptomyces* DnaA protein to DNA. The location, spacing and orientation of the DnaA boxes are conserved.

Although specialized RNA polymerases may recognize features of the −10 and/or −35 regions of these genes, other features of the promoter regions also may be involved in temporal or induction/repression mechanisms. DNA within several *streptomycete* promoter regions has significant potential for forming secondary structures (*i.e.*, hairpin loops). Some *streptomycete* promoters thus far studied are clearly regulated temporally. Those temporally regulated promoter do not share significant sequence similarities from −40 to +1.

Nevertheless, conserved −10 and −35 hexameric sequences have been shown to have significant contributions to promoter activities in most cases.

(2) Shine Dalgarno (SD) sequences from *Streptomyces* sp (链霉菌的 SD 序列)

Relationship of transcription start site and translation initiation codon

Of 48 *streptomycete* genes Strohl analyzed, the distance from the transcription start site to the coding region (not including the eleven genes containing leaderless mRNAs) ranged from 9 to 345 nucleotides. With most of the *streptomycete* genes analyzed, the transcription start sites were within 100 nucleotides of the apparent coding regions. This compares to an average distance of ca. 23 nucleotides separating the transcription start site from the coding region in a typical *E. coli* gene.

The apparent Shine-Dalgarno sequences of 44 *streptomycete* genes, chosen to reflect genes encoding a wide range of functions, were analyzed for their complementarity to the 3′ end of the 16S rRNA of *S. lividans* and for their distance upstream of the initiation codon. These Shine-Dalgarno sequences ranged from 5 to 12 nucleotides (average of 8.5 nucleotides) upstream of the initiation codons. *E. coli* Shine-Dalgarno sequences are typically 5 to 9 nucleotides upstream of the initiation codon (AUG or GUG), and *B. subtilis* Shine-Dalgarno sequences are 7 to 14 nucleotides upstream of the AUG. McLaughlin *et al.* proposed that the Shine-Dalgarno sequences of Gram-positive bacterial mRNAs are typically able to form strong complexes with the 3′ end of 16S rRNA, whereas *E. coli* Shine-Dalgarno sequences are more variable. The conserved Shine-Dalgarno sequence for these 44 *streptomycete* genes was (a/g)-G-G-A-G-G. *Streptomycete* ribosomes do not require extensive complementarity between the Shine-Dalgarno sequences and the 3′ end of the 16S rRNA in order to initiate translation.

In the case of eleven actinomycete genes, *i.e.*, streptothricin acetyltransferase (*sta*)（链丝菌素乙酰转移酶）from *S. lavendulae*（淡紫灰链霉菌）, the erythromycin resistance gene (*ermE*)（红霉素抗性基因）from *Saccharopolyspora erythraea*（糖多孢红霉菌）(formerly *Streptomyces erythreus*), the aminoglycoside phosphotransferase gene (*aph*)（氨基糖苷类磷酸转移酶基因）from *S. fradiae*（弗氏链霉菌）, ribostamycin phosphotransferase (*rph*)（核糖霉素磷酸转移酶）from *S. ribosidificus*（核糖苷链霉菌）, aminocyclitol acetyltransferase (*aacC7*)（氨基环醇乙酰转移酶）from *S. rimosus* forma *paromomycinus*（核糖体链霉菌属假丝酵母菌）, the nosiheptide（诺西肽）resistance (*nshR*) gene of *S. actuosus*（活跃链霉菌）, *afsA* from *S. griseus*（灰色链霉菌）, chloramphenicol acetyltransferase（氯霉素乙酰转移酶）from *S. acrimycini*, *korB* from plasmid pIJ101, as well as *aacC9* from *Micromonospora chalcea*（青铜小单孢菌）and *cdh* from *Norcardia* spp.（诺卡氏菌）, transcription from the nearest promoter and translation are proposed to be initiated at the same nucleotide (or in one case one nucleotide removed from the promoter). In the case of the *cdh* gene from *Nocardia*, transcription was initiated from the same nucleotide in both *Nocardia* and *S. lividans*（变铅青链霉菌）.

Similarly, at least seven different RNA polymerase holoenzymes already have been found in the *Streptomyces*, suggesting that the sigma factors play an active role in regulation of gene expression in these complex microorganisms.

(3) The secretory signal peptide from *Streptomyces* sp.（链霉菌的分泌信号肽）

The secretory signal peptide is located at the N-terminal region of the presecretory protein of *Streptomyces sp.*, which would be cleaved off by signal peptidase when the preprotein is transfering towards outside membrane or soon after. The secretory signal peptide sequence is not very conserved in the primary structure, while possessing the structure of a typical signal peptide.

Streptomyces has much longer signal peptides than that of other organisms, with an average length of 29~31 amino acids. It has been reported that the longest signal peptides of *Streptomyces* have reached 70 amino acids. It is believed that the long signal peptides those *Streptomyces* possess may just have evolved to provide a more effective secretion mechanism.

(4) Protein secretion pathways in *Streptomyces* spp.

In most instances, the Sec-dependent pathway has been used with variable success. In some instances, the **twin-arginine-dependent translocation (Tat)** pathway was required such as for the secretion of eGFP.

The Sec pathway constitutes the main protein secretion pathway in *Streptomyces*. Proteins secreted via this pathway are initially synthesized as preproteins with an N-terminal hydrophobic signal peptide (SP) with a positively charged N-domain followed by a longer, hydrophobic H-domain and a C-terminal part containing at the end three amino acids which form the signal peptidase recognition site.

It is generally believed that the signal peptide (SP) is required for targeting the preprotein to the Sec translocon（易位子）consisting of SecY, SecE and SecG, which mediates the translocation of the proteins. During or after translocation, the SP is cleaved off and degraded, and the mature protein is then released in the culture medium. Recent data suggest, however, that the mature domain of the preprotein adds a significant contribution to the targeting, rendering the signal peptide less critical in bacterial secretory proteins than generally assumed. They should rather function as allosteric activators of the translocase that makes signal peptides essential for protein secretion. Once preproteins are bound to the translocase, the ATPase motor SecA drives stepwise the translocation of the unfolded proteins across the membrane. During or shortly after translocation, secretory preproteins are processed by a type I signal peptidase (SPase I) removing the signal peptide.

Streptomycetes also contain a functional **Tat** pathway. The Tat machinery exports fully folded proteins across the cytoplasmic membrane and the energy for translocation is provided by the proton-motive force (PMF). Similarly to Gram-negative bacteria, in actinomycetes TatA , TatB and TatC are the essential components for this pathway.

Signal peptides that target proteins to the Tat pathway resemble Sec signal peptides, but with a conserved S/T-R-R-x-F-L-K consensus motif, where the twin arginines are invariant and normally essential for efficient export by the Tat pathway. However, the Tat-specific signal sequence with two arginine residues may not be an absolute prerequisite for the Tat pathway. Whereas for most bacteria with an identified Tat pathway, only few proteins are transported via this pathway, for *Streptomyces* species investigated the *in silico*（经由电脑模拟）Tat substrate prediction programs (TATFIND 1.4 and TatP) revealed an exceptionally high number of Tat substrates.

(5) Approaches to improve heterologous protein secretion
Screening for and modulation of proper signal peptide
Signal peptidases

Overexpression of a SPase which efficiently cleaves the precursors may result in increased secretion of a particular protein. Deletion of a SPase which binds efficiently, but cleaves the substrate poorly allows the binding of the precursor to a better processing SPase as such resulting in improved secretion of that particular protein. The finding that SPases compete for binding preproteins and have different substrate-processing efficiencies *in vivo*, opens perspectives for the rational engineering of improved secretion of heterologous proteins.

Towards metabolic flux analysis

As extensively described above, protein yield can be improved by the modulation, co-overexpression or deletion of key proteins involved in the secretion pathway such as the signal peptide, signal peptidases, Tat components.

A transcriptomics-based approach represents a useful tool for a rational optimization of heterologous protein secretion in *Streptomyces*. Transcriptomics is a systems biology approach that examines the global pattern（总体模式）of gene expression at the mRNA level. This technique allows systematic determination of the effects of heterologous protein secretion at genomic level by identifying genes that are differentially expressed under secretion stress conditions. Relevant genes can be selected for strain engineering to reduce stress during secretion process and thus, optimize recombinant protein production in *S. lividans*. Among the proteins with a known or predicted functions, several of these are linked to stress regulation (cold shock proteins, sigma factors), while others are involved in metabolic processes such as energy production and conversion, and general metabolism.

Streptomyces deserves its own place in the array of production systems. It has been shown in several cases to be a valuable alternative, or even a necessary substitute. As for other Gram-positive bacteria, and other secretory systems, a main advantage is that it secretes the proteins directly into the culture medium, eventually producing the heterologous protein in the right conformation as such avoiding expensive refolding processes. Some heterologous proteins can be expressed at commercially attractive levels, but unfortunately — like for other hosts — not all proteins can be secreted in sufficiently high amounts and yield optimization is pressing（难以推却的，不容忽视的）. To improve yield, several successful approaches have become available, but a general observation in these efforts for strain optimization, with the intention to increase heterologous protein yield, is that, no predictions on the success can be made so far, nor for *Streptomyces* nor for any other host cell, and that, up-to-now these efforts are based on empirical grounds. Study of differential expression of genes through transcriptomics as well as study of the metabolic burden through metabolic flux analysis will open new paths to enhance protein production in *S. lividans* (as well as in other hosts).

(6) Streptomyces plasmid vectors（链霉菌的质粒载体）

The main plasmids found in *Streptomyces* spp. and developed into vector series are pIJ101 (Fig. 2-68), pJV1, pSG5, SCP2*, SLP1, pSAM2, *etc.*, and on this basis, a large number of plasmid vectors were constructed.

Most of the plasmid vectors used for gene expression are derivatives of **pIJ101** (*e.g.*, **pIJ702**), which carry both the thiostrepton（硫链丝菌素） resistance gene (*tsr*) (mel) and the tyrosinase（酪氨酸） gene. There are three single restriction endonuclease sites within the tyrosinase gene regulatory region, hence the recombinants can be determined by the loss of enzyme activity after the introduction of exogenous genes. **pFD666**, a high copy *Escherichia coli-Streptomyces* shuttle cosmid vector with neomycin resistance gene (*neo^r*) (marker gene) was constructed based on **pJV1**. **PUWL** series shuttle plasmids such as

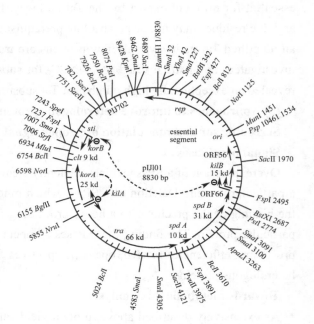

Fig. 2-68   Plasmid pIJ101.

pUWL218 and pUWL219 were obtained by connecting pIJ699, a pIJ101 derived plasmid containing *tsr* gene replication region, with pUC18 and pUC19. LacZ gene was inserted into those plasmids to construct more convenient shuttle plasmids.

pIJ101

pIJ101, is one of the small high copy number plasmids contained in *Streptomyces lividans* ISP5434. The plasmid is of size 8.9 kb, the largest member of the family of autonomous plasmids present in this strain. The copy number of plasmids of the pIJ101 family (40 to 300 per chromosome, appearing to vary with the age or physiological state of the culture) is among the highest (without artificial amplification) so far described in any bacterium. The pIJ101 family has a broad host range and possesses several convenient restriction sites for DNA insertion.

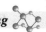

Several properties of the pIJ101 series of plasmids are useful for incorporation into such vectors. These include high copy number (making for ease of study of the DNA and, probably, useful amplification of some products of cloned genes); broad host range; and the ability to manipulate the plasmid to give conjugal or non-conjugal vectors. The non-conjugative property is advantageous in the use of these high copy number plasmids for shotgun cloning since presumptive clones are harder to purify in the presence of a conjugative plasmid which can superinfect（双重感染，重复感染）the clones on the protoplast regeneration plates.

Many variants of pIJ101 were constructed *in vitro* by inserting DNA fragments determining resistance to neomycin, thiostrepton（硫链丝菌素）or viomycin（紫霉素）, and having *Bam*HI termini, into *Mbo*I or *Bcl*I sites on the plasmid, sometimes with deletion of segments of plasmid DNA.

Knowledge of dispensable（可有可无的，非必要的）DNA segments and the availability of restriction sites for the insertion of DNA, deduced from the properties of plasmids carrying the *E. coli* plasmid PACYC184 introduced at various sites, was used in the construction of several derivatives of pIJ101 suitable as DNA cloning vectors. These were mostly designed to be non-conjugative and to carry pairs of resistance genes for selection. They include a bifunctional shuttle vector for *E coli* and *Streptomyces*; a *Streptomyces* viomycin resistance gene of this plasmid is expressed in both hosts.

pIJ702

Interest in the biology of the *Streptomyces* and application of these soil bacteria to production of commercial antibiotics and enzymes has stimulated the development of efficient cloning techniques and a variety of *streptomycete* plasmid and phage vectors.

The *streptomyces* plasmid pIJ702 has been used widely in cloning experiments. The *mel* gene on it provides a very convenient marker for insertional inactivation.

Plasmid pIJ702 is an effective vector for cloning and expression of *Streptomyces* genes and mammalian genes in *Streptomyces lividans*. Vector pIJ702 was constructed from a variant of a larger autonomous plasmid and is often used as a cloning vehicle in conjunction with *S. lividans*. The host range of vector pIJ702 extends beyond *Streptomyces* spp. — pIJ702 or its derived plasmids have a wide host range and can be replicated in many *Streptomyces* and other actinomycetes, and its high copy number has been exploited for the overproduction of cloned gene products. This combination of host and vector has been used successfully to investigate antibiotic biosynthesis, gene strucrure and expression, and to map various *Streptomyces* mutants.

Origin of vector pIJ702

The ability to synthesize melanin or melanin-like pigments is a common property among *streptomycetes*. The enzyme responsible, tyrosinase (Phenoloxidase), inducible by different amino acids, is synthesized intracellularly, and is then secreted into the culture medium. The *mel* sequence provides a convenient cloning marker for insertional or replacement inactivation because the altered gene cannot confer pigmentation（色素沉着，天然颜色）to its host. pIJ350, the nonconjugative high copy number plasmid carrying the thiostrepton resistance determinant, was subsequently employed for subcloning the tyrosinase gene (*mel*) originating in *S. antibioticus*（抗生链霉菌）. The vector was linearized by partial digestion with *Bcl*I and ligated with fragments obtained from a *Bcl*I-cleaved plasmid carrying *mel*. After transformation and regeneration of *S. lividans* 1326 protoplasts, colonies were isolated that were melanin (+) and thiostrepton-resistant. Characterization of the new plasmid (pIJ702; 5.65 kb) revealed that the tyrosinase

DNA insert (1.55 kb) had three single sites upstream of the structural gene for *Sst*I, *Bgl*II, or *Sph*I (Figure 2-69). The melanin operon has also been used to construct shuttle vectors for the Gram-negative bacterial *Escherichia coli*, *Erwinia carotovora*（欧文菌）, and *Xanthomonas campestris*（野油菜黄单胞菌）.

The advantages offered by this cloning vehicle include the fact that its host range extends beyond the genus *Streptomyces*. It is well documented that few *Streptomyces* promoters function in *E. coli*. However, two promoters from the *Streptomyces* plasmid pIJ101 (parent of pIJ702) are recognized by *E. coli* RNA polymerase. Another pIJ101 DNA fragment demonstrated *in vivo* promoter activity in both *S. lividans* and *E. coli*.

A second useful feature of pIJ702 is the presence of the two genetic elements, that facilitate screening of clones. **Selection** of transformants is based on their resistance to the antibiotic thiostrepton (*tsr*⁺). Insertional inactivation of the melanin phenotype (*mel*⁻) at any of three unique cloning sites serves as the basis of recognition of recombinant plasmids (Fig. 2-69). Furthermore, the nonconjugative ability of pIJ702 is beneficial during shotgun cloning because putative clones are easier to purity in the absence of a conjugal vector, which can superinfect the clones during protoplast regeneration. Plasmid pIJ702 occurs at an unusually high copy number (40 to 300 per chromosome). This characteristic enables the efficient production of extracellular enzymes, and it reduces the phenomenon or genetic instability during subsequent rounds of bacterial growth and sporulation.

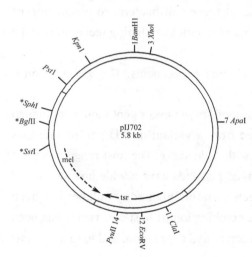

Fig. 2-69 Plasmid pIJ702. This plasmid includes *S. coelicolor* in its wide host range and its high copy number(40 to 300 per chromosomal equivalent) offers the potential advantage of enhanced product formation of cloned genes. The plasmid carries genes for thiostrepton resistance(*tsr*), conveniently used for the selection of transformants, and for melanin（黑色素）production (*mel*) by the action of tyrosinase. The regulatory region of the *mel* gene(*) has unique sites for the restriction endonucleases *Sph*1, *Bgl*II, and *Sst*I, allowing easy recognition of colonies containing recombinant plasmids on primary transformation plates by their inability to convert tyrosine to black melanin pigment.

Benefits of using *Streptomyces lividans* as a host. *Streptomyces lividans* is routinely employed as a host for gene cloning, largely because this species recognizes a large number of promoters and appears to lack a restriction system.

S. lividans has several advantages as an alternative host to *E. coli* for the cloning and expression of exogenous DNA. These include their ability to secrete foreign proteins and to recognize a large number of promoters. Successful cloning of foreign genes to achieve high level expression requires a host that is capable of supporting efficient secretion of the overproduced protein. *Streptomycetes* are rich producers of exoenzymes（胞外酶）, of which many [proteases, amylases, lipases, xylanases（木聚糖酶）, agarase（琼胶酶）, chitinases, and nucleases] are related to their ecology（生态学）as saprophytic（腐生的）decomposers of macromolecules in soil and compost（堆肥，混合物）habitats. These organisms export enzymes (and antibiotics) efficiently, which is fundamental to their importance in industrial microbiology. *S. lividans* is no exception and is routinely employed as the host for high-copy-vector-derived gene products. It is fortuitous that *S. lividans* secretes insignificant（无足轻重的）quantities of protease.

Applications for the cloning vector pIJ702

A. *In vitro* Manipulation of *Streptomyces* DNA. Cloning of exogenous DNA using vector pIJ702 facilitates the detection of recombinants among a population of *Streptomyces* transformants. Clones containing a DNA insert at any of the three unique sites in *mel* are readily scored by their inability to convert tyrosine into the diffusible black pigment. pIJ702 has been successfully employed in a variety of cloning applications within the genus *Streptomyces*.

B. Gene Amplification for Overproduction of Proteins. As described earlier, pIJ702 contains the pIJ101 replicon, which has been estimated to exist at 40 to 300 copies per genome in *S lividans*. This feature has been exploited for the overproduction of a variety of gene products. A final outstanding example of amplified expression involved the agarase gene from *S. coelicolor* A3(2) strain M130. The initial *S. lividans* transformant carried a 7-kb DNA insert in the *Bgl*II site of pIJ702 (pMT605) and produced sixfold more agarase than *S. coelicolor*. The agarase gene was subsequently localized to a 1.9-kb DNA segment by deletion and subcloned into *S. lividans*. One isolate (harboring pMT608) overproduced and efficiently exported at least 500 times more agarase into the medium, while the enzyme accounted for nearly 50% of the total extracellular protein.

pJV1

The 11-kb circular plasmid pJV1, isolated from *Streptomyces phaeochromogenes*（暗产色链霉菌），replicates via single-stranded intermediates by a rolling-circle mechanism. Intermycelial plasmid transfer requires the products of the pJV1 *traA* and *traB* genes, whose expression is regulated by the product of *traR*; in addition, the products of the PJV1 *spdB* genes are required for colonization of the recipient mycelium（菌丝体），leading to a "pock" formation. *clt*, another pJV1 locus, which is also necessary for efficient plasmid transfer. The pJV. *clt* locus resembles in function, but not in sequence, the *clt* locus of pIJ101 and shows some structural similarity to an *oriT*. Since it resembles in function the *clt* locus of pIJ101, this region, therefore, is best described as the pJV1 *cis* locus for transfer (*clt*).

pFD666 — A versatile shuttle cosmid vector for use in *Escherichia coli* and actinomycetes

pFD666 is a shuttle cosmid vector constructed for *Escherichia coli* and Actinomycetes. This vector, utilizes the origin of replication (*ori*) of the broad-host-range plasmid, pJV1, from *Streptomyces phaeochromogenes*, for replication in Actinomycetes. The *ori* of pJV1 is compatible with vectors based on the pIJ101 origin of replication, the resultant pFD666 absorbed the merit and became compatible with those vectors accordingly.

The pFD666 vector (Fig. 2-70) has a relatively small size (5.25 kb) and possesses nine unique restriction sites useful for cloning, The polylinker cloning site is flanked by bacteriophage SP6 and T7 promoters, allowing the *in vitro* synthesis of RNA probes that can be used to identify overlapping clones in a cosmid library. Terminators on both sides of the polylinker protect the vector from transcription originating from cloned inserts.

The pFD666 vector employs the neomycin phosphotransferase-encoding gene (*neo*)（新霉素磷酸转移酶编码基因）from transposon Tn5 as the selective marker. To achieve this, the native promoter

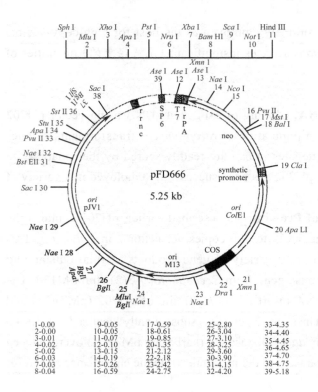

Fig. 2-70 Physical map of pFD666. Locations of the *neo* gene, the synthetic promoter, ColEl *ori*, cohesive end site of λ (COS), M13 *ori*, pJV1 *ori*, promoters for the T7 and SP6 RNA polymerase (T7, SP6) and transcription terminators (*rrnC*, *trpA*) are shown. The polylinker cloning sites that are underlined are unique in the vector. The coordinates given are in kb. There are no *Afl*II, *Avr*II, *Bcl*I, *Bgl*II, *Bsp*HI, *Bst*BI, *Eco*RI, *Eco*RV, *Kpn*I, *Hpa*I, *Nde*I, *Nhe*I, *Nsi*I, *Sma*I, *Sna*BI, *Spe*I, *Ssp*I sites in the vector. There are multiple *Aat*II, *Bss*HII, *Eag*I, *Nar*I, *Pvu*I, *Sal*I sites in the vector.

1-0.00	9-0.05	17-0.59	25-2.80	33-4.35
2-0.00	10-0.05	18-0.61	26-3.04	34-4.40
3-0.01	11-0.07	19-0.85	27-3.10	35-4.45
4-0.02	12-0.10	20-1.35	28-3.25	36-4.65
5-0.02	13-0.15	21-2.12	29-3.60	37-4.70
6-0.03	14-0.19	22-2.18	30-3.90	38-4.75
7-0.03	15-0.26	23-2.42	31-4.15	39-5.18
8-0.04	16-0.59	24-2.75	32-4.20	

of *neo* was replaced by one optimized for expression in both hosts (*E. coli* and *Streptomyces*). The presence of the synthetic promoter in the vector has allowed the direct selection of transformants with kanamycin on regeneration plates with both hosts, which was impossible with the native promoter of the *neo* gene.

An M13 *ori* allows the production of single-stranded DNA. Single-stranded DNA is 10~100 times more efficient for gene disruption in *Streptomyces* than is double-stranded DNA.

Applications and properties of pFD666

Plasmid pFD666 was successfully used to transform *E. coli*, *S. lividans*, or *Sa. erythraea* using standard procedures;

Since gene cloning in Actinomycetes is time-consuming compared to cloning in *E. coli*, the use of shuttle vectors can speed up routine sub-cloning experiments. The construction and applications of pFD666 facilitates the cloning, restriction mapping, DNA sequencing, and functional analysis of actinomycete genes. Actually, the pFD666 plasmid was used for the sub-cloning, restriction mapping and localization of a chitosanase gene isolated from *Kitasatosporia* (北里孢菌属) N174; sub-clones were shuttled many times between *E. coli* and *S. lividans* without encountering any stability problems.

Furthermore, *S. lividans* was cotransformed with pFD666 and pIJ702 and both plasmids could be isolated from the transformants in an apparently unaltered form.

In short, the pFD666 vector, a small, high-copy-number, broad-host-range cosmid, is a valuable genetic tool available for the molecular study of Actinomycetes. Moreover, it is compatible with commonly used vectors derived from pIJ101, and could be used in complementation studies involving multiple cloned genes in one host. Its extensive polylinker and its capacity to be used to produce ssDNA can facilitate localization and sequence analysis of cloned genes.

Characteristics

As a recently developed system for foreign gene expression, *Streptomyces* has the following characteristics.

Its advantages include:

① Bacteria of *Streptomyces* exhibit no pathogenicity towards human being and livestock.

② A significant advances have been made in the studies on molecular genetics in recent years, and a host of vector plasmids with considerable practical value have been developed.

③ The whole-Genome sequencing of the bacterium *Streptomyces coelicolor* has almost been completed.

④ The secretory ability of *Streptomyces* is great, and this is conducive（有助的，有益的）to the subsequent separation and purification of recombinant proteins.

⑤ The proteins being expressed in *Streptomyces* would usually fold properly, and do not form inclusion body.

⑥ *Streptomyces lividans*（变铅青链霉菌）is a kind of strain with a weak restriction and modification capability, hence more suitable for heterogenous gene expression.

⑦ *Streptomyces* is an important genus of industrial microorganisms, and its downstream technology is mature.

The disadvantages are as follows:

① The molecular biology of *Streptomyces* is not as intensely studied as that of *E. coli*, still need to be further intensified;

② The factors affecting exogenous gene expression, and furthermore, the secretion mechanism, still needs to be systematically studied.

2.5.2　Eukaryotic expression systems（真核表达体系）

Eukaryotic expression system（真核生物表达体系）

2.5.2.1　Yeast expression system（酵母表达体系）

Saccharomyces cerevisiae（酿酒酵母），*Pichia Pastoris*

Expression systems in yeast typically use the common and well known *Saccharomyces cerevisiae*, but also *Pichia pastoris*（毕赤酵母）. Systems using *Pichia pastoris* allow stable and lasting production of proteins closer to mammalian cells, at high yield, in chemically defined media of proteins.

Saccharomyces cerevisiae

Saccharomyces cerevisiae is particularly widely used for protein expression studies in yeast, for example in **yeast two-hybrid system**（酵母双杂交系统）for the study of protein-protein interaction. The vectors used in yeast two-hybrid system contain fusion partners for two cloned genes that allow the transcription of a reporter gene when there is interaction between the two proteins expressed from the cloned genes.

Pichia pastoris

Pichia pastoris is a species of methylotrophic yeast（甲醇酵母，甲基营养型酵母）. *Pichia* is widely used for protein expression using recombinant DNA techniques. Hence it is used in biochemical and genetic research in academia（学术界）and the biotechnical industry.

Yeast expression vector in *Pichia*

A yeast commonly used for protein expression is *Pichia pastoris*（毕赤酵母）. Examples of yeast expression vector in *Pichia* are the pPIC series of vectors, and these vectors use the *AOX1* promoter which is inducible with methanol. The plasmids may contain elements for insertion of foreign DNA into the yeast genome and signal sequence for the secretion of expressed protein. Proteins with disulphide bonds and glycosylation can be efficiently produced in yeast.

Pichia pastoris as an expression system

Pichia pastoris is frequently used as an expression system for the production of proteins. A number of properties makes *P. pastoris* suited for this task: *P. pastoris* has a high growth rate and is able to grow on a simple, inexpensive medium. *P. pastoris* can grow in either shake flasks or a fermenter, which makes it suitable for both small and large scale production.

Pichia pastoris has two alcohol oxidase genes, *Aox1* and *Aox2*, which have a strongly inducible promoter. These genes allow *Pichia* to use methanol as a carbon and energy source. The *AOX* promoters are induced by methanol and are repressed（抑制）by *e.g.*, glucose. Usually the gene for the desired protein is introduced under the control of the *AOX1* promoter, which means that protein production can be induced by the addition of methanol. In a popular expression vector, the desired protein is produced as a fusion product to the secretion signal of the α-mating factor from *Saccharomyces cerevisiae* (baker's yeast). This causes the protein to be secreted into the growth medium, which greatly facilitates subsequent protein purification. There are commercially available plasmids that have these features incorporated (such as the pPICZα vector).

Comparison to other expression systems

In standard molecular biology research, the bacterium *Escherichia coli* is the most frequently used organism for production of recombinant DNA and proteins. This is due to *E. coli*'s fast growth rate, good protein production rate and undemanding growth conditions. Protein expression in *E. coli* is usually faster than in *Pichia pastoris* for several reasons: competent *E. coli* cells can be stored frozen, and thawed immediately before use, whereas *Pichia* cells have to be produced immediately before use. Expression yields in *Pichia* vary between different clones, and usually a large number of clones needs to be screened for protein expression before a good producer is found. Optimal induction times of *Pichia* are usually on the order of days, whereas *E. coli* usually reaches optimal yields within hours of induction. The major advantage of *Pichia* over *E. coli* is that *Pichia* is capable of producing disulfide bonds and glycosylations in proteins. This means that in cases where disulfides are necessary, *E. coli* might produce a misfolded protein that is usually inactive or insoluble.

The well-studied *Saccharomyces cerevisiae* (baker's yeast) is also used as an expression system with similar advantages over *E. coli* as *Pichia*. However *Pichia* has two main advantages over *S. cerevisiae* in laboratory and industrial settings:

Firstly, *Pichia*, as mentioned above, is a methylotroph（甲基营养生物）, meaning it can grow with the simple alcohol methanol as its only source of energy — *Pichia* can easily be grown in cell suspension in reasonably strong methanol solutions that would kill most other microorganisms, a system that is cheap to set up and maintain.

Secondly, *Pichia* can grow to very high cell densities, and under ideal conditions can multiply to the point where the cell suspension is practically a paste. As the protein yield from expression in a microbe is roughly equal to the product of the protein produced per cell and the number of cells, this makes *Pichia* of great use when trying to produce large quantities of protein without expensive equipment.

Compared to other expression systems such as S2-cells from *Drosophila melanogaster*（果蝇，黑腹果蝇）or Chinese Hamster Ovary cells, *Pichia* usually gives much better yields. Cell lines from multicellular organisms usually require complex rich media, including amino acids, vitamins and growth factors. These media significantly increase the cost of producing recombinant proteins. Additionally, since *Pichia* can grow in media containing only one carbon source and one nitrogen source, it is suitable for isotopic（同位素的）labeling applications in *e.g.,* protein NMR. However, a number of proteins require chaperonins（伴侣蛋白）for proper folding. Thus, *Pichia* is unable to produce a number of proteins for which the host lacks the appropriate chaperones. In 2006 a research group has managed to create a strain that produces Erythropoietin（促红细胞生成素）in its normal glycosylation form. This was achieved by exchanging the enzymes responsible for the fungal-type glycosylation, with the mammalian homologs. Thus, the altered glycosylation pattern allowed the protein to be fully functional.

Pichia pastoris as a model organism

Another advantage of *Pichia pastoris* is its similarity to the well-studied *Saccharomyces cerevisiae* (also known as baker's yeast). As a model organism for biology, and having been used by man for various purposes throughout history, *S. cerevisiae* is well studied, to say the least. The two yeast species (*Pichia*, *Saccharomyces*) have similar growth conditions and tolerances, and thus the culturing of *Pichia pastoris* can be readily adopted by labs without specialist equipment.

The *Pichia pastoris* GS115 genome has been sequenced by the Flanders Institute for Biotechnology (VIB) and Ghent University (UGent) and published in *Nature Biotechnology*. The genome sequence and gene annotation can be browsed（浏览，查看网络信息）through the ORCAE（真核生物社区注释网络资源）system.

Pichia pastoris expression system possesses following advantages:

① *Pichia pastoris* is a eukaryotic expression system, hence the expressed protein can be subject to folding and post-translational modification.

② The expression level of exogenous protein is high in *Pichia pastoris*.

③ The production cost of this expression system is low as compared with that of other eukaryotic expression system, just a simple salt-containing medium is enough.

④ *Pichia pastoris* is suitable for high-density culture.

⑤ The protein products would be purified easily, since there are less "other proteins".

Kluyveromyces lactis（乳酸克鲁维酵母）

Another yeast used for protein expression is *Kluyveromyces lactis*（乳酸克鲁维酵母）and the protein is expressed driven by a variant of the strong lactase *LAC4* promoter.

2.5.2.2 *Insect cell expression system*（昆虫细胞表达体系）

Baculovirus（杆状病毒）

Baculovirus, a rod-shaped virus which infect insect cells, is used as the expression vector in this system. Insect cell lines derived from *Lepidopterans*（鳞翅目昆虫）(moths and butterflies), such as *Spodoptera frugiperda*（草地夜蛾，秋黏虫）, are used as host. The shuttle vector is called bacmid（杆状病毒质粒，杆粒，杆状病毒穿梭载体）, and protein expression is under the control of a strong promoter P$_{polh}$.

Baculovirus has also been used with mammalian cell lines in the BacMam system.

Baculovirus is normally used for production of glycoproteins, although the glycosylations may be different from those found in vertebrates. In general, it is safer to use than mammalian virus as it has a limited host range and does not infect vertebrates without modifications.

When insect cell is chosen to be the expression host, *Spodoptera frugiperda*（草地夜蛾）cell sf9, sf21, *etc.* are mostly adapted. In addition, silkworm larvae were also used for expression. The main expression vector of this system is baculoviral vector, which was constructed from the strong polyhedrin (*polh*)（多角体蛋白）promoter of the *Autographa california*（苜蓿银纹夜蛾，苜蓿尺蠖）multiple nuclear polyhedrosis virus (AcMNPV) and *Bombyx mori* nuclear polyhedrosis virus（BmNPV, 家蚕核型多角体病毒）.

Baculoviruses are the most prominent viruses known to affect the insect population. They are double-stranded circular, supercoiled DNA molecules in a rod-shaped capsid. More than 500 baculovirus isolates (based on hosts of origin) have been identified, most of which originated in arthropods（节肢动物），particularly insects of the order（目）Lepidoptera（鳞翅类，鳞翅目）. Two of the most common isolates used in foreign gene expression are *Autographa californica* multiple nuclear polyhedrosis virus (AcMNPV) and *Bombyx mori* (silkworm) nuclear polyhedrosis virus (BMNPV).

Infection by viral vectors emerged as the dominant method of choice to deliver genes into primary cells. An ideal viral vector for multigene delivery should have virtually unlimited foreign DNA cargo capacity allowing for integration of a multitude of independent expression cassetes functionalities and regulatory elements. Moreover, such an optimal viral vector should exhibit low cytotoxicity in mammalian cells and should enable transduction of dividing and non-dividing mammalian cells alike. Currently used lenti- and other retroviruses, as well as adeno- and adeno-associated viruses have a limitation on DNA cargo size due to spatial constraints imposed by the tight geometry of their capsids.

Baculoviral vectors, in contrast, can accommodate very large DNA cargo insertions. The *Autographa californica* multiple nuclear polyhedrosis virus (ACMNPV), is a baculovirus with a large (134 kb) double-stranded circular DNA genome that normally infects specific moth larvae. Transgene capacity of AcMNPV is very large, extending probably beyond 100 kbp. Replication of AcMNPV is highly insect-cell specific; however, AcMNPV is capable of efficiently transducing not only insect but also mammalian cells. Transduction is usually transient without DNA integration into the target cell genome and such viruses are replication deficient. In baculoviruses used for mammalian cell transduction (Bacmam) heterologous genes are placed under the control of mammalian promoters and inserted into the baculoviral genome, and viral stocks are produced in insect cells. Once the baculovirus enters mammalian cells, these genes are actively transcribed within 9 h and the cells produce the heterologous gene product. In the last decade, baculovirus has emerged as a useful and safe technology to deliver heterologous genetic material to mammalian cell types both *in vitro* and *in vivo*.

Plasmid vector pTriEx-1 contains p10 (baculovirus) promoter, which make it express in insect cells. In addition, it also contains T7*lac* promoter, which make it express in *Escherichia coli*.

Therefore, pTriEx-1 is an insect-cell-*E. coli* shuttle plasmid. Meanwhile, it can be expressed in mammal cells.

Since 1983, when Baculovirus Expression Vector System (BEVS) Technology was introduced, the baculovirus system has become one of the most versatile and powerful eukaryotic vector systems for recombinant protein expression. More than 600 recombinant genes have been expressed in baculoviruses

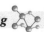

up to 2002. Since 1985, when the first protein (IL-2) was produced in large scale from a recombinant baculovirus, use of BEVS has increased dramatically. BEVS technology offers the following advantages over other expression vector systems.

(1) ***It has intact infectivity.*** Virions are quite stable in standard serum-supplemented growth media, they maintain their integrity and infectious competency for days at elevated temperatures, weeks at room temperature, and months to years at 4℃. The recombinant region of insect virus vector is an unnecessary region of the genome, even the deletion of this part will not affect the replication and expression of the virus, thus maintains the intact infectivity of the baculovirus vector.

(2) ***It has large cargo capacity.*** Due to its flexible envelop structure, very large heterologous DNA cargo can be incorporated into the baculoviral genome, up to 100 kb.

(3) ***It has a noticeable marker.*** After inserting exogenous gene into the gene region of polyhedral protein, the plaque would not appear without polyhedral protein produced, thus it is easy to select the recombinants.

(4) ***The expressed protein products can be secreted extracellularly.***

(5) ***High Levels of Recombinant Gene Expression:*** The expression level is high. The exogenous gene is placed under the control of the polyhedrin promoter, which is a strong promoter. The expression level of the exogenous protein can reach 50% of the total protein of the cell, with the highest reaching several mg/ml. In many cases, the recombinant proteins are soluble and easily recovered from infected cells late in infection when host protein synthesis is diminished.

(6) ***Insect cell-pathogenic viruses expression system can be applied to the expression of cytotoxic recombinant proteins.***

(7) ***Accuracy:*** Baculoviruses can be propagated（繁殖）in insect hosts which are able to modify peptides post-translationally in a manner similar to that of mammalian cells. The post-translational processing can be conducted effectively in this system, *e.g.*, glycosylation.

(8) ***Safety:*** Baculoviruses have a restricted host range, which is often limited to specific invertebrate species. They are essentially nonpathogenic to vertebrates (especially mammals) and plants, so is environmentally safe. Because the insect cell lines are not transformed by pathogenic or infectious viruses, they can be cared for under minimal containment（遏制，控制）conditions. Helper cell lines or helper viruses are not required because the baculovirus genome contains all the genetic information.

(9) ***Insect cells can be serially passaged.*** When cultured at 25~30℃, no CO_2 is needed.

(10) ***Use of Cell Lines Ideal for Suspension Culture:*** Insect cell can be subject to suspension cultivation, hence is suitable for large-scale cell cultivation. BmNPV has a narrow host range, while silkworm is easy to raise, can be subject to large-scale sterile feeding, hence it is convenient to express a large amount of heterologous genes. AcNPV is usually propagated in cell lines derived from the fall armyworm（黏虫，行军虫）*Spodoptera frugiperda* or from the cabbage looper（粉纹夜蛾）*Trichoplusia ni*（粉纹夜蛾）. Cell lines are available that grow well in suspension cultures, allowing the production of recombinant proteins in large-scale bioreactors.

(11) ***Ease of Scale Up:*** Baculoviruses have been reproducibly scaled up for the large-scale production of biologically active recombinant products.

Generating a Recombinant Virus by Homologous Recombination

Using homologous recombination to generate a recombinant baculovirus is outlined in Fig. 2-71. The most common baculovirus used for gene expression is AcMNPV. AcMNPV has a large (130-kb), circular, double-stranded DNA genome. The gene of interest is cloned into a transfer vector containing a baculovirus promoter flanked by baculovirus DNA derived from a nonessential locus — in this case, the polyhedrin gene. The gene of interest is inserted into the genome of the parent virus (such as AcMNPV) by homologous recombination after transfection into insect cells. Typically, 0.1% to 1% of the resulting progeny are recombinant. The recombinants are identified by altered plaque morphology. For a vector with the polyhedrin promoter, as in this example, the cells in which the nuclei do not contain occluded virus (多角体病毒，包含体病毒), contain recombinant DNA. Detection of the desired occlusion-minus plaque phenotype against the background of greater than 99% wild-type parental viruses is difficult.

Generating a Recombinant Virus by Site-Specific Transposition

A faster approach for generating a recombinant baculovirus uses site-specific transposition with Tn7 to insert foreign genes into bacmid DNA propagated in *E.coli*. The gene of interest is cloned into a pFASTBAC™ vector, and the recombinant plasmid is transformed into DH10BAC™ competent cells which contain the bacmid with a mini-*att*Tn7 target site and the helper plasmid. The mini-Tn7 element on the pFASTBAC plasmid can transpose (转换，对调，调换) to the mini-*att*Tn7 target site on the bacmid in the presence of transposition proteins (转座蛋白) provided by the helper plasmid. Colonies containing recombinant bacmids are identified by antibiotic selection and blue/white screening, since the transposition results in disruption of the lacZα gene. High molecular weight mini-prep DNA is prepared from selected *E. coli* clones containing the recombinant bacmid, and this DNA is then used to transfect insect cells.

A variety of pFASTBAC donor plasmids are available which share common features. The plasmid pFASTBAC 1 is used to generate viruses which will express unfused (未融合的，非融合的) recombinant proteins. The pFASTBAC HT series of vectors are used to express polyhistidine-tagged proteins which can be rapidly purified on metal affinity resins. The pFASTBAC DUAL vector has two promoters and cloning sites, allowing expression of two genes, one from the polyhedrin promoter and one from the p10 promoter.

Cell Lines

The most common cell lines used for BEVS applications are listed in Table 2-9. Of these, Sf9, a clonal isolate of the *Spodoptera frugiperda* cell line IPLB-Sf21-AE, is probably the most widely used. Sf9 was

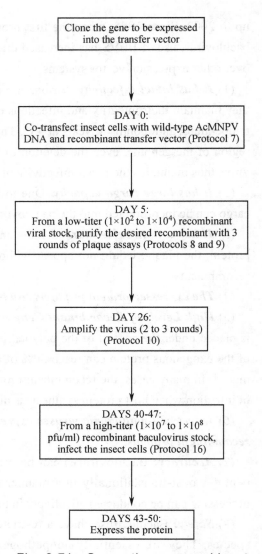

Fig. 2-71 Generating a recombinant baculovirus by homologous recombination.

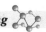

originally established from ovarian tissue of the fall armyworm. Although there is significant scientific data on the characteristics of this *Lepidopteran* cell line, it remains to be confirmed whether it is the best line for virus or recombinant protein production. Ongoing research suggests that different insect cell lines may support, varying levels of expression and differential glycosylation with the same recombinant protein.

Table 2-9　Insect cell lines commonly used in BEVS applications.

Insect Species	Cell Line
Spodoptera frugiperda	Sf9
Spodoptera frugiperda	Sf-21
Trichoplusia ni	Tn-368
Trichoplusia ni	High-five BTI-TN-5B1-4

Note: Each of these cell lines has been successfully adapted to suspension cultures.

Baculovirus-infected cells（杆状病毒感染的细胞）

Infected insect cells (Sf9, Sf21, High Five strains) or mammalian cells (HeLa, HEK 293) allows expression of glycosylated proteins that cannot be expressed using yeast or prokaryotic cells (like *E. coli*). It is a very useful system for expression of proteins in high quantity. Genes are not expressed continuously because infected host cells will eventually lyse and die during each infection cycle.

Non-lytic insect cell expression

Non-lytic insect cell expression is an alternative to the lytic baculovirus expression system. In non-lytic expression, vectors are transiently or stably transfected into the chromosomal DNA of insect cells for subsequent protein expression. This is followed by selection and screening of recombinant clones. The non-lytic system has been used to give higher protein yield and quicker expression of recombinant proteins compared to baculovirus-infected cell expression. Cell lines used for this system include: Sf9, Sf21 from *Spodoptera frugiperda* cells, Hi-5 from ***Trichoplusia ni***（粉纹夜蛾）cells, and Schneider 2 cells and Schneider 3 cells from *Drosophila melanogaster*（果蝇）cells. With this system, cells do not lyse and several cultivation modes can be used. Additionally, protein production runs are reproducible. This system gives a homogeneous product. A drawback of this system is the requirement of an additional screening step of selecting viable clones.

Sf9

Sf9 cells, a clonal isolate of *Spodoptera frugiperda* Sf21 cells　(IPLB-SF21-AE), are commonly used for recombinant protein production using baculovirus. They can be grown in the absence of serum, and can be cultured attached or in suspension.

Sf21

Sf21 (officially called **IPLB-Sf21AE**) is a continuous cell line developed from ovaries of the fall armyworm（草地夜蛾），*Spodoptera frugiperda*, a moth species that is an agricultural pest on corn and other grass species. It was originally developed in the United States at the Henry A. Wallace Beltsville Agricultural Research Center. Sf9 is a substrain (clone) of these cells that was isolated from Sf21 by researchers at Texas A&M University.

Both the clone and parent strains of the cells have been extensively used in research on viruses, especially baculoviruses in their use for producing recombinant proteins.

This is just one of the over 500 insect cell lines that have been developed from more than 125 insect species.

High Five cells

High Five Cell Line (officially called **BTI-TN-5B1-4**) is an insect cell line that originated from the ovarian cells of the cabbage looper（粉纹夜蛾）, *Trichoplusia ni*（粉纹夜蛾）. It was developed by the Boyce Thompson Institute for Plant Research, Ithaca, NY.

High Five cells have become one of the most commonly used cell lines for recombinant protein expression using baculovirus or transfection, and have been demonstrated, in a number of cases, to express more recombinant protein than other lepidopteran（鳞翅类的）cell lines, such as Sf9 cells. They can be grown in the absence of serum, and can be cultured in a loose attached state or in suspension.

Schneider 2 cells

Schneider 2 cells, usually abbreviated as **S2 cells**, are one of the most commonly used *Drosophila melanogaster* cell lines. S2 cells were derived from a primary culture of late stage (20~24 hours old) *Drosophila melanogaster* embryos, likely from a macrophage-like lineage.

S2 cells can be grown at room temperature either as a semi-adherent monolayer or in suspension, and they can be grown in the absence of serum.

Media and Growth Supplements

Fetal bovine serum (FBS) has been the primary growth supplement used in insect cell culture medium.

Second-generation serum-free formulations such as Sf-900 II SFM and EXPRESS-FIVE SFM are specifically designed for large-scale production of recombinant proteins. They contain optimized concentrations of amino acids, carbohydrates, vitamins, and lipids that reduce or eliminate the effect of rate-limiting nutritional restrictions or deficiencies. Both Sf-900 II SFM and EXPRESS-FIVE SFM support faster population doubling times and higher saturation cell densities than do traditional media. Thus, you can obtain both higher wild-type or recombinant baculovirus titers and increased levels or yields of recombinant protein expression by using these formulations. The optimized formulations offer the following advantages over sera:

- ◇ Eliminate the need for costly fetal bovine and other animal sera supplements
- ◇ Increase cell and product yields
- ◇ Eliminate adventitious（偶然的，外来的）agents
- ◇ Have lot-to-lot consistency

Presence of a Cystine Protease

Ambient medium（周围介质）of baculovirus infected cells may contain a cystine protease. Proteolysis is a serious issue in serum-free cultures. Because SFM are low in protein or protein-free, they provide little competitive substrate for the protease activity. Secreted proteins have demonstrated a variable sensitivity to ambient proteases. Researchers have examined a variety of protease inhibitors with variable success. A report using pCMBS (p-chloromercuribenzene) appears promising. The best way to reduce the chance of significant proteolysis is to keep post-infection culture supernatants refrigerated, to harvest the product before significant cell lysis occurs, and to process the product as soon as possible after harvest. Addition of 0.1% to 1% BSA can provide a competitive substrate for the protease.

In the three decades since their inception baculovirus-based expression systems have become well-established and widely used for recombinant protein production in insect cells. Later, it was discovered that baculoviruses not only infect insect cells but can also drive heterologous protein expression in mammalian cells if appropriate mammalian regulatory elements are provided in the recombinant baculovirus genome. This so-called 'BacMam' method has been applied to produce heterologous proteins in academic and industrial research and development, notably for pharmacological screening. Today, it is becoming increasingly evident that most physiological activities are mediated by multiple proteins forming complex assemblies.

Co-expression of protein complexes in insect cells

Expression and co-expression of proteins in baculovirus-infected insect cells has been in use for some time. Initially, most experiments were performed with multiple viruses, each one bearing a single gene to be overexpressed. Since no selection can be performed on these viruses, the major problem of this approach is that it gives partial as well as full co-infection and often very careful quantification of the virus titer is required to obtain reasonable results. However, large complexes have been obtained and purified using this technique, albeit in small amounts. The use of a single vector with multiple promoters, in a fashion similar to *E. coli*, clearly increases the yields and has also been used in a number of cases.

2.5.2.3   *Mammalian cell expression system* （哺乳动物细胞表达体系）

Mammalian expression vectors offer considerable advantages for the expression of mammalian proteins — proper folding, post-translational modifications, and relevant enzymatic activity — over bacterial expression systems. Furthermore, proteins expressed in other eukaryotic non-mammalian systems may not contain the correct glycosylations. It is of particular use in producing membrane-associating proteins that require chaperones for proper folding and stability as well as containing numerous post-translational modifications. The downside （缺点）, however, is the low yield of product in comparison to prokaryotic vectors as well as the costly nature of the techniques involved. Its complicated technology, and potential contamination with animal viruses of mammalian cell have also restricts the use of mammalian cell expression in large-scale industrial production.

Cultured mammalian cell lines such as the Chinese hamster ovary (CHO，中国仓鼠卵巢细胞)，HEK（人胚肾细胞），HeLa, and COS cell lines may be used to produce protein. Vectors are transfected into the cells and the DNA may be integrated into the genome by homologous recombination in the case of stable transfection, or the cells may be transiently transfected. Examples of mammalian expression vectors include the adenoviral vectors（腺病毒载体），the pSV and the pCMV series of plasmid vectors, vaccinia（牛痘）and retroviral vectors, as well as baculovirus. The promoters for cytomegalovirus (CMV，巨细胞病毒) and SV40（猿猴空泡病毒40）are commonly used in mammalian expression vectors to drive protein expression. Non-viral promoter, such as the elongation factor (EF)-1 promoter, is also known.

Mammalian systems

➢ *Bos primigenius* (Bovine)
➢ *Mus musculus* (Mouse)
➢ Chinese Hamster Ovary
➢ Human Embryonic Kidney cells
➢ Baby Hamster Kidney

Chinese hamster ovary cell（中华仓鼠卵巢细胞）

Chinese hamster ovary (CHO) cells are a cell line derived from the ovary of the Chinese hamster, often used in biological and medical research and commercially in the production of therapeutic proteins. They were introduced in the 1960s, are grown as a cultured monolayer and require the amino acid proline in their culture medium.

CHO cells are used in studies of genetics, toxicity screening, nutrition and gene expression, particularly to express recombinant proteins. Today, CHO cells are the most commonly used mammalian hosts for industrial production of recombinant protein therapeutics.

History

The use of the Chinese hamster in research began in 1919 where they were used in place of mice for typing（分型）*pneumococci*（肺炎双球菌）. They were subsequently found to be excellent vectors for transmission of kala-azar（黑热病，利什曼病）[a.k.a. visceral leishmaniasis（内脏型利什曼病）], facilitating research in epidemiology.

In 1948, the Chinese hamster was brought to the United States for breeding in research laboratories. In the following years, the Chinese hamster became noteworthy for the cell lines that were derived from its tissues. Having a very low chromosome number (2n=22) for a mammal, the Chinese hamster is an ideal model for radiation cytogenetics（辐射细胞遗传学）and tissue culture.

In 1957, Theodore T. Puck obtained a female Chinese hamster from Dr. George Yerganian's laboratory at the Boston Cancer Research Foundation and used it to derive the original Chinese hamster ovary (CHO) cell line. Since then, CHO cells have been a cell line of choice because of their rapid growth and high protein production. They have become the mammalian equivalent of *E. coli* in research and biotechnology today, especially when long-term, stable gene expression and high yields of proteins are required.

Properties

CHO cells do not express the Epidermal growth factor receptor (EGFR), which makes them ideal in the investigation of various EGFR mutations.

The first CHO cell line was derived from the original cell lines in Dr. Puck's laboratory through single cell cloning in 1957. CHO-K1 was later derived from this ancestral cell line, and it contains a slightly lower amount of DNA than the original CHO. CHO-K1 was mutagenized to generate CHO-DXB11 (also referred to as CHO-DUKX), a cell line lacking DHFR（二氢叶酸还原酶）activity. These cells have a deletion of one *dhfr* allele and a Missense mutation（错义突变）in the other. Subsequently, the proline-dependent CHO-pro3- strain, another derivative of the original CHO cell line, was mutagenized to yield CHO-DG44, a cell line with deletions of both *dhfr* alleles. These two DHFR-minus strains require glycine, hypoxanthine（次黄嘌呤）, and thymidine (GHT) for growth. Although not initially intended for recombinant protein manufacture, DHFR-minus CHO cells were used for a number of pioneering experiments demonstrating stable transfection with an exogenous *dhfr* gene via selection in GHT-minus medium. This genetic selection scheme remains one of the standard methods to establish stably transfected CHO cell lines for the production of recombinant therapeutic proteins. The multistep process begins with the molecular cloning of the **gene of interest (GOI)** and the *dhfr* gene in a single or in separate mammalian expression vectors. The plasmid DNA(s) carrying the two genes are then delivered into cells by transfection, and the cells are grown under selective conditions in GHT-minus medium. Each surviving cell will have one or more copies of the exogenous *dhfr* gene, usually along with the

---

GOI, integrated in its genome. The integrated plasmid copy number varies widely from one recombinant cell to another, but there is almost always only one integration site per cell even if multiple plasmids are transfected. The growth rate and the level of recombinant protein production of each cell line also vary widely. To obtain a few stably transfected cell lines with the desired phenotypic characteristics, it may be necessary to evaluate several hundred candidate cell lines.

The CHO and CHO-K1 cell lines can be obtained from a number of biological resource centers such as the European Collection of Animal Cell Cultures (ECACC，欧洲细胞株保藏中心) which is part of the Health Protection Agency Culture Collections. CHO-K1 data, such as growth curves, timelapse（间隔拍摄，定时拍摄）videos of growth, images and subculture routine information are available from ECACC.

HEK 293 cells

Human Embryonic Kidney 293 cells, also often referred to as **HEK 293**, **HEK-293**, **293 cells**, or less precisely as **HEK cells**, are a specific cell line originally derived from human embryonic kidney cells (from an aborted human embryo) grown in tissue culture and from stillborn（死产的）animals. HEK 293 cells are very easy to grow and transfect very readily and have been widely used in cell biology research for many years. They are also used by the biotechnology industry to produce therapeutic proteins and viruses for gene therapy.

Applications

HEK 293 cells are straightforward to grow in culture and to transfect, and so have been widely used as hosts for gene expression. Typically, these experiments involve transfecting a gene (or combination of genes) of interest, and then analyzing the expressed protein. The widespread use of this cell line is due to its extreme transfectability by the various techniques, including calcium phosphate method, achieving efficiencies approaching 100%.

Examples of such experiments include:

➤ A study of the effects of a drug on sodium channels
➤ Testing of an inducible RNA interference system
➤ Testing of an isoform-selective protein kinase C agonist
➤ Investigation of the interaction between two proteins
➤ Analysis of a nuclear export signal（核输出信号，出核信号）in a protein

A more specific use of HEK 293 cells is in the propagation of adenoviral vectors. Viruses offer an extremely efficient means of delivering genes into cells, since this is what they have evolved to do, and are thus of great use as experimental tools. However, as pathogens, they also present a degree of danger to the experimenter. This danger can be avoided by the use of viruses which lack key genes, and which are thus unable to replicate after entering a cell. In order to propagate such viral vectors, a cell line that expresses the missing genes is required. Since HEK 293 cells express a number of adenoviral genes, they can be used to propagate adenoviral vectors in which these genes (typically, E1 and E3) are deleted, such as AdEasy.

An important variant of this cell line is the 293T cell line that contains the SV40 Large T-antigen, that allows for episomal（附加型的）replication of transfected plasmids containing the SV40 origin of replication. This allows for amplification of transfected plasmids and extended temporal expression of the desired gene products. Note that any similarly modified cell line can be used for this sort of work; HeLa, COS and Chinese Hamster Ovary cell are common alternatives. HEK 293, and especially HEK 293T, cells are commonly used for the production of various retroviral vectors. Various retroviral packaging cell lines are also based on these cells.

Native proteins of interest

Depending on various conditions, the gene expression of HEK 293 cells may vary. The following proteins of interest (among many others) are commonly found in untreated HEK 293 cells:

➤ Corticotrophin（促肾上腺皮质激素）releasing factor type 1 receptor

➤ Sphingosine-1-phosphate（1-磷酸鞘氨醇）receptors EDG1, EDG3 and EDG5

➤ Muscarinic（毒蕈碱的）acetylcholine receptor M3

➤ Transient receptor potential TRPC1, TRPC3, TRPC4, TRPC6

Mammalian Cell Expression System possesses following advantages:

The main advantage of Mammalian Cell Expression System is that it can recognize introns in the pre-mRNA (also known as a "primary transcript") of the exogenous gene and excise them, and process the pre-mRNA to form the mature mRNA (using various forms of post-transcriptional modification).

(1) Characterization of artificially constructed mammalian cell expression system. 人工构建的哺乳动物细胞表达载体条件

Mammalian Cell Expression System contains

① Prokaryotic gene sequence, meanwhile possesses selectable markers for eukaryotic gene.

② Mammalian promoters and enhancer elements.

③ A stop coden and the conserved AAUAAA motif, the polyadenylation signal.

④ More than one unique restriction enzyme recognition sites.

⑤ If introns are unfavorable for exogenous gene expression, use cDNA instead; while if introns are favorable for exogenous gene expression, selectable cleavage signal should be retained.

(2) Main vectors of mammalian cells（哺乳动物细胞主要载体）

Viral technology of gene transfer harness（利用）the method of entry and integration with the host genome used by the wild-type organism. They provide a useful alternative to non-viral methods, which have low transfer efficiencies in certain cell types — for example, primary culture and epithelial cells. The most frequently used vectors are adenoviral or retroviral; however, others include adeno-associated virus (AAV), herpes virus, vaccinia virus, and several RNA viruses. Currently, AAVs are the safest to use clinically.

① SV40-Based Vectors

SIMIAN VIRUS 40

Simian virus-40 (SV40), is a small non-enveloped virus — papovavirus（乳多空病毒）. First described in 1960, SV40 is one of the best characterized viruses and its DNA genome has been extensively studied. The natural animal host for SV40 infection is monkeys. Uniquely among gene transfer vectors, the SV40 minichromosome is circular, a single molecule of covalently closed, superhelical, double-stranded DNA of 5243 bp associated to histones. It therefore lacks terminal repeat regions that characterize many other viral vectors with linear genomes.

SV40 virion. The SV40 viral capsid, formed by three virus-encoded proteins (VP1, VP2, and VP3), packages the SV40 minichromosome in an icosahedral（二十面体的）symmetric structure. One SV40 capsid has 360 molecules of VP1 arranged as 72 pentamers that face the outside of the virion. Each VP1 pentamer is associated with either VP2 or VP3, that bridge VP1 to the SV40 DNA. VP1 monomers

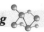

associate in pentamers via interlocking tertiary structures. VP1 pentamers [$(VP1)_5$] are tied together through the insertion of carboxyterminal arms into the cores of neighboring pentamers. Calcium ions are required to stabilize pentamer/pentamer interactions and play a role in virus cell entry, intracellular trafficking, virus uncoating, and capsid assembly. Deletion mapping has shown that a region close to the C-terminus of VP2 or VP3 is joined to the inner cavity of a VP1 pentamer. This $VP1_5$-VP2/VP3 complex is the basic building block of the viral capsid.

SV40 genome. SV40 genome regulatory sequences comprise an origin of replication (*ori*), an encapsidation signal (*ses*), and early and late transcriptional promoters and enhancers in a region of approximately 500 bp. The origin of replication (core origin and two auxiliary elements) binds to the cellular replication machinery. The origin is composed of inverted repeats (IR), a 27-bp sequence repeated four times (27 bp × 4) and a 17-bp AT rich sequence (A/T). The 200-bp encapsidation signal (*ses*) includes part of the origin of replication, GC-boxes, and 26 bp of the enhancer element and confers specificity for the encapsidation of viral genomes. The transcriptional enhancer is formed by a sequence of 72 bp that has been duplicated in some laboratory-adapted strains. Both early and late promoters and polyadenylation sequences are in opposite strands; thus, the transcription extends bidirectionally. Transcription starts at the SV40 early promoter that drives the expression of alternatively spliced mRNAs that encode for the **large tumor antigen** (Tag, 708 AA), **small tumor antigen** (tag), and 17 kT proteins. The 17 kT protein, detected in some Tag expressing cells, is identical to Tag for the first 131 amino acids followed by four different residues before the stop codon is reached in a different reading frame. Tag is essential for regulation of early promoter, activation of replication and late promoter transcription, and virion assembly. SV40 late promoter drives the expression of the three structural proteins, VP1, VP2, and VP3, and the agnoprotein (LP1). Alternative splicing produces two mRNA species that give rise to the four proteins. Translation of VP3 starts in an internal in-frame AUG codon of VP2 mRNA, so VP2 and VP3 share the same carboxyterminal domains that contain the DNA binding domain and the nuclear localization signal. LP1 mediates efficient localization of VP1 into the nucleus, and facilitates spread of the virus to neighboring cells.

SV40 infection cycle. SV40 genome is released into the nucleus as nucleosome-associated minichromosome capable of binding the cellular transcription machinery. Transcription starts from the early promoter to express the *Tag* genes. Soon the cell nucleus contains high concentrations of Tag proteins that bind to several regulatory SV40 sequences. First, Tag binds to the early promoter sequences to repress its own transcription. Then, Tag proteins bind to the 27-bp regions of the origin of replication forming two hexamers capable of recruiting the cellular replication apparatus and initiating structural alterations that result in the opening of the DNA core region. Each Tag hexamer acts as a DNA helicase that facilitates replication bidirectionally. After replication, Tag activates transcription from the SV40 late promoter by binding components of the cellular transcription machinery. The activated late promoter allows expression of capsid proteins that move to the nucleus after being translated. Once in the nucleus, capsid proteins participate in SV40 DNA nucleosomal rearrangement. As capsid proteins recognize DNA nonspecifically, specificity mediated by the transcription factor Sp1 that binds the capsid proteins VP1 and VP2/3. Interaction between Sp1 and $(VP1)_5$-VP2/VP3 inhibits viral promoter activity and allows recruitment of capsid complexes to *ses*. There, encapsidation starts by gradual addition of $(VP1)_5$-VP2/VP3 complexes around the SV40 minichromosome. In addition, VP3-activated PARP, a poly(ADP-ribose) polymerase nuclear enzyme, facilitates the release of mature virions. VP2 seems to be dispensable for the formation of infective particles.

Tropism（生物向性，嗜性）. SV40 infects virtually all mammalian species and nucleated（成核的）cell types. Its ability to infect cells is the same whether cells are cycling or quiescent. Some species' cells permit wild type (wt) SV40 replication optimally (monkeys, "permissive"); some support wt SV40 replication, but not as effectively (*e.g.*, human, "semi-permissive"); and some do not support wt SV40 replication at all (*e.g.*, mouse, "nonpermissive").

SV40 can undergo two types of interactions with cultured mammalian cells. In African green monkey kidney cells, which are the permissive host, the virus undergoes a productive cycle. Few days after infection, cells are killed and a burst of infectious virus is released. Interestingly, SV40 does not shut off the synthesis of host cell macromolecules during the productive cycle. Even late in infection, normal or increased amounts of cellular DNA, RNA and proteins are produced. In other types of cells, termed non-permissive or semi-permissive, this cycle is aborted prior to the onset of viral DNA replication. Instead, part or all of the viral genome becomes stably associated with the host cell, usually through random integration into the chromosomal DNA.

Integration, transformation & persistence. Like oncoretroviruses（致癌反转录病毒）, SV40 integrates at random into cellular genomes. Depending on the nature of the activated gene, cellular proliferation and oncogenesis potentially could result. Cellular genes would thus only be activated if virus sequences at an integration site were just downstream from the early promoter.

SV40 normally infects differentiated cells that are growth arrested, and these quiescent cells must be stimulated to enter the S phase for efficient viral DNA replication to occur. When SV40 infects a cell that is unable to support viral replication, continuous cell division will be activated so cell immortalization may occur. The viral early gene region encodes the viral tumor antigens. Tag is involved in both the initiation of viral DNA synthesis and in transformation, and is required for both productive and non-productive infection. Although Tag is sufficient for the immortalization of growing cells, efficient transformation of growth-arrested cells also depends on the expression of tag. SV40 transformation has been observed in several mammalian species including rat, mouse, hamster, and human. However, SV40 is probably harmless to man.

Wt SV40 can persist in infected cells in two ways: either integrated into the genome, or as a self-replicating minichromosome. The latter requires Tag expression. This long-term expression seems to be mediated by integration.

rSV40 VIRUSES AS VECTORS

SV40 has recently been modified to SV40 recombinant viruses (rSV40) to serve as vectors for expression in mammalian cells since the late 1970s. Actually, it was utilized as vector in the first attempts to apply recombinant DNA technology to introduce DNA into animal cells.

Production of rSV40 virus using a packaging cell line

The methods of producing rSV40 vectors can be divided in those that use a packaging cell line or the *in vitro* packaging system.

Different protocols are used to produce rSV40 vectors using a packaging cell line, which share several common features in that the packaging cell line that provides Tag in *trans* must be transfected with a Tag deleted SV40 plasmid. To accommodate a transgene, for safety, and sometimes for other reasons, viruses

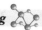

are made replication-incompetent — some necessary and/or pathogenic viral genes are deleted.

Tag is excised in new generations of SV40 recombinants, or rSV40 viruses (Fig. 2-72), to ensure the production of replication incompetent vectors incapable of late gene expression, as Tag is necessary for virus genome replication, and able to activate SV40-LP, hence is needed for expression of the late (structural) virus genes. An SV40 genome lacking Tag should therefore be incapable of replicating itself and also incapable of producing the capsid proteins necessary for packaging. Tag deletion also results in nononcogenic, and non-immunogenic rSV40 vectors —Tag binds and inactivates two important tumor suppressor proteins, p53 and pRb. It therefore can immortalize cells *in vitro*; Tag is the main SV40 antigen that the immune system recognizes on infected cells — a small amount of Tag is expressed on the cell surface of transformed cells, removing Tag from SV40 vectors also virtually abolishes cellular and humoral immune responses targeted towards transduced cells. Removal of the *Tag* gene also leaves 2.5 kb of available space in SV40 genome, making room to clone exogenous genomic material.

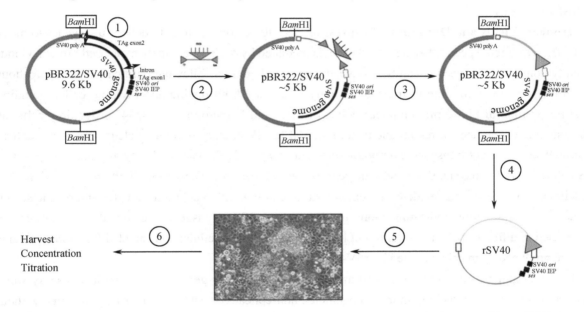

Fig. 2-72 Molecular cloning of recombinant SV40 vectors. 1. The first step in cloning recombinant SV40 vectors consists in removing large T antigen exon 1 and 2 from wild type SV40 genome carried by pBR322 backbone using adequate restriction enzymes (double arrows). 2. Next, a multiple cloning site (mcs + priming site for T7 and sp6 (triangles)) is cloned. SV40 immediate early promoter (triangle*), *ori*, *ses* and polyA (square) are conserved. 3. The mcs allows the cloning of any given therapeutic cassette comprising promoter and transgene of interest. 4. pBR322 backbone containing the bacterial sequences essential to plasmid replication in *E. coli* is removed using *Bam*H1 restriction enzyme, before self ligation of the recombinant SV40 genome. 5. Recombinant SV40 genomes are transiently transfected in either COS-1, CMT-4, COS-7 cells, which provide large T antigen in *trans*. 6. Following foci of replication formation, COS-7 lysates are harvested, sonicated, and subjected to 3 cycles of freezing at −80℃ followed by incubation at 37℃. SV40 vectors are purified, concentrated and titrated before further manipulation.

Generation of rSV40 genomes has been performed by substitution of *Tag* genes by an ampicillin resistance gene (*amp*^r). that allows the rSV40 plasmid to be selected in bacteria and amplified for further modifications. Different polylinkers, that share some restriction enzyme target sites, have been cloned at the 5′ and 3′ ends of the *amp*^r gene. Most of the constructs carry a polylinker downstream from the early promoter (EP), and retain the viral late genes intact. These polylinkers facilitate both cloning of different transgenes under the control of the early SV40 promoter and the necessary removal of the *amp*^r gene.

These modifications generate a rSV40 genome capable of producing rSV40 virus. Curiously, Tag deleted rSV40 viruses cannot support the expression of some reporter genes.

Resulting avirulent（无致病力的）viruses may only reproduce in specific (packaging) cells that supply in *trans* those deleted functions that are necessary for the virus to be packaged. Packaging cells should therefore yield replication-defective recombinant virus in useful quantities, free of contaminating wild type (wt) or other viruses. COS-1 and COS-7 cell lines are commonly used for rSV40 production, as they constitutively express Tag.

The recombinant virus genome carrying the transgene is then excised from the carrier plasmid, purified, recircularized, and transfected into COS-7 cells. These cells carry an integrated copy of the wt SV40 genome that is defective at the origin of replication [and so cannot produce virus on their own]. Tag was supplied in *trans*. The rSV40 that is produced in this fashion is prepared from lysates of these COS-7 cells. rSV40 is then amplified by infecting COS-7 cells with rSV40 virus. No helper virus or additional transfection is used.

Tropism, Yields and Durability of expression. rSV40 vectors are able to deliver transgenes to many cells from different species, because viral entry is mediated by MHC-I, a widely expressed protein. Good-quality nonreplicative vectors can be produced with very high titer following purification (10^{12} infectious units/ml), and they are able to transduce highly efficiently both resting and dividing cells, including resting peripheral blood mononuclear cells (PBMC) and hematopoietic CD34$^+$ progenitor cells, as disassembly of the nuclear membrane is not required for SV40 entry into the nucleus. Furthermore, they can deliver persistent transgene expression to a wide range of cell types and they are nonimmunogenic. rSV40-delivered transgene DNA and transgene expression persist for long times, both *in vitro* and *in vivo*. Luciferase expression was evident in mononuclear and polymorphonuclear leukocytes and platelets even at day 105 postinfection, indicating a long-term expression of the transgene. Functional transgenes can be expressed in different cell lines to different levels. Also, both intracellular and secreted functional proteins can be produced from cells infected by rSV40 vectors.

Recombinant SV40 vectors (rSV40) are good candidates for gene transfer, as they display some unique features: stable, lacking in immunogenicity, nonreplicative vectors can be easily prepared without helper viruses, and concentrated to high titers. SV40 infects a wide range of cell types from humans and other mammals, ensuring that recombinant SV40 vectors can deliver transgenes to almost any type of mammalian cell. They also efficiently transduce both resting and dividing cells, capable of providing sustained high levels of transgene expression in a wide range of cell types. The principle limitation of SV40-derived vectors is the size of the packageable insert ($\leqslant 5$ kb). Another disadvantage of rSV40 vectors for gene therapy is the possible risks related to random integration of the viral genome into the host genome. Considerable efforts have been devoted to modifying this virus and setting up protocols for viral production.

Improvements

Huge amounts of effort have been made to improve the overall structure of the vector, to make it safer in its potential applications. In addition, packaging cell line efficiency and safety has been optimized. Other novel methods have also been invented.

Improving capacity of rSV40 vectors. Since circular DNA from 3.5 kb to 5.7 kb can be encapsidated, transgenes up to 2.5 kb can be packaged in Tag-deleted rSV40 vectors, making transgene size limitation

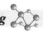

one of the major drawbacks of the system. To accommodate larger inserts, constructs have been made from which more of the SV40 genome has been removed. Different approaches have been developed to overcome the cloning space restriction problem. Expanded polylinkers have been made, to provide greater flexibility in cloning. David Strayer and coworkers produced rSV40 vectors without the capsid genes. These "gutless" rSV40 vectors can be obtained with the same protocol as Tag-deleted vectors, since some packaging cell lines provide in *trans* both Tag and capsid proteins. Also, recombinant adenovirus or wild-type SV40 as helper viruses can provide in *trans* the capsid proteins for the production of pseudovirions. Gutless SV40 can pack transgenes of up to 5 kb. According to David Strayer, rSV40 DNA as much as 5.7 kb has been packaged into the SV40 capsid without compromising yields. Using pT7A5D4.2, which lacks most of the late virus genome besides the removed virus early genome, 4.7 kb of foreign DNA have been packaged by using COS-7 cells with the theoretical capacity of the rSV40 viruses about 5.2 kb of foreign DNA. Using a different packaging system, Sandalon and coworkers could encapsidate up to 7.5 kb of DNA into SV40, carrying as little as 150 bp of SV40 genome.

Improving packaging cells. In order to eliminate the generation of viable SV40, packaging cell-lines that can express the Tag but contain minimal sequence identity with the SV40 vector have been constructed by Oppenheim *et al*. These packaging cell-lines eliminated the generation of T-antigen positive revertants. One of the cell-lines, COT-18, allowed significant propagation of high titer stocks with minimal loss of transducing activity.

The use of the complementation cells has been extended to make SV40 vectors delivering multiple moieties (cDNA, RNAi, proteins⋯.) to multiple targets (tissues, cell lines, primary cells), to treat multiple pathologies [cancer, HIV infection, Crigler-Najjar syndrome, β- thalassemia（地中海贫血）⋯] with irrefutable（无可辩驳的）successes.

***In vitro* system to package recombinant DNA.** The group of Ariella Oppenheim developed an *in vitro* system to package recombinant DNA into SV40 capsids. In the *in vitro* packaging system, capside proteins are expressed in baculovirus infected Sf9 insect cells. Incubation of VP1 alone or in combination with VP2 and VP3 proteins can form capsids. Incubation of capsids with naked DNA, amplified in *Escherichia coli*, allows the formation of pseudovirions. This method has several advantages. First, plasmids, as large as 17 kb can be efficiently packaged in VP1 capsides, which seem to be more flexible than capsids produced from the three VP proteins. Second, wild-type SV40 sequences are not required for *in vitro* production of pseudovirions, so wild-type revertants cannot arise, thus increasing the safety of the system. Furthermore, replication occurs in bacteria, DNA quality can be easily tested, and DI (defective interfering) particles are not selected. Finally, any sequence that could affect SV40 replication can be included and any gene (including reporter genes) can be expressed from SV40 vectors packaged *in vitro*. In short, these vectors combine the advantages of SV40 as a viral gene delivery vehicle and the safety of nonviral vectors. However, low yields are obtained with this method: 10^6 IU/ml compared to 10^{12} IU/ml using the *in vivo* packaging system.

Making viral vectors without viral sequences. In 2004, Ariella Oppenheim's group proposed a patent to make so called "virus-like particle" based on SV40 virus. These so called nanoparticles made of recombinant SV40 capsid protein are capable of infecting mammalian cells to express an exogenous DNA. This has been later extended to the transfer of RNA, protein, peptide, antisense RNA, ribozyme RNA or any RNA or DNA which inhibits or prevents the expression of undesired protein(s) in the mammalian cell.

First, Oppenheim *et al.* designed plasmids to express the complete VP1, VP2 and VP3 polypeptides as fusion proteins to glutathione-S-transferase (GST) in *E. coli.* As an alternative, SV40 capsids might be produced in Sf9 cells from recombinant baculovirus. Viral packaging *in vivo* occurs by gradual addition and organization of capsid proteins around the SV40 chromatin. The three capsid proteins VP1, VP2 and VP3 bind to DNA nonspecifically. Recombinant capsid proteins self-assembled to form SV40-like structures of various sizes. The pseudoviral nanoparticles are prepared by encapsidating plasmids that carry the SV40 *ori* and *ses.* These nanoparticles have been very efficient in DNA and RNAi transfer into a wide range of cells, including human bone marrow cells, and are therefore potential vectors for gene therapy. In addition, large sized DNA can be packaged efficiently, thus circumventing the size limitation of gene delivery using recombinant SV40 viral vectors.

② **Retroviral vectors**

Although adenoviral vectors are useful in transient assays, retroviral vectors stably integrate into the dividing target cell genome so that the introduced gene is passed on and expressed in all daughter cells.

Traditionally, the retrovirus is regarded as an enemy to be overcome. However. for the past four decades retroviruses have been harnessed as vehicles for transferring genes into eukaryotic cells, a process known as transduction.

The retrovirus consists of two copies of a single stranded RNA genome with sequences known as *gag, pol*, and *env*, which encode viral structural and catalytic proteins. These are surrounded by a glycoprotein envelope. At the onset of infection, the surface glycoprotein envelope interacts with receptors, on the surface of the target cell to gain entry. When inside the cell, the single stranded viral genome is converted into linear double stranded DNA by a virus encoded reverse transcriptase. As the target cell undergoes mitosis, the viral DNA integrates with the target cell DNA — at which point it is known as a provirus. It is this proviral DNA that is manipulated to form retroviral vectors for gene transfer. The provirus then undergoes transcription and translation with the rest of the genome, resulting in the assembly of new viral particles that bud off the surface of the target cell to infect others cells.

During virus assembly, retroviruses package two copies of viral RNA into virions as genetic material. Viral RNAs are specifically selected to be packaged; the specificity of RNA packaging is determined by the interactions between the packaging signal in the viral RNA and the viral polyprotein Gag. Deletion of the packaging signal can drastically reduce viral RNA packaging, whereas mutations in the Gag polyprotein can affect packaging specificity. The Gag polyproteins of all retroviruses have three common domains: matrix (MA), capsid (CA), and nucleocapsid (NC). Among these domains, NC plays an important role in RNA recognition and packaging, although other domains in Gag have also been suggested previously to contribute to RNA packaging specificity. Mutations in NC can result in decreased viral RNA packaging, whereas swapping (交换，用······替换) the NC domain from different viruses can alter packaging specificity.

Packaging signals in many retroviruses have been identified; the major packaging signals are generally located in the 5′ untranslated regions of the viral RNA, with some signals extending into the group-specific antigen gene (*gag*). Sequences elsewhere in the viral genome have also been suggested previously to affect RNA packaging.

Vector technology

A retroviral vector consists of proviral sequences that can accommodate the gene of interest, to allow incorporation of both into the target cells. The vector also contains viral and cellular gene promoters, such as the CMV promoter, to enhance expression of the gene of interest in the target cells. The most important advance in vector technology has been the use of the packaging cell.

Packaging cells are typically fibroblast derivatives that contain sequences of independently coding DNA sequences, known as DNA plasmids, expressing viral gene products such as gag and pol, but are *cis*-acting packaging domain-defective — their RNA components cannot be assembled into virions. Whereas in the retroviral vector, most retroviral gene sequences, *i.e.*, *gag*, *pol*, and *env* genes have been replaced by exogeneous genes, only the retroviral package signal ψ and related sequences are retained. In that way, the recombinant retroviral vector and the packaging cell line can compensate for each other's loss of functionality upon transfection. When the retroviral vector with the gene of interest is introduced into the packaging cells by non-viral transfection techniques, virions containing the vector genome are produced, which bud off into the culture medium (Fig. 2-73). These are then allowed to infect and stably integrate with the genome of dividing target cells. The retroviral vector is not able to replicate further because the vector construct lacks retroviral gag/pol or *env* coding sequences, *i.e.*, it does not encode the viral structural proteins, which had been provided by the packaging cell.

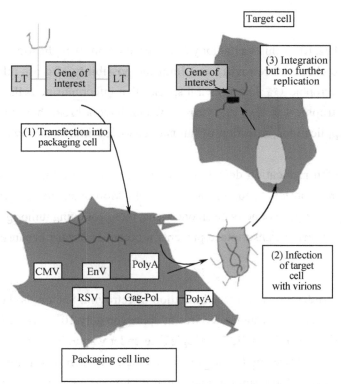

Fig. 2-73 The production of retrovirus and infection of target cells.

Tissue-specific promoters, such as CEA promoters, have been used to construct targeted vectors to enable targeted gene expression in CEA positive tumor cells. In CEA producing cells, the CEA promoter has been shown to be as efficient as the SV40 enhancer/promoter in driving expression of therapeutic genes.

Clinical applications

Retroviral vectors have been used to introduce a drug susceptibility or "suicide" gene, such as *herpes simplex* thymidine kinase (TK), to target cells. When the patient is treated with a particular drug, such as gancyclovir（丙氧鸟苷）, the target cells containing TK are killed selectively. The suicide gene approach has been used with some success for the treatment of recurrent malignancy. For example, when T cells, which have been previously harvested, are administered to patients with melanoma on the development of a recurrence, they are effective in destroying malignant cells. Unfortunately, the T cells can go on to damage normal tissue. Therefore, the harvested T cells are retrovirally transduced with a suicide gene, so that they can be removed after they have eliminated the recurrent tumor.

A more corrective（矫正的）approach has been used to restore apoptotic pathways in tumor cells by introducing apoptosis related genes, such as p53 and bcl-xs via retroviral vectors. However, experimentally both p53 and bel-xs were unable to induce apoptosis in certain tumors, and it may be that a more complex set of signals is necessary to trigger this pathway.

Retroviral vectors have also been used in alternative efforts to enhance the body's own immune response to tumors; this treatment involves reinjecting tumor cells that have been UV irradiated, genetically manipulated, or admixed（混合，掺合）with non-specific adjuvants. Combinations of these strategies are under way.

Limitations

Safety

The main potential hazard of this technology is the production of replication competent virus, which can infect humans. The choice of retrovirus can limit the possibility of cross infection in the laboratory set up. For example, ecotrophic（嗜亲性的）viral species that infect murine cells only are less hazardous compared with amphotrophic（兼嗜性的）viruses, which have a broad host range including humans. However, in clinical applications, infection of human cells is desirable, meanwhile the potential hazard remains real.

Furthermore, even with replication defective vectors, it is possible that integration of the retroviral vector occurs within an important locus in the target cell. Moreover, the integration could potentially inactivate a tumor suppressor gene or activate an oncogene, thus promoting tumorigenesis of the target cell.

In addition, the viral reverse transcriptase presents a potential hazard because it is characteristically highly error prone.

Retroviral titer

Apart from safety considerations, a major limitation of retroviral vectors is the low titer produced by the packaging cells. At present, they generate virus at approximately 10^6 to 10^7 infectious particles/mL of tissue culture supernatant. Several technical strategies are under way to improve this "real" titer. However. the "effective" titer is even lower owing to several factors. First, most murine retroviruses on which gene therapy vectors are based are rapidly inactivated by human complement. At present, viruses with modified envelopes to resist complement inactivation are being developed. Another main drawback is that murine retroviral vectors infect actively dividing cells only. A future possibility is that the lentiviruses (for example human immunodeficiency virus (HIV)) might overcome the inability of retroviral vectors to infect quiescent cells. The ability of HIV to infect non-dividing cells might result in part from a nuclear transport signal that allows transport of the provirus to the nucleus in the absence of mitosis. It is not clear at present whether incorporation of these sequences into traditional retroviral vectors will allow similar division independent infection to occur.

Gene expression

Although the retrovirus stably integrates into the target cell genome, it is clear that the choice of promoter chosen to drive expression of the therapeutic gene is crucial. Although the promoter drives high levels of gene expression *in vitro*, there is often a lack of gene expression *in vivo* because of the methylation of viral promoters. At present, vectors that have cellular promoters are being developed; these might be less susceptible to transcriptional shutdown than viral promoters. In the future, self inactivating vectors, which remove all viral promoters after integration with the target cell, leaving the cellular promoter alone, might combat this problem.

Future developments

The future development of retroviral technology to overcome these limitations might hinge on（取决于）the targeting of vectors.

Two main possibilities include cell surface targeting or transcriptional targeting. In principle, cell surface targeting should be the easier to achieve because of the well defined packaging system and current detailed knowledge of retroviral receptor structure. Several groups have shown that the tropism of retroviral vectors can be altered by the incorporation of hybrid proteins into the envelope of the virus; however, this is not yet advanced enough to produce high titer stocks. Transcriptional targeting could be achieved by incorporating transcriptional control elements that restrict expression of the inserted gene in target cells. Although several such retroviral vectors have been described, in many cases different interacting promoter elements have resulted in a partial loss of cell type specific gene expression.

In conclusion, far from being a foe, retroviruses have been harnessed so that they are used routinely for gene transfer in the laboratory setting and in clinical trials of gene therapy. The main drawbacks at present centre around potential safety, retroviral titer and gene expression. In the future, it might be that powerfully hybrid delivery systems that utilize the desirable properties of different vectors can be synthesized according to individual laboratory and clinical requirement.

③ Adenovirus vector (AdV).

All adenovirus (Ad) genomes are linear, double-stranded DNA molecules. They vary in length (26 163~48 395 bp) containing an inverted terminal repeat (ITR) of 30-371 bp at its termini [*e.g.*, the terminal repeats of human adenovirus type 5 (Ad5) are 103 bp], with the 5′ ends of each DNA strand linked covalently to a virus-coded protein, known as the terminal protein (TP), which plays an important role in the initiation of viral DNA replication. This linkage is a consequence of the mechanism of DNA replication. ITR sequences enable circularization of single-stranded DNA, leading to base paired panhandle regions（柄状的的狭长区域）that can also function as DNA replication origins. These sequences are followed by the viral packaging sequences (Ψ) at the left end of the genome, which direct viral DNA encapsidation.

Although there are some small differences between various adenoviruses, the overall content and organization of adenovirus genomes is very similar. All share genes encoding the major proteins required for viral DNA replication and major structural components. The genetic organization of the central part of the genome (where the structural proteins and replication proteins are coded) is conserved throughout the family, whereas the terminal parts show large variations in length and gene content. The nucleotide composition is 33.6%~67.6% G+C.

Adenovirus genes are organized into transcription units. The five early transcription units include early region 1A (E1A), E1B, E2, E3, and E4. Intermediate transcription units, including IX, IVa2, L4 intermediate, and E2 late, are transcribed at the onset of DNA replication. A single late transcription unit (major late) generates five populations of late mRNAs, L1-L5. Early (*E1* through *E4*) transcriptional units, function in part as master transcriptional regulators, and late transcripts code for structural proteins. Most of the adenovirus transcription units are transcribed by RNA polymerase II and give rise to multiple mRNAs that are differentiated by alternative splicing or alternative poly(A) sites.

Splicing was first discovered in AdVs, and is a common means of expressing mRNAs in this virus family. In the conserved region, most late genes are expressed by splicing from the rightward-oriented major late promoter located in the DNA-dependent DNA polymerase gene (*pol*). The early genes encoding pol, the precursor of TP (pTP), and the DNA-binding protein (DBP) are spliced from leftward-oriented promoters. Where it has been examined, splicing is also a common feature of genes in the nonconserved regions.

The capsid (衣壳) is composed of three major proteins (II, III, and IV) and five minor proteins (IIIa, IVa2, VI, VIII, and IX). Proteins V, VII, and X/mu are associated with the DNA and form the core within the virion. These proteins are believed to condense the Ad DNA and mediate interactions between the core and the capsid. Ad protease is required for the maturation of the assembled particle to form fully infectious virus.

Ads are excellent example of viruses that efficiently use limited genetic space and information to maximize their protein production for optimal virus propagation. Expression of the viral genes is temporally regulated at many different levels to produce a stepwise, logical progression of gene expression in order to take full advantage of the cellular machinery to direct virus production. As an example, the late viral genes are not expressed to a full extent until after viral replication takes place and, even then, late gene expression is tightly controlled at both the transcriptional and the posttranscriptional level.

Adenovirus as a Gene Therapy Vector

The ease with which the adenovirus genome can be manipulated using recombinant DNA techniques, along with its tissue promiscuity (混乱) and ability to infect postmitotic (有丝分裂后期的), nondividing cells, has led to the use of adenoviruses as vectors for expression of heterologous genes, and as delivery systems for gene therapeutics and recombinant vaccines. Adenovirus is not associated with serious illness in immunocompetent (免疫活性的) individuals. For more than *four* decades unattenuated (未变弱的) adeno-viruses have been used successfully as oral vaccines, offering strong evidence of the safety of such vectors as potential gene therapy tools, and attenuated adenoviruses have already been used as vaccines with few side effects.

Adenoviruses are used as vaccine delivery vehicles to deliver genes from pathogens into a host, which in turn stimulates that host to generate a protective immune response against the disease-causing pathogen. Adenovirus vectors are proving exceptionally useful delivery platforms for the next generation of vaccines for prevention of infectious diseases. They are also being used in the treatment of cancer and for gene therapy.

As a minimum, three regions of the viral genome can accept insertions or substitutions of DNA to generate helper-independent viruses: a region in *E1* (including *E1A* and *E1B*), a region in *E3*, and a short region between *E4* and the end of genome. Since the *E1A* gene is indispensable for virus replication, in the first generation of Ads, the modification of the Ad genome was based on deletion of the entire *E1A* and/or partial deletions of *E1B* and *E3* genes to produce replication-incompetent vectors providing appropriate space to insert transgenes. However, even in the absence of *E1* gene products, there was low-level viral replication of these vectors inducing CD4$^+$- and CD8$^+$-dependent immune responses leading to a reduced duration of gene expression in *in vivo* systems. To decrease toxicity and prolong gene expression, newer second-generation Ad vectors have been created which lack *E2A* and contain mutations and/or deletions of the viral *E4* gene. In another approach, "gutted" or "gutless" Ad vectors were formed by removing the complete viral coding regions leaving only the inverted terminal repeats (ITR). Therapeutic genes transmitted by gutless virus have been successfully transported to the liver of mouse models for various human diseases, such as hemophilia（血友病）A and B, obesity, familial hypercholesterolemia（血胆固醇过多）, diabetes, and chronic viral hepatitis, with encouraging consequences in the context of long-term expression with reduced and transient cellular immune responses. However, in most cases, stimulating a noticeable and durable antitumor response necessitates multiple administrations of replication-incompetent Ads, which can stimulate an immune response, promoting viral clearance.

Initial clinical studies with replication-selective adenoviruses have shown that this type of therapy is relatively safe and holds promise as a feasible approach in cancer treatment. It even appears that a combination treatment regimen involving replication-sensitive adenoviruses, along with standard chemotherapy, is synergistic over either treatment alone. The optimal use of these types of adenoviruses in the clinic will undoubtedly require several different strains tailored to the specific therapeutic application. Adenoviruses will be engineered to contain transgenes that augment antitumor response and suppress the antiviral response.

Replication-defective adenoviruses have been used for the delivery of genes encoding immune-modulating cytokines and growth factors to tumor sites to increase tumor susceptibility to host defenses. Because adenovirus infects terminally differentiated postmitotic cells, it represents an attractive vector system for delivery of these cytokines into normal cells juxtaposed（并列）to the tumor, ensuring constant cytokine production to stimulate the host cellular defense system. In addition, adenoviruses have been used as vectors to deliver therapeutic cell cycle-regulating genes intratumorally to attempt to restore proliferative control as well as to deliver genes encoding factors that augment and sensitize tumors to various chemotherapeutic regimens, thereby providing the additive effect of a multidrug regimen consisting of viral-mediated cell lysis and standard cytotoxic drug-mediated cell killing.

Another approach to the treatment of tumors is the use of replication-competent adenoviruses. An adenovirus EIB-55-kDa gene deletion mutant (dl1520) was the first genetically constructed adenovirus to be administered to humans. The E1B-55-kDa product is required to inactivate the p53 cellular tumor suppressor and to enable subsequent adenoviral replication in host cells. It follows that an adenovirus harboring a mutation in the E1B-55-kDa gene is unable to replicate in normal host cells that contain a functional p53 gene product, but can replicate very efficiently in host tumor cells that have defective p53. Thus, such a virus has the potential to lyse tumor cells without killing normal cells.

Adenoviral (Adv) vectors have a number of positive and negative attributes（特性）. The positive attributes include the transduction of a wide profile of cellular phenotypes, including not only epithelial and carcinoma cells but also hematopoietic cells. Further, the use of Adv vectors results in a high frequency of transduction and high levels of transgene expression. A negative attribute of Adv vectors is transient expression, although for appropriate targets, such transitory（短暂的）infection is a positive attribute. The transient expression is due, in part, to the high level of innate vector immunogenicity, which can limit multiple cycles of transduction and chronic transgene expression. The resulting Adv profile of activity is ideal for the transduction of dendritic cells as vaccines, the purging（清除）of tumor cells from stem cell products, and intralesional（病灶内的）injection of carcinomas. Further, the ability to develop Adv vectors that are conditionally replicative has great potential for the treatment of neoplastic disease.

China has granted its first COVID-19 vaccine patent to the adenovirus vector vaccine developed by Chen Wei of the Academy of Military Medical Sciences and Chinese biotech company CanSino Biologics in 2020. And this vaccine, dubbed "Ad5-nCoV", with a full name "Recombinant novel coronavirus vaccine (adenovirus type 5 vector) (CanSinoBio), was approved on Feb. 25, 2021 in China by NMPA, and later in other countries. The vaccine uses an attenuated adenovirus (replication-defective adenovirus serotype 5 vector) to introduce genetic material from the novel coronavirus into the human body （Expression system: CHO cells）. The goal is to train the body to produce antibodies that recognize the coronavirus's spike (S) protein and fight it off.

④ **Adeno-associated viral (AAV) vector**

Adeno-associated virus (AAV) is a small, non-enveloped virus that contains a single-stranded DNA genome of approximately 4.7 kb, enwrapped with a 25 nm icosahedral（二十面体的）capsid which is composed of 60 viral protein subunits arranged on a T = 1 icosahedral lattice. AAV is a member of the parvovirus（细小病毒）family that require a helper virus such as adenovirus (Ad) or *herpes simplex* virus（HSV，单纯孢疹病毒）for replication.

Biological features. The AAV genome encodes three open reading frames (ORFs), *rep*, *cap*, and *AAP*, which are flanked by the 145 nucleotide long inverted terminal repeat sequences (ITR). The 5′ ORF *rep* controlled by two different promoters (P5, P19) encodes four overlapping functional proteins (Rep78, Rep68, Rep52, and Rep40), which play a part in viral replication, transcriptional control, and accumulation of single-stranded progeny genomes. Rep78 and Rep68 have site-specific endonuclease, DNA helicase, and ATPase activities that are required for adeno-associated virus (AAV) DNA replication. Rep52 and Rep40 contain helicase activity and are required for packaging AAV DNA into the capsids. The 3′ ORF *cap* encodes three capsid proteins driven by promoter P40, VP1 (90 kD), VP2 (72 kD) and VP3 (60 kD), which are responsible for the assembly of infectious particles. To maintain a 1 ∶ 1 ∶ 10 ratio of VP1 ∶ VP2 ∶ VP3 for virus particle assembly, AAV uses an alternative splicing mechanism for VP1 and a less efficient start codon (ACG) for VP2 to lower their protein levels, yet keeps high efficiency start codon for VP3. The N-terminal sequence present in VP1 contains a phospholipase A2 domain that is required for AAV infectivity. In addition, the VP2/VP3 mRNA codes for an assembly-activating protein (AAP) from a weak CTG start codon but in a different reading frame. AAP facilitates nuclear import of the major VP3 capsid protein and promotes assembly and maturation of the capsid, but AAP is not present in the mature capsid.

AAVs can infect both dividing and non-dividing cells via interaction of the AAV capsid proteins with cell receptors. The AAV is internalized by endocytosis whereupon it enters the nucleus and is converted to double stranded DNA for expression of the transgene. It remains episomal（游离的，附加的，非整合的）to the chromosomes but does occasionally randomly integrate with the DNA.

The infection of permissive cells to AAV is a multi-step process. AAV enters host cells *via* specific receptors on the cell surface. AAV first binds to the primary or attachment receptor heparan sulfate proteoglycans（HSPG，硫酸乙酰肝素蛋白聚糖）on the cell surface. Subsequently, AAV interacts with αVβ5 integrin, fibroblast growth factor receptor 1 (FGFR1), dynamin（发动蛋白）, Racl and phosphatidylinositol-3 kinase (PI3K) as AAV co-receptors, and then AAV is rapidly internalized via clathrin-coated pits. After endocytosis, AAV enters intracellular trafficking. Then, AAV is released from the endosome（内体，内涵体，核内体）into the cytoplasm and is located around the perinuclear. Once inside the cell, AAV uncoats and releases its genome, which is transported into the nucleus.

During endosomal endocytosis, low pH-triggered structural and autoproteolytic changes to the viral capsid are believed to be necessary for endosome escape and virus uncoating. AAV and other endosome-dependent viruses rely on the gradual pH decrease during endosome maturation to time（为……安排时间）their escape. A pH-triggered change in AAV capsid conformation that is necessary, but not sufficient, to enable endosomal escape. Similarly, low pH-triggered structural changes in AAV capsid proteins are believed to activate an autolytic function that has been hypothesized to be associated with eventual virus uncoating and endosomal escape mechanisms.

Finally, AAV slowly enters the nucleus via nuclear pore complexes (NPC) and then integrates into the chromosome to mediate the transgene expression. A main feature of AAV is that it is capable of site-specific integration. The AAV genome integrates into the host chromosome 19 AAVS1 site when no helper virus is present, or it replicates to produce progeny when a helper virus, such as adenovirus or herpes virus, is present.

Ideal candidate drug vector and manufacture platform

The benefits of AAVs is that they have low background integration and have the potential to be a good *in vivo* gene delivery vector. Without the presence of an adenovirus, AAVs are unable to replicate. Gutless AAVs with the replication machinery provided in *trans* can transduce dividing and postmitotic cells. Once an AAV has entered a cell and a second strand of DNA is produced, it forms a circular DNA structure that can remain in postmitotic cells for years.

Adeno-associated virus (AAV) is a promising viral vector and meets most requirements of being a safe biological agent. Wild-type AAV is not considered to be pathogenic and has not been known to cause any human disease, which satisfies the principal safety demands of biological products. rAAV virions are icosahedral parvovirus（细小病毒）without envelope, making them physically robust and able to withstand harsh treatment during processing. Accordingly, the physiochemical properties of AAV are amenable to industry accepted manufacturing methodologies, longtime storage, and *in vivo* administration. Also, no adverse events in clinical trials have been directly attributed to rAAV. Additionally, rAAV vectors have low immunogenicity compared to other viral vectors used in clinical trials, assuring more reliable clinical curative effects. All the aforementioned features make AAV an ideal candidate drug vector.

The commonly used AAV serotypes and variants are AAV1, AAV2, AAV3A, AAV3B, AAV4, AAV5, AAV6, AAV7, AAV8, AAV9, AAVShH10, AAV7m8, AAVDJ, and scAAV. With their diverse tissue tropism, transduction efficiency and immunological profiles, these AAV vectors can be used to target various tissues for a variety of applications. Among all the AAV serotypes discovered, AAV2 has the best transduction efficiency in cell culture and therefore is the best tool for *in vitro* studies. Nearly all serotypes of AAV vectors use the AAV2 ITRs for AAV manufacture, and AAV2 requires heparan sulfate proteoglycan (HSPG) for cell attachment.

AAV vector production

To make an AAV vector, the *rep* and *cap* sequences are removed and replaced with an expression cassette containing the target gene. When the AAV vector containing the target gene and regulatory sequences, together with the *rep* and *cap* sequences provided *in trans* — the packaging plasmid, and helper virus (adenovirus, HSV, or baculovirus, *etc.*) are introduced into host cells under proper conditions, AAV vectors will be produced.

There are several technologies available for production of AAV vectors. These include transient plasmid transfection, adenovirus infection, stable-cell lines harboring AAV helper functions, HSV infection/transfection, and baculovirus infection technologies. All these technologies have the common elements for AAV vector manufacturing: (1) target gene flanked by ITRs, which in most cases are derived from AAV2; (2) AAV *rep* and *cap* genes provided *in trans*, in which the *rep* gene is derived from AAV2 while the *cap* gene can be of any serotypes; and (3) helper functions from adenovirus, HSV, or baculovirus. When these three components are introduced into a host cell under proper conditions, AAV vectors will be produced. Each of the technologies has unique properties to suit specific applications. In adenovirus complementation system, Hela cell lines, A549 cell lines, Vero cell lines, and HEK293 cell lines were all engineered to consolidate (合并) *Rep/Cap* gene in their cellular genomes to complement Rep/Cap proteins. Infection of these cells with the Ad/AAV hybrid virus resulted in the rescue and appropriate packaging of rAAV genomes. Adenovirus *E1*, *E2a*, *E4*, and *VARNA* genes are critical helper genes for AAV replication and packaging.

Assembling mechanism disclosure in insect cell

The dynamic process of AAV packaging has been widely studied in mammalian cell systems. Ad and HSV have long been utilized as helper viruses for AAV assembly. HSV and Ad supply help in different ways. Replication associated proteins of HSV (UL5, UL8, UL52, and UL29) can be directly used by AAV for virus DNA replication and packaging, in which UL5, UL8, and UL52 offer helix release (松开) and primer forming functions, while UL29 serves as a single strand DNA-binding protein. In addition, polymerase UL30, polymerase cofactor UL42, and initial binding protein UL19 are also functional in virus packaging. In Ad complementation system, Ad genes *E1*, *E2a*, *E4*, and *VARNA* are essential for AAV assembly. In contrast to HSV, Ad promotes AAV replication both directly through *trans*-activators that stimulate *AAV Rep* gene expression and indirectly by forcing the cell to enter S phase that provides AAV with active cellular replication machinery. Furthermore, dramatic episomal (游离基因的) amplification of *Rep/Cap* genes in the presence of this helper function, which is supplied by *trans*-acting factors *E1*, host cellular DNA polymerase, *E2B*, *Rep*, and *cis*-acting Rep-dependent element (CARE), is strongly correlated with high yield of rAAV production.

AAV purification technologies

There are several methodologies to purify AAV vectors from cell cultures. They include density gradient ultracentrifugation, column chromatography, and chloroform extraction/polyethylene glycol (PEG) precipitation partitioning. They can be used either alone, or in combination with each other.

Even in highly purified AAV, there are probably small amounts of different impurities, such as residual

Cap DNA. One trillion（万亿）AAV particles in clinical trials would be the minimal dosage. Thereby, theoretical risk remains even at the trace levels (*e.g.*, 10^{-10}) of **replication competent AAV (rcAAV)** present in clinical-grade AAV formulation, as they would be toxic and may incite immune responses. Many methods have been developed to purify clinic-grade AAV virions.

History & Progress

AAV was initially discovered during adenovirus preparation in 1965. Since then, there have been over 100 AAV serotypes and variants isolated from adenovirus stocks or from human/nonhuman primates tissues and even some other mammals, and at least partially characterized.

The first infectious clone was constructed in 1982, and in 1984 recombinant adeno-associated virus (rAAV) vector was firstly used to transfer the neomycin resistance gene into mammalian cells. In the wild, AAV virions infect and replicate in mammalian cells. They are AAV's natural host, while AAV could replicate in its homologous viral host insect cells. In 2002, Urabe *et al* demonstrated for the first time that the AAV genome could replicate in insect cells, and AAV virions could then be packaged in insect cells when full complemental AAV structural and nonstructural proteins were provided by the baculovirus. Years later, several modifications have been made to improve the infectivity of AAV vectors including phospholipase A2 domain (PLA2) swapping（交换）, supplementation of VP1, and the optimization of the VP1 initial codon and its surrounding nucleotide sequence.

Today, AAV has been successfully applied in Hemophilia B, HIV, Leber's congenital amaurosis（利伯氏先天性黑蒙症）, Parkinson's disease, Duchenne muscular dystrophy, *etc*. In 2009, AAV was ranked among *Science*'s "Top 10 breakthroughs of the year" for its use in treatment of Leber's Congenital Amaurosis. AAV was used to express antibody against HIV *in vivo*, and was shown to eradicate HIV virions in mouse and monkey models. Trials of miR-26a delivered by sc-rAAV8 to treat hepatocellular carcinoma also produced encouraging results. Impressively, AAV encapsulating the ZFN gene directly corrected the mutant *Factor IX* gene in genome, and restored hemostasis（止血）in hemophilia B（B型血友病）mouse model. Glybera®, an adeno-associated viral (AAV) vector has become the first gene therapy drug approved by European Commission in 2012 for the treatment of lipoprotein lipase deficiency（LPLD）and spurred huge excitement in the gene therapy field.

However, the commercialization of AAV had been hampered due to the limitation of large-scale production. In recent years, progresses in scalable manufacturing of AAV have dramatically improved AAV-based clinical researches, and have assisted the development of investigational drug products. For instance, the production process of Glybera, involves a scalable baculovirus-insect cell system. However, many problems still need to be solved to improve the productivity and quality of AAV. Novel AAV-producing platforms in *Saccharomyces cerevisiae* and *vaccinia virus* complementation system have also been developed for scalable AAV production.

⑤ Vaccinia virus vector (VV)

Vaccinia virus（牛痘病毒）is a kind of DNA virus with the most complicated virus structure. The most thoroughly studied member of the poxvirus family, was successfully used as a live vaccine to eradicate smallpox. Medical interest in vaccinia virus subsequently declined but was restimulated when live recombinants were shown to be capable of expressing foreign genes and of protectively immunizing animals against infections with influenza virus, herpes simplex virus types 1 and 2, hepatitis B virus, rabies virus and vesicular stomatitis virus. The ability to incorporate large amounts of foreign DNA without a loss of infectivity (exogenous genes of 25~40 kb can be inserted, furthermore, multiple foreign genes can be inserted simultaneously), the correct processing of expressed proteins, and the wide host range of vaccinia virus also make this expression system of special value for research purposes. One novel application has been to identify target antigens for cell-mediated immune responses to viruses.

Vaccinia virus promoters, which are found immediately upstream of early and late vaccinia virus genes, are necessary because of the specificity of the viral transcription system and the cytoplasmic site of replication. Flanking segments of vaccinia virus DNA are used for homologous recombination, the most practical way of inserting foreign sequences into the large 187 000-base-pair (187-kilobase) vaccinia virus genome, which is linear and double-stranded.

The exogenous gene expressed was cDNA, because the DNA sequence of vaccinia virus itself is continuous, and it does not have the ability to cut and process eukaryotic genes after transcription.

Transient expression was previously shown to be dependent on vaccinia virus *cis*-regulatory signals contained in plasmids and on *trans*-acting factors present in vaccinia virus-infected cells.

The advantages of vaccinia virus vectors include the retention of infectivity, the large capacity for DNA, the wide host range (they can grow and reproduce in a variety of cells), and the correct processing of many proteins. Vaccinia virus recombinants have already proven their value for research purposes and may eventually be used for the immunoprophylaxis (免疫预防, 接种免疫) of infectious diseases.

Cell-free systems

Cell-free expression of proteins is performed *in vitro* using purified RNA polymerase, ribosomes, tRNA and ribonucleotides. These reagents may be produced by extraction from cells or from a cell-based expression system. *E. coli* cell lysate containing the cellular components required for transcription and translation are used in this *in vitro* method of protein expression. The advantage of such system is that protein may be produced much faster than those produced *in vivo*, but it is also more expensive. Vectors used for *E. coli* expression can be used in this system although specifically designed vectors for this system are also available. Eukaryotic cell extracts may also be used in other cell-free systems, for example, the wheat germ (麦芽) cell-free expression systems. Mammalian cell-free systems have also been produced.

Due to the low expression levels and high cost of cell-free systems cell-based systems are more widely used.

2.5.3 Transgenic animals (转基因动物)

Transformation of animal and plant cells was also investigated with the first transgenic mouse being created by injecting a gene for a rat growth hormone into a mouse embryo in 1982.

Transgenic animals, especially farm animals such as cattle, sheep, goats, pigs, and even rabbits offer particularly attractive possibilities for the preparation of recombinant proteins with pharmaceutical properties.

Among the many potentially exploitable expression systems for the production of biopharmaceuticals, the animal platform, based on the use of animals as bioreactors, has been shown to be highly competitive by adding critical value to low cost implementation (低成本实现), production and scale up, as well as high productivity and quality of the synthesized proteins, and the flexibility of increasing production by simple breeding. These advantages led to the development of the "gene pharming" concept, which has now advanced to commercial application.

Transgenic animal platforms — Sites of Production

Many valuable therapeutic proteins have been produced over the past 30 years from transgenic animal models such as goats, sheep, cows, pigs, and rabbits.

Four potential sources of recombinant proteins have been studied in mammals, each of which is a body fluid: milk, urine, seminal fluid, and blood. Fluids are more suitable than solid tissues for this purpose because they are renewable and can be obtained from animals without harm or excessive invasion. Furthermore, many biomedically important proteins are themselves secreted into body fluids. Milk is by far the best-studied production system and the only method that has been examined on a large scale. Biopharmaceutical production in birds has focused exclusively on protein production in the white of eggs, specifically egg albumen（白蛋白）.

The choice of a suitable method for expressing a desired protein will depend on its features and intended application. In such context, the mammary gland of transgenic animals is the main bioreactor path for recombinant protein production, although other relevant alternative systems are also available, such as blood, urine, seminal plasma and eggs. Such expression systems can result in high level of recombinant protein production. Moreover, such recombinant proteins are easy to harvest and animals can be used as more cost-effective bioreactors than cell culture-based bioreactors.

Milk

Thus far, milk is the most mature and proven transgenic system for the production of recombinant pharmaceutical proteins. The mammary gland is a promising site because of the ease of milk collection and the high quantities of protein that can be produced using specific gene promoters. The lactating mammary gland has an enormous capacity to synthesize proteins and other biochemicals for infant nutrition. Besides, GMP methods have been established for extraction and purification of proteins from milk.

Many recombinant human therapeutic proteins require post-translational modifications for bioactivity, immunological or pharmacokinetic properties. Glycosylation is perhaps the best known post-translational modification, but there are many other possible critical modifications, including propeptide cleavage, multi-chain assembly, disulfide bonding, phosphorylation, hydroxylation, amidation（酰胺化）, methylation, hydroxylation, γ-carboxylation, acylation, and lipid attachment. The repertoire of enzymes that carry out these functions varies considerably between mammalian tissue types. Ideally, the protein processing capability of the producing cells should match the requirements of the desired protein, or be readily modifiable to carry out the appropriate processing. The main reason to express a particular protein in a mammalian mammary gland system is because the mammary gland tissue glycosylation pattern seems to be similar to human native proteins.

In 1989 John Clark of the Roslin Institute, Edinburgh (UK), demonstrated that the BLG promoter could be used to direct the expression of the human blood clotting Factor IX gene in sheep and that the product was secreted during lactation. Since then, promoters and regulatory sequences of almost all major milk genes have been utilized and investigated for their suitability in driving the expression of potentially useful proteins. And a large number and wide variety of foreign proteins have been expressed in the milk of transgenic animals. This work has included: complex multi-chain proteins, for example, fibrinogen; combinations of transgenes designed to supplement the natural protein processing abilities of the lactating mammary gland, for example, prolyl hydroxylase coexpressed with type 1 procollagen; and coexpression of transgenes to improve the stability of secreted protein in milk, for example, α1-antitrypsin protease inhibitor with fibrinogen. Expression levels as high as 35 g/L have been achieved using the ovine (绵羊的) BLG promoter to express human α-antitrypsin (α- 抗胰蛋白酶) in sheep. In each case, the foreign protein is secreted as part of the whey (乳清，乳浆) fraction.

Currently, the use of milk as a vehicle for production of biopharmaceuticals has reached a valuable step with the approval of two drugs — ATryn, a recombinant human antithrombin, the first commercial biopharmaceutical recombinant protein produced in transgenic animals and approved (by EMA in 2006 and by FDA in 2009) for human use for the treatment of patients with hereditary antithrombin deficiency developed by GTC Biotherapeutics (currently rEVO Biologics Inc.), was produced in goat mammary gland. And RUCONEST or RHUCIN, the human recombinant C1 inhibitor from Pharming BV, The Netherlands, approved (by EMA in 2010 and by FDA in 2014) for treatment of acute angioedema attacks in patients with hereditary angioedema, was produced in transgenic rabbit milk. The approval of these two mammary gland-derived recombinant proteins for commercial and clinical use has boosted the interest for more efficient, safer and economic ways to generate **transgenic founders** to meet the increasing demand for biomedical proteins worldwide, paving the way for new approvals for drugs produced by the transgenic animal platform.

Therapeutic antibody production in the milk. The production of monoclonal antibodies (Mabs) in the milk promises to become an important platform for biomedical applications due to its economic prospects. Thus far, available Mabs are produced in mammalian cells in culture, but the mammary gland is particularly suitable for the expression of monoclonal antibodies (Mabs), particularly for the production not only of biosimilars, but especially for enhanced (biobetter) proteins. Over 40 g/L of a Trastuzumab-like Mab had been expressed from a line of animals, while goats can produce 500~800 L per year, each of these animals can produce kilograms of product yearly.

The Mabs expressed in goat milk have all been shown to have target-binding characteristics equivalent to the commercial products. This was demonstrated with Adalimumab (阿达木单抗), Trastuzumab (曲妥珠单抗), and Cetuximab (西妥昔单抗). The glycosylation profile on these IgG1 molecules provided equivalent and even enhanced effector (biobetter) functions. Interestingly, the Cetuximab, produced in goat milk was devoid of the immunogenic 1,3-alpha-galactose sugar moiety found in the commercial product, rendering the protein potentially less immunoreactive upon use for treatment.

Transient protein expression in the milk. Transient gene expression in the mammary gland is consisting of intramammary injection via the teat canal (乳头管) of high titer recombinant adenoviral particles containing the gene of interest.

In 2004, the adenoviral system was used to produce recombinant proteins in large scale, through the transient expression of human growth hormone (hGH) in the milk of non-transgenic mice and goats. Since then, levels ranging from mg/L to g/L of another five recombinant proteins were obtained in different animal species transduced with adenovirus into the mammary gland: human erythropoietin, human lactoferrin, human nerve growth factor beta, E2 antigen for classical swine fever (猪瘟) and human antithrombin.

Blood

The physiology and development of the animal are intimately exposed to any adverse effects of bioactive proteins circulating in the blood; therefore the range of suitable products is very restricted. Besides, purification of human therapeutic proteins from blood, as in the case of tissue extracts, is an inefficient, expensive, labor- and time-consuming process that can also incur considerable risk of contamination with human pathogens.

Nevertheless, production of recombinant human proteins in the blood of transgenic livestock is likely to become more important as a source of human polyclonal antibodies. Progress is being made towards the production of humanized immune systems in cattle, pigs, and rabbits. Using this biological system, genetically engineered transchromosomic cattle were generated to produce fully human polyclonal antibodies, carrying a human artificial chromosome comprising the entire unrearranged human immunoglobulin (Ig) heavy-chain (hIGH), kappa-chain (hIGK), and lambda-chain (hIGL) germline loci, with both of the bovine immunoglobulin (bIGHM and bIGHML1) homozygously inactivated after double knockouts. Such animals could be immunized against a wide range of antigens to provide an abundant source of human polyclonal antibodies, which could play an important role in passive immunotherapy and offer considerable advantages over monoclonal antibodies.

Urine

For the sake of production and secretion of desired proteins into the urine, urothelium（膀胱上皮，尿道上皮）is to be engineered.

The main advantages of the urinary system when compared to the mammary gland, for instance, are that animals produce urine much earlier than lactation, and the recombinant protein can mature in a more proper manner. In comparison with blood, the effect of the foreign protein store is less deleterious for the animal's health, but the limiting factor of using this system is the yield, as the rates of protein secretion from bladder epithelial cells are usually low.

Seminal fluid

Seminal fluid is an abundant male body fluid in some animal species, mainly in pigs, and can be easily collected, posing a low risk to the animal's health. Therefore, it has been considered as an effective site for recombinant protein expression in transgenic animals. Accessory sex glands such as prostate and bulbourethral glands（尿道球腺）are responsible for most of the protein production and secretion in semen. Seminal plasma should be a suitable source for bioactive protein production since protein secretion is strictly exocrine, without adversely affecting the animal health, and this tissue has a great capacity for protein processing, stability and purification.

Bird Eggs

Chickens may be more suitable than mammalian systems for certain proteins. For example, some bioactive proteins with toxic effects in mammals may not affect birds. There is also evidence that chickens and human proteins have similar glycosylation patterns. The secretory cells of the chicken oviduct（输卵管）certainly have a high protein synthetic capacity. Each egg contains approximately 4 g protein in the white, of which more than 54% is ovalbumin（卵白蛋白，卵清蛋白）. Production is also very flexible, large flocks of birds can be rapidly produced from a single transgenic male. Furthermore, the use of eggs for pharmaceutical purposes is already established for the production of vaccines, providing a framework of regulatory guidelines for Good Manufacturing Practice (GMP).

Over recent years, sebelipase alfa (Kanuma™). a recombinant human **lysosomal acid lipase** (LAL) produced in egg whites of transgenic hens, has progressed through clinical development and, on 28

August 2015 the agent received its first global approval, in the EU, for long-term enzyme replacement therapy in patients of all ages with LAL deficiency.

Transgenic Constructs

Usually, these transgenes are fusions of the target protein gene with mammary gland specific regulatory sequences (Fig. 2-74). In addition to the regulatory and coding elements, transgenic constructs may harbor signal sequences to facilitate secretion of the protein and untranslated exons and introns to enhance expression levels. Ideally, the transgenes should stably integrate into the host genome, be inherited in Mendelian fashion, and direct the abundant expression and secretion of a desired protein to the target organ without affecting the health or well being of the producing animal.

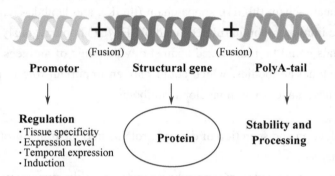

Fig. 2-74   Schematic drawing of the main components of a gene construct.

The first requirement is a region of cloned DNA that encodes the amino acid sequence to be expressed (the structural gene). This may be a fragment of genomic DNA, cDNA, or chemically synthesized DNA. It may be necessary to alter the coding sequence to optimize expression in a transgenic animal.

An important factor in the success of transgene expression is the location within the host genome. Transgenes integrated at different sites can exhibit wide variations in expression, due to the influence of different chromatin (染色质) environments.

Several strategies are available to either minimize or circumvent the position effect. The level, specificity, and consistency of transgene expression can sometimes be improved by flanking the transgenic construct with insulator elements. Insulators of various types have been demonstrated to block the spread of heterochromatin (异染色质) effects into the transgene and to isolate transgenic promoters from the influence of adjacent endogenous enhancers and other regulatory elements. Alternatively, the uncertainties of random integration can be avoided by placing the transgenic construct in a well-characterized permissive site in the host genome using gene targeting.

Organ Specific Expression Vectors

Production of a biopharmaceutical in a transgenic animal requires transcription and protein expression of the transgene to be directed to the site of production. This is commonly achieved using a gene promoter expressed specifically and preferably abundantly in the chosen tissue, such as the lactating mammary gland. The DNA sequences of most of milk proteins are known. The promoter elements from the bovine αs1-casein gene, the caprine (山羊的) β-casein gene, the rodent WAP genes, the ovine (绵羊的) β-lactoglobulin (β-乳球蛋白) gene, and the bovine α-lactalbumin gene have been used to direct expression into milk. The ovalbumin gene promoter is used for production in the white of chicken eggs.

Inducible Expression

An inducible system can also be used to improve control over recombinant protein production. Inducible promoter elements responsive to heavy metals, steroid hormones, IPTG, RU-486, ecdysone（蜕皮激素）, or tetracycline derivatives have been tried.

Non-integrating Vectors

The position effect can be avoided by using vectors that do not integrate into the host genome, but nevertheless efficiently express the transgene. To achieve this, the foreign DNA must replicate autonomously and be stably maintained after multiple cell divisions. Artificial chromosome vectors that carry DNA regions responsible for stable chromosome behavior are promising. A second form of non-integrating, or episomal（游离的，附加体的）vector has been developed that contains an attachment site for the system of structural proteins within the nucleus, termed the nuclear matrix or scaffold (MAR or SAR).

Methods for the Production of Transgenic Animals

The methods divide into two broad categories: DNA transfer directly into embryos and cell-mediated transgenesis.

DNA transfer into embryos, for example, by DNA microinjection or viral transduction, is more straightforward than cell-mediated transgenesis. Until recently, this approach was limited to transgene addition and allowed no control over where the transgene integrates into the genome, but emerging technologies based on highly specific DNA endonucleases (see Section ***Highly Specific DNA Endonucleases***) have now overcome this limitation.

The various methods of cell-mediated transgenesis each have in common the feature that genetic manipulation and analysis of the transgenic genotype are carried out in cells in the laboratory, rather than in animals "on the farm". These cells are then used to produce the modified genotype in whole animals.

Pronuclear DNA Microinjection

DNA microinjection into fertilized oocytes was developed originally in mice and extended to transgenic livestock more than 30 years ago. It is technically straightforward but inefficient. Nevertheless, DNA microinjection has been used to produce a broad range of genetically modified large animals for applications in both agriculture and biomedicine.

Collection of Fertilized Eggs. Oocytes fertilized *in vivo* can be collected from animals after spontaneous ovulation or hormonal treatment to induce a superovulatory（超排的）response by means of laparoscopy（腹腔镜术）or surgery under general anesthesia. Alternatively, oocytes can be withdrawn from ovarian follicles collected from commercial slaughterhouses and embryos are produced by *in vitro* maturation of oocytes and fertilization *in vitro* by co-incubation with motile sperm (IVM/IVF), followed by a variable period of *in vitro* culture. For DNA microinjection, well defined developmental stages are required that harbor the maternal and paternal pronucleus, called zygotes（受精卵，合子）. These stages are found for a short period of time (18~20 h) approximately 18~26 h after fertilization, depending on the species.

Preparation of DNA. Preparation of a DNA construct for microinjection entails purifying linear fragments of the transgene portion away from the plasmid DNA backbone, residual bacterial material, and chemical reagents. Purified linear fragments are dissolved in microinjection buffer at a concentration between 1~6 ng/μl. Within this range, lower concentrations result in higher embryo viability but a lower proportion of transgenic embryos, higher concentrations produce more transgenic embryos but viability may be reduced.

Injection of DNA. Morphologically normal fertilized oocytes with visible pronuclei are selected for microinjection. The next developmental step is fusion of the two pronuclei with the recombination of the two parental genomes. This incre ases the chances that a foreign DNA is readily integrated into the host genome. In pigs and cattle, pronuclei can be visualized using gentle centrifugation to shift the lipids to one pole (Fig. 2-75). In sheep, interference phase contrast microscopy is required to visualize the pronuclei (Fig. 2-75a). Microinjection is carried out on the stage of an inverted microscope at ~ 200 × magnification, with the fertilized oocytes contained within microdrops into which are inserted a blunt-ended, glass holding pipette and a sharp, glass microinjection needle containing the DNA solution. Movements of the pipettes are controlled by micromanipulation arms. Individual zygotes are held in place on the holding pipette by gentle suction, and oriented such that one of the pronuclei is adjacent to the needle. The needle is inserted into the pronucleus and the DNA solution injected. Injected zygotes can then be either immediately transferred to recipients, or cultured *in vitro*, sometimes as far as blastocyst (囊胚) stage (cattle), to reveal those that would sustain further development.

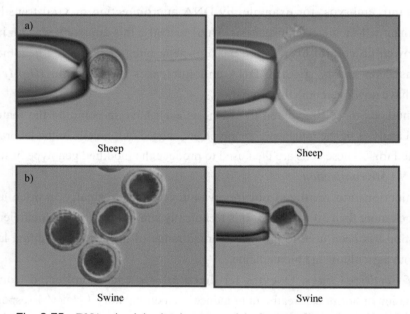

Fig. 2-75 DNA microinjection into pronuclei of zygotes from sheep (a) and pigs (b). Ovine pronuclei are visualized by DIC; porcine zygotes have to be centrifuged to visualize the pronuclei.

Transfer and Gestation in Recipients. Microinjected fertilized oocytes are either immediately transferred to suitable recipients or cultured *in vitro* for a certain period of time. Viable embryos are selected and inserted into the oviducts or uterus of hormonally synchronized recipients depending on the developmental stage of the early embryos to maintain gestation.

Identification of Founders and Subsequent Breeding. Microinjection is an inefficient process. On average, between 5%~20% of mice and 1%~5% of large animals born after microinjection carry the transgene, and an even smaller proportion of these express the transgenic product. Therefore there is a strong incentive to reduce the number of animals gestating non-transgenic fetuses. One approach has been

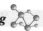

to screen embryos for the presence of a transgene prior to transfer. This can be achieved by extracting a portion of the embryo, often a single blastomere (卵裂球，胚叶细胞), and detecting the transgene by polymerase chain reaction (PCR) amplification. This procedure is however labor-intensive, can reduce embryo viability, and the presence of non-integrated DNA may result in false positives. Alternatively, a gene encoding a non-toxic fluorescent protein can be either co-injected, or incorporated into the transgene construct to identify intact living transgenic embryos. Expression of a non-integrated reporter construct may however produce a false positive signal, and the presence of additional DNA may be undesirable.

Transgenic fetuses can be identified *in utero* by analysis of cells obtained by amniocentesis (羊膜穿刺术) or allantocentesis. However, these procedures carry a significant risk of inducing abortion. The most common practice is therefore to screen animals shortly after birth by either PCR or Southern hybridization, using small samples taken from the blood, tail or ear tips. Transgenic animals are then analyzed in more detail to identify those most suitable for further breeding.

In the case of biopharmaceutical production, the amount and properties of the recombinant protein will be determined, and an analysis conducted to identify whether the physiology of the animal is affected in any way. It should be emphasized that the health of transgenic animals is of foremost importance for both ethical and practical reasons.

Obtaining milk expression data requires that female animals must be produced, reach sexual maturity, breed, and lactate. This is necessarily time-consuming in livestock, especially if the founder is male. Protocols for artificial hormone-induced lactation in virgin females and even males have therefore been developed.

In summary, DNA microinjection is a straightforward method of producing transgenics, and was the dominant technology for more than two decades. The limitations of random transgene addition and the inefficient use of animals are major drawbacks. Significant improvements are now being made by combining microinjection with highly specific DNA endonucleases (see Section *Highly Specific DNA Endonucleases*), and also integration systems such as φ C31.

Viral Mediated Gene Transfer

In 1976, Rudolf Jaenisch reported that mouse embryos could be infected with a retrovirus that stably integrated into their genome. These animals incorporated the proviral DNA into their somatic tissues and germ line and passed it on to their progeny in Mendelian fashion. Since then a number of viruses have been used to produce transgenic animals with varying degrees of success. By far the most commonly used are retroviruses.

Mammalian embryos may be infected either by removing the *Zona pellucida* (透明带) and culturing in culture medium containing the virus, or a small volume of viral supernatant may be microinjected into the perivitelline space (卵周隙). The virus vector can infect and incorporate into the host genome, but is incapable of further replication. Procedures for embryo collection and transfer are basically those described for DNA microinjection.

Lentiviral (慢病毒) transduction may allow more efficient production of transgenic animals.

Sperm-Mediated Gene Transfer

Mouse spermatozoa exposed to exogenous DNA could be used as a vector to produce transgenic mice by artificial insemination.

A variation of this technique is based on **intracytoplasmic sperm injection (ICSI，卵泡浆内单精子注**

射) of DNA associated with frozen-thawed, or detergent-treated sperm. Several groups have used ICSI to produce transgenic mice, rats, and pigs. In mice it offers a lower incidence of founder mosaicism（镶嵌性，镶嵌现象）and a greater efficiency of transgenesis than standard DNA microinjection, particularly for large transgenes.

Sperm-mediated gene transfer by natural fertilization is not yet a reliable method of producing transgenic animals. Variations based on ICSI may offer greater success, but their potential in large animal transgenesis has yet to be fully explored.

Transposon-Mediated Gene Transfer

Transposons have been developed as important tools for transgenesis in flies, fish, frogs, mice, rats, and pigs. DNA-based, or class II, transposons are mobile genetic elements that move around the host genome via a "cut-and-paste" mechanism. Most DNA transposons are simply organized; they encode a transposase protein flanked by inverted terminal repeats (ITRs), which carry transposase binding sites. It has been possible to separate the transposase coding sequence from the ITR sequences. Any DNA flanked by the ITRs will be recognized by the transposase and become enzymatically integrated into nuclear DNA. Apparently, no cellular cofactors are required. The size of the integrated foreign DNA can exceed 10 kb, but may reduce the efficiency of transgenesis. In a two-component system, the transposon is integrated solely by the *trans*-supplementation activity of the transposase.

Transposition-mediated gene delivery offers efficient chromosomal integration and a high proportion of single-copy insertion events. However, the main advantage of transposon-mediated transgenesis is that the integration of foreign DNA is directed to accessible euchromatic（常染色质的）rather than heterochromatic regions, reducing transgene silencing.

Injection of *in vitro* synthesized mRNA coding for transposase can enhance the efficiency of this technique due to the rapid availability of the transposase and circumvents the danger of integrated transposase sequences. Transposon-mediated transgenesis for farm animal species is as yet（至今仍）at an early stage, but transgenic pigs produced using Sleeping Beauty and piggyBAC transposon systems have been reported.

Pluripotent Stem Cells

Embryonic Stem Cells. Embryonic stem (ES) cells are pluripotent cells derived from early mammalian Embryos. ES cells made it possible to engineer genetic modifications in culture and then study the effects in whole animals. DNA can be introduced into cultured mammalian cells by a wide range of chemical, electrical, mechanical, and viral methods, often collectively referred to as "transfection". In ES cells, transfection can be used to randomly add DNA sequences to the genome, but the most potent application has been the precise modification of genes *in situ*, termed gene targeting. Gene targeting exploits the ability of cells to support recombination between exogenous DNA molecules and their cognate chromosomal sequences at regions of shared homology. Typically, ES cells are transfected with a DNA construct carrying an engineered modification flanked by 2~15 kb "arms" homologous to the target locus. At a certain, usually low frequency, transfected cells undergo homologous recombination with the construct and seamlessly incorporate the engineered modification at the target locus. Targeted cell clones can be selected and identified amongst a background of random integrants（组成部分）by a variety of methods.

Embryonic Germ Cells. Primordial germ cells（PGCs, 原生殖细胞）are the undifferentiated embryonic precursors of germ cells and arise outside the embryo and migrate through the body during mid-stage development to the urogenital（泌尿生殖器官的）ridges where the gonads develop. Embryonic germ cells （EGCs，胚胎生殖细胞）were first derived from explanted mouse PGCs and shown to possess all pluripotent characteristics of murine ES cells, including the ability to re-enter the germ line. Murine PGCs become EGCs in culture when the medium is supplemented with specific growth factors such as stem cell factor (SCF), leukemia inhibitory factor (LIF), and basic fibroblast growth factor (bFGF). EGCs resemble ES cells, in that they can be cultured and transfected *in vitro* and then contribute to（促成）somatic and germ cells of a chimera. Mammalian EG cells are now rarely used.

Avian EG cells have been more successful, and have produced transgenic chickens on several occasions. The typical technique has been to isolate primordial germ cells from the blood of chick fetuses two to three days after laying and convert them into EG cells. Cultured EG cells can be reintroduced into the blood stream of fetuses at the same stage, where they migrate to the gonads and form functional gametes （配子）. The efficiency of chimera production and incidence of germ line transmission is increased if recipient eggs are chemically pre-treated to deplete endogenous primordial germ cells.

Induced Pluripotent Stem Cells (iPS Cells). Fully differentiated fibroblasts both from mouse and human could be reprogrammed into pluripotent state by ectopic（异位的，异常的）expression of four transcription factors such as OCT4, SOX2, c-MYC, and KLF4 or by OCT4, SOX2, NANOG, and LIN28. Today such cells have been generated from various mouse and human cell types including liver cells, neural stem cells, blood cells, cord blood cells, pancreatic beta cells, mesenchymal stem cells（间充质干细胞）, and stomach cells.

Most iPS cell lines established today have been produced using retroviral or lentiviral vectors, which integrate in the host genome. Alternative approaches have been explored, by which the virus vectors are substituted and thereby integration of viral sequences in the host genome is avoided. This has been achieved using small molecules, non-integrating adenoviral vectors, proteins, plasmids, mRNA, miRNA, or transposon based reprogramming systems.

The iPS cells were functionally indistinguishable from ES cells derived from *in vitro* fertilized embryos, but had retained epigenetic（后生的，外成的，表观遗传的）marks characteristic of their tissue of origin (epigenetic memory).

Spermatogonial Stem Cells

Spermatogonial stem cells (SSCs，精原干细胞) are precursors of male gametes, which reside in the seminiferous tubules（生精小管）of the postnatal testis. The SSC population is small, ~35 000 stem cells per mouse testis, comprising 0.03% of all germ cells in testis. Mouse SSCs can be derived from adult and neonatal testis and proliferate for extended periods *in vitro* in the presence of growth factors such as glial cell line-derived neurotrophic factor (GDNF), leukemia inhibitory factor (LIF，白血病抑制因子), bFGF, and epidermal growth factor (EGF). SSCs have been successfully used for insertional mutagenesis in mice. *In vivo*, spermatogonial stem cells are unipotent（单能性的）, giving rise only to spermatozoa（精子）. After transplantation into seminiferous tubules of infertile mice, SSC can resume spermatogenesis（精子发生）and produce offspring. Unipotent murine SSCs can be converted *in vitro* into pluripotent cells by modifying the culture conditions, and have been termed germ line-derived pluripotent stem (gPS) cells.

After transplantation, spermatogonial stem cells can be identified in the host tissue. Only spermatogonial stem cells can repopulate （使重新入驻）sterile （不育的）testes when injected into seminiferous tubules of infertile recipients.

Germ cell transplantation offers an exciting new method of producing genetically modified animals, providing culture conditions under which SSCs can be expanded, undergo DNA transfection, and selection, while remaining genetically and epigenetically（后成说的，表观遗传的）intact for transplantation. Because modifications are introduced directly into the male germ line, without embryo manipulation, the time required for gestation and maturing founder animals is avoided, a significant factor in large animals. SSC technology is at an early stage.

Somatic Cell Nuclear Transfer (SCNT)

The technical aspects of nuclear transfer in mammals had already been established in the 1980s using blastomeres（分裂球，胚叶细胞）from early stage embryos as donor cells. Cell-mediated transgenesis using nuclear transfer became possible when live sheep were produced from cells that had been cultured for several weeks. "Dolly" was the first cloned mammal generated from an adult cell.

Common somatic cloning protocols involve the following steps:

1) *Enucleation of the recipient oocyte:* Oocytes at the metaphase II (MII) stage of meiosis are the most appropriate recipients for the production of viable cloned mammalian embryos. Oocytes need to be matured *in vitro* to the MII stage, which in cattle requires a 24 h incubation period. *In vitro* maturation (IVM) protocols have advanced to the extent that *in vitro* matured oocytes can be used for somatic cloning with similar success rates as their *in vivo* matured counterparts. Oocytes are enucleated（从……摘除细胞核）by sucking or squeezing out a portion of the oocyte cytoplasm closely apposed（放……在近处）to the first polar body（极体）where the MII chromosomes are usually located (Fig. 2-76).

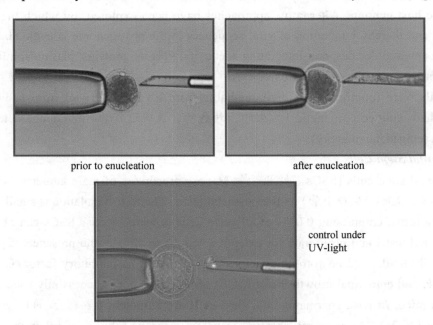

prior to enucleation   after enucleation

control under
UV-light

Fig. 2-76 Enucleation（去核）of an *in vitro* matured bovine oocyte in the process of somatic cell nuclear transfer.

2) *Preparation and subzonal transfer of the donor cell:* The intact donor cell is isolated by enzymatic disaggregation and inserted under the *Zona pellucida*（透明带）in intimate contact to the cytoplasmic membrane of the oocyte using a micropipette (Fig. 2-77). Various somatic cells, including mammary

epithelial cells, cumulus cells（卵丘细胞）, oviductal（输卵管）cells, leucocytes（白细胞）, hepatocytes, granulosa cells（粒层细胞）, epithelial cells, myocytes（肌细胞）, neurons, lymphocytes, and germ cells, have successfully been used as nuclear donors. Fetal cells, such as fibroblasts, have frequently been used in somatic cloning experiments, because they are thought to have less genetic damage and higher proliferative capacity than adult somatic cells.

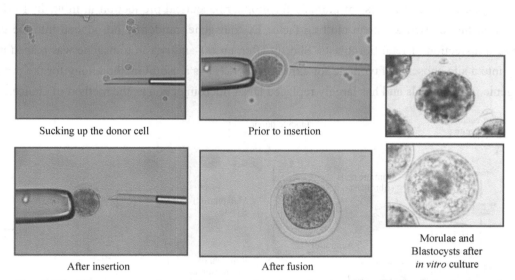

Fig. 2-77　The process of somatic cell nuclear transfer; transfer of a somatic donor cell into an enucleated（从……摘除细胞核，无核的）oocyte, fusion, and development to reconstructed morulae（桑葚胚）and blastocysts.

In most experiments, donor cells are induced to exit the cell cycle by serum deprivation, which arrests cells at the G0/G1 cell cycle stage. Nevertheless, unsynchronized somatic donor cells have been successfully used to clone offspring in mice and cattle.

3) ***Fusion of the two components:*** The enucleated oocyte and donor cell are fused, usually by short, high voltage pulses through the point of contact between the two cells.

4) ***Activation of the reconstructed complex:*** Activation is achieved either by short electrical pulses, or brief exposure to calcium ionophores（离子载体）, such as ionomycin（离子霉素）, or cell cycle regulators, such as dimethylaminopurine（DMAP，二甲基氨基吡啶）.

5) ***Temporary culture of reconstructed embryos:*** Cloned embryos can be cultured *in vitro* to the blastocyst stage (5~7 days) to assess the initial developmental competence prior to transfer into a foster mother. Culture systems for bovine embryos are well advanced and allow routine production of 30%~40% blastocysts from *in vitro* fertilized oocytes isolated from abattoir（屠宰场）ovaries.

6) ***Transfer to a foster（代养的，寄养的）mother or storage in liquid nitrogen:*** Bovine embryos at morula （桑葚胚）and blastocyst stages can be transferred non-surgically to the uterine horns of synchronized recipients using established procedures. Whereas in pigs, activated nuclear transfer complexes are transferred immediately into recipients because *in vitro* embryo culture systems are not yet as effective as in cattle. This requires surgical intervention under general anesthesia.

To date, somatic cell nuclear transfer (SCNT，体细胞核移植) has been successful in more than 16 mammalian species and holds the greatest promise for improving the production of transgenic livestock.

Nuclear transfer from somatic cells opened a new path to produce transgenic livestock, lifting（解除）the requirement for ES cells for cell-mediated transgenesis (Fig. 2-78). "Ordinary" cells such as primary fetal fibroblasts can be obtained in large quantities, manipulated in culture, and then converted into whole animals by nuclear transfer. This could potentially generate large numbers of genetically modified animals without conventional breeding. Initial work in the area was inspired by the possibility of producing such "instant flocks" of animals for biopharmaceutical production in milk. In 1997 lambs were reported that carried a human clotting factor IX transgene, randomly introduced into the genome by *in vitro* transfection of fetal fibroblasts. Shortly after, an α1-antitrypsin transgene was placed by gene targeting into a site chosen as favorable for expression. SCNT is a useful methodology for the production of transgenic farm animals and has largely replaced DNA microinjection as the method of choice.

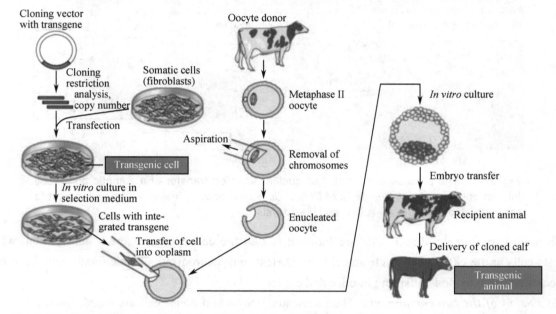

Fig. 2-78 Schematic drawing of the steps involved in the production of transgenic animals (here cattle) via somatic cell nuclear transfer.

In summary, nuclear transfer from somatic cells is currently the major means of producing transgenic large animals and until recently was the only method of achieving gene targeting in mammals other than rodents. Clone viability remains a problem, but technical refinements may yet resolve this. Nuclear transfer requires relatively few experimental animals because oocytes are obtained from animals slaughtered for other purposes.

Highly Specific DNA Endonucleases & site-specific nucleases

A new technology based on synthetic endonuclease enzymes such as **zinc-finger nucleases (ZFNs)** and **transcription activator-like effector（TALE，转录激活因子样效应因子）** nucleases is making a significant impact on the field of transgenic mammals. It is applicable to both direct and cell-mediated transgenesis and enables both gene inactivation by mutagenesis and precise sequence deletion, replacement, or insertion by gene targeting.

These "molecular scissors" make it possible to introduce a double-strand break at a single predetermined site in the genome. ZFN cleavage can stimulate, by several orders of magnitude, homology-directed genetic exchange between a conventional DNA gene targeting construct and the chromosomal locus. This is now significantly streamlining the production of animals carrying sequence replacements by enabling gene targeting directly in early embryos, effectively removing the need for a cell intermediate for many purposes. Efficient ZFN-mediated gene targeting by homologous recombination in embryos has been achieved in mice, rats, and most recently in rabbits.

With the advance of the ability for targeted genome engineering via site-specific nucleases, such as TALENs (transcription activator like effectors nucleases) and the CRISPR-Cas9 system, cell engineering and animal transgenesis have gained a new breath. These programmable nucleases are a powerful tool for the genetic engineering arsenal（军械库）, especially to improve site specific insertions, giving the possibility of manipulating any gene or inserting DNA sequences at specific sites with great precision.

Analysis of Transgenic Animals

Guidelines have been produced for potential products from transgenic sources. These include sequence validation of the gene construct, characterization of the isolated recombinant protein, and monitoring of the genetic stability of the transgenic animals.

Future perspectives

The legalized trade of Atryn, Ruconest and Kanuma™ (sebelipase alfa) for therapeutic use revolutionized the landscape of scientific and marketing possibilities of biopharmaceuticals and added much to the reliability of recombinant protein production system through animal platforms using the milk expression system and chicken oviduct expression system.

The development of new biopharmaceutical, biosimilar or biobetter drugs is a colossal（巨大的，庞大的）undertaking and a lot has been accomplished since the emergence of recombinant DNA technology, especially regarding therapeutic protein production. In a rapidly expanding market, representing a segment of the industry with the highest growth rate, the biopharmaceutical segment is in need of new ways to increase productivity and minimize costs. The animal platform for production of therapeutic protein in the milk can offer an economic, efficient way to meet the demands of a growing and hungry market, with the advantage of a sophisticated refolding and glycosylation machinery of the mammalian cells, including not only genetic but also the glycoengineering. Similarly, chicken oviduct expression system has its own advantages, such as high protein synthetic capacity, similar glycosylation patterns as human being's, cooperated with the mature, highly productive, easily scaled and cost effective virtues of poultry industry.

The therapeutic proteins to treat human illnesses from transgenic animals became a solid reality, with the approval of three commercial drugs purified from milk or eggs of transgenic animals in recent years representing an important step towards the consolidation of the animal platform for future use and for a wide range of applications. Still, new ideas, insights, innovations, and discoveries are urged to ameliorate life, to better eradicate biological diseases and social maladies, and to promote health and well being in a more equal and sustainable world.

2.5.4 Transgenic plants（转基因植物）

Plant

Many plant expression vectors are based on the Ti plasmid of *Agrobacterium tumefaciens*（*A. tumefaciens*，根癌农杆菌，致瘤农杆菌）. In these expression vectors, DNA to be inserted into plant is cloned into the T-DNA（T-DNA 二元体系）, a stretch of DNA flanked by a 25-bp direct repeat sequence at either end, and that can integrate into the plant genome. The T-DNA also contains the selectable marker. The *Agrobacterium* provides a mechanism for transformation, integration into the plant genome, and the promoters for its *vir* genes may also be used for the cloned genes.

In 1907 a bacterium that caused plant tumors, *Agrobacterium tumefaciens*, was discovered and in the early 1970s the tumor-inducing agent was found to be a DNA plasmid called the Ti plasmid. By removing the genes in the plasmid that caused the tumor and adding in novel genes, researchers were able to infect plants with *A. tumefaciens* and let the bacteria insert their chosen DNA into the genomes of the plants. Not all plant cells are susceptible to infection by *A. tumefaciens*, so other methods were developed, including electroporation and micro-injection. Particle bombardment was made possible with the invention of the Biolistic Particle Delivery System (gene gun) by John Sanford in the 1980s.

Methods for transfering DNA into plant cells

A number of methods are available to transfer DNA into plant cells. Some vector-mediated methods are:

Agrobacterium-mediated transformation is the easiest and most simple plant transformation. Plant tissue (often leaves) are cut into small pieces, *e.g.*, 10 mm × 10 mm, and soaked for 10 minutes in a fluid containing suspended *Agrobacterium*. The bacteria will attach to many of the plant cells exposed by the cut. The plant cells secrete wound-related phenolic（酚的）compounds which in turn act to upregulate the virulence（毒性，致命性）operon（操纵子）of the *Agrobacterium*. The virulence operon includes many genes that encode for proteins that are part of a Type IV secretion system (delineated by specific recognition motifs called border sequences and excised as a single strand from the virulence plasmid) that exports from the bacterium into the plant cell through a structure called a pilus. The transferred DNA (called T-DNA) is piloted（指引）to the plant cell nucleus by nuclear localization signals present in the *Agrobacterium* protein VirD2, which is covalently attached to the end of the T-DNA at the Right border (RB). Exactly how the T-DNA is integrated into the host plant genomic DNA is an active area of plant biology research. Assuming that a selection marker (such as an antibiotic resistance gene) was included in the T-DNA, the transformed plant tissue can be cultured on selective media to produce shoots. The shoots are then transferred to a different medium to promote root formation. Once roots begin to grow from the transgenic shoot, the plants can be transferred to soil to complete a normal life cycle (make seeds). The seeds from this first plant (called the T1, for first transgenic generation) can be planted on a selective soil (containing an antibiotic), or if an herbicide resistance（除草剂抗性）gene was used, could alternatively be planted in soil, then later treated with herbicide to kill wildtype segregants（分离子）. Some plants species, such as *Arabidopsis thaliana*（拟南芥）can be transformed by dipping the flowers or whole plant, into a suspension of *Agrobacterium tumefaciens*, typically strain C58 (C=Cherry, 58=1958, the year in which this particular strain of *A. tumefaciens* was isolated from a cherry tree in an orchard at Cornell University in Ithaca, New York). Though many plants remain recalcitrant to transformation by this method, research is ongoing that continues to add to the list the species that have been successfully modified in this manner.

Other plant viruses may be used as vectors since *Agrobacterium* does not work for all plants. Examples of plant virus used are the tobacco mosaic virus (TMV, 烟草花叶病毒), potato virus X（马铃薯 x 病毒）, and cowpea mosaic virus（豇豆花叶病毒）. The protein may be expressed as a fusion to the coat protein of the virus and is displayed on the surface of assembled viral particles, or as an unfused protein that accumulates within the plant. Expression in plant using plant vectors is often constitutive, and a commonly used constitutive promoter in plant expression vectors is the cauliflower mosaic virus (CaMV, 花椰菜花叶病毒) 35S promoter.

Gene guns used in plants

The target of a gene gun is often a callus (愈伤组织，胼胝体) of undifferentiated plant cells growing on gel medium in a Petri dish. After the gold particles have impacted (撞击) the dish, the gel and callus are largely disrupted. However, some cells were not obliterated (彻底破坏或毁灭) in the impact, and have successfully enveloped a DNA coated gold particle, whose DNA eventually migrates to and integrates into a plant chromosome.

Cells from the entire Petri dish can be re-collected and selected for successful integration and expression of new DNA using modern biochemical techniques, such as using a tandem (串联的) selectable gene and Northern blots.

Selected single cells from the callus can be treated with a series of plant hormones, such as auxins (植物生长素，植物激素) and gibberellins (赤霉素), and each may divide and differentiate into the organized, specialized, tissue cells of an entire plant. This capability of total regeneration is called totipotency (全能，全能性). The new plant that originated from a successfully shot cell may have new genetic (heritable) traits.

The use of the gene gun may be contrasted with the use of *Agrobacterium tumefaciens* and its Ti plasmid to insert genetic information into plant cells.

Chapter 3
The Downstream Technology for the Production of Biopharmaceuticals Made by Genetic Engineering
第 3 章　基因工程制药的下游技术

The downstream techniques of genetically engineered pharmaceuticals include not only the expression of the target gene in the host systems, but also the separation and purification, the biological activity determination, and the structure analysis and determination of the expressed products.

The downstream technology for the production of biopharmaceuticals made by genetic engineering include:

(1) Expression of target gene in host cell;

(2) Isolation and purification of the expressed protein/peptide;

(3) Determination of Biological activity of the purified product of the expressed protein/peptide;

(4) Structural analysis and determination of the product.

From the current range of applications, the commonly used host systems are mainly microorganism, they also include some animal cells. The separation, purification and identification of the expressed products are all key stages in downstream processing.

The method and process of separation, purification, analysis and identification are different for each specific expressed product. Regarding the current technical availability, there is no fixed means and approaches to model the process of separation, purification and identification of expressed products. Speaking of the separation and purification of certain products, it is not only an engineering science in the strict sense, but also an exquisite art science. The purpose of this chapter is to make readers gain some sense through the following simple introduction of downstream technology.

3.1　Cultivation of genetically engineered bacteria（基因工程菌的培养）

3.1.1　Large-scale cultivation of genetically engineered bacteria（基因工程菌的规模化培养）

Today, *Escherichia coli* is still the main host bacteria in the field of genetically engineered pharmaceuticals. In this chapter, we mainly discuss the downstream techniques of *Escherichia coli*. At the same time, other hosts such as genetically engineered yeast are also taken into consideration.

3.1.1.1　*Medium for recombinant Escherichia coli*（重组大肠埃希菌培养基）

1. Chemical composition of microbial cells

Analysis of the chemical composition of microbial cells is an important basis for the preparation of

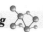

culture media, especially synthetic ones. Microbial cells contain approximately 80% of water and 20% of dry-matter. The composition of common microbial cells on a dry matter basis is shown in Table 3-1. Carbon, hydrogen, oxygen, nitrogen and other elements account for 90% to 97% of total dry matter, of which the carbon nitrogen ratio is about 5 : 1. Inorganic minerals account for 3% to 10% of the dry weight, among which phosphorus content is the highest and 50% of the total ash content, followed by sulfur, potassium, sodium, calcium, magnesium, and there are still traces of iron, zinc, manganese, boron, molybdenum（钼）, silicon and so on.

Table 3-1　Chemical composition of microbial cells

Element	% (dry weight)
C	50
O	20
N	14
H	8
P	3
S	1
K	1
Na	1
Ca	0.5
Mg	0.5
Cl	0.5
Fe	0.2

2. Medium composition for culture of recombinant *Escherichia coli*

Basic components: carbon source, nitrogen source, mineral salts, trace element, vitamins, biotins, *etc.*

Nitrogen sources generally used:

Organic nitrogen source: yeast powder, peptone（蛋白胨）, casein hydrolysate（酪蛋白水解物）, corn steep liquor（玉米浆）

Inorganic nitrogen source: ammonia（氨水）, ammonium sulfate, ammonium nitrate, ammonium chloride

Carbon sources generally used: glucose, glycerol, lactose, mannose, fructose, *etc.*

Appropriate nutrients should be replenished to the media culturing auxotroph（营养缺陷型）. According to the composition of media, they can be classified as: synthetic culture medium, semisynthetic culture medium, and complex culture medium（复合培养基）. Semisynthetic culture medium is usually adopted for high density cell culture, in which the concentrations of all constituents and their ratio should be appropriate. Various medium components should be selected according to the metabolic characteristics of the genetically modified individual's, *e.g.*, different carbon sources have different impacts on the growth of bacteria and on the expression of an exogenous gene.

3.1.1.2　*Basic cultivation methods*（基本培养方式）

1. Batch cultivation（分批培养）

A large-scale closed system cultivation in which cells are grown in a fixed volume of nutrient culture medium under specific environmental conditions (*e.g.*, nutrient type, temperature, pressure, aeration, etc.) up to a certain density in a tank or airlift fermentor (气升式发酵罐), harvested and processed as a batch, especially before all nutrients are used up.

2. Fed-batch cultivation (补料分批培养)

A "fed-batch" is a biotechnological batch process which is based on feeding of a growth limiting nutrient substrate to a culture (Fig. 3-1). The fed-batch strategy is typically used in bio-industrial processes to reach a high cell density in the bioreactor. Mostly the feed solution is highly concentrated to avoid dilution of the bioreactor. The controlled addition of the nutrient directly affects the growth rate of the cultivation and allows to avoid overflow metabolism (溢出代谢) (formation of side metabolites, such as acetate for *Escherichia coli*, lactic acid in cell cultures, ethanol in *Saccharomyces cerevisiae* (酿酒酵母), oxygen limitation (供氧受限，缺

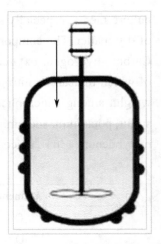

Fig. 3-1　Sketch of a Fed-batch reactor.

氧) (anaerobiosis 厌氧生活). In most cases the growth-limiting nutrient is glucose which is fed to the culture as a highly concentrated glucose syrup (600~850 g/L).

Why is the fed-batch principle (理念) used? — Substrate limitation offers the possibility to control the reaction rates to avoid technological limitations connected to the cooling of the reactor and oxygen transfer, it also allows the metabolic control, to avoid osmotic (渗透的，渗透性的) effects, catabolite repression and overflow (溢出) metabolism of side products.

Different strategies can be used to control the growth in a fed-batch process:

Control Parameter	Control Principle
DOT (PO$_2$)	DOstat (DOT = constant), F~DOT
Oxygen uptake rate (OUR)	OUR = constant, F~OUR
Glucose	on-line measurement of glucose (FIA), glucose = constant
Acetate	on-line measurement of acetate (FIA), acetate = constant
pH (pHstat)	F~pH (acidification is connected to high glucose)
Ammonia	on-line measurement of ammonia (FIA), ammonia = constant
Temperature	T adapted according to OUR or PO$_2$

DOT——Dissolved Oxygen Tension

3. Continuous cultivation (连续培养)

An alternative to the liquid batch culture system is **continuous cultivation** in a liquid medium.

This involves the **continuous addition of fresh culture medium** to the vessel and the withdrawal (by means of an overflow device) of a corresponding volume of **old**, **spent medium**, which will contain some of the microbial cells. The apparatus used is called a **chemostat** (培养微生物的恒化器) (Fig. 3-2).

Many environmental factors (*e.g.*, pH, oxygen levels, nutrients and temperature) can be controlled very precisely throughout the incubation period. The culture is stirred continuously, ensuring nutrients and oxygen reach the cells and metabolic products are distributed away from them.

Chemostats may be used to culture **yeasts** or **mycelial** (菌丝体的) fungi. When culturing a mycelial fungus, the stirrer consists of blades which prevent large mycelial pellets from forming.

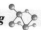

In this system the fungus continues growing exponentially because it's continuously supplied with fresh nutrients and oxygen, and the pH is controlled. However the actual **exponential growth rate** will depend upon the **flow rate of the culture medium** through the culture vessel, *i.e.*, the **dilution rate**.

The exponential growth rate = specific growth rate = μ = dilution rate D.

$\mu = D = f/v$, where f = flow rate ($ml \cdot h^{-1}$) and v = volume of the culture (ml).

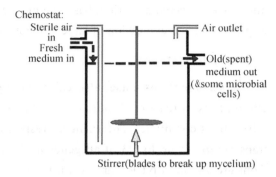

Fig. 3-2   Sketch of a chemostat.

If all environmental factors are optimal for growth then the maximum specific growth rate (μ_{max}) will be achieved.

Continuous cultivation is a cultivation approach of microorganisms in a liquid medium which is maintained under constant conditions and with a constant nutrient supply so that it can grow steadily for an extended period of time.

Continuous cultivation is a technique used to grow microorganisms or cells continually in a particular phase（阶段）of growth. For example, if a constant supply of cells is required, a cell culture maintained in the log phase is best; the conditions must therefore be continually monitored and adjusted accordingly so that the cells do not enter the stationary phase. Growth may also have to be maintained in a particular growth phase if an enzyme or metabolite product is produced only during that phase.

4. Continuous dialysis cultivation

Continuous dialysis cultivation is an approach in which a population of growing microorganisms is nurtured within a dialysis-membrane-enclosed environment, while outside the membrane fresh culture media flows freely. Using this method, microorganisms is incessantly replenished with fresh nutrients, while the old waste is ceaselessly being got rid off. Therefore, the phase of logarithmic growth was prolonged, and the number of cells is increased in the cell resting stage（静止期）. Furthermore, a microorganism's optimal nutrient environment may gradually undergo some changes by changing the nutrient content in culture medium outside the dialysis membrane little by little as scheduled. Besides, two kinds of microorganisms can be cultured simutaneously with only one dialysis membrane in between, in the hope of disclosing the relationship between them through studying their metabolites.

3.1.1.3   *The relationship between bacteria growth and progenitor supply*（菌体生长和前体供应的关系）

The addition of some amino acids to the basic culture medium increases the specific growth rate of bacteria and protein synthesis. According to Jonsen, the availability of small molecular precursors and catalytic structures is limited in bacteria, which puts the synthesis of biological macromolecules in a state of subsaturation（半饱和）, thus restrict limits the specific growth rate of bacteria. Competition among gene expressions at various levels is the result of competition among genes for the same precursors and the same catalytic structures. For genetically engineered bacteria, replication of plasmid and transcription and translation of exogenous gene(s) would compete with the survival of the host bacteria for common precursors and catalytic structures, which would exacerbate the shortage. Therefore, the specific growth rate of an engineered bacterium is often lower than that of the plasmid-free host strain. It is especially true after the engineered bacterium has been induced — the specific growth rate would even drop to cessation of growth, due to expression of large amounts of foreign genes.

Stringent response

The **stringent response**, also called **stringent control**, is a stress response of bacteria and plant chloroplasts in reaction to amino-acid starvation, fatty acid limitation, iron limitation, heat shock and other stress conditions. The stringent response is signaled by the alarmone (p)ppGpp, and modulates transcription of up to 1/3 of all genes in the cell. This in turn causes the cell to divert resources away from growth and division and toward amino acid synthesis in order to promote survival until nutrient conditions improve.

In *Escherichia coli*, (p)ppGpp production is mediated by the ribosomal protein L11 (*rplK* resp. *relC*) and the ribosome-associated (p)ppGpp synthetase I, RelA; deacylated tRNA bound in the ribosomal A-site is the primary induction signal. RelA converts GTP and ATP into pppGpp by adding the pyrophosphate from ATP onto the 3′ carbon of the ribose in GTP, releasing AMP. pppGpp is converted to ppGpp by the *gpp* gene product, releasing Pi. ppGpp is converted to GDP by the *spoT* gene product, releasing pyrophosphate (PPi). GDP is converted to GTP by the *ndk* gene product. Nucleoside triphosphate (NTP) provides the Pi, and is converted to Nucleoside diphosphate (NDP).

In other bacteria, the stringent response is mediated by a variety of RelA/SpoT Homologue (RSH) proteins, with some having only synthetic, or hydrolytic or both (Rel) activities.

During the stringent response, (p)ppGpp accumulation affects the resource-consuming cell processes — replication, transcription, and translation. (p)ppGpp is thought to bind RNA polymerase and alter the transcriptional profile, decreasing the synthesis of translational machinery (such as rRNA and tRNA), and increasing the transcription of biosynthetic genes. Additionally, the initiation of new rounds of replication is inhibited and the cell cycle arrests until nutrient conditions improve. Translational GTPases involved in protein biosynthesis are also affected by ppGpp, with Initiation Factor 2 (IF2) being the main target.

Chemical reaction catalyzed by RelA:

$$ATP + GTP \rightarrow AMP + pppGpp$$

Chemical reaction catalyzed by SpoT:

$$ppGpp \rightarrow GDP + PPi \text{ or } pppGpp \rightarrow GTP + PPi$$

3.1.1.4 *Impact of cell cultivation technology and culture condition on exogenous gene expression* (细胞培养工艺条件对外源基因表达的影响)

Temperature

Two-stage temperature control strategy. For a recombinant host cell with **temperature sensitive plasmids** (Ts plasmid), a lower temperature (*e.g.*, 30℃) is adopted at first, enabling the bacteria to proliferate, then the temperature is raised to above 35℃, *e.g.*, 42℃, allowing the copy number of plasmids to be significantly increased (uncontrollably), and therefore the protein yield is increased.

pH

The optimal pH range for the product synthesis stage may be different from that for bacterial growth stage.

Dissolved oxygen (DO)

Oxygen saturation or dissolved oxygen (DO) is a relative measure of the amount of oxygen that is

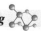

dissolved or carried in a given medium. It can be measured with a dissolved oxygen probe such as an oxygen sensor or an optode (光纤化学传感器，光极) in liquid media, usually water.

In order to increase oxygen enrichment capability of bacteria, researchers have cloned *Vitreoscilla hemoglobin* (VHb) gene into recipient bacteria by means of genetic engineering.

Vitreoscilla haemoglobin (**VHb**) is a type of haemoglobin found in the Gram-negative aerobic (需氧的) bacterium, *Vitreoscilla* (透明颤菌). It is the first haemoglobin discovered from bacteria, but unlike classic hemoglobin it is composed only of a single globin molecule.

VHb was first discovered by Dale A Webster in 1966 from a *Vitreoscilla* species. Being a soluble protein, and its close similarities of its spectral properties to those of bacterial cytochrome oxidase (cytochrome o), it was initially identified as "soluble cytochrome o". The real nature of VHb as a hemoglobin rather than a soluble cytochrome was resolved (解决) only after the amino acid sequence was determined in 1986. The amino acid sequence revealed that it is made up of a single globin domain without additional structural elements, in contrast to typical hemoglobin. Yet the solution of its crystal structure confirmed that the three-dimensional structure of VHb is remarkably similar to the classic globin fold.

VHb is the best understood of all the bacterial hemoglobins, possessing a number of cellular functions. Its main role is likely the binding of oxygen at low concentrations and its direct delivery to the terminal respiratory oxidase(s) such as cytochrome o.

The VHb is thought to aid *Vitreoscilla*'s obligately (绝对) aerobic host's survival in the microaerobic (微好氧的) environments. *Vitreoscilla* Hb is a homodimeric molecule, consisting of two identical subunits of 15.7 kDa along with two protohemes IX per molecule. It may function to enable the organism to survive in oxygen-limited environments by acting as an oxygen storage-trap or to facilitate oxygen diffusion. The whole and functioning VHb consists of hemoglobin subunits and hemes. The gene *vgb* encodes the hemoglobin subunit.

The gene encoding VHb, *vgb*, has been isolated, sequenced, cloned and characterized in *Escherichia coli* in 1988. Researchers have integrated heterologous bacterial hosts with *vgb* for purpose of enhancing production of recombinant protein and fermentation products. The *vitreoscilla* hemoglobin co-expressed in the recipient bacteria can increase the rate of ATP synthesis, thereby promoting the growth of cells and increasing the production of target products (proteins, pigments, antibiotics, *etc.*) in the recombinant host bacteria/fungi/cells (Fig. 3-3), *e.g.*, *Pichia pastoris* (毕赤酵母), *Bacillus subtilis* (枯草芽孢杆菌), *Streptomyces lydicus* (利迪链霉菌), recombinant Chinese hamster ovary (CHO) cells, *Chlorella vulgaris* (小球藻). Meanwhile VHb transgenic plants have shown enhanced growth and altered metabolite production when VHb is expressed in plants. In this way, VHb has been demonstrating its usefulness as a genetic engineering tool.

Specific growth rate

Specific growth rate is defined as the increase in cell mass per unit cell mass per unit time, *e.g.*, grams cells (g) per gram cells (g) per hour (h). The specific growth rate is commonly given by the symbol, μ (mu), and the most common units are in reciprocal hours (h^{-1}); however, it can also be expressed in reciprocal seconds (s^{-1}) or minutes (m^{-1}) or any other units of time.

Specific growth rate can be calculated from

$$\mu = K' = \frac{\ln(m_{t_2}/m_{t_1})}{t_2 - t_1} ; \quad t_2 > t_1$$

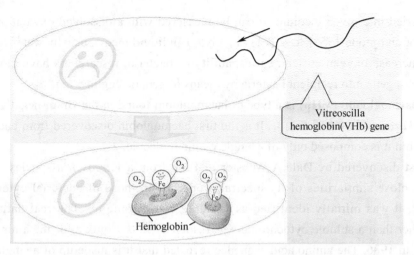

Fig. 3-3   Illustration of the role of recombinant *Vitreoscilla* hemoglobin in heterologous bacterial hosts.

where m_t are biomasses at the different timepoints (t_1 and t_2) respectively.

When looking for doubling time, then use that $m_{t2}/m_{t1}=2$ and the doubling time t_d is t_2-t_1.

3.1.1.5   *Impact of culture condition on activity, existing form and release of product*（培养条件对产物活性、存在形式及释放的影响）

1. Impact on product activity and existing form
Temperature

Culture temperature and pH have impact on product activity and inclusion body formation. When Jensen *et al.* studied the expression of rMAE-HGH, they found that the products mainly existed in soluble form when cultured at 30℃, and in inclusion form when cultured at 37℃. Chalmers *et al.* studied the existence forms of β-lactamase induced by IPTG at different temperatures (37, 30, 25, and 20℃), and the results showed that the lower temperature greatly reduced the formation of periplasmic β-lactamase inclusion bodies, increased significantly the total amount of β-lactamase activity, and increased the purity of extracellular β-lactamase approximately from 45% to 90%. Strandberg *et al.* studied the existence form of a fused protein consisting of protein A from *Staphylococcus aureus* and β-galactosidase from *E. coli,* which was placed under the control of the temperature-inducible P_R promoter, and found that only 15%~20% of the produced recombinant protein appearing as inclusion bodies when induced at 39~44℃. The authors found that when induced at 42℃, inclusion bodies were formed only during the first hours after induction, and thereafter all the recombinant protein that was further produced appeared in a soluble and active state.

Gram-negative bacteria sense and respond to extracytoplasmic stress via at least two distinct regulatory systems, the Cpx two-component system and the heat shock regulon（调节子）σ^E. Sabine Hunke *et al* found that (i) overproduction of MalE31, which forms inclusion bodies in the periplasm, is lethal for *E. coli* only at 37℃; (ii) under mild heat shock conditions (42℃) or by overproducing DegP at 37℃, this lethality is suppressed by the degradation of inclusion bodies; and (iii) the Cpx two-component regulatory system is activated by the presence of unfolded periplasmic MalE. Their research has demonstrated that MalE31 overproduction at 30℃ or 37℃ stimulates *degP* transcription by activating the Cpx two-

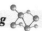

component system and has no effect on the heat-shock σ^E pathway. However, at 37°C, increased amounts of periplasmic DegP via the Cpx response are not sufficient to suppress the lethal phenotype caused by MalE31 aggregation while a temperature shift-up to 42°C, which induced the heat shock σ^E pathway and doubled the rate of DegP synthesis, led to the degradation of MalE31.

pH

Sugimoto *et al.* studied the impact of pH on inclusion body formation of salmon growth hormone (under the control of the *E. coli* tryptophan promoter), and the results showed that inclusion body ratio was 45% at pH6.6 and 85% at pH7.6. Researchers proposed that most inclusion bodies were derived from intermediates in protein folding pathways — nascent chains are forming sequentially on the ribosome and must reach their native state with some factors, such as chaperone. Elevation of culture pH may interrupt protein folding process or promote the aggregation of folding intermediates of SGH.

In addition, Bowden found that the aggregation (the formation of inclusion bodies) of β-lactamase in the periplasmic space was inhibited when non-metabolizable sugars, such as sucrose and raffinose（棉子糖，蜜三糖）, were added into the growth medium. A four-fold increase in the amount of soluble protein was obtained under optimal conditions. This effect depends on the type and concentration of sugar. Raffinose is more effective than sucrose.

It is accepted that kinetic mechanism for protein folding *vs.* aggregation *in vivo* is similar to *in vitro* folding process. Other key factors that can facilitate protein aggregation in addition to environmental stress, are charge average and turn forming residue fraction of proteins.

2. Impact on extracellular release of the product

The outer membrane of *Escherichia coli* acts as a permeable barrier, which only allows limited diffusion of hydrophobic substances. With so many outer membrane lipopolysaccharides, macromolecules cannot penetrate through the outer membrane. Therefore, many products produced via secretory expression can only enter the periplasmic space and cannot be released out of the cell. Extracellular release of proteins is related to the hydrophobicity and conformation of proteins, as well as the integrity of the outer membrane.

The outer membrane transport of proteins is different from its plasma membrane transport in that:

(1) The protein may have formed a tertiary or quaternary structure before passing through the outer membrane;

(2) There may be no signal peptide left for a protein to cross the outer membrane, and its transport mechanism may be related to the accepted secretory mechanism.

(3) There may be molecular recognition between the outer membrane transporter and the protein being transported, which involves the surface groups.

Therefore, factors affecting the spatial structure and surface groups of a protein, as well as the integrity of the outer membrane have impacts on extracellular release of that protein. Adding some chemical reagents (such as EDTA, toluene, polysorbate and Triton X-100) to the cultivation medium can affect the structure of cell membrane and promote the release of intracellular enzymes.

3.1.1.6   *Strategies for high density culture and high-level expression*（高密度和高表达培养对策）

1. High-cell-density cultivation

Fed-batch strategy is the key technique in the high cell density fermentation of a recombinant *E.*

coli strain, *i.e.*, an appropriate cell culture feeding strategy should be formulated according to the growth characteristics of recombinant cells and the mode of protein expression. Carbon source and nitrogen source are two commonly used nutritionally limiting substrates, and glucose is widely used as a nutritionally limiting substrate for high cell density fermentation of recombinant bacteria due to its high utilization efficiency, lower cost and easy availability. While **"Glucose Effect"** happens in a glucose excess and oxygen deficient condition. Under such condition, *Escherichia coli* will subject to "glucose effect", accumulate considerable amount of organic acids, hence affect the growth of recombinant bacteria and the effective expression of exogenous proteins.

Crabtree effect/Glucose Effect（"葡萄糖效应"）

The **Crabtree effect** describes the observation that respiration is frequently inhibited when high concentrations of glucose or fructose are added to the culture medium — a phenomenon observed in numerous cell types, particularly in proliferating cells, not only in tumor cells, but also in bacteria, and yeast. The Pasteur effect (suppression of glycolysis by oxygen) is the converse（相反的，逆向的，颠倒的）of the Crabtree effect (aerobic glycolysis to lactate or ethanol).

The **Crabtree effect,** mentioned for the first time by the English biochemist Herbert Grace Crabtree in 1929 (then named after him), originally describes the phenomenon whereby the yeast, *Saccharomyces cerevisiae*（酿酒酵母）, produces ethanol (alcohol) in aerobic（含氧）conditions and high external glucose concentrations rather than producing biomass via the tricarboxylic acid (TCA) cycle, the usual process occurring aerobically in most yeasts, *e.g., Kluyveromyces spp*（克鲁维酵母菌属）. Increasing concentrations of glucose accelerates glycolysis (the breakdown of glucose) which results in the production of appreciable（可观的）amounts of ATP through substrate-level phosphorylation. This reduces the need of oxidative phosphorylation done by the TCA cycle via the electron transport chain and therefore decreases oxygen consumption. The phenomenon is believed to have evolved as a competition mechanism (due to the antiseptic nature of ethanol) around the time when the first fruits on Earth fell from the trees.

The "glucose effect" is not the only mechanism controlling the activity of alcohol dehydrogenase. Oxygen strongly inhibits the formation of this enzyme when glucose is not present in the growth medium.

The Crabtree effect, considered an inherent peculiarity（特点，奇特）of the majority of malignant tissues, was found in all examined strains of *Escherichia* and *Proteus*（变形杆菌属）and was absent in *Micrococcus*（微球菌属）and *Serratia*（沙雷氏菌属）. The maximal value of the Crabtree effect in *E. coli* cultures occurred at the time of the initial period of log multiplication. The finding of the Crabtree effect in the examined bacteria strains indicates an analogy（类比）existing between the metabolic behavior of malignant tissues and certain facultatively anaerobic bacteria（兼性厌氧性细菌）.

Therefore, in high cell density fermentation of *Escherichia coli*, reasonable carbon source feeding to reduce the glucose effect is the key to success. There are three commonly used fed-batch fermentation strategies: Constant fed batch cultivation（恒速流加）(also called Constant feeding), Variable fed batch cultivation（变速流加）(also called Variable feeding) and Exponential feeding（指数流加）.

Constant fed batch cultivation. In constant fed batch cultivation, glucose, as the limiting substrate, is added at a constant rate. In proportion to the bacteria in the fermentation tank, the nutrient concentration is gradually reduced, and the specific growth rate of the bacteria also slows down. The total mass of the bacteria increases linearly during the culture process.

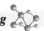

Variable fed batch cultivation. When bacteria multiply to high cell density, more nutrients can be added in this way to facilitate cell growth and target gene expression.

Variable fed batch cultivation can be categorized as:

➢ Gradient fed batch cultivation (梯度流加)

➢ Multi-step fed-batch cultivation (阶段流加)

➢ Linear fed batch/Linear gradient fed cultivation (线性流加)

Exponential feeding technique. It is a simple and effective feeding technique, which controls the concentration of the substrate in the reactor at a lower level, hence greatly reduce the formation of harmful metabolites such as acetic acid. Bacteria increase exponentially at certain specific growth rate. Meanwhile, the growth rate of bacteria can be controlled by regulating the flow rate, allows bacteria to express exogenous proteins adequately while they grow stably. This technique has been widely used in high cell density cultivation of recombinant *Escherichia coli* to produce exogenous proteins.

In addition, in order to fit the actual growth of bacteria in the fermenter and further reduce the generation of harmful metabolites, many feasible feeding techniques have been developed according to the feedback information of cell metabolism with online or offline detection methods, such as constant pH cultivation, constant DO cultivation, bacteria concentration feedback approach, CER feedback approach, DO-stat approach, *etc*.

2. High-level expression

If a culture medium is only suitable for the growth of a host microbe, it is far from enough for high cell density fermentation of a genetically engineered microbe.

High cell density cultivation of microbes can be easily achieved by using synthetic medium, but often accompanied with no expression of exogenous genes. Results showed that the main factors affecting the expression level at high cell density were hypertonic inhibition (高渗抑制), acetic acid inhibition, feeding composition, degradation by proteinases and the difference in amino acid compositions between the target protein and microbial cell proteins.

Hypertonic inhibition. High concentration of nutrients, especially high concentration of inorganic salts, is required in high cell density cultivation, which may negatively affect the growth and gene expression of microbes.

Inhibition by acetic acid. Another issue for high cell density and high level expression is how to overcome the inhibition effect upon growth and expression of microbes by the accumulation of large amounts of acetic acid (HAc). When the HAc content ≥ 6 g/L, the growth of microbes was completely inhibited, whereas when HAc content ≥ 2.4 g/L, the specific yield was significantly reduced.

Glycine and methionine can eliminate the inhibition effect of acetic acid upon microbes, and increase the specific growth rate. Under 2 g/L acetic acid, 0.5 g/L glycine or methionine eliminated the inhibition effect of acetic acid on the growth of wild strain and improved the specific production rate. Addition of 0.6 g/L methionine eliminated the inhibition effect of acetic acid on the growth of recombinant microbe and produced β-lactamase in large quantities. The effect of methionine on the expression of recombinant microbes was related to dilution rate D. When $D > 0.4 \text{ h}^{-1}$, the addition of methionine promoted β-lactamase synthesis and reduced acetic acid production rate. When $D < 0.3 \text{ h}^{-1}$, the addition of methionine inhibited the synthesis rate of β-lactamase and promoted the generation of acetic acid. In order to reduce the generation of acetic acid, the following strategies are usually adopted in the fermentation process — selecting an appropriate recipient microbe, changing the composition of the medium, reducing the specific growth rate, reducing the culture temperature, restricted feeding of glucose in a fed-batch process, and even dialysis cultivation.

Effects of various feeding components. Many studies have shown that continuous or intermittent addition of composite organic nitrogen source (*e.g.*, casein hydrolysates) can improve the expression level of recombinant microbes. Changing C/N ratio after induction significantly affects the efficiency of exogenous gene expression, while changing C/N ratio at the growth stage has little effect.

Degradation by proteinases. Either heat shock or stringent response would induce protease generation, resulting in degradation of target protein expressed.

Difference of amino acid compositions between the target protein and microbial cell proteins. The more difference there is between the amino acid composition of the target protein and that of the microbial cell proteins, it is more likely for the target protein to be degraded. If one or more types of amino acids are added to meet the specific needs of a target protein synthesis, the expression level and stability of the product might be improved.

Strategies for feeding during the growth phase, the induction and the expression phases in high cell density cultivation of engineered yeast strains (*e.g.*, *Pichia pastoris*)：

Phase I：the growth phase similar to what happened in an underway batch culture

Phase II：Increasing cell density by feeding glycerol

Phase III：Inducing protein expression by feeding methanol

Strategies for improving the stability of the products include:

Choosing appropriate pH — pH 2.8~6.5 is the pH range suitable for microbe growth;

Feeding composite nutritional supplement, such as casamino acid（酪蛋白水解物）, yeast extract and peptone（蛋白胨）；

Adding EDTA;

Using protease-deficient host strains.

3.1.2 Basic fermentation equipments and applications（基本发酵设备及其应用）

3.1.2.1 *Bioreactor design fundamentals*（生物反应器基本结构）(Fig. 3-4)

Housing（壳体）

Temperature control system（控温部分）

Agitation system（搅拌部分）

Ventilation system（通气部分）air inlet/outlet system

Entry-exit holes（进出料口）

Charge inlet, discharge outlet, feed supplement hole

Measuring system/Sensors（测量系统）

Anti-foam control system（消泡装置）

Accessory system（附属系统）

3.1.2.2 *Measurement and detection of parameters during the fermentation process and process optimization*（发酵过程参数的测量和过程优化）

Devices for the optimization of bioprocesses — monitoring and controlling various fermentation

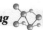

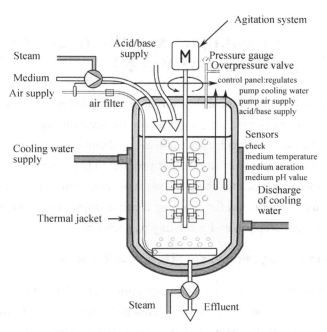

Fig. 3-4   A schematic of a bioreactor as how it works in real life.

parameters — are equipped.

1. Temperature measurement（温度测量）

The optimal temperature for protein expression is not always the optimal temperature for bacterial growth. Thermal resistance detector is commonly used for detecting fermentation temperature.

2. Agitation-speed measurement（搅拌转速测量）

Agitation-speed is usually measured by using Magnetic Inductive Tachometer（转速计，流速计），Optical Sensing Tachometer or Techo-generator（测速发动机）.

3. Ventilation measurement（通气量的测量）

Rotameter（转子流量计）and Thermal mass flowmeter（热式质量流量计）are two commonly used gas flow meters.

4. pH measurement（pH 测量）

The formation of acidic/alkaline metabolites, as well as the utilization of physiological acids/bases in a fermentation process changes the pH of the fermentation culture, which can be detected with a pH detection system and adjusted accordingly.

5. Dissolved Oxygen (DO) Measurement（溶解氧的测量）

Dissolved Oxygen (DO) concentration in the fermentation culture has a direct impact on the metabolic properties of microbes, hence it is another key parameter to be detected and adjusted.

6. On-line analysis of tail gas（尾气的在线分析）

The concentrations of carbon dioxide and oxygen in the tail gas should be analyzed on-line.

A tail gas sampling system（取样系统）branched from the exhaust pipe（排气管，发酵尾气管）connects both the Carbon Dioxide Analyzer and the Oxygen Analyzer.

7. The calculation of indirect parameters（间接参数的计算）

Oxygen Utilization Rate（OUR，耗氧速率），Carbon Dioxide Evolution Rate（CER，二氧化碳释放率）and Respiration Quotient（RQ，呼吸商）can be calculated according to certain formulas. They are very important indirect parameters.

3.2 Cell disruption techniques specific to genetically engineered microbes（基因工程菌细胞的破碎技术）

Cell disruption is an essential step in the utilization of accumulated intracellular products, which can be embodied in cell permeation or cell cracking, and this can be done through various means, which can be categorized as physical, chemical, or mechanical. Not all methods are suitable for large-scale processing, while each one has different impacts on the target product. This section discusses the need for cell permeation or cell cracking, demonstrates the methods most commonly used in laboratory and industry, highlights aspects that must be evaluated for choosing a cell disruption method, and briefly comments on the necessary steps following disruption and preceding purification.

3.2.1 Prokaryotic and eukaryotic cells（原核细胞与真核细胞）

Cells in our world come in two basic types, prokaryotic and eukaryotic. Prokaryotic cells have no nuclei, while eukaryotic cells do have true nuclei. This is far from the only difference between these two cell types, however. The cells of animals, plants, fungi and protists（原生生物）are all eukaryotic. According to the degree of a microbial evolution and the degree of cell structural differentiation, microbes can also be classified as prokaryotes and eukaryotes. Bacteria and cyanobacteria belong to prokaryotes. Fungi, algae and protozoa belong to eukaryotes.

3.2.2 Structural features of the microbial cell wall（微生物细胞壁结构特点）

A **cell wall** is a structural layer that surrounds some types of cells, situated outside the cell membrane. It can be tough, flexible, and sometimes rigid. Cell walls are present in plants, fungi and prokaryotic cells, In microbial kingdom, the vast majority of prokaryotic bacterial and eukaryotic fungi and algae do possess cell wall, except for funginite（真菌体）(fungus), the thermoplasma（热源体属）(archaea), and protozoa. Meanwhile, cell wall is absent from mycoplasmas（支原体）.

The cell wall is a crucial extracellular organelle that surrounds cells, responsible for cell shape and osmotic stability, and acts as a filter for large molecules. They provide cells with both structural support and protection. They may give cells rigidity and strength, offering protection against mechanical stress. In multicellular organisms, they permit the organism to build and hold certain shape (morphogenesis). Cell walls act as a natural barrier, separating the cell contents from the extracellular environment. Cell walls also limit the entry of large molecules that may be toxic to the cell. They further permit the creation of stable osmotic environments by preventing osmotic lysis（渗透性溶解）.

Their composition, properties, and form may change during the cell cycle and depend on growth conditions. The **chemical composition** of the cell walls is very complex and varies between species, it depends not only on cell type, but also on developmental stage. An important gist for the classification and identification of microorganisms is according to the differences in their cell wall structures and chemical compositions. Cell wall usually consists of two kinds of material — one is used to form the skeleton of cell wall, the other is used to form the matrix of cell wall. Although all microbial cell walls are composed of polysaccharides, lipids, and proteins embedded on the three-dimensional structure, but they are different in their chemical composition and the unit structure arrangement. The primary cell wall of land plants is composed of the polysaccharides cellulose, hemicellulose and pectin （果胶，胶质）. In bacteria, the cell wall is composed of peptidoglycan （肽聚糖）. Archaean cell walls have various compositions, and may be formed of glycoprotein S-layers, pseudopeptidoglycan （假肽聚糖）, or polysaccharides （多聚糖）. Fungi possess cell walls made of the glucosamine （葡萄糖胺，氨基葡萄糖） polymer chitin （几丁质）, and algae typically possess walls made of glycoproteins and polysaccharides. Unusually, diatoms （硅藻） have a cell wall composed of biogenic silica （生物硅）. Often, other accessory molecules such as lignin （木质素） or cutin （角质，蜡状质，表皮素） are found anchored （使固定） to the cell wall. All these differences can be reflected on the variation in sensitivity during cell disruption.

At present, the major microbes involved in the study of genetically engineered microbes are bacteria, yeast and algae.

3.2.2.1　Bacteria （细菌）

Bacteria are microscopic organisms whose single cells have neither a membrane-bounded nucleus nor other membrane-bounded organelles like mitochondria and chloroplasts. They belong to prokaryotes and reproduce via binary fission. Traditionally, bacteria have been grouped based on their Structure, Physiology, Molecular Composition, and Reaction to specific types of stains — Gram Stain — rather than on their evolutionary relationships.

By comparing **ribosomal RNA sequences**, scientists have found that there are **two vastly** different types of Bacteria:

➢ The Bacteria that we generally refer to as "**germs**" are classified in the **kingdom** （界） **Eubacteria**, or **Eubacteria** （真细菌）, or simpler yet **Bacteria**.

➢ The **other type** of bacteria are called **Archaebacteria** （古细菌）, and belong to the **Kingdom Archaebacteria**. These are the more ancient bacteria.

Structural features of the bacterial cell envelope （细菌细胞被膜结构特点）

The DNA is carried on the genophore （基因带）, a circular chromosome, in an ill-defined area of the cytosol called the nucleoid （类核）. The chromosome is attached to the cell membrane during cell division （fission 裂殖）, frequently at a point called the mesosome （间体）.

Bacterial cell wall

Most bacteria have cell walls. The cell wall forms a boundary around the cell, to support and protect the cell. It protects the cell from dryness and infection. The cell wall is very important because it allows bacteria to survive.

The bacterial cell wall is a tough and elastic layer of cystic structure surrounding the cell, around the outside of the cell membrane. The walls of prokaryotic cells range from 5 to 80 nm along a diameter.

In bacteria, there are two types of cell walls each from the Gram-positive bacteria and the Gram-negative bacteria (Fig. 3-5). The Gram-positive cell walls are much thicker than the Gram-negative ones.

The **Gram-positive** cell wall is usually between 20 and 80 nm thick, with 15~50 layers of peptidoglycan （肽聚糖）, each 1 nm thick, containing 20% ~ 40% teichoic acid （磷壁酸） and some containing small amounts of proteins. The thickest cell wall among prokaryotic cells is that of *Lactobacillus acidophilus* （嗜酸乳杆菌）, up to 80 nm.

In contrast, **Gram-negative** cell wall is usually thinner and between 5 and 10 nm thick. However, the structure of the cell envelope of Gram-negative bacteria is more complex — it has a distinctly layered appearance, containing three layers.

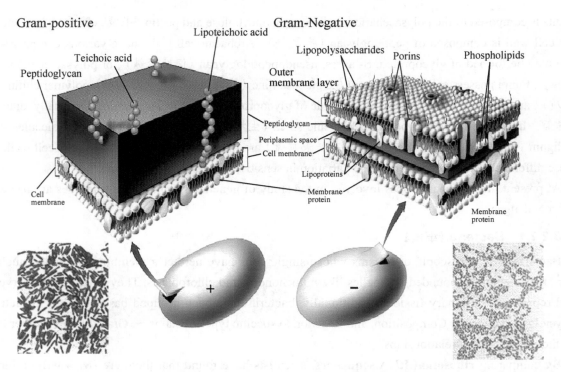

Fig. 3-5 Structures associated with Gram-positive and Gram-negative cell walls. Gram-positive bacteria have a thicker layer of peptidoglycan in their cell walls, made of a protein-sugar complex that takes on the purple color during Gram staining. Gram-negative bacteria have an extra layer of lipid on the outside of the cell wall and appear pink after Gram staining. The extra lipid layer stops the purple stain from entering the cell wall. They do absorb the pink stain, so they are easily distinguished with a microscope.

In Gram-negative bacteria, a further outer membrane containing **lipopolysaccharides** and **lipoproteins** surrounds the plasmalemma（质膜）, with a thin cell wall and periplasmic space trapped between them. When ultrathin sections of bacteria are detected through electron microscopy, multilayers were observed on cell wall, and distinguished as outer layer and inner layer. The peptidoglycan wall is a rigid framework around which is built an elaborate membrane structure (Fig.3-6).

Gram-Negative Envelope

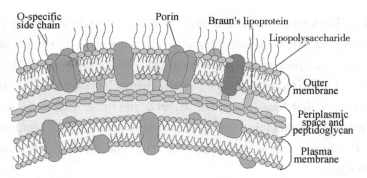

Fig. 3-6 The cell surface of Gram negative bacteria has a distinctly layered appearance. The peptidoglycan wall is a rigid framework around which is built an elaborate membrane structure.

The outer layer of the cell wall, *i.e.*, the outer membrane, about 8 ± 2 nm thick, is composed of **lipopolysaccharides** on the outside and phospholipids on the inside. It also contains various proteins. Those lipopolysaccharides can determine the antigenicity of the bacteria, and are referred to as "O antigens". While proteins, including most of the enzymes, are embedded in the outer layer of the cell wall.

Peptidoglycan is the second thinner layer. The inner layer of cell wall in Gram-negative bacteria is also composed of **peptidoglycan** polysaccharides, but the content is lower, only 2~3 layers of peptidoglycan exist. The peptidoglycan of Gram-negative cells is similar to the Gram-positive cell, except that the tetrapeptide units cross-link directly and not through a glycine pentapeptide.

The **inner** and **outer layers** of the cell wall are connected by **lipoproteins** covalently. The peptidoglycan layer is attached to the **outer bilayer** membrane by the **Braun lipoprotein** (an intrinsic membrane protein of the outer cell membrane).

The best example of this type of cell is *Escherichia coli*, a major prokaryote host organism in biotechnology. Many recombinant products have been produced by using *E. coli.*

Most bacteria have the Gram-negative cell wall and only the Firmicutes（厚壁菌门）and Actinobacteria（放线菌门）(previously known as the low G+C and high G+C Gram-positive bacteria, respectively) have the alternative Gram-positive arrangement. These differences in structure can produce differences in antibiotic susceptibility, for instance vancomycin（万古霉素）can kill only Gram-positive bacteria and is ineffective against Gram-negative pathogens, such as *Haemophilus influenzae* or *Pseudomonas aeruginosa*（铜绿假单胞菌）.

The plasma membrane — a bilayer

The innermost layer, called the plasma lemma, the plasma membrane or the inner membrane, is common to both Gram-positive and Gram-negative organisms. It is a typical unit membrane structure, about 8 ± 2 nm thick, close to the cell wall on the outside. It consists largely of phospholipids, the building blocks of the cell membranes, but also contains dispersed proteins and metal ions. Phospholipids are both hydrophilic and hydrophobic — they are zwitterions (Fig.3-7).

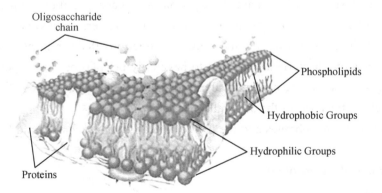

Fig. 3-7   A more detailed picture of the plasma membrane（细胞膜结构）. The membrane consists largely of zwitterionic phospholipids, but it also contains a significant amount of protein.

The cell membrane is made of two layers of phospholipids, *i.e.*, a lipid bilayer. In the bilayer, the hydrophobic fatty acid tails of each layer are held together by weak van der Waals forces in the center of the membrane and the hydrophilic phosphates project outward forming hydrogen bonds with tight, organized layers of water on each face (the cytoplasmic and outer surfaces) of the membrane.

Cell membrane has many important functions closely related to cell material exchange, cell recognition, secretion, excretion, immunity and so on.

Functions each layer performs

In Gram-negative bacteria, the outer membrane, the peptidoglycan layer and plasma membrane, these three layers have different functions.

The outer membrane and the peptidoglycan layer provide the mechanical strength to the cell. The bacterial cell wall helps protect bacterial cell, maintain cell shape and keep cell's integrity. It has the function of preventing the external physiological active substances from damaging the bacteria body, so as to maintain the life of bacterial cells, and resisting the infiltration of water into the cell from its surroundings. It can prevent the contents of different cells from contacting and mixing with each other and genetic information from recombination.

The cell wall is essential to the survival of many bacteria, although L-form bacteria（L 型细菌） can be produced in the laboratory that lack a cell wall. The antibiotic penicillin is able to kill bacteria by preventing the cross-linking of peptidoglycan and this causes the cell wall to weaken and lyse. The lysozyme enzyme can also damage bacterial cell walls.

The cytoplasmic membrane may be considered the biochemical boundary of the cell and the major player in permeability. It lets water, certain ions and substrates enter the cell; it is vital for the cell's energy budget and it excretes substances. It protects the cell — without it would the cell contents diffuse into their surroundings, information containing molecules would be lost and the metabolic pathways would seek a thermal equilibrium — the death of each living system.

Periplasmic space

The peptidoglycan layer encloses the periplasmic space — a "gap" between the cell membrane (the inner bilayer membrane) and the cell wall (the peptidoglycan layer), which is 10~25 nm thick — particularly evident in Gram-negative bacteria. Once secreted through the plasma membrane, some of the protein and glycoprotein species will remain at the periplasmic space, possibly playing enzymatic roles.

Periplasmic spaces are rarely observed in Gram-positive bacteria. However, such bacteria must accomplish many of the same metabolic and transport functions that Gram-negative bacteria do. At present most Gram-positive bacteria are thought to have only periplasms — not periplasmic spaces — where metabolic digestion occurs and new cell wall peptidoglycan is attached（连接，结合）. The periplasm in Gram-positive cells is thus part of the cell wall.

Destruction of the outer membranes and the peptidoglycan layer is what should be focused on in this context.

Various bacterial wall constituents

(1) *Peptidoglycans*

Peptidoglycans, the macromolecules of cell wall are arranged in layers. A polysaccharide chain is composed of N-acetylglucosamine and N-acetylmuramic acid（乙酰胞壁酸）, covalently connected with β-1,4 linkage, and repeated successively, thus forming a long linear copolymer molecular chain. **Peptidoglycans** are made up of those polysaccharide chains cross-linked by peptide bridges, which are unusual oligopeptides, forming a network structure, hence called peptidoglycan. It is the main skeletal component of bacterial cell wall.

The amino acids that make up those oligopeptides are mainly D-amino acids, which are usually arranged in the order of L-alanine, D-glutamate, DA, D-alanine, and (L-alanine). DA is a diamino acid, such as DAP (diaminopimelic acid), L-lysine, L-ornithine（鸟氨酸）, *etc*. Among them, D-alanine is involved in the synthesis of peptidoglycan, which is hydrolyzed off in the process of crosslinking between the oligopeptides on the adjacent polysaccharide chains to form the tetrapeptide side chain. However, some bacteria use L-serine or glycine instead of L-alanine, while some others use D-glutamine instead of D-glutamic acid.

All Gram-negative bacteria contain diaminopimelic acid in their cell-wall oligopeptides. However, most Gram-positive bacteria contain lysine, and only a small number of Gram-positive bacteria contain diaminopimelic acid in their cell-wall peptides, and a few others contain other amino acids.

Not all peptide chains on N-acetylmuramic acid participate crosslinking. The crosslinking degree of peptide chain in the cell wall of **Gram-positive bacteria** is much higher than that of **Gram-negative bacteria**. In addition, the **content of peptidoglycan** in the cell wall of Gram-positive bacteria is much higher than that of Gram-negative bacteria, with the former accounts for about 30% to 85% of the cell dry weight, while the latter accounts for 5% to 20%. But some other bacteria, such as methanogen（产甲烷细菌）, halobacteria（嗜盐细菌）and sulfolobus（硫化叶菌）, do not have a peptidoglycan layer at all in their cell walls.

(2) *Teichoic acid*（磷壁酸）

In addition to the peptidoglycan as its main component, teichoic acid is another important component found within the cell wall of most Gram-positive bacteria such as species in the genera *Staphylococcus*, *Streptococcus*, *Bacillus*, *Clostridium*, *Corynebacterium*, and *Listeria*, and appears to extend to the surface of the peptidoglycan layer. **Teichoic acids** are bacterial copolymers of glycerol phosphate or ribitol phosphate（磷酸核糖醇）and carbohydrates linked via phosphodiester bonds.

Teichoic acid can be classified into three categories: glycerophosphoric acid（甘油磷壁酸）, phosphoinosidic acid（核醇磷壁酸）and lipoteichoic acid（脂磷壁酸）. They can be covalently linked to *N*-acetylmuramic acid or a terminal D-alanine in the tetrapeptide crosslinkage between *N*-acetylmuramic acid units of the peptidoglycan layer, or they can be anchored in the cytoplasmic membrane with a lipid anchor. Teichoic acids that are covalently bound to peptidoglycan are referred to as wall teichoic acids (WTA), whereas teichoic acids that are anchored to the lipid membrane are referred to as lipoteichoic acids (LTAs).

Generally speaking, there is only one kind of teichoic acid in the cell wall of each type of bacteria, but there are also some bacteria that take one type of teichoic acids as primary one, whereas the other as auxiliary one. The most common **structures** (in wall teichoic acids) are a ManNAc (β1→4)GlcNAc disaccharide with one to three glycerol phosphates attached to the C4 hydroxyl of the ManNAc residue followed by a long chain of glycerol- or ribitol phosphate repeats.

Teichoic acid is an acidic polymer and contributes negative charge to the cell surface of Gram-positive bacteria, and the main function of teichoic acids is to **provide rigidity** to the cell-wall by **attracting cations** such as magnesium and sodium. Teichoic acids give the molecule zwitterionic properties, which make teichoic acids suspected ligands for toll-like receptors 2 and 4.

Another function of teichoic acid is that it is involved in the **regulation of cell wall extension** during the cell growth and cell division. It is responsible for hydrolizing the cell wall which has already been synthesized so that the cell wall can accommodate new subunits. Teichoic acids assist in **regulation of cell growth** by limiting the ability of **autolysins**（自溶素）(produced by the cell itself, responsible for participating in the process of cell growth) to break the β (1-4) bond between the *N*-acetyl glucosamine and the *N*-acetylmuramic acid. The function of teichoic acid is to regulate the time of action of **autolysin** and keep it in balance with the synthesis of cell wall.

The cell wall can also be opened before the completion of cell wall synthesis, followed by cytolysis or cell death.

Lipoteichoic acids（脂磷壁酸）may also act as receptor molecules for some Gram-positive bacteriophage; however, this has not yet been conclusively supported.

(3) *Lipopolysaccharides*（脂多糖）

Most Gram-negative bacteria have the outermost part of their cell wall composed of lipopolysaccharides (LPS), which are the principal components of the outer membrane of Gram-negative bacteria. Lipopolysaccharides are composed of O-antigen oligosaccharides, core oligosaccharides and lipid A. O-antigen oligosaccharide is a polymer composed of repeating units of four or five monosaccharides. The types and arrangement of its residues vary from strain to strain. It possesses antigen-specificity, hence called O-antigen. Core oligosaccharides (or Core-OS) is a short chain of sugar residues within Gram-negative lipopolysaccharide (LPS). Core-OS are highly diverse among bacterial species and even within strain of species. The sugar residues of core oligosaccharides do not vary much in different strains, mainly composed of hexose, heptose（庚糖）, octose（辛糖）, phosphoric acid and ethanolamine. The basic structure of lipid A is disaccharide, which consists of two glucosamine residues. The hydroxyl group of this sugar residue is replaced by some fatty acids and phosphoric acids. The fatty acids include lauric acid, myristic acid, palmitic acid, and 2-hydroxytetradecanoic acid（2-羟基十四烷酸）. Lipid A is toxic, it is a kind of endotoxin.

(4) *Lipoproteins*（脂蛋白）

Lipoprotein forms the outer side of the outer layer of the cell wall of Gram-negative bacteria, while the inner side is composed of lipoprotein and phospholipids. The lipid part of lipoprotein forms the inner part of the outer layer of the cell wall, and the protein part covalently bound to the lipid part may be covalently bound with its opposite end (the C-terminal end) to the peptidoglycan molecules in the inner layer of the cell wall. Hence the outer layer of the cell wall of Gram-negative bacteria is also a bilayer membrane, with various proteins embedded in it. An important function of Gram-negative bacteria cell wall is selective permeation. It only allows small molecules with molecular weight between 600~1 000 Da to penetrate freely, while enzymes or other large molecules cannot. Therefore, only after EDTA was added to destroy the cell wall and to increase the permeability of the outer layer of cell wall, can lysozyme penetrate into the cell wall, and act on the peptidoglycan, hence can protoplasts be prepared. In addition, the cytoplasmic space between the cell wall and the cytoplasmic membrane of Gram-negative bacteria has various proteins responsible for solute transportation and various hydrolases. The hydrolases produced by Gram-positive bacteria are mostly secreted out of the cell.

Internal Structures（膜内结构）

Ribosomes — are complexes of RNA and protein that are found in all cells. The ribosome functions in the expression of the genetic code from nucleic acid into protein, in a process called translation.

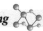

Inclusions（包涵物）(Cytoplasmic) — are chemical substances that may or may not be present in a cell, depending on the cell type. Inclusions are stored nutrients, secretory products, and pigment granules.

Inclusion bodies — Most of the proteins are soluble in naturally occurring prokaryotes; however, some proteins are insoluble in genetically engineered species.

Cytoplasm — a dense, gelatinous solution and is a prominent site for many of the cell′s biochemical and synthetic activities. Its major component is water (70%~80%), which serves as a solvent for a complex mixture of nutrients including sugars, amino acids, and other organic molecules and salts.

Plasmids — These are tiny strands that exist as separate double-stranded circles of DNA. During bacterial reproduction they are duplicated and passed on to the offspring.

Nucleoid（类核）— This is where the DNA is aggregated in a central area of the cell. It is an extremely long molecule of DNA that is tightly coiled to fit inside the cell compartment. Arranged along its length are genetic units that carry information required for bacterial maintenance and growth.

Destruction of the outer membranes and the peptidoglycan layer is what should be focused on in this context.

3.2.2.2   *Yeast*（酵母）

Fungal cell walls

Chemical structure of a unit from a chitin polymer chain.

Yeast is widely distributed in nature and mainly grows in an acidic sugar-containing environment. It is a typical eukaryotic microbe. Its cell diameter is generally 10 times larger than that of a bacterium. Structure differentiation of the cell can be observed under an optical microscope.

In fungi, the cell wall is the outer-most layer, external to the plasma membrane. The yeast cell wall is tough and about 70 nm thick (varying with the growth conditions, especially the type of carbon source). The fungal cell wall is a matrix of three main components. The main components of yeast cell wall are β-1,3 and β-1,6-glucans, mannoproteins and chitin, with β-1,3-glucan being the principal cell wall component, to which the components are crosslinked (Fig. 3-8). Altogether they account for 90% of the cell dry weight, with the relative proportions of these constituents varying with growth conditions and the cellular developmental program. Mannose is covalently bound to proteins in the outer layer of the cell wall. The inner layer is composed of glucan, which are complex branched polymers while a layer of protein molecules is located in the middle, accounting for 10% of the cell dry weight.

Cell wall composition changes during growth, budding, mating, and sporulation（孢子形成）, and those dynamic processes require remodeling of the crosslinking of β-1,3- and β-1,6-glucans to themselves and to other cell wall components.

In addition, they contain a small amount of lipids.

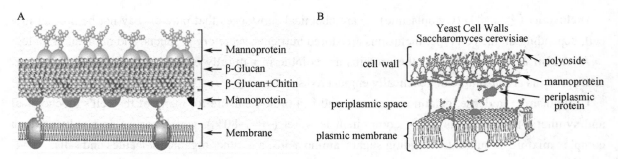

Fig. 3-8　Structure of the yeast cell wall. A. The wall is primarily composed of mannoproteins and β-glucan that is linked (1→3) and (1→6). Ergosterol（麦角固醇）is the major lipid component of the underlying plasma membrane. B. Model structure of cell wall of *saccharomyces cerevisiae*.

(1) *Glucan (glucans)*

Glucans（葡聚糖）are glucose polymers that function to cross-link chitin（几丁质）or chitosan（壳聚糖，聚氨基葡糖，脱乙酰几丁质）polymers. β-glucans are glucose molecules linked via β- (1,3)- or β-(1,6)- bonds and provide rigidity to the cell wall while α-glucans are defined by α- (1,3)- and/or α- (1,4) bonds and function as part of the matrix.

There are two kinds of glucan in *Saccharomyces cerevisiae* cell wall, one is β-1,3-glucan, another is β-1, 6-glucan, which is highly branched. The cell wall of yeast organisms are mainly composed of β-linked glucan, a polysaccharide comprised of a backbone chain of β- (1,3) glucose units with a low degree of inter- and intra- molecular branching through β- (1,6) linkages.

A β-1,3-glucan chain is long and twisted, hydrophilic at one end, and hydrophobic at the other. Two such long chains form a double helix with their hydrophobic sides attracting each other. Many such double helices are so parallelly layed out that it is possible for the cell wall to expand moderately. β-1, 6-glucan has a reticular appearance and is soluble in dilute acids.

A minor component that consists mainly of highly branched β-1,6-glucan is closely associated with the main component, and both together comprise the alkali-insoluble glucan fraction.

(2) *Proteins/Mannoproteins*（甘露糖蛋白）

Most of the structural proteins found in the cell wall are glycosylated and contain mannose, thus these proteins are called mannoproteins（甘露糖蛋白）or mannans（甘露聚糖）. Actually, mannoprotein is a complex formed by the covalently binding of mannose and protein(s), forming a network structure on the outer layer of the cell wall. It has antigenicity. The mannose part in the mannoprotein is a branched polysaccharide. It connects several glycine residues with α-1,2 linkage and α-1,3 linkage to their side chain. Enzymes necessary for cell wall synthesis and lysis in addition to structural proteins are all present in the cell wall.

(3) *Chitin*（几丁质）

Chitin is a linear polymer consisting mainly of β- (1,4)-linked-N-acetylglucosamine in the Ascomycota（子囊菌门）and Basidiomycota（担子菌门）, or poly-β-(1,4)-linked-N-acetylglucosamine (chitosan) in the Zygomycota（接合菌门）. It is unbranched and mainly exists around the bud scars on the yeast cell wall, that is, the synthesis of chitin occurs only when and where the yeast is budding.

Most yeast cell walls contain glucan, but not all contain mannose. Generally speaking, yeast cell walls which are lack of mannose usually contain more chitin. Both chitin and chitosan are synthesized and extruded at the plasma membrane.

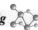

3.2.2.3   *Algae*（藻类）

Algal cell walls

Like plants, algae have cell walls. The cell wall structure of algae is quite complex. Algal cell wall contains either polysaccharides such as cellulose [a glucan（葡聚糖）] or a variety of glycoproteins (Volvocales（团藻目）) or both as its structural skeleton. They appear as fibrous microfibrils（微纤维） layed out in layers within the cell wall, generally about 10~20 nm thick, but the cell wall of *Chorella pyrenoides* is rather thin, only 3~6 nm.

The algae cell wall matrix is mainly composed of heteroglycan, some of which also contain a small amount of proteins and lipids. For example, alginic acid（褐藻酸） is a heteroglycan of the brown algal cell wall, which is a polymer composed of D-mannose and L-glucuronic acid. Agar-agar is the main matrix polysaccharide of red algae *Gelidium amansii*（石花菜）. It is a polymer composed of galactose and galacturonic acid（半乳糖醛酸）. These are still some other algae with silicon and calcium carbonate deposited in their cell wall.

In some algal cell walls, xylose（木糖） and mannose replace cellulose as the skeleton.

The inclusion of additional polysaccharides in algal cells walls is used as a feature for algal taxonomy（分类）.

- Mannans: They form microfibrils in the cell walls of a number of marine green algae including those from the genera, *Codium*（绿藻类的松藻属）, *Dasycladus*（绒枝藻属）, and *Acetabularia*（伞藻） as well as in the walls of some red algae, like *Porphyra*（紫菜属） and *Bangia*（红毛菜）.

- Xylans（木聚糖）:
  - **Xyloses** is another monosaccharide residue exist in the cell wall of **green algae**, **red algae**, **blue-green algae**, and one of the components composing the sulfated polysaccharides in some kinds of **brown algae**, such as *Spatoglossum schroederi*（海篦藻）.

- Alginic acid（海藻酸，褐藻酸）:
  - Alginic acid, also called algin（褐藻酸，褐藻胶） or alginate（藻酸盐）, a common and abundant polysaccharide in the cell walls of brown algae, is a viscous gum. It is a linear copolymer with homopolymeric blocks of (1-4)-linked β-D-mannuronate（甘露糖醛酸）(M) and its C-5 epimer（差向（立体）异构体）α-L-gluronate（葡（萄）糖盐（或酯））(G) residues, respectively, covalently linked together in different sequences or blocks. The monomers can appear in homopolymeric blocks of consecutive G-residues (G-blocks), consecutive M-residues (M-blocks), alternating M and G-residues (MG-blocks), or randomly organized blocks.

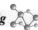

- Sulfonated polysaccharides: They occur in the cell walls of most algae; those common in red algae include agarose（琼脂糖）, carrageenan（卡拉胶，角叉菜胶）, porphyran（金属卟啉）, furcelleran（红藻胶） and funoran [海萝聚糖（胶）].
  - Agarose（琼脂糖） is the polysaccharide agarose which forms the supporting structure in the cell walls of certain species of algae. These algae are known as agarophytes（洋菜植物，产琼胶原藻）and

belong to the Rhodophyta（红藻，红藻植物门，红藻门）(red algae) phylum.

○ Agar is actually the resulting mixture of two components: the linear polysaccharide **agarose**（琼脂糖）, and a heterogeneous mixture of smaller molecules called **agaropectin**（琼脂胶）. Agarose, the predominant component of agar, is a linear polymer of molecular weight about 120 000, made up of the repeating monomeric unit of agarobiose（洋菜二糖，琼脂二糖）. Agarobiose is a disaccharide made up of D-galactose and 3,6-anhydro-L-galactopyranose. Agaropectin is a heterogeneous（非均质）mixture of smaller molecules that occur in lesser amounts, and is made up of alternating units of D-galactose and L-galactose heavily modified with acidic side-groups, such as sulfate and pyruvate（丙酮酸）.

Other compounds that may accumulate in algal cell walls include sporopollenin（孢子花粉素，孢粉素）and calcium ions.

The group of algae known as the diatoms synthesize their cell walls [also known as frustules（硅藻细胞壳）or valves（瓣）] from silicic acid（硅酸）[specifically orthosilicic acid（原硅酸）, H_4SiO_4]. The acid is polymerized intracellularly, then the wall is extruded（挤压，突出）to protect the cell. Significantly, relative to the organic cell walls produced by other groups, silica frustules（硅藻细胞壳）require less energy to synthesize (approximately 8%), potentially a major saving on the overall cell energy budget and possibly an explanation for higher growth rates in diatoms.

In brown algae, phlorotannins（褐藻多酚）may be a constituent of the cell walls.

3.2.3 Cell disruption（细胞的破碎）

In many cases, the expressed products, especially the proteins produced by genetically engineered bacteria, are always concentrated and deposited within the cell, rather than secreted into the culture broth. *i.e.*, they are intracellular. Lipids and some antibiotics are also trapped in the biomass. In order to perform biochemical analysis of intracellular molecules (*i.e.*, proteins, lipids, and nucleic acids), or subject them to further extraction, isolation and purification for producing biopharmaceutical products, the cells have to be disrupted at first, releasing the biomolecules from inside the cell. The molecules of interest can then be separated or purified from the cell lysate using affinity purification, charge- and size-based separation, filtration, precipitation, *etc*.

By reviewing the structure of the cell wall and the existing cell disruption methods, more cell disruption techniques would be devised, useful on a large scale.

Cell disruption techniques commonly used（常用破碎技术）

Microbial cells are very tough. For example, the osmotic pressures in both *Micrococcus lysoleikticus* （溶壁微球菌）and *Sarcina lutea* Schroeter（藤黄八叠球菌）are about 2.0 MPa, which can give you an idea of how tough the cell structure is to tolerate this pressure.

There are many ways to crush down such tough cell walls and cytomembranes so as to make the cells release their contents. According to whether an applied force is used, the existing cell disruption methods can be divided into two categories, "**mechanical**" and "**non-mechanical**".

The **mechanical methods** are dominated by homogenization（匀浆法）and ball mill grinding（研磨法）. In both cases, cells are broken by high mechanical shear（高速机械剪切力）. Heat generation is a weak point hence scale-up is difficult — If we find a method that works at a laboratory scale, we usually have no idea about whether it works on a large scale.

In the **non-mechanical methods**, the cell membrane is ruptured by osmotic pressure（渗透冲击法）, dissolved by detergents（表面活性剂增溶法）, or enfeebled by organic solvents（有机溶剂溶解法）. Usually these reactions are mild and the products are not irreversibly denatured even while the cells are ruptured, and easy to do at scale.

Except for some mechanical methods such as ball mill (already miniaturized as bead mill or beadbeating) methods and high pressure homogenization methods, which have been applied not only in laboratories but also in industry, the ultrasonic methods and the non-mechanical methods, in general, are still in the stage of laboratory applications, with their industrial applications being limited by many factors, thus people are still looking for new approaches for crushing cells, such as laser-assisted crushing method, high-speed opposite direction impinging（冲击）stream method, cryogenic（低温）jet-spray method and so on.

Cell Disruption and Primary Recovery Methods

The production of biologically-interesting molecules using cloning and culturing methods allows the study and manufacture of relevant molecules. The first step in the purification of a recombinant protein is to harvest it from the cell suspension used in its production.

Except for the case of secretory molecules, cells cultured for producing exogeneous proteins are to be disrupted. In the case of a secretory systems, this means gently removing the cells and recovering the product in the resulting supernatant. However, for intracellular proteins, the cells must first be disrupted. Various methods are used. An overview of some commonly used cell disruption techniques is shown in Table 3-2. Selection of the appropriate method must balance economic and operational considerations with situation involving cell breakage, product release and stability, and the impact on downstream processing. Disruption of prokaryotic and yeast cells at the industrial scale is almost always carried out by one of the mechanical methods, with the most common being solid-shear (bead-mill) and high pressure homogenization. Non-mechanical methods offer a gentler and sometimes more selective alternative that is based on physical, chemical, or enzymatic lysis. However, these methods are typically used only for laboratory experiments or to supplement mechanical disruption.

Table 3-2   Methods for cell disruption in the recovery of intracellular proteins.

Mechanical	Non-Mechanical		
	Physical	**Chemical**	**Enzymatic**
Bead Mill	Osmotic shock	Detergents	Lytic Enzymes
Cryopulverization	"cell bomb"	Chelating Agents	Autolysis
Rotor-stator Processors and blenders	Freeze-thawing	Chaotropes	
Valve-type processors	Thermolysis	Solvents	
Fixed-geometry fluid processors	Freeze-fracturing		
Fixed Orifice and Constant Pressure			
Ultrasonicator			

The primary recovery step constitutes a solid-liquid separation in which the cells and cellular debris are removed from the liquid phase. For soluble proteins, the product is recovered in the liquid medium; however, for inclusion bodies produced by *E. coli*, the insoluble protein fraction must first be differentially recovered from the other cellular solids and then the soluble form of the protein renatured from these inclusion bodies. Primary recovery is typically carried out by centrifugation, sedimentation, filtration, or microfiltration. Flocculation（絮凝）and filter aids are sometimes used to enhance the efficiency of these techniques. The choice of the specific technique and its operating conditions depends on the expression system, the solubility of the expressed protein, and whether or not whole cells or cellular debris are being removed.

Some commonly used cell disruption techniques

Various cell disruption methods have proven useful in releasing biomolecules from inside a cell (Table 3-2).

The cell disruption methods have been widely used in biochemistry, but only on a small scale. For larger scale operations, especially in gene engineering, their application is still limited. The equipment being used is not designed for biotechnology.

In addition to these techniques, **expanded-bed adsorption**（扩张床吸附）[**EBA**, also known as **fluidized bed chromatography**（流化床层析）] has been developed as a way of combining primary recovery with the initial **capture chromatography**（捕获色谱）. In EBA, a distribution of chromatographic particle diameters with varying densities is operated in a fluid field（流场，流体场，流动场），resulting in an expansion of the bed by a factor of two- to three-fold. This expanded bed has a significantly increased void volume, allowing cellular debris and whole-cell broth to move through the column more easily as long as the feed（进料）is diluted to around 10%~15% wet cell weight. Although EBA has been demonstrated at the pilot scale（中试，中试规模），its deployment（部署，展开）in industrial-scale production is still not commonplace due to concerns about fluid distribution, cleaning validation（清洁验证），and chromatographic performance.

Major factors

Several factors must be considered.

Sample size of cells to be disrupted

If only a few milliliters or milligrams of sample are available, care must be taken to minimize loss and avoid cross-contamination. Disruption of microbial cells, when hundreds or even thousands of liters of material are being processed in a production environment, presents different challenges. Here, throughput（某一时期内的生产量），efficiency, and reproducibility are key factors.

Number of samples to be disrupted at one time

Frequently when sample sizes are small [10 mg to 10 g (wet weight)]，methods and equipment are available to process many samples at the same time. Mechanical cell disrupters are available that can batch process 192 samples at a time. Other machines are capable of automated sequential processing of multiple samples. Some issues to consider when processing multiple samples are cross-contamination, speed of processing, equipment availability and cost and ease of cleaning and decontaminating of equipment between cell samples.

Toughness of cells to be disrupted

Some cells are relatively easy to disrupt (*e.g.*, *E. coli*, blood cells, brain tissue). More difficult samples (*e.g.*, yeast, fungi, animal connective tissue), often require increased mechanical power or more aggressive chemical treatments. The most difficult samples (*e.g.*, spores) may require mechanical forces combined with chemical or enzymatic methods. Samples with a strong extracellular matrix, such as animal connective tissue, biopsy samples, venous tissue, cartilage（软骨）, seeds, *etc.*, are often disrupted by impact pulverization（粉碎）in liquid nitrogen. This technique, also known as cell lysis in liquid nitrogen, is based on the fact that samples containing water become very brittle at extremely cold temperatures.

Efficiency of cell disruption method

Disruption conditions may impact the desired product. For example, if subcellular fractionation studies are undertaken, it is often more important to have an optimal yield of intact subcellular components, while sacrificing overall disruption efficiency. In another example, extreme extraction conditions such as high or low pH, heat formation, or the presence of detergents and other denaturing chemicals may increase the yield of disrupted cells but destroy the intracellular component being sought.

For production scale processes, the timing of disruption and the reproducibility of the method become more important factors.

Stability of the molecule(s) or component being isolated

In general, the cell disruption method is closely matched with the material that is desired from the cell studies. It is usually necessary to establish the minimum force of the disruption method that will yield the best product. Additionally, once the cells are disrupted, it is often essential to protect the desired product from biological degradation processes (*e.g.*, proteases), from oxidation or other chemical events and from putrefaction（腐败）.

Purification methods to be used following cell disruption

It is rare that a cell disruption process produces a directly usable material; in almost all cases, subsequent purification events are necessary. Thus, when the cells are disrupted, it is important to consider what components are present in the disruption media so that efficient purification is not impeded.

Is the sample or its cell contents biohazardous?

Preparation of cell-free extracts of pathogens or recombinant cells expressing potentially toxic material presents unique difficulties. Several mechanical disruption techniques are not suitable because of potential biohazard problems associated with the contamination of equipment and the generation of aerosols（雾，悬浮颗粒，气溶胶，气雾剂）during processing.

3.2.4 Methods to break down cell walls（细胞壁的破碎方法）

3.2.4.1 Mechanical methods of cell disruption（机械法）

Mechanical cell disruption is really just that: forcing open the cell wall and spilling（溢漏，泄漏）the contents. The advantage of to mechanical disruption is that no chemicals are introduced that might interfere with the substance you want to extract. The drawback however is that the method has to be carefully adjusted so as not to destroy that molecule of interest.

(1) Mortar and pestle

Cryo-pulverization（冷冻研磨法）

Just give the cells a good old grinding by using mortar（研钵）and pestle（杵，碾槌）. This does not have to be in suspension and is often done with plant samples frozen in liquid nitrogen. When the material has been disrupted, metabolites can be extracted by adding solvents.

Samples with a tough extracellular matrix, such as animal connective tissue, some tumor biopsy samples, venous tissue, cartilage（软骨）, seeds, *etc.*, are reduced to a fine powder by impact pulverization（粉碎，研磨）at liquid nitrogen temperatures. This technique, known as cryo-pulverization, is based on the fact that biological samples containing a significant fraction of water become brittle at extremely cold temperatures. This technique was first described by Smucker and Pfister in 1975, who referred to the technique as cryo-impacting（冷冻冲击法）. The authors demonstrated cells are effectively broken by this method, confirming by phase and electron microscopy that breakage planes cross cell walls and cytoplasmic membranes.

The technique can be carried out using a mortar and pestle cooled to liquid nitrogen temperatures, but the use of this classic apparatus is laborious and sample loss is often a concern. Specialized stainless steel pulverizers（粉碎机，研磨机）generically known as Tissue Pulverizers are also available for this purpose. They require less manual effort, give good sample recovery, and are easy to clean between samples.

The major advantages of this technique are higher yields of proteins and nucleic acids from small, hard tissue samples — especially when used as a preliminary step to mechanical or chemical/solvent cell disruption methods.

(2)Beadbeating method（高速珠磨法）

Another common laboratory-scale mechanical method for cell disruption uses tiny glass, ceramic or steel beads mixed with a sample suspended in aqueous media (Fig. 3-9). Glass or ceramic beads are used to crack open cells — it might not sound like it, but this kind of mechanical shear is gentle enough to keep organelles intact. It can be used with all kinds of cells, just add beads to an equal amount of cell suspension and vortex!

First developed by Tim Hopkins in the late 1970s, the sample and bead mix（混合体）is subjected to high-level agitation by stirring or shaking. Beads collide with the cellular sample, cracking open the cell to release intracellular components. Unlike some other methods, mechanical shear is moderate during homogenization resulting in an excellent membrane or subcellular preparations. The method, often called "beadbeating", works well for all types of cellular material — from spores to animal and plant tissues. It is the most widely used method of yeast lysis and can yield breakage of over 50%. It has the advantage over other mechanical cell disruption methods of being able to disrupt very small sample sizes, process many samples at a time with no cross-contamination concerns, and does not release potentially harmful aerosols in the process.

In the simplest example of the method, an equal volume of beads is added to a cell or tissue suspension in a test tube and the sample is vigorously mixed on a common laboratory vortex（涡旋）mixer. While processing times are slow, taking 3~10 times longer than that in specialty（专用，专门）shaking machines, it works well for easily disrupted cells and is inexpensive.

In most laboratories, beadbeating is done in sealed, plastic vials, centrifuge tubes, or deep well microtiter plates（微量滴定板）. The sample and tiny beads are agitated（摇动）at about 2 000 oscillations（振荡，摆动）per minute in specially designed vial shakers driven by high power electric motors. Cell disruption is complete in 1~3 minutes of shaking. Machines are available that can process hundreds of samples simultaneously inside deep well microplates（微孔板）.

Successful beadbeating is dependent on not only design features of the shaking machine (which take into consideration shaking oscillations per minute, shaking throw (摆度) or distance, shaking orientation and vial orientation), but also the selection of correct bead size (0.1~6 mm diameter), bead composition (glass, ceramic, steel) and bead load in the vial.

All high energy beadbeating machines warm the sample about 10 degrees per minute. This is due to frictional collisions of the beads during homogenization. Cooling of the sample during or after beadbeating may be necessary to prevent damage to heat-sensitive proteins such as enzymes. Sample warming can be controlled by beadbeating for short time intervals with cooling on ice between each interval, by processing vials in pre-chilled aluminum vial holders or by circulating gaseous coolant (冷却剂) through the machine during beadbeating.

A different beadbeater configuration, suitable for larger sample volumes. uses a fluorocarbon rotor inside a 15, 50 or 200 ml chamber to agitate the beads. In this configuration, the chamber can be surrounded by a static cooling jacket. Using the same rotor/chamber configuration, large commercial machines are available to process many liters of cell suspension. Currently, these machines are limited to processing monocellular organisms such as yeast, algae and bacteria.

A number of manufacturers produce machines that can be used for bead beating. These products include the Beadbeater and the FastPrep-24.

Bead/Ball Mill — These mills use small grinding media to act against cells by one of two methods. The DYNO®-MILL and BeadBeater series use agitator discs (阀瓣) inside an enclosed chamber to whip (搅打) the beads into a high-shear frenzy which then collide with the cells and produce breakage. The other mills listed here use a violent shaking action (either side-to-side or up-and-down) to bring about rapid cell disruption.

- DYNO®-MILL
- BeadBeater
- MiniBeadBeater
- Mini-BeadBeater-16
- Mini-BeadBeater-96
- High-Speed Mixer Mill (MM400)

Ball mills and varieties — tracking the archetypes

A ball mill (球磨粉碎机) is a type of grinder used to grind (磨碎，碾) and blend materials for use in mineral dressing processes (选矿生产工艺), paints (油漆，涂料，颜料), pyrotechnics (烟火材料), ceramics (陶瓷) and selective laser sintering (选择性激光烧结).

A ball mill consists of a hollow cylindrical shell rotating about its axis. The axis of the shell may be either horizontal or at a small angle to the horizontal. It is partially filled with balls. The grinding medium is the balls, which may be made of steel (chrome steel 铬钢), stainless steel, flint (燧石) pebbles, ceramic, or rubber. The inner surface of the cylindrical shell is usually lined with an abrasion-resistant material such as manganese steel (锰钢) or rubber. Less wear (磨损) takes place in rubber lined mills. The length of the mill is approximately equal to its diameter.

Ball mills rotate around a horizontal axis, partially filled with the material to be ground plus the grinding medium. Mill rotation speeds are set such that the balls are lifted nearly to the top of the jar before tumbling to the bottom. **It works on the principle of impact and attrition (摩擦)：size reduction**

is done by impact as the balls drop from near the top of the shell. An internal cascading effect（级联效应）reduces the material to a fine powder (Fig. 3-9B).

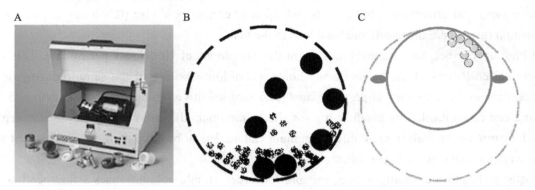

Fig. 3-9   A. Laboratory scale ball mill. B. Illustration of working principle of Ball mill. C. Illustration of working principle of High-energy ball milling.

Large to medium-sized ball mills are mechanically rotated on their axis, but small ones normally consist of a cylindrical capped container that sits on two drive shafts（轴）[pulleys（滑轮）and belts are used to transmit rotary motion]. A rock tumbler（磨石机）functions on the same principle. High-quality ball mills are potentially expensive and can grind mixture particles to as small as 5 nm, enormously increasing surface area and reaction rates.

Industrial ball mills can operate continuously, fed at one end and discharged at the other end. In case of a continuously operated ball mill, the material to be ground is fed from the left through a 60° cone（圆锥体）and the product is discharged through a 30° cone to the right. As the shell rotates, the balls are lifted on the rising side of the shell and then they cascade down (or drop down on to the feed), from near the top of the shell. In doing so, the solid particles in between the balls and ground are reduced in size by impact.

The general idea behind the ball mill is an ancient one, but it was not until the industrial revolution and the invention of steam power that an effective ball mill could be built. It is reported to have been used for grinding flint for pottery in 1870.

The grinding works on the principle of critical speed. Critical speed can be understood as that speed after which the steel balls (which are responsible for the grinding of particles) start rotating along the direction of the cylindrical device; thus causing no further grinding.

There are two kinds of ball mill, grate type（算式，炉排式）and overfall type（溢流型）due to different ways of discharging material. Many types of grinding media are suitable for use in a ball mill, each material having its own specific properties and advantages. Key properties of grinding media are size, density, hardness, and composition.

The grinding chamber can also be filled with an inert shield gas that does not react with the material being ground, to prevent oxidation or explosive reactions that could occur with ambient air inside the mill.

Advantages of the ball mill

Ball milling boasts（拥有）several advantages over other systems: the cost of installation and grinding medium is low; it is suitable for both batch and continuous operation, similarly it is suitable for open as well as closed circuit grinding and is applicable for materials of all degrees of hardness.

Varieties

Aside from common ball mills there is a second type of ball mill called a planetary ball mill (行星式球磨机) (Fig. 3-10). Planetary ball mills are smaller than common ball mills and mainly used in laboratories for grinding sample material down to very small sizes. A planetary ball mill consists of at least one grinding jar (缸) which is arranged eccentrically (离开中心) on a so-called sun wheel. The direction of movement of the sun wheel is opposite to that of the grinding jars (ratio: 1:-2 or 1:-1). The grinding balls in the grinding jars are subjected to superimposed (重叠, 叠加) rotational movements, the so-called Coriolis forces (科里奥力). The difference in speeds

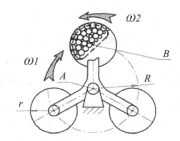

Fig. 3-10   Illustration of working principle of planetary ball mill.

between the balls and grinding jars produces an interaction between frictional and impact forces (冲击力), which releases high dynamic energies (Fig. 3-9C). The interplay between these forces produces the high and very effective degree of size reduction of the planetary ball mill.

High-shear mechanical methods.

High-shear mechanical methods for cell disruption fall into four major classes: rotor-stator disruptors, valve-type processors, fixed-geometry processors and fixed orifice and constant pressure processors. (These fluid processing systems also are used extensively for homogenization and deaggregation of a wide range of materials.) These processors all work by placing the bulk aqueous media under shear forces that literally tear the cells apart. These systems are especially useful for larger-scale laboratory experiments (over 20 ml) and offer the option for large-scale production.

Homogenizer

Homogenizers use shearing forces on the cell similar to the bead method. Homogenization can be performed by squeezing cells through a tube that is slightly smaller than them, thereby shearing away the outer layer (French Press), or by using a rotating blade like in a blender (Rotor-Stator Processors).

(1) *Rotor-Stator Homogenizer* (转子 - 定子式匀浆器)

Rotor-Stator Homogenizers — This type of homogenizer employs a high-speed, tightly fitted rotor inside a many-toothed stator. The samples to be homogenized are drawn into the center of the rotor having been mixed, accelerated and pressed through the narrow gap between the rotor and stator. The Polytron and Tissue Tearor units are batch models and the Megatron is continuous.

➢ Polytron

➢ Megatron

➢ Tissue Tearor

Rotor-stators consist of a fast-spinning inner rotor with a stationary outer sheath (stator) to homogenize samples through mechanical tearing, shear fluid forces, and/or cavitation (气穴现象, 空穴作用) (the rapid forming and collapsing of bubbles). Rotor-stators are broadly capable of homogenizing a wide variety of tissues or cells, although very tough tissue can be a problem. Most rotor-stators homogenize a single sample at a time, although some high-throughput models and continuous in-line (在线的) models are available.

Keep in mind: rotor-stator homogenizers require a probe (探头) to operate and not all rotor-stators come with a probe.

Rotor-stator homogenization uses a rotating metal shaft（轴）— the rotor — inside a stationary metal casing（套管，外壳）— the stator. The rotation of the rotor creates a suction（吸力，抽吸）effect which draws the sample into the space between the rotor and stator, in which it is subject to（使经受，使经历）very high shear forces due to an extreme change in velocity in the small space between the rotor and stator — the laws of fluid mechanics state that the velocity in the fluid immediately adjacent to the rotor is the same as the velocity of the rotor, while the velocity of the fluid immediately adjacent to the stationary stator is zero. Centrifugal forces then push the material out through slots（狭缝）in the stator, and the rapid motion of the fluid caused by the rotor-stator ensures that the process is repeated as the liquid and sample repeatedly cycle through it.

The rotor/stator homogenizer is commonly used for small volumes of tissue suspended in 3 to 10 times its volume of homogenizing media (1~100 ml total). Larger volumes of tissue in homogenization media (100~2000 ml total) are processed either by larger rotor/stator machines or by blade blenders（叶片搅拌机）(often called a drink blender). Both of these homogenizers rely on rotary cutting and/or chopping action using compact blades or paddles turning at speeds of 10 000 to 30 000 rpm.

Benefits & Drawbacks

There are a number of benefits and drawbacks to any instrument which uses a probe to homogenize samples, including rotor-stators. Because you can switch（转换）between probes, the volume range which can be processed is greater than with other methods. There are rotor-stator homogenizers that, using different probes, can homogenize volumes between 30 microliters and 30 liters. Additionally, there is effectively no maximum volume — rotor-stator homogenizers exist for laboratory, pilot（试验的）, and industrial scale applications.

Rotor-stator homogenizers are very fast and efficient for single samples. Because of the use of probes, however, rotor-stator homogenizers are not as well suited for multi-sample, high-throughput applications. If cross-contamination is a concern, the probe must be washed between each use. Some manufacturers who provide packs（一组，一套）of lower-cost probes or disposable, limited-use probes which are intended to allow you to process a number of samples using a different, clean probe each time (such as the PRO Multi-Gen Generator Probes). There are also a number of automated, higher-throughput rotor-stator homogenizers. These are generally more expensive than a bead mill of equivalent throughput（确定时间内的生产量）, but allow for processing larger samples. There are also a number of rotor-stator homogenizers that allow semi-continuous in-line [（生产过程）顺序连接的] processing, and can therefore handle very large volumes. Along with high-pressure homogenizers, these are the only kinds of homogenizers where true industrial-scale units exist.

Other disadvantages include:

➢ Does not work with microorganisms like bacteria, yeast and fungi and most monocellular tissue cultures.

➢ Often variable in product yield.

Tips（秘诀，技巧，小窍门）for Using Rotor-Stator Homogenizers

Rotor-stator homogenizers are very well suited for liquid applications, such as mixing or creating emulsions. They are also very good for breaking open cells and homogenizing relatively soft tissue. If homogenizing solids, keep in mind that the particles need to fit between the rotor and stator to be homogenized. While for soft solids (such as most soft tissue) the suction effect can partially overcome the shape of the tissue, for harder tissue (for example tablets or fibrous tissue) the sample may need to be pre-processed such that the particle size is sufficiently small. Probes with saw-toothed（锯齿状的）heads can help tear apart and break down fibrous samples and many other solids.

For best results with a rotor-stator, the probe should be moved around inside the sample during use. This helps ensure that the sample is uniformly and completely homogenized. It can also help reduce the necessary run time, especially when operating near the maximum operating volume for the instrument.

Rotor-Stators impart a moderate amount of heat into the sample during use, mostly due to frictional forces. If your application is heat-sensitive, consider methods to cool your sample. For most laboratory scale applications, attaching the sample container to a clamp（夹钳，夹器）and placing it in an ice bath is appropriate.

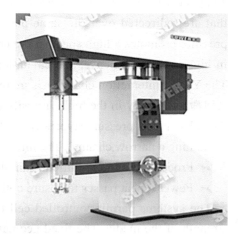

To help maximize the useful life of your probes, ensure they are cleaned after each use. Cleaning the probes in a volatile cleaner, such as 70% ethanol, will help them dry faster.

(2) *Valve-type processors*

A kind of high pressure homogenization technology（高压匀浆法）

Valve-type processors disrupt cells by forcing the media with the cells through a narrow valve under high pressure (20 000~ 30 000 psi or 140~210 MPa). As the fluid flows past the valve, high shear forces in the fluid pull the cells apart. By controlling the pressure and valve tension, the shear force can be regulated to optimize cell disruption. Due to the high energies involved, sample cooling is generally required, especially for samples requiring multiple passes through the system. Two major implementations of the technology exist: batch processors French pressure cell press（挤压设备）and pumped-fluid processors.

The French pressure cell press uses an external hydraulic pump to drive a piston within a larger cylinder that contains the sample. The pressurized solution is then squeezed past a needle valve. Once past the valve, the pressure drops to atmospheric pressure and generates shear forces that disrupt the cells (Fig. 3-11).

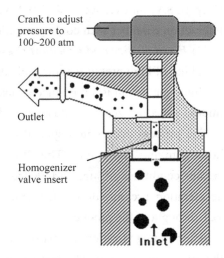

Fig. 3-11   Schematic diagram of a high pressure homogenizer.

Disadvantages include:

➢ Not well suited to larger volume processing.

➢ Awkward to manipulate and clean due to the weight of the assembly (about 30 lb or 14 kg).

Mechanically pumped-fluid processors function by forcing the sample at a constant volume flow past a spring-loaded valve.

Disadvantages include:

> Requires 10 ml or more of media.

> General sample heating. Very high transient heating at valve interface.

> Prone to valve-clogging events.

> Due to variations in the valve setting and seating, less reproducible than fixed-geometry fluid processors.

(3) *Fixed-geometry fluid processors*

A kind of high pressure homogenization technology.

Fixed-geometry fluid processors are marketed under the name of Microfluidizer processors, which is equipped with Y-Type Interaction Chamber. In these chamber, the flow stream is split into two channels that are redirected over the same plane at right angles and propelled into a single flow stream. High pressure promotes a high speed at the crossover（混合，交叉，转线路）of the two flows, which results in high shear, turbulence, and cavitation over the single outbound（向外去的，向外的）flow stream. The Y-type interaction chamber is more powerful than valve and orifice type processors in spite of block （阻滞）tendency in the high viscosity condition. The processors disrupt cells by forcing the media with the cells at high pressure (typically 20 000~30 000 psi or 140~210 MPa) through an interaction chamber containing a narrow channel. The ultra-high shear rates allow for:

> Processing of more difficult samples.

> Fewer repeat passes to ensure optimum sample processing.

The systems permit controlled cell breakage without the need to add detergent or to alter the ionic strength of the media. The fixed geometry of the interaction chamber ensures reproducibility. Especially when samples are processed multiple times, the processors require sample cooling. The Microfluidics Corp (USA) and Genizer LLC (USA) are two providers for Y-type interaction chamber. The Y-type interaction chamber with cooling function are provided by Genizer LLC (USA).

(4) *Fixed Orifice and Constant Pressure*

A kind of high pressure homogenization technology.

Homogenization is a fluid mechanical process that involves the subdivision of particles or droplets into micron（微米）sizes to create a stable dispersion（分散）or emulsion for further processing.

The process occurs in a special homogenizing valve（阀）, the design of which is the heart of the homogenizing equipment. The fluid passes through a minute gap in the homogenizing valve. This creates conditions of high turbulence（湍流）and shear（剪切）, combined with compression（挤压）, acceleration, pressure drop, and impact. Causing the disintegration（崩解）of particles and dispersion（分散）throughout the product.

After homogenization, the particles are of a uniform size, typically from 0.2 to 2 micron, depending on the operating pressure. The homogenizer（匀浆器）is the most efficient device for particle and droplet size reduction. The actual properties of the product vary with pressure and product type in a complex relationship. In general, higher processing pressure produces smaller particles, down to a certain limit of micronization（微粉化）.

Constant Cell Disruption Systems by Constant Systems part of Score Group plc — these systems are fully contained and operate using a finely controlled hydraulic system powered by electricity only. The sample is taken in and instantly pressurized up to a maximum of 40 000 psi before being passed through a very small and fixed orifice and then returned to atmospheric pressure. As the sample is being processed this type of cell disruptor ensures that the pressure is maintained throughout the process, ensuring repeatability throughout the sample run.

Both fluid and non fluid samples can be processed through this type of cell disruptor, plant leaves and skin samples being a good example of non fluid samples. Having a maximum process pressure achievable of 40 000 psi enables this type of unit to process more difficult sample types with fewer repeat passes. A built-in cooling jacket ensures temperature control of the sample (Water Bath or Chiller Unit is required) .

High Pressure Homogenizer — Both these units utilize high pressure to burst (使爆裂) cell walls. The French Press G-M™ uses a hydraulic press and carefully machined (精心加工的) pressure cells (压力受感装置) to produce pressures up to 40 000 psi. The MicroMincer is a small hand operated unit.

- French Press G-M™
- Micro Mincer

(5) *High pressure extrusion method* (高压挤压法)

X-press〔X-press 法〕

X-press is a kind of instrument that exploits the phase-changes in ice under pressure for the disintegration (碎裂) of cells in the frozen state. By forcing the frozen cells contained in a cylinder through a hole much smaller than the diameter of the cylinder but much larger than the size of the cells, a satisfactory disintegration can be obtained. It has been named the "X-press", originally because it was a purely experimental press (压榨机，压力机) but later also because of the rapidity (快捷) of disintegration (=express).

The X-press consists of two heavy-walled steel cylinders, which were separated by a disc with a central hole (or several holes), of which may be of different sizes, and held together by a threaded ring (螺纹环) or bolts (Fig. 3-12).

The material to be disintegrated is forced from the frozen state through this hole. By moving the piston, on which pressure is applied, from one chamber to the other, the material could be pressed through the hole in one or other direction.

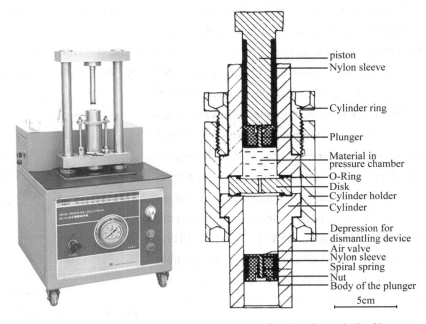

Fig. 3-12   An X-press and its schematic diagram. Section through the X-press.

In the standard X-press the material to be disintegrated can be freeze-pressed several times by simply inverting the press after each press cycle. By forcing the cells through the hole repeatedly rather than once, a higher degree of disintegration can be achieved. By making the receiver identical to the charge chamber, repeated operations are possible without uncoupling the press. While repeated pressings not only increased the disintegration with regard to the percentage of cells disrupted but also the degree of disintegration of the cellular constituents.

Usually the disintegration process has been performed at around −25°C with a standard X-press (1976), since an increase in temperature above −25°C seemed to reduce the disintegration effect, whereas more extensive disintegration is achieved by a lower temperature, −35°C, and by a high velocity of flow through the orifice, such that more than 95% of the *S. cerevisiae* is disrupted by one pressing at less than 2×10^8 Pa.

The freeze-pressing technique has found a wide application for the disintegration of biological material, such as microorganisms (*i.e.*, bacteria, yeasts, moulds) and other different cells (plant and animal cells) and tissues.

The Freeze-Pressing Process

Before freeze-pressing, the press was precooled to the desired temperature in an alcohol bath and then filled with material. Then it was temperature equilibrated either by reimmersing it in the alcohol bath or by circulating alcohol around it. The pressure was generated with a hydraulic jack or a motor-driven pump and applied directly via a piston to the specimens. By moving the piston forward toward the sample, the latter was extruded through the hole in the disc. With manual pumping the speed of the piston was 0.02~0.03 cm/sec and with motor-pumping, 0.9~1.0 cm/sec.

The pressing operation was performed by increasing the pressure until suddenly, at a certain pressure, depending on the hole(s) and the temperature, a loud crack was heard and some material flowed through the hole(s) and the pressure fell. The pressure was then again increased and the procedure repeated until all the material had been forced through the hole. In those cases where it was considered desirable to force the material through the hole(s) of the disc many times, the large piston was moved to the hole on the other side of the press which was turned upside-down.

At first (1951~1960), it was suggested that shearing forces, phase transition, pressure gradient or all of the three mentioned above participate(s) disintegration in the X-press, with crystal transformations of the water, actually ice I, being the main determinant of flow in the X-press (1960). Experiments in the following years (1973~1977) have substantiated the phase transition story and indicated that the flow of material is preceded and initiated by a liquid state of the specimen in the vicinity of the hole, where the stress concentrations are greatest, and the phase transitions (*e.g.*, from ice I to liquid and/or ice III) may be induced even between −25 °C and −35°C (1974, 1976) (Fig. 3-13). Whereas internal friction or shear, the grinding effect of ice crystals, which increases at lower temperatures, and increasing cell concentrations, is another main cause of cell disruption.

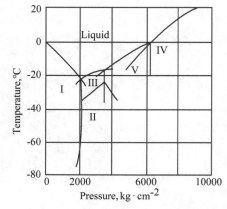

Fig. 3-13　A part of the phase diagram of water in the liquid-solid region.

For the disruption of larger quantities of cells (microorganisms and other biological), a semicontinuous X-press has been constructed. At a sample temperature of −35℃ and a press temperature of −20℃, about 90% disruption is achieved in a single passage of undiluted baker's yeast (*Saccharomyces cerevisiae*, 270 mg/g) through the orifice of the pressure chamber, with this press about 10 kg of material can be freeze-presses per hour.

Concerning that the degree of disintegration would be increased by repeated pressing in a standard X-press, whereas the same strategy could not be used in a semicontinuous X-press, the procedure had been optimized with regard to the temperature at freeze-pressing, the concentration of biological material in the sample to be freeze-pressed, the dimensions of the pressure cylinder, and the hole of the disc, to achieve the same degree of disruption of biological material **in a single passage** of the orifice of the pressure chamber.

The general mechanisms shown for the standard X-press were recognized with this semicontinuous press. The flow of material is preceded by phase changes into liquid, initiated in the vicinity of the orifice. Such phase changes also seem to occur in this semicontinuous press.

The extrusion ratios, *i.e.*, the ratio between the diameter of the pressure cylinder and the hole, are designed to be around 8 and 40 for the larger and narrower hole, respectively, with a value of 11 (obtained with a hole diameter of 2.5 mm) for the standard X-press. Since the extrusion ratio to a large extent (在很大程度上) determines the velocity field and the strain rate (应变率，应变速率) distribution, one may expect similar disruption efficiency. Further stepping-up (增加，递升) of the freeze-pressing process by using pressure chambers of great diameters might, therefore, make still wider orifices (5 mm or above) convenient.

Sonication method（超声破碎法）— deflation（放气）with sonication

Another common laboratory-scale method for cell disruption applies ultrasound (typically 20~50 kHz) to the sample (*sonication*).

Sonication is the act of applying sound (usually ultrasound) energy to agitate（搅动）particles in a sample, for various purposes. In biological applications, sonication may be sufficient to disrupt（破坏）or deactivate a biological material. For example, sonication is often used to disrupt cell membranes and release cellular contents. This process is called sonoporation（声孔效应）.

In principle, the high-frequency is generated electronically and the mechanical energy is transmitted to the sample via a metal probe that oscillates（振荡）with high frequency. The probe is placed into the cell-containing sample and the high-frequency oscillation causes a localized low pressure region resulting in cavitation（空穴现象）and impaction（碰撞，冲击），ultimately breaking open the cells.

Ultrasonic homogenizers work by inducing vibration in a titanium（钛）probe that is immersed in the cell solution. A process called cavitation occurs, in which tiny bubbles are formed and explode, producing a local shockwave（冲击波）and disrupting cell walls by pressure change. This method is very popular for plant and fungal cells but comes at a disadvantage: It's very loud and has to be performed in an extra room, otherwise you will be very unpopular.

Ultrasonic Liquid Processor — High frequency oscillations of a piezoelectric（压电的）crystal are translated into very small movements of a submerged probe. As the probe moves in it "pushes" the sample away, as it moves in a void（空隙）is created which collapses and creates localized cavitation. This cavitation causes rapid homogenization of many types of cells. The Sonicator is a batch model and the Sonitube is continuous.

➢ Sonicator

➢ Sonitube

Although the basic technology was developed over 50 years ago, newer systems permit cell disruption in smaller samples (including multiple samples under 200 μl in microplate wells) and with an increased ability to control ultrasonication parameters.

Disadvantages include:

➢ Heat generated by the ultrasound process must be dissipated（散逸）.

➢ High noise levels [most systems require hearing protection and sonic enclosures（围隔）].

➢ Yield variability.

➢ Free radicals are generated that can react with other molecules.

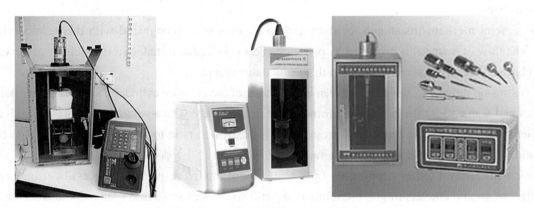

Ultrasonicator （超声发生器，超声破碎仪）

3.2.4.2　*Non-mechanical cell disruption methods*（非机械法）

Non-mechanical methods involve the addition of enzymes or chemicals that specifically break down cell wall components. They are often used in combination with mechanical force to ensure complete disruption of the cell. The disadvantage to their use is that they often have to be removed from the sample afterwards.

Physical

1. Osmotic shock（渗透冲击）

Osmotic shock or osmotic stress（渗透胁迫）is a sudden change in the solute concentration around a cell, causing a rapid change in the movement of water across its cell membrane. Under conditions of high concentrations of either salts, substrates or any solute (*e.g.*, glycerol or sucrose) in the supernatant, water is drawn out of the cells through osmosis（渗透，渗透作用）. This also inhibits the transport of substrates and cofactors into the cell thus "shocking" the cell. Alternatively, at low concentrations of solutes, water enters the cell in large amounts, causing it to swell and either burst or undergo apoptosis (Fig. 3-14).

All organisms have mechanisms to respond to osmotic shock, with sensors and signal transduction networks providing information to the cell about the osmolarity（渗量，容积渗克分子浓度）of its surroundings, these signals activate responses to deal with extreme conditions. Although single-celled organisms are more vulnerable to osmotic shock, as they are directly exposed to their environment, cells in large animals such as mammals still suffer（承受）these stresses under some conditions.

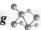

Calcium acts as one of the primary regulators of osmotic stress. Intracellular calcium levels rise during hypo-osmotic and hyper-osmotic stresses. During hyper-osmotic stress extracellular albumin (白蛋白) binds calcium.

This method only applies to cells with vulnerable cell wall, cells treated with some enzymes, or with some inhibitors (*e.g.*, antibiotics) during cell culturing, hence became defective and fragile.

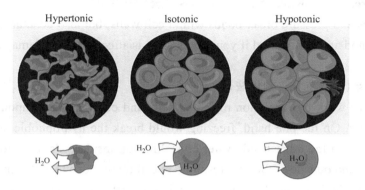

Fig. 3-14　Principle of Osmotic shock.

Mild Lysis

For easily disrupted cells such as blood cells and insect or animal cells grown in culture media, a mild osmosis-based method for cell disruption (lysis) is commonly used. Quite frequently, simply lowering the ionic strength of the media will cause the cells to swell and burst. In some cases it is also desirable to add a mild surfactant and some mild mechanical agitation to completely disassociate (使分离) the cellular components. Because these mild lytic methods are performed under chemically mild conditions, they are often used for subcellular fractionation (分级分离) studies.

Most biological cells are more difficult to disrupt. This includes most bacteria, yeast, algae and many plant and animal tissues. In these cases, mild lysis methods such as osmotic shock are insufficient to open the cell. Further, cost and relative effort to grow and harvest these cells, combined with the often small quantity of cells available to process, have favored cell disruption methods utilizing laboratory-scale manual mechanical devices such as bead mills (beadbeaters), rotor-stator homogenizers, ultrasonicators or high pressure homogenizers.

'Cell bomb'

Another laboratory-scale system for cell disruption is rapid decompression (解压, 降压) or the "cell bomb" method. In this process, cells in question are placed under high pressure (usually nitrogen or other inert gas up to about 25 000 psi) and the pressure is released rapidly. The rapid pressure drop causes the dissolved gas to be released as bubbles that ultimately lyse the cell.

Disadvantages include:

Only easily disrupted cells can be effectively disrupted [stationary phase (静止期，稳定期) *E. coli*, yeast, fungi, and spores do not disrupt well by this method].

Large scale processing is not practical.

High gas pressures have a high risk of personal hazard if not handled carefully.

2. Thermolysis (热裂解)

Thermolysis method is used to disrupt *E. coli* cells to release recombinant thermostable proteins/

peptides. Heat treatment of *E. coli* is highly effective to destroy the integrity of bacterial cell walls and release recombinant thermostable proteins/peptides at temperatures above 60℃. The most effective temperature for cell disruption was at 80℃, while the pH and cell concentration have only minor effect on the release of the thermostable proteins/peptides. In addition, the recombinant proteins/peptides could be purified at the early stage of the thermolysis, which is a major advantage of the thermolysis method.

High temperatures (Microwave, Autoclave) （高压蒸汽灭菌器）

High temperatures and pressure break bonds within cell walls, but also denature proteins. Although it is quick, you better find another method if your application is affected by the damage heat does to the rest of the cell.

3. Freeze-thawing （反复冻结 - 融化法）

Freeze-thaw cycles work by formation of ice crystals and cell expansion upon thawing, ultimately leading to cell rupture. On the one hand, freezing would break the hydrophobic bonds in the structure of plasma membrane. On the other hand, water crystallization inside cells leads to changes of solution concentrations inside and outside of the cell, resulting in cell rupture due to cell expansion.

Freeze-thawing method is usually used for algae and soft plant material, and suitable for some microbes with a fragile cell wall. The drawback is that it is very time-consuming. The broken rate is usually low, thus repetition of freeze-thaw cycles is needed. Furthermore, those cycles tend to cause denaturation of some proteins.

Chemical Cell Disintegration Techniques

Chemical permeabilization method （化学渗透法）

Chemical permeabilization works by using some chemicals to disassemble （分解） cell wall, solubilize membranes and/or denature proteins, bringing about release of some bioactive constituents out of these cells and harvest them.

Some chemicals [*e.g.*, organic solvents, chaotropes （离液剂，离散剂）, surfactants, antibiotics, metal chelator, *etc.*] are capable of changing the permeability of cell wall or cell plasma membrane, thus the constituents in a cell can diffuse out of the cell selectively. The resulting average pore size and pore number vary according to the type and concentration of the chemicals used, and the nature of the organisms (with different structure and composition of cell wall and plasma membrane) being treated (Table 3-3).

Table 3-3　Different chemical penetration enhancers can be adopted for different kind of cells
（不同细胞可采用的化学渗透处理方式）

Cell Types	Chaotropes/ Denaturants 变性剂	Surfactants/ Detergents 清洁剂	Organic Solvents 有机溶剂	Enzymes 酶	Antibiotics 抗生素	Biological reagents/ Bioreagents 生物试剂	Chelating Agents 螯合剂
G⁻ Bacteria	*	*	*	*	*		*
G⁺ Bacteria		*	*	*			
Yeast Cells	*	*	*	*	*	*	
Plant Cells		*	*		*	*	
Macrophages		*	*			*	

* represent "being applicable"

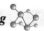

Chemical permeabilization can be classified as cell membrane **solubilization approaches** （增溶法） and cell membrane **lipid dissolution approaches** （脂溶法）. Solubilization approaches are to use the solubilization effects of some chemicals such as surfactants, chelating agents, chaotropes to increase the permeability of the cell walls and plasma membrane, causing the cellular contents to leak out. While lipid dissolution approaches utilize the interaction between some organic solvents such as toluene （甲苯） and octanol （辛醇） and lipids on the cell wall and cell membrane to make the cells swell and then disrupt.

It is very possible to disrupt a biological sample using nothing more than water and a blender （搅拌器）. This would be considered a mechanical approach to sample disruption. However, most methods use lysis buffers/solutions instead of water as they provide a degree of stability when isolating specific biomolecules. Virtually all lysis solutions address （考虑处理） pH (which is why they are usually called lysis buffers) but they may also control ionic strength, osmotic strength （渗透浓度，克分子渗透压浓度）, and the activity of nucleases and proteases. When isolating membrane proteins, surfactants are normally used to partition the membrane proteins from the membrane to surfactant particles, called micelles （胶束，胶团）. Other common lysis buffer additives include lytic enzymes, that which can liberate cellular contents from cell wall envelopes, and chaotropes that disrupt the ordered structure of biological systems which protects biomolecules from enzymatic degradation.

Lysis buffers in many instances can be used to lyse cells and tissues without the assistance of mechanical homogenizers. Indeed one of the most common disruption methods relies on lysing *Escherichia coli* with an alkaline solution of SDS (the detergent sodium dodecylsulfate，十二烷基硫酸钠) for plasmid isolation. Similarly, adherent tissue culture cells （贴壁组织培养细胞） can be lysed with high concentrations of chaotropic guanidine （胍） salts [*e.g.*, chloride or isothiocyanate （异硫氰酸盐）]. For solid and resilient （有弹力的） samples, lysis buffers are commonly used in combination with a mechanical disruption method. This is particularly true for tissues that are very dense, like organs （脏器，器官） and seeds. Some microorganisms which are resistant to chemical and enzymatic lysis, such as members of the genus *Mycobacterium* （分支杆菌）, must also be disrupted mechanically.

Other additives protect liberated biomolecules from denaturation, oxidation and enzymatic degradation. Reducing agents protect free thiol groups from oxidation, especially cysteine located in the active site. Protease inhibitors are regularly added to prevent protein degradation by proteases released from cells during homogenization.

The most commonly used chemical lysis methods include the use of detergents, such as Triton-X, SDS, *etc.*, and chaotropic agents, such as guanidinium thiocyanate (GUSCN), guanidine hydrochloride (GUHCL), ethanol, *etc.*

(1) *Detergents*

Detergent-based lysis is the easiest and mildest form for cell lysis. Detergents disrupt the lipid bilayer surrounding cells by solubilizing proteins and disrupting lipid-protein interactions. This solubilization and disrupting might contribute to cell lysis, and facilitate some constituents of cells to solubilize. Triton X-100, a nonionic detergent, has strong affinity towards hydrophobic constituents. It can bind phospholipids, dissolve them, destroy phospholipid bilayer of the inner membrane, resulting in release of the intracellular contents out of the cells. Other surfactants, *e.g.*, sodium taurocholate (ST) （牛磺胆酸钠）, SDS, can also be used to disrupt cells.

Detergent-based cell lysis is an alternative to physical disruption of cell membranes, although it is sometimes used in conjunction with homogenization and mechanical grinding. Detergents disrupt the lipid barrier surrounding cells by disrupting lipid : lipid, lipid : protein and protein : protein interactions. The ideal detergent for cell lysis depends on cell type and source and on the downstream applications following cell lysis. Animal cells, bacteria and yeast all have differing requirements for optimal lysis due to the presence or absence of a cell wall. Because of the dense and complex nature of animal tissues, they require both detergent and mechanical lysis to effectively lyse cells.

Surfactants（表面活性剂）, which are commonly called detergents（清洁剂，去垢剂）, have the characteristic of disrupting the distinct（明显的，明确的）interface between hydrophobic and hydrophilic systems. Biological membranes, the most obvious hydrophobic/hydrophilic interfaces, are the primary target of detergents. Indeed with the example of *E. coli* and SDS, the detergent completely (and effectively) obliterates（消除，除去）the distinct interface separating the cell from its environment, *i.e.*, the membrane. However, SDS also has the ability to unfold (denature) cytosolic proteins and partition membrane proteins into small detergent droplets (micelles). Depending upon the detergent used and its concentration, the impact these surfactants have on biological systems will vary greatly.

Detergents have at least two fundamental properties, namely a water soluble hydrophilic head and a hydrophobic (oil soluble) tail. These properties allow detergents to insert into and then disperse membranes, in addition to unfolding proteins. Depending upon the chemical makeup（组成）of the hydrophilic and hydrophobic ends its action on proteins and membranes will vary. Not all surfactants are chemically equal as some are capable of completely solubilizing（使溶解，使增溶）membranes and denaturing proteins while others, like mild surfactants, will disassociate loosely bound proteins (Table 3-4).

Table 3-4　Detergents used for sample preparation and their properties.

Detergent	Type	Characteristics	Use Level
SDS (sodium dodecylsulfate)	Anionic	Strong detergent used to disrupt membranes and denature proteins	Commonly used between 1%~10%
Sodium Deoxycholate	Anionic	Derived from bile salts. Effective at solubilizing proteins and disrupting protein-protein interactions	Common use level is 0.5%
CTAB (cetyltrimethylammonium bromide) 溴化十二烷基三甲烷	Cationic	Popular cationic detergent used for the isolation of DNA from plants. Polysaccharides associated with plants are insoluble in CTAB and high concentrations of NaCl. This can be used to effectively separate DNA from plant carbohydrates	For DNA isolation buffers, typical use level is 2%
NP-40 (nonyl phenoxypolyethoxyl ethanol) 壬基苯氧基聚羟乙基乙醇	Non-ionic	Generally mild surfactant which can dissolve cytoplasmic membranes but not nuclear membranes. Useful for isolating nuclei	Use at 0.1% to 1%
Nonidet P-40 (octylphenoxy polyethoxyethanol) 诺乃清洁剂 P-40，辛基苯氧基聚羟乙基乙醇	Non-ionic	This mild surfactant is useful for disrupting cytoplasmic membranes of cultures cells, but lacks the strength to emulsify nuclear membranes. Consequently it can be used to harvest cytoplasmic proteins and analytes	Use at 0.1% to 1%
Triton X-100	Non-ionic	This is a mild surfactant/surfactant that has polyethylene oxide as a hydrophilic group and a tetramethylbutyl phenyl group as the hydrophobic portion	For lysis solutions, up to 5%. In wash solutions, 0.1%~0.5%

continued

Detergent	Type	Characteristics	Use Level
Polysorbate 20 [Tween 20, Polyoxyethylene (20) sorbitan monolaurate] 聚山梨醇酯 20，吐温 20，去水山梨糖醇月桂醇酯聚乙二醇 20	Non-ionic	This surfactant is a heavily modified sorbitol in which polyoxyethylenes serve as the hydrophilic group and a 12 carbon lauric acid as the hydrophobic end. It is a very biomolecule friendly surfactant, being used in foods, pharmaceuticals, and in wash solutions for assays	

Detergents are comprised of a polar hydrophilic head and a nonpolar hydrophobic tail. The nature of the head group is used to categorize the detergent as either ionic (cationic or anionic), nonionic, or zwitterionic. Nonionic detergents (such as the Triton-X series) and zwitterionic detergents (such as CHAPS) are less denaturing than ionic detergents and retain native protein functions. Ionic detergents (such as SDS) are strong solubilizing agents and tend to denature proteins.

A major characteristic of surfactants is whether the hydrophilic group is ionic or non-ionic. Ionic surfactants tend to be better at solubilizing membranes and denaturing proteins. With ionic surfactants, the hydrophilic moiety is typically a sulfate or carboxylic group for anionic surfactants or ammonium group for cationic surfactants. SDS, is an anionic detergent with a sulfate hydrophilic head and 12 carbon tail [dodecyl（十二烷基）or lauryl（月桂基，十二烷基）] which is important not only in the lab but also in many household detergents. Sodium deoxycholate（脱氧胆酸钠）is a carboxylic（羧基的）based anionic detergent derived from bile salts（胆汁盐）which is commonly used in many lysis buffers. CTAB [cetyltrimethylammonium bromide（溴化十六烷基三甲铵）] is a cationic detergent widely used in the isolation of DNA from plants.

In addition to detergents with a net charge, zwitterionic（两性离子的，兼性离子的）detergents are a class of surfactants that possess both anionic and cationic groups and have a net charge of zero. The zwitterionic detergent CHAPS（3-〔3-（胆酰胺基丙基）二甲氨基〕丙磺酸内盐），a derivative of cholic acid（胆酸），is effectively used for isolating membrane proteins.

Non-ionizing detergents have a head which is polar, but uncharged, such as a glycoside（糖苷）(sugar) or polyethylene chain, tend to be milder and less likely to denature proteins, but still capable of dispersing（分散，使散开）some membranes. They often act to dissociate loosely interacting molecules. These surfactants, such as Triton X-100, Brij-35, NP-40 and Nonidet P-40, are widely used in immunoassay wash solutions at low concentrations, but also in lysis buffers at higher concentrations.

The value of detergents when applied to isolating membrane proteins is related to their ability to form micelles. In aqueous environments and at the correct concentrations, detergents will spontaneously form small particles called micelles where the hydrophilic heads orient outward and the hydrophobic tails congregate inwards. The concentration at which this occurs is called "critical micelle concentration" or CMC. Depending upon the detergent, the molecular weight of the micelles can range from 1 200 to 80 000 daltons.

Micelles dissolve into and disrupt cell membranes which then disperse into membrane/micelle hybrids particles. Proteins embedded in cellular membranes are picked up by these micelles. A constant equilibrium between monomer detergent molecules and micelles ideally lead to a dispersion of membrane proteins so that each micelle contains one protein. For protein purification, the protein/micelle acquires characteristics which allow it to be separated from other membrane proteins/micelles.

In general, nonionic and zwitterionic detergents are milder, resulting in less protein denaturation upon cell lysis, than ionic detergents and are used to disrupt cells when it is critical to maintain protein function or interactions. CHAPS, a zwitterionic detergent, and the Triton X series of nonionic detergents are commonly used for these purposes. In contrast, ionic detergents are strong solubilizing agents and tend to denature proteins, thereby destroying protein activity and function. SDS, an ionic detergent that binds to and denatures proteins, is used extensively for studies assessing protein levels by gel electrophoresis and Western blotting.

Detergents and their use are application specific and not always predictable.

In addition to the choice of detergent, other important considerations for optimal cell lysis include the buffer, pH, ionic strength and temperature. Salts, chelating agents [e.g., EDTA), and reducing agents (e.g., dithiothreitol (DTT)] can be added for more efficient lysis.

(2) *Chelators*（EDTA 螯合剂）

EDTA can be used specifically to disrupt the outer membrane of Gram-negative bacteria, which contain lipopolysaccharides and various proteins that are stabilized by cations like Mg^{2+} and Ca^{2+}. EDTA would chelate those cations, resulting in some lipopolysaccharides falling off, leaving holes on the outer cell envelop membrane. Some phospholipids on the inner membrane (plasma membrane) will leave there to fill in those holes on the outer cell envelop membrane, while in this way the permeability of the plasma membrane will increase.

(3) *Chaotropes*（离液剂）

Chaotropes are strong protein denaturants and induce cell permeabilization by weakening the hydrophobic interactions of the membrane. In case of bacterial cells, chaotropic agents also inhibit the assembly of cross-linked peptidoglycans in the cell wall.

Where surfactants are used to disrupt the interface between hydrophobic and hydrophilic systems, chaotropes are used to disrupt the weak interactions between molecules, like hydrogen bonding in water and hydrophobic interactions between proteins. By interacting with hydrogen bonding in water and weakening the hydrophobic interaction between any solutes (*e.g.*, protein molecule), chaotropes can facilitate the dissolution of hydrophobic compounds in an aqueous solution. Chaotropes are effective at denaturing proteins that can cause havoc（大破坏）on freshly homogenized samples, which is the rationale（基本原理）for adding chaotropes to RNA lysis buffers. Common chaotropes used in lysis buffers include sodium iodide, guanidine hydrochloride, guanidine isothiocyanate（异硫氰酸胍）, and urea.

Unlike surfactants which are used at relatively low concentrations, chaotropes are used at high molarities（摩尔浓度）. Guanidine salts, used extensively for RNA isolation, is used at 6 M concentrations. Sodium iodide, which at times is used like guanidine, is also used at 6 M. Urea is often used at 8 M or 9.5 M. Very often chaotropes are used in combination with detergents so that biological systems can not only be denatured, but emulsified as well.

Chaotropes are widely used and applicable to nucleic acid isolation procedures which use silica based resins/gels for purification. Nucleic acids liberated from tissues lysed（溶解）in chaotropic agents, such as 6 M guanidine, supplemented with Proteinase K [an unusually hearty（强健的）protease that is active in both denaturing conditions and elevated temperatures] will adsorb to silica gel upon the addition of ethanol. The very clean nucleic acids can be eluted with water or TE buffer.

(4) *Organic solvents* (有机溶剂)

Solvent Use

Organic solvents like alcohols, ether, benzene, methylbenzene, dimethylbenzene or chloroform can disrupt the cell wall by permeabilizing (使通透性增加) cell walls and membranes. They are capable of dissociating the lipids (类脂) in cell walls, therefore make the cytoplasmic membrane swell and finally the cell burst, releasing intracellular contents. It is a simple and rapid method for disruption of bacteria for protein studies. They are especially handy if you want to extract hydrophobic molecules (like plant pigments) because they can be collected in a solvent. Organic solvents are often applied on plants in combination with shearing forces.

Advantages and disadrantages of chemical permeabilization (化学渗透法优缺点)

This method has some selectivity in product releasing. Low-molecular-mass solutes such as peptides and low-molecular-mass enzymes would diffuse out of the cell through the pores formed on the fragile lipid bilayer, whereas high-molecular-mass substances such as nucleic acids would remain in the cell.

Using this approach, the cell morphology would remain almost intact, with reduced debris and cell lysate viscosity, thus it would be handy to do the liquid-solid separation and further extraction.

Shortcomings primarily include its poor universality and its inefficiency. The releasing rate for intracellular contents is usually no more than 50%. And it is time-consuming. Meanwhile, some proteins would be denatured. Furthermore, some of the solvents applied are poisonous.

Biological disruption techniques — Enzymatic method (生物破碎法 —— 酶溶法)

1. Addition of exogenous lytic enzymes (外加酶)

Another common method for disrupting microbial cell walls is the enzymatic digestion of cell walls (*e.g.*, using lysozymes to hydrolyze the polysaccharide component of the bacterial cell wall).

The use of enzymatic methods to remove cell walls is well-established for cell disruption, for preparation of protoplasts (原生质体) (cells without cell walls) and for other uses such as introduction of cloned DNA into living cells or subcellular organelle isolation. The enzymes are generally commercially available and, in most cases, were originally isolated from biological sources [*e.g.*, snail gut enzymes (蜗牛肠酶) and lysozyme from hen egg white].

When it comes to enzymatic cell disruption, appropriate enzymes must be selected according to the structure and chemical composition of the cell wall and the corresponding order of steps should also be determined. Depending on what organism you work with, that can be cellulases (纤维素酶，木纤维质酵素), chitinases (几丁质酶，壳多糖酶), bacteriolytic enzymes (细菌溶解酶) like lysozymes (destroys peptidoglycans), mannase (甘露聚糖酶), glycanases (聚糖酶). The most commonly used enzymes also include lysostaphin (溶葡球菌素，溶葡球菌酶), zymolase (消解酶，溶细胞酶), mutanolysin (变溶菌素), lyticase (溶壁酶，溶细胞酶), proteases, *etc*. Naturally occurring enzymes can be used to remove the cell wall specifically, for example when preparing the protoplast.

Enzymatic treatment of tissues and cells can be a very effective first step in processes where cell walls and extracellular matrices may introduce unwanted contaminants into a cell lysate. On the one hand, primary hepatocytes can be generated from sacrificed rats where the liver has been perfused (灌注) with a combination of trypsin and collagenase. This allows for the harvesting of viable, intact cells from a tissue that releases vast amounts of proteolytic enzymes when homogenized mechanically. Similarly, yeast cells can be treated with cell wall degrading enzymes to yield protoplasts (naked cells) and cell wall shells, or what is commonly referred to as ghosts（空胞，菌蜕）. This is a common step in traditional transformation procedures used with yeast, but it can also be used to selectively harvest periplasmic enzymes, cell wall mannans or similar component.

Proteases are used in sample disruption to disaggregate tissues and release individual cells, or in the case of genomic DNA isolation, attack other proteins that may either bind up the DNA (histones) or threaten the final product (nucleases). Proteases such as trypsin, dispase（分散酶，中性蛋白酶）, and collagenase are used to release cells from tissues and culture plates（培养皿）. However outside of this application, they are undesirable in disrupting samples as they also degrade receptors and other surface proteins. Proteinase K is extensively used in DNA isolation as it is resistant to SDS and heat, both of which are used in the typical genomic DNA isolation procedure.

Highly specific lytic enzymes are very useful in sample preparation protocols. With plant, yeast, and molds, cell wall degrading enzymes can be used to either rupture cells in hypertonic buffers or generate protoplasts in isotonic（等渗的）lysis buffers. Most cell wall degrading enzyme preparations are a complex of several enzymes as cells walls are typically composed of a mixture of polymers. Yeast cell walls contain glucans and mannans, molds contain chitin, glucan, and galactomannans（半乳甘露聚糖）, and plants have a combination of cellulose and xylans（木聚糖）.

Enzyme-containing cell lysis solutions require a (proper) buffer at a minimum. When it comes to generating protoplasts, cells are typically treated with buffered enzyme in the presence of an osmotic（渗透性的，渗透的）stabilizer, such as 1 M sorbitol（山梨醇）. The enzymes tend to degrade the cell wall components leaving some holes which then allow the protoplast to escape. Gentle centrifugation of protoplasts allows for the separation of empty shells from the cell membrane and its contents. This can be an effective method of separating periplasmic enzymes from other cell associated proteins.

When enzymatic methods are applied to yeast cells, protease(s) were supposed to be firstly added to act on the protein part of mannoproteins in the outermost layer of the cell wall to let them dissociate from the cell wall, then glucanase(s)（葡聚糖酶）added to act on the naked glucan layers, and finally a change of osmotic pressure would act on the protoplasts, rupture the plasma membrane and release the intracellular products. Likewise, plants can be treated with cellulases to yield protoplast while filamentous fungi can be treated with chitinase(s).

Advantages（酶溶法的优点）:

Comparing with that of mechanical methods, the exogenous cell wall lytic enzyme methods possess advantages such as mild lysis conditions; less release of nucleic acids, improved cell integrity, and recombinant products can be selectively released.

Disadvantages:

Firstly, since cell wall lytic enzymes are expensive, large scale applications of lytic enzymes tend to be costly; Besides, enzymatic cell disruption has poor universality, different enzymes should be chosen for different strains; Furthermore, the process is not always reproducible. Hence, enzymatic cell disruption is not usually applicable to large scale.

Secondly, the phenomena known as product inhibition, is a bottleneck to efficient biomass breakdown.

During cell disruption processes, mannose inhibits proteases and dextran inhibits glucanases（葡聚糖酶）.

In addition to potential issues with the enzyme stability, the susceptibility of the cells to the enzyme is dependent on the metabolic profile of the cells. For example, yeast cells grown to maximum density (stationary phase) possess cell walls that are notoriously difficult to remove whereas cells in midlog growth phase are much more susceptible to enzymatic removal of the cell wall.

2. Autolysis（自溶）

In biology, autolysis, or more commonly known as self digestion refers to the destruction of a cell through the action of its own enzymes. It may also refer to the digestion of an enzyme by another molecule of the same enzyme. The term derives from the Greek words αυτó（"self"）and λύσις（"splitting"）.

In a biopharmaceutical process, autolysis is often achieved by inducing the microbe to generate excess cytases（细胞溶解酶，溶胞酶）or stimulate the activity of cytases.

The main factors affecting the process of autolysis include temperature, time, pH, agonist and the cell's metabolic pathway.

Disadvantages: For some microbes, autolysis may lead to protein denaturation, increased viscosity of cell suspension, hence a decreased filtration rate.

Other Additives

Aside from buffers, there are several other important components of homogenization buffers that warrant（使…显得必要，使…显得适当）discussing. When the objective is to purify an active protein, homogenization buffers may contain many additional components. These can generally be viewed as additives that will help to retain the active form of the protein and those that prevent the degradation of the protein.

The cytosol contains high concentrations of solutes in a reduced environment. Protein concentrations have been estimated to be as high as 30 mg/ml. Liberating the contents of cytosols causes the solutes to become rapidly diluted that not only can cause non-associated solutes to diffuse, but also protein subunits and co-factors. Osmotic stabilizers, such as sucrose or sorbitol, can be added to help bind up water and prevent dissociation of related solutes.

With many homogenization methods, high volumes of air are also introduced into the system, where the oxygen can shift（转换）the environment from reduced to oxidized. Within cells, oxygen tension（氧张力，氧含量）is extremely low, essentially anaerobic, thus the introduction of oxygen and their related radicals can lead to deleterious effects. Reducing agents such as glutathione, dithiothreitol（二硫苏糖醇），and ß-mercaptoethanol can react with oxidized species and prevent their negative consequences.

For protein isolation procedures, it is very common to add protease inhibitors to the homogenization buffer and/or homogenate（匀浆）. In animal cells, proteases are contained in lysosomes where their function is to recycle the amino acids and breakdown foreign material. Dependent upon the cell and tissue type, the concentration of lysosomes and associated enzymes can be high. The proteases contained within are heterogeneous（由很多种类组成的）and capable of degrading proteins at many different locations. Generally there are exoproteases（外切蛋白酶）which cleave both the amino and carboxyl terminal residues, as well as endoproteases（内切蛋白酶）that can attack specific peptide bonds.

Plants are generally believed to lack lysosomes, but rather use vacuoles in much the same manner.

Microorganisms also have proteases, but these are usually located in the periplasmic space. Similar to animal cells, disruption of plant and microbial cells releases the proteases which then can degrade proteins in the homogenate.

The deleterious action of proteases can be reduced by keeping samples cold while processing and by adding protease inhibitors. Though it is impractical to inhibit every type of proteases, several inhibitors can drastically reduce proteolytic activity. These inhibitors are summarized in Table 3-5.

Table 3-5　Protease inhibitors commonly used during sample processing.

Inhibitor	Specificity	Use Level	Comment
PMSF	Cysteine and serine proteases	0.1~1 mM (24~240 μg/ml)	PMSF has a short half life in water. Dissolve in ethanol and addjust before processing
EDTA	Metalloproteases	1 mM (0.37 mg/ml)	EDTA chelates divalent cations which are required by metalloproteases
Pepstatin A 胃酶抑素,抑肽素	Acid Proteases (aspartyl peptidase)	1~2 μM (0.5~1.0 μg/ml)	Prepare 1 mg/mL in ethanol (stable at −20℃). Use by diluting 1 μl/ml
Leupeptin 亮抑酶肽,亮抑蛋白酶肽	Serine and thiol proteases	10~100 μM (5~50 μg/ml)	Prepare 25 mg/ml stock and use 0.2-2 μl/ml
Aprotinin 抑酞酶	Serine proteases	0.1~0.8 μM (0.65~5.2 μg/ml)	Use 1 μl/ml of 5 mg/ml stock in water (0.76 mM)

When homogenizing plants, the disruption of the vacuole is much like disrupting a lysosome. Proteases are released in addition to phenolic oxidases. Plants contain substantial concentrations of phenolic compounds which when oxidized can react with proteins. Plant homogenate turns black as a result of these reactions. The addition of a phenolic scavenging reagent, such as polyvinylpyrrolidone (聚乙烯吡咯烷酮) used at a concentration of 0.5%~2%, can bind the phenolics and prevent their oxidation and subsequent reaction with proteins.

3.3　Isolation and purification of recombinant proteins（基因重组蛋白的分离和纯化）

Since the 1980s, with the widespread application of gene recombination technology, a large number of genetically engineered products have emerged. These recombinant products are cloned and expressed in the host cells (*e.g.*, *E. coli* and yeast cells), and most of them are intracellular substances. Therefore, the separation and purification of recombinant proteins is of great significance in modern biotechnology, which determines the purity, yield and safety of those products.

Concerning the separation and purification of recombinant proteins, the separation and purification methods and the choice of purification approach would be varying according to the nature of the target product and the requirements for the degree of purification of the product, but are mainly divided into two aspects:

(1) The coarse separation of the target products. This mainly includes the separation of cells from the culture medium after cell cultivation, and the following cell crushing to release coarse protein/peptide products, dissolution of inclusion bodies and protein renaturation to remove most of the impurities;

(2) Purification of the target product. This is to purify the protein/peptide product according to the requirements on the basis of separation, with a variety of high selectivity precision instruments.

The recombinant proteins obtained by using genetic engineering usually have the following issues: low product concentration, compositional complexity (containing cells, cell debris, proteins, nucleic acids, lipids, carbohydrates and inorganic salts, *etc*.), unstable physicochemical properties, liability to inactivation in the process of separation (such as the influence of pH and temperature, the effect of proteolytic enzymes), *etc*. Therefore, in the process of separation and purification of recombinant proteins, the separation and purification procedures should be minimized, the separation and purification time should be shortened, and the exposure of the desired product to the environmental pollutants should be avoided. Only in this way can the purity and recovery rate of the target product be improved.

3.3.1   Major isolation techniques of recombinant proteins（基因重组蛋白的主要分离技术）

3.3.1.1   Centrifugation and precipitation（离心及沉淀）

Centrifugation

Centrifugation is a process that involves the use of the centrifugal force for the separation of mixtures, used in industry and in laboratory settings（设置）. More-dense components of the mixture migrate away from the axis of the centrifuge, while less-dense components of the mixture migrate towards the axis. Chemists and biologists may increase the effective gravitational（引力，重力）force on a test tube so as to more rapidly and completely cause the precipitate（沉淀）("pellet") to gather on the bottom of the tube. The remaining solution is properly called the "supernate（上清液）" or "supernatant liquid". The supernatant liquid is then either quickly decanted（轻轻倒出）from the tube without disturbing the precipitate, or withdrawn with a Pasteur pipette.

The rate of centrifugation is specified（明确要求）by the acceleration applied to the sample, typically measured in revolutions per minute (rpm) or g. The particles' settling velocity（沉降速度）in centrifugation is a function（函数）of their size and shape, centrifugal acceleration, the volume fraction of solids present, the density difference between the particle and the liquid, and the viscosity.

In the chemical and food industries, special centrifuges can process a continuous stream of particle-laden（颗粒负载）liquid.

Centrifugation in Biotechnology

Microcentrifuges and Superspeed Centrifuges

In microcentrifugation（微量离心）, centrifuges are run in batch to isolate small volumes of biological molecules or cells (prokaryotic and eukaryotic). Nuclei is also often purified via microcentrifugation. Microcentrifuge tubes generally hold 1.5~2 ml of liquid, and are spun（旋转）at maximum angular speeds of 12 000~13 000 rpms. Microcentrifuges（微量离心机）are small and have rotors（转子）that can quickly change speeds. Superspeed（超高速）centrifuges work similarly to microcentrifuges, but are conducted via larger scale processes. Superspeed centrifuges are also used for purifying cells and nuclei, but in larger quantities. These centrifuges are used to purify 25~30 ml of solution within a tube. Additionally, larger centrifuges also reach higher angular velocities (around 30 000 rpm) and also use a larger rotor.

Ultracentrifugation

Ultracentrifugation (超速离心法) makes use of high centrifugal force for studying properties of biological particles. While microcentrifugation and superspeed centrifugation are used strictly to purify cells and nuclei, ultracentrifugation can isolate much smaller particles, including ribosomes, proteins, and viruses. Ultracentrifuges can also be used in the study of membrane fractionation. This occurs because ultracentrifuges (Fig. 3-15) can reach maximum angular velocities in excess of 70 000 rpm. Additionally, while microcentrifuges and supercentrifuges separate particles in batch, ultracentrifuges can separate molecules in batch and continuous flow systems.

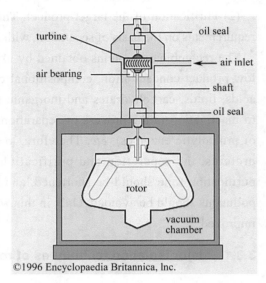

©1996 Encyclopaedia Britannica, Inc.

Fig. 3-15   Sketch of an ultracentrifuge.

In addition to purification, analytical ultracentrifugation (AUC) can be used for determination of macromolecular properties, including the amino acid composition of a protein, the protein's current conformation (构象), or properties of that conformation. In analytical ultracentrifuges, concentration of solute is measured using optical calibrations (校准). For low concentrations, the Beer-Lambert law (比尔 - 朗伯定律) can be used to measure the concentration. Analytical ultracentrifuges can be used to simulate physiological conditions (correct pH and temperature).

In analytical ultracentrifuges, molecular properties can be modeled (模拟) through sedimentation (沉降) velocity analysis or sedimentation equilibrium analysis. In sedimentation velocity analysis, concentrations and solute properties are modeled continuously over time. Sedimentation velocity analysis can be used to determine the macromolecule's shape, mass, composition, and conformational properties. During sedimentation equilibrium analysis, centrifugation has stopped and particle movement is based on diffusion. This allows for modeling of the mass of the particle as well as the chemical equilibrium properties of interacting solutes.

Protein precipitation

Precipitation is widely used in downstream processing of biological products, such as proteins. This unit operation serves to concentrate and fractionate the target product from various contaminants. For example, in the biotechnology industry protein precipitation is used to eliminate contaminants commonly contained in blood. Academic research on protein precipitation explores new protein precipitation methods. The underlying mechanism of precipitation is to alter the solvation (溶剂化) potential of the solvent and thus lower the solubility of the solute by addition of a reagent.

Isoelectric point precipitation

The isoelectric point (pI) is the pH of a solution at which the net primary charge of a protein becomes zero. At a solution pH that is above the pI, the surface of the protein is predominantly negatively charged and therefore like-charged molecules will exhibit repulsive forces. Likewise, at a solution pH that is below the

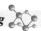
pI, the surface of the protein is predominantly positively charged and repulsion between proteins occurs. However, at the pI the negative and positive charges cancel, repulsive electrostatic forces are reduced and the dispersive (分散) forces predominate. The dispersive forces will cause aggregation and precipitation. The pI of most proteins is in the pH range of 4~6. Mineral acids, such as hydrochloric and sulfuric acid (硫酸) are used as precipitants. The greatest disadvantage to isoelectric point precipitation is the irreversible denaturation caused by the mineral acids. For this reason isoelectric point precipitation is most often used to precipitate contaminant proteins, rather than the target protein. The precipitation of casein (酪蛋白) during cheesemaking, or during production of sodium caseinate (酪蛋白酸钠), is an isoelectric precipitation.

Salting out

Salting out is the most common method used to precipitate a target protein. Addition of a neutral salt, such as ammonium sulfate, compresses (压缩) the solvation layer and increases protein-protein interactions. As the salt concentration of a solution is increased, more of the bulk water becomes associated with the ions. As a result, less water is available to partake (分担) in the solvation layer around the protein, which exposes hydrophobic patches on the protein surface. Proteins may then exhibit hydrophobic interactions, aggregate and precipitate from solution.

Hofmeister series (霍夫迈斯特序, 感胶离子序)

Kosmotropes or "water structure makers" are salts which promote the dissipation (消散) of water from the solvation layer around a protein. Hydrophobic patches are then exposed on the protein's surface, and they interact with hydrophobic patches on other proteins. These salts enhance protein aggregation and precipitation. Chaotropes or "water structure breakers" have the opposite effect of Kosmotropes. These salts promote an increase in the solvation layer around a protein. The effectiveness of the kosmotropic salts in precipitating proteins follows the order of the Hofmeister series:

Most precipitation $PO_4^{3-} > SO_4^{2-} > COO^- > Cl^-$ least precipitation

Most precipitation $NH_4^+ > K^+ > Na^+$ least precipitation

The ideal salt for protein precipitation is most effective for a particular amino acid composition, inexpensive, non-buffering, and non-polluting. The most commonly used salt is ammonium sulfate. There is a low variation in salting out over temperatures 0℃ to 30℃. Protein precipitates left in the salt solution can remain stable for years — protected from proteolysis and bacterial contamination by the high salt concentrations. Ammonium sulfate salt cannot be used in solutions that have pH>8 because the ammonium ion has a buffering effect on the solution. Sodium citrate (柠檬酸钠) is a good alternative for solutions above pH 8.

Precipitation with organic solvents

Addition of miscible (可混合的, 能混溶的) solvents such as ethanol or methanol to a solution may cause proteins in the solution to precipitate. Miscible organic solvents decrease the dielectric constant (介电常数) of water, which in effect allows two proteins to come close together. Meanwhile, the solvation/ hydration layer around the protein will decrease in thickness as the organic solvent progressively robs the protein of the hydration water away from the protein surface by attracting water molecules as its own hydration layers. With thinner solvation/hydration layers, the proteins would aggregate via attractive electrostatic interaction and dipole forces. Important parameters to consider are temperature — which should be less than 0℃ to avoid denaturation, pH and protein concentration in solution.

3.3.1.2 *Membrane separation*（膜分离）

Membrane separation processes

Membrane separation processes have very important role in separation industry. Nevertheless, they were not considered technically important until mid-1970. Membrane separation processes differ based on separation mechanisms and size of the separated particles. The widely used membrane processes include microfiltration, ultrafiltration, nanofiltration（纳米过滤）, reverse osmosis（反渗透）, electrolysis（电解）, dialysis（透析）, electrodialysis（电渗析）, gas separation, vapor permeation（蒸汽渗透）, pervaporation（全蒸发，过蒸汽化）, membrane distillation（膜蒸馏）, and membrane contactors（接触器）. All processes except for pervaporation involve no phase change. All processes except (electro) dialysis are pressure driven. Microfiltration and ultrafiltration are widely used in food and beverage processing (beer microfiltration, apple juice ultrafiltration), biotechnological applications and pharmaceutical industry (antibiotic production, protein purification), water purification and wastewater treatment, microelectronics（微电子学）industry, and others. Nanofiltration and reverse osmosis membranes are mainly used for water purification purposes. Dense membranes are utilized for gas separations (removal of CO_2 from natural gas, separating N_2 from air, organic vapor removal from air or nitrogen stream) and sometimes in membrane distillation. The later process helps in separating of azeotropic（共沸的，恒沸的）compositions reducing the costs of distillation processes.

3.3.1.3 *Aqueous two-phase extraction*（双水相萃取）

Two phase liquid extraction

Two phase liquid extraction, also known as aqueous two phase extraction, is a unique form of solvent extraction. In standard liquid extraction, an aqueous liquid（水溶液）is brought into contact with an organic solvent, and compounds in the aqueous solution are separated based on their relative solubility in the two phases. In an aqueous two phase extraction, compounds are still separated based on their solubility, but the two immiscible（不混溶的）phases are both water-based, an aqueous two phase system.

Aqueous two phase extractions can have a number of advantages over traditional solvent extraction. Solvents are often destructive to proteins, making the traditional extraction impossible for purifying proteins. In addition, organic solvents can be flammable, and their use can cause both environmental and health concerns. Aqueous two phase extractions do not require solvents, and so avoid these concerns.

Types of Aqueous Two Phase Extractions

Polymer/Polymer systems

In a Polymer/Polymer system, either phase is generated by a water-soluble polymer. The heavy phase will generally be Polyethylene glycol（PEG, 聚乙二醇）, and the light phase is generally a polysaccharide（多糖）. Traditionally, the polymer used is dextran（葡聚糖，右旋糖酐）. However, dextran is relatively expensive, and research has been exploring using less expensive polysaccharides to generate the light phase.

If the target compound being separated is a protein or enzyme, it is possible to incorporate a ligand to the target into one of the polymer phases. This improves the target's affinity to that phase, and improves its ability to partition from one phase into the other. This, as well as the absence of solvents or other denaturing agents, makes polymer/polymer extractions an attractive option for purifying proteins.

Unlike standard solvent extractions, where the two phases are generally highly immiscible, the two phases of a polymer/polymer system often have very similar densities, and very low surface tension between them. Because of this, demixing（分层）a polymer/polymer system is often much more difficult than demixing a solvent extraction. Methods to improve the demixing include centrifugation, and application of an electric field.

Polymer/Salt systems

Aqueous two phase systems can also be generated by introducing a high concentration of salt to a polymer solution. The polymer phase used is generally still PEG. Generally, a kosmotropic salt, such as Na_3PO_4 is used, however PEG/NaCl systems have been documented when the salt concentration is high enough.

Polymer/salt systems are less expensive than polymer/polymer systems. They are also easier to use, due to the fact that polymer/salt systems demix readily. However, at high salt concentrations, proteins generally either denature, or precipitate from solution. Thus, polymer/salt systems are not as useful for purifying proteins.

Ionic Liquids（离子液体）

Ionic liquids are ionic compounds with low boiling points. While they are not technically aqueous, recent research has experimented with using them in an extraction that does not use organic solvents.

Applications

DNA Purification: The ability to purify DNA from a sample is important for many modern biotechnology processes. However, samples often contain nucleases that degrade the target DNA before it can be purified. It has been shown that DNA fragments will partition into the light phase of a polymer/salt separation system. If ligands known to bind and deactivate nucleases are incorporated into the polymer phase, the nucleases will then partition into the heavy phase and be deactivated. Thus, this polymer/salt system is a useful tool for purifying DNA from a sample while simultaneously protecting it from nucleases.

Food Industry: The PEG/NaCl system has been shown to be effective at partitioning small molecules, such as peptides and nucleic acids. These compounds are often flavorants（食用香料）or odorants（有气味的东西）. The system could then be used by the food industry to isolate or eliminate particular flavors.

3.3.1.4 *Reversed micellar extraction*（反胶团萃取）

Micellar liquid chromatography (MLC)

Micellar liquid chromatography (MLC) is a form of reversed phase liquid chromatography that uses an aqueous micellar solutions as the mobile phase.

Theory

The use of micelles in high performance liquid chromatography was first introduced by Armstrong and Henry in 1980. The technique is used mainly to enhance retention and selectivity of various solutes that would otherwise be inseparable or poorly resolved. Micellar liquid chromatography (MLC) has been used in a variety of applications including separation of mixtures of charged and neutral solutes, direct injection of serum and other physiological fluids, analysis of pharmaceutical compounds, separation of enantiomers [镜像体, 对映（异构）体], analysis of inorganic-organometallics, and a host of others.

One of the main drawbacks of the technique is the reduced efficiency that is caused by the micelles. Despite the sometimes poor efficiency, MLC is a better choice than ion-exchange LC or ion-pairing LC for separation of charged molecules and mixtures of charged and neutral species.

Reverse phase high-performance liquid chromatography (RP-HPLC) involves a non-polar stationary phase（固定相）, often a hydrocarbon chain, and a polar mobile or liquid phase. The mobile phase generally consists of an aqueous portion with an organic addition, such as methanol or acetonitrile. When a solution of analytes is injected into the system, the components begin to partition out of the mobile phase and interact with the stationary phase. Each component interacts with the stationary phase in a different manner depending upon its polarity and hydrophobicity. In reverse phase HPLC, the solute with the greatest polarity will interact less with the stationary phase and spend more time in the mobile phase. As the polarity of the components decreases, the time spent in the column increases. Thus, a separation of components is achieved based on polarity. The addition of micelles to the mobile phase introduces a third phase into which the solutes may partition.

Micelles

Micelles are composed of surfactant, or detergent, monomers with a hydrophobic moiety, or tail, on one end, and a hydrophilic moiety, or head group, on the other. The polar head group may be anionic, cationic, zwitterionic, or non-ionic. When the concentration of a surfactant in solution reaches its critical micelle concentration（CMC，临界胶束浓度）, it forms micelles which are aggregates of the monomers. The CMC is different for each surfactant, as is the number of monomers which make up the micelle, termed the aggregation number（AN，聚集数目）.

Applications

Despite the reduced efficiency verses reversed phase HPLC, hundreds of applications have been reported using MLC. One of the most advantageous is the ability to directly inject physiological fluids. Micelles have an ability to solubilize proteins which enables MLC to be useful in analyzing untreated biological fluids such as plasma, serum, and urine. The main advantage of the use of MLC with this type of sample, is the great time savings in sample preparation. Alternative methods of analysis including reversed phase HPLC require lengthy extraction and sample work up procedures（样品加工程序）before analysis can begin. With MLC, direct injection is often possible, with retention times of less than 15 minutes for the separation of up to nine antagonists [拮抗物（药）].

3.3.2 Purification method for recombinant proteins（基因重组蛋白的纯化方法）

Recombinant proteins are purified mainly by chromatographic methods. The most commonly used include ion exchange chromatography, gel filtration chromatography, reversed phase chromatography, hydrophobic interaction chromatography and affinity chromatography.

3.3.2.1 Ion-exchange chromatography（离子交换层析）

Ion-exchange chromatography (or **ion chromatography**) is a process that allows the separation of ions and polar molecules based on their charge. Dionex Corp introduced commercial systems in the early 1970's that used revolutionary（革新性的）suppression technology to reduce background conductivity（导电性）, thus enhancing ion detection capabilities. It can be used for almost any kind of charged molecule including large proteins, small nucleotides and amino acids. The solution to be injected is usually called a sample, and the individually separated components are called analytes（分析物）. It is often used in protein purification, water analysis, and quality control.

History

Ion methods have been in use since 1850, when H. Thompson and J. T. Way, researchers in England, treated various clays（粘土）with ammonium sulfate or carbonate（碳酸钙）in solution to extract the ammonia and release calcium. In 1927, the first zeolite（沸石）mineral column was used to remove interfering calcium and magnesium ions from solution to determine the sulfate content of water. The modern version of IEC was developed during the wartime Manhattan Project（曼哈顿计划）. A technique was required to separate and concentrate the radioactive elements needed to make the atom bomb. Researchers chose adsorbents that would latch（附着）onto charged transuranium elements（超铀元素）, which could then be differentially eluted. Ultimately, once declassified（解密）, these techniques would use new IE resins to develop the systems that are often used today for specific purification of biologicals and inorganics. In the early 1970s, ion chromatography was developed by Hamish Small and co-workers at Dow Chemical Company as a novel method of IEC usable in automated analysis. This later lead to the formation of Dionex Corp (Dow-Ion Exchange) who lead the market in IC equipment and developments. IC uses weaker ionic resins for its stationary phase and an additional neutralizing stripper（剥离器）, or suppressor（抑制器）, column to remove background eluent（洗脱剂）ions. It is a powerful technique for determining low concentrations of ions and is especially useful in environmental and water quality studies, among other applications.

Principle

Ion exchange chromatography retains analyte molecules on the column based on coulombic（库仑的）(ionic) interactions. The stationary phase surface displays ionic functional groups (R-X) that interact with analyte ions of opposite charge. This type of chromatography is further subdivided into cation exchange chromatography and anion exchange chromatography. The ionic compound consisting of the cationic species M^+ and the anionic species B^- can be retained by the stationary phase.

Cation exchange chromatography retains positively charged cations because the stationary phase displays a negatively charged functional group:

$$R\text{-}X^-C^+ + M^+B^- \rightleftharpoons R\text{-}X^-M^+ + C^+ + B^-$$

Anion exchange chromatography retains anions using positively charged functional group:

$$R\text{-}X^+A^- + M^+B^- \rightleftharpoons R\text{-}X^+B^- + M^+ + A^-$$

Note that the ion strength of either C^+ or A^- in the mobile phase can be adjusted to shift the equilibrium position and thus retention time.

Ion Chromatogram

The ion chromatogram shows a typical chromatogram obtained with an anion exchange column (Fig. 3-16).

Typical technique

A sample is introduced, either manually or with an autosampler（自动进样器）, into a sample loop of known volume. A buffered aqueous solution known as the mobile phase carries the sample from the loop onto a column that contains some form of stationary phase material. This is typically a resin or gel matrix consisting of agarose（琼脂糖）or cellulose beads with covalently bonded charged functional groups. The

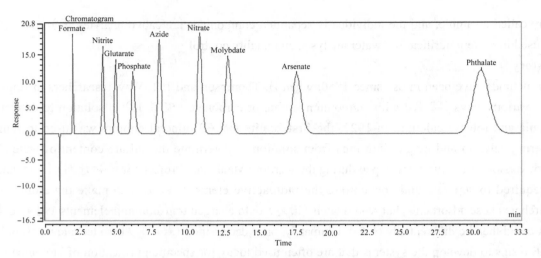

Fig. 3-16　A typical chromatogram obtained with an anion exchange column.

target analytes (anions or cations) are retained on the stationary phase but can be eluted by increasing the concentration of a similarly charged species that will displace the analyte ions from the stationary phase. For example, in cation exchange chromatography, the positively charged analyte could be displaced by the addition of positively charged sodium ions. The analytes of interest must then be detected by some means, typically by conductivity（电导率）or UV/Visible light absorbance.

In order to control an IC system, a chromatography data system (CDS) is usually needed. In addition to IC systems, some of these CDSs can also control gas chromatography (GC) and HPLC systems.

Separating proteins

Proteins have numerous functional groups that can have both positive and negative charges. Ion exchange chromatography separates proteins according to their net charge, which is dependent on the composition of the mobile phase. By adjusting the pH or the ionic concentration of the mobile phase, various protein molecules can be separated. For example, if a protein has a net positive charge at pH 7, then it will bind to a column of negatively-charged beads, whereas a negatively charged protein would not. By changing the pH so that the net charge on the protein is negative, it too will be eluted.

Elution by changing the ionic strength of the mobile phase has a more subtle（微妙的）effect — it works as ions from the mobile phase will interact with the immobilized ions in preference over those on the stationary phase. This "shields" the stationary phase from the protein, (and *vice versa*) and allows the protein to elute.

3.3.2.2　*Gel filtration chromatography*（凝胶过滤层析）

Size exclusion chromatography (SEC) is a chromatographic method in which molecules in solution are separated based on their size [more correctly, their hydrodynamic volume（流体力学体积）]. It is usually applied to large molecules or macromolecular complexes such as proteins and industrial polymers （工业树脂）. Typically, when an aqueous solution is used to transport the sample through the column, the technique is known as gel filtration chromatography, versus the name gel permeation chromatography （凝胶渗透色谱法）which is used when an organic solvent is used as a mobile phase. SEC is a widely used Polymer characterization（高分子表征）method because of its ability to provide good MW results for polymers.

Application and usage

The main application of gel filtration chromatography is the fractionation (分离) of proteins and other water-soluble polymers, while gel permeation chromatography is used to analyze the molecular weight distribution of organic-soluble polymers. Either technique should not be confused with gel electrophoresis, where an electric field is used to "pull" or "push" molecules through the gel depending on their electrical charges.

SEC is a widely used technique for the purification and analysis of synthetic and biological polymers, such as proteins, polysaccharides and nucleic acids. Biologists and biochemists typically use a gel medium — usually polyacrylamide (聚丙烯酰胺), dextran (葡聚糖) or agarose — and filter under low pressure. Polymer chemists typically use either a silica (硅胶) or crosslinked polystyrene (聚苯乙烯) medium under a higher pressure. These media are known as the stationary phase.

Advantages and Disadvantages

The advantages of this method include good separation of large molecules from the small molecules with a minimal volume of **eluent** (洗提液), and that various solutions can be applied without interfering with the filtration process, all while preserving the biological activity of the particles to be separated. The technique is generally combined with others that further separate molecules by other characteristics, such as acidity, basicity, charge, and affinity for certain compounds. With size exclusion chromatography there are short and well-defined separation times, narrow bands which demonstrate good sensitivity. There is also no sample loss because solutes (溶质) don't interact with the stationary phase.

Disadvantages are for example that only a limited number of bands can be accommodated because the time scale of the chromatogram is short, and generally there has to be a 10% difference in molecular mass to have a good resolution.

Discovery

The technique was invented by Grant Henry Lathe and Colin R Ruthven, working at Queen Charlotte's Hospital, London. They later received the John Scott Award for this invention. While Lathe and Ruthven used starch gels as the matrix (基质), Jerker Porath and Per Flodin later introduced dextran gels; other gels with size fractionation properties include agarose and polyacrylamide.

Theory and method

The underlying principle of SEC is that particles of different sizes will elute (filter) through a stationary phase at different rates. This results in the separation of a solution of particles based on size. Provided that all the particles are loaded simultaneously or near simultaneously, particles of the same size should elute together. Each size exclusion column has a range of molecular weights that can be separated. The exclusion limit defines the molecular weight at the upper end of this range and is where molecules are too large to be trapped in the stationary phase. The permeation limit defines the molecular weight at the lower end of the range of separation and is where molecules of a small enough size can penetrate into the pores of the stationary phase completely and all molecules below this molecular mass are so small that they elute as a single band.

This is usually achieved with an apparatus called a column, which consists of a hollow tube tightly packed with extremely small porous polymer beads designed to have pores of different sizes. These pores may be depressions (凹陷) on the surface or channels through the bead. As the solution travels down the column some particles enter into the pores. Larger particles cannot enter into as many pores. The larger the particles, the faster the elution (Fig. 3-17).

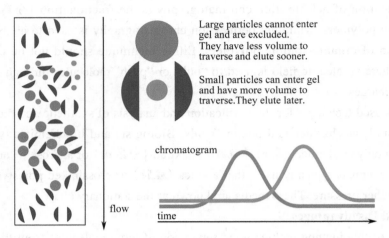

Fig. 3-17   A cartoon illustrating the theory behind size exclusion chromatography.

The filtered solution that is collected at the end is known as the **eluate**（洗脱液，洗出液）. The **void volume** includes any particles too large to enter the medium, and the **solvent volume** is known as the column volume.

Factors affecting filtration

In real-life situations, particles in solution do not have a fixed size resulting in the probability that a particle which would otherwise be hampered by a pore passing right by it. Also, the stationary phase particles are not ideally defined; both particles and pores may vary in size. Elution curves therefore resemble Gaussian distributions（高斯分布）. The stationary phase may also interact in undesirable ways with a particle and influence retention times, though great care is taken by column manufacturers to use stationary phases which are inert and minimize this issue（问题）.

Like other forms of chromatography, increasing the column length will enhance the resolution, and increasing the column diameter increases the capacity of the column. Proper column packing is important to maximize resolution: an overpacked column can collapse the pores in the beads, resulting in a loss of resolution. An underpacked column can reduce the relative surface area of the stationary phase accessible to smaller species, resulting in those species spending less time trapped in pores. Unlike affinity chromatography techniques, a solvent head at the top of the column can drastically diminish resolution as the sample diffuses prior to loading, broadening the downstream elution. The **void volume** is the total space surrounding the gel particles in a packed column.

Analysis

In simple manual columns the **eluate** （洗出液） is collected in constant volumes, known as fractions （部分）. The more similar the particles are in size, the more likely they will be in the same fraction and not detected separately. More advanced columns overcome this problem by constantly monitoring the **eluate**.

The collected fractions are often examined by spectroscopic techniques to determine the concentration of the particles eluted. Common spectroscopy detection techniques are **refractive index**（**RI**，折射率）and **ultraviolet (UV)**. When eluting spectroscopically（利用分光设备）similar species (such as during biological purification) other techniques may be necessary to identify the contents of each fraction. It is also possible to analyze the eluent flow continuously with RI, LALLS（小角激光光散射）, Multi-Angle Laser Light Scattering（MALS，多角度激光光散射光度计）, UV and/or viscosity measurements.

The elution volume (Ve) decreases roughly linearly with the logarithm（对数）of the molecular hydrodynamic volume（流体力学体积）. Columns are often calibrated （标定，校准）using 4~5 standard samples (*e.g.*, folded proteins of known molecular weight), and a sample containing a very large molecule such as thyroglobulin （甲状腺球蛋白）to determine the void volume. [Blue dextran is not recommended for Vo determination because it is heterogeneous（非均质）and may give variable results]. The elution volumes of the standards are divided by the elution volume of the thyroglobulin (Ve/Vo) and plotted against the log of the standards' molecular weights (Fig. 3-18).

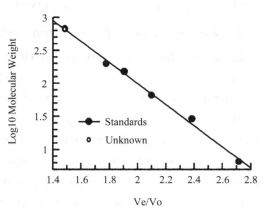

Fig. 3-18　Standard curve used to calculate molecular weight of a biomacromolecule after size exclusion chromatography.

Applications

Biochemical applications

SEC is generally considered a low-resolution chromatography as it does not discern（分辨，识别）similar species very well, and is therefore often reserved for the final "polishing" step of a purification. The technique can determine the quaternary structure of purified proteins which have slow exchange times, since it can be carried out under native solution conditions, preserving macromolecular interactions. SEC can also assay protein tertiary structure as it measures the hydrodynamic volume (not molecular weight), allowing folded and unfolded versions of the same protein to be distinguished. For example, the apparent hydrodynamic radius（流体力学半径）of a typical protein domain might be 14 Å and 36 Å for the folded and unfolded forms respectively. SEC allows the separation of these two forms as the folded form will elute much later due to its smaller size.

Polymer synthesis

SEC can be used as a measure of both the size and the polydispersity（多分散性）of a synthesized polymer — that is, the ability to be able to find the distribution of the sizes of polymer molecules. If standards of a known size are run previously, then a calibration curve（标准曲线）can be created to determine the sizes of polymer molecules of interest in the solvent chosen for analysis [often THF（四氢呋喃）]. Alternatively, techniques such as light scattering and/or viscometry（黏度法）can be used online with SEC to yield absolute molecular weights that do not rely on calibration with standards of known molecular weight. Due to the difference in size of two polymers with identical molecular weights, the absolute determination methods are generally more desirable. A typical SEC system can quickly (in about half an hour) give polymer chemists information on the size and polydispersity of the sample. The preparative SEC can be used for polymer fractionation（聚合物分级）on an analytical scale.

Drawback

In SEC, mass is not measured so much as the hydrodynamic volume of the polymer molecules, that is, how much space a particular polymer molecule takes up when it's in solution. However, the approximate molecular weight can be calculated from SEC data because the exact relationship between molecular weight and hydrodynamic volume for polystyrene（聚苯乙烯）can be found. For this, polystyrene is used as a standard. But the relationship between hydrodynamic volume and molecular weight is not the same for all polymers, so only an approximate measurement can be arrived at.

3.3.2.3 *Reversed-phase chromatography*（反相层析）

Reversed-phase chromatography (RPC) includes any chromatographic method that uses a non-polar stationary phase. The name "reversed phase" has a historical background. In the 1970s most liquid chromatography was done on non-modified silica or alumina（氧化铝）with a hydrophilic surface chemistry and a stronger affinity for polar compounds, hence it was considered "normal"（正）. The introduction of alkyl chains bonded covalently to the support surface reversed the elution order. Now polar compounds are eluted first while non-polar compounds are retained, hence "reversed phase". All of the mathematical and experimental considerations used in other chromatographic methods apply (*i.e.*, separation resolution proportional to the column length). Today, reversed-phase column chromatography accounts for（占）the vast majority of analysis performed in liquid chromatography.

Stationary Phases

Silica Based Stationary Phases

Any inert non-polar substance that achieves sufficient packing can be used for reversed-phase chromatography. The most popular column is a C18 bonded silica (USP classification L1) with 297 columns commercially available. This is followed by C8 bonded silica (L7-166 columns), pure silica (L3-88 columns), cyano（氰基）bonded silica (L10-73 columns) and phenyl bonded silica (L11-72 columns). Note that C18, C8 and phenyl are dedicated reversed-phase packings while cyano columns can be used in a reversed phase mode depending on analyte and mobile phase conditions. It should be noted at this point that not all C18 columns have identical retention properties. Surface functionalization（官能化）of silica can be performed in a monomeric（单体的）or a polymeric（聚合的）reaction with different short-chain organosilanes（有机硅烷）used in a second step to cover remaining silanol（硅烷醇）groups (end-capping [封端（反应）]). While the overall retention mechanism remains the same, subtle differences in the surface chemistries of different stationary phases will lead to changes in selectivity.

Mobile Phase Considerations

Mixtures of water or aqueous buffers and organic solvents are used to elute analytes from a reversed-phase column. The solvents have to be miscible with water and the most common organic solvents used are acetonitrile, methanol or tetrahydrofuran (THF). Other solvents can be used such as ethanol, 2-propanol [iso-propyl alcohol（异丙醇）]. Elution can be performed isocratic（等度）(the water-solvent composition does not change during the separation process) or by using a gradient (the water-solvent composition does change during the separation process). The pH of the mobile phase can have an important role in the retention of an analyte and can change the selectivity of certain analytes. Charged analytes can be separated on a reversed-phase column by the use of ion-pairing（离子对）(also called ion-interaction). This technique is known as reversed phase ion-pairing chromatography.

3.3.2.4 *Hydrophobic interaction chromatography*（疏水相互作用层析）

Hydrophobic Interaction Chromatography (HIC) is a separation technique that uses the properties of hydrophobicity to separate proteins from one another. In this type of chromatography, hydrophobic groups such as phenyl, octyl（辛基）, or butyl (Fig. 3-19), are attached to the stationary column. Proteins that pass through the column that have hydrophobic amino acid side chains on their surfaces are able to interact with and bind to the hydrophobic groups on the column.

phenyl   octyl   butyl

Fig. 3-19   Commonly used hydrophobic groups to covalently attached to the stationary phase in hydrophobic interaction column.

HIC separations are often designed using the opposite conditions of those used in ion exchange chromatography. In this separation, a buffer with a high ionic strength, usually ammonium sulfate, is initially applied to the column. The salt in the buffer reduces the solvation (溶剂化) of sample solutes thus as solvation decreases, hydrophobic regions that become exposed are adsorbed by the medium (Fig. 3-20).

The more hydrophobic the molecule, the less salt is needed to promote binding. To elute the proteins, the salt concentration is gradually decreased in order of increasing hydrophobicity. Additionally, elution can also be achieved through the use of mild organic modifiers (改性剂) or detergent.

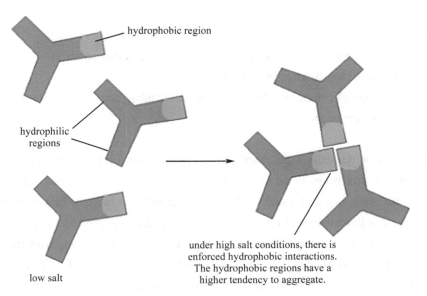

Fig. 3-20   The diagram illustrates how an increase in salt concentration can result in enforced hydrophobic interactions.

The stationary phase is designed to form hydrophobic interactions with other molecules. These interactions are too weak in water. However, addition of salts to the buffer results in hydrophobic interactions. The following is a list of salts that increase hydrophobic interactions in the order of their ability to enhance interactions:

$$
\begin{array}{c}
\text{increase} \Big\uparrow \quad
\begin{array}{l}
Na_2SO_4 \\
K_2SO_4 \\
(NH_4)_2SO_4 \\
NaCl \\
NH_4Cl \\
NaBr \\
NaSCN
\end{array}
\Big\downarrow \text{decrease}
\end{array}
$$

Although reversed-phase chromatography and hydrophobic interaction chromatography are very similar, the ligands in reversed-phase chromatography are much more hydrophobic than the ligands in hydrophobic interaction chromatography. This enables hydrophobic interaction chromatography to the use of more moderate elution conditions, which do not disrupt the sample nearly as much.

3.3.2.5 Affinity chromatography（亲和层析）

Affinity chromatography is a method of separating biochemical mixtures, based on a highly specific biological interaction such as that between antigen and antibody, enzyme and substrate, or receptor and ligand. Affinity chromatography combines the size fractionation capability of gel permeation chromatography（凝胶渗透色谱）with the ability to design a Chromatography that reversibly binds to a known subset（子集）of molecules. The method was by Cuatrecasas P, Wilchek M, and Meir Wilchek for which the Wolf Prize in Medicine was awarded in 1987. Due to its interdisciplinary（跨学科）nature, affinity chromatography has been the means by which many scientists from different disciplines have been introduced to the field of modern biology.

Uses

Affinity chromatography can be used to:

➢ Purify and concentrate a substance from a mixture into a buffering solution

➢ Reduce the amount of a substance in a mixture

➢ Discern what biological compounds bind to a particular substance, such as drugs

➢ Purify and concentrate an enzyme solution.

Principle

The immobile phase is typically a gel matrix, often of agarose; a linear sugar molecule derived from algae. Usually the starting point is an undefined（不明确的）heterogeneous（多样化的）group of molecules in solution, such as a cell lysate（溶解产物）, growth medium, or blood serum. The molecule of interest will have a well-known and defined property that can be exploited（利用）during the affinity purification process. The process itself can be thought of as an entrapment, with the target molecule becoming trapped on a solid or stationary phase or medium（基质，介质）. The other molecules in solution will not become trapped as they do not possess this property. The solid medium can then be removed from the mixture, washed and the target molecule released from the entrapment in a process known as elution. Possibly the most common use of affinity chromatography is for the purification of recombinant proteins.

Batch and column setup

Binding to the solid phase may be achieved by column chromatography whereby the solid medium is packed onto a column, the initial mixture run through the column to allow binding, a wash buffer run through the column and the elution buffer subsequently applied to the column and collected. These steps are usually done at ambient (环境) pressure. Alternatively binding may be achieved using a batch treatment, by adding the initial mixture to the solid phase in a vessel, mixing, separating the solid phase (for example), removing the liquid phase, washing, re-centrifuging, adding the elution buffer, re-centrifuging and removing the **eluate**.

Sometimes a hybrid method is employed, the binding is done by the batch method, then the solid phase with the target molecule bound is packed onto a column and washing and elution are done on the column.

A third method, expanded bed adsorption (扩张床吸附), which combines the advantages of the two methods mentioned above, has also been developed. The solid phase particles are placed in a column where liquid phase is pumped in from the bottom and exits at the top. The gravity of the particles ensures that the solid phase does not exit the column with the liquid phase.

Specific uses

Affinity chromatography can be used in a number of applications, including nucleic acid purification, protein purification from cell free extracts, and purification from blood.

Immunoaffinity chromatography

Another use for the procedure is the affinity purification of antibodies from blood serum. If serum is known to contain antibodies against a specific antigen (for example if the serum comes from an organism against the antigen concerned) then it can be used for the affinity purification of that antigen. This is also known as Immunoaffinity Chromatography. For example, if an organism is immunized against a GST-fusion protein it will produce antibodies against the fusion-protein, and possibly antibodies against the GST tag as well. The protein can then be covalently coupled to a solid support such as agarose.

For thoroughness, the GST protein and the GST-fusion protein can each be coupled separately. The serum is initially allowed to bind to the GST affinity matrix. This will remove antibodies against the GST part of the fusion protein. The serum is then separated from the solid support and allowed to bind to the GST-fusion protein matrix. This allows any antibodies that recognize the antigen to be captured on the solid support. Elution of the antibodies of interest is most often achieved using a low pH buffer such as glycine pH 2.8. The **eluate** is collected into a neutral Tris or phosphate buffer, to neutralize the low pH elution buffer and halt any degradation of the antibody's activity. This is a nice example as affinity purification is used to purify the initial GST-fusion protein, to remove the undesirable anti-GST antibodies from the serum and purify the target antibody.

A simplified strategy is often employed to purify antibodies generated against peptide antigens. When the peptide antigens are produced synthetically, a terminal cysteine residue is added at either the N- or C-terminus of the peptide. This cysteine residue contains a sulfhydryl (巯基) functional group which allows the peptide to be easily conjugated (结合) to a carrier protein [*e.g.*, Keyhole limpet hemocyanin (KLH, 匙孔血蓝蛋白, 一种免疫球蛋白, 可作辅助抗原和示踪分子)]. The same cysteine-containing peptide is also immobilized onto an agarose resin through the cysteine residue and is then used to purify the antibody.

Immobilized metal ion affinity chromatography

Immobilized metal ion affinity chromatography (IMAC) is based on the specific coordinate (配位) covalent bond of amino acids to metals, particularly histidine. This technique works by allowing proteins with an affinity for metal ions to be retained in a column containing immobilized metal ions, such as cobalt, nickel（镍）, copper for the purification of histidine containing proteins or peptides, iron, zinc or gallium（镓）for the purification of phosphorylated proteins or peptides. Many naturally occurring proteins do not have an affinity for metal ions, therefore recombinant DNA technology can be used to introduce such a Protein tag into the relevant gene. Methods used to elute the protein of interest include changing the pH, or adding a competitive molecule, such as imidazole（咪唑）.

Recombinant proteins

Possibly the most common use of affinity chromatography is for the purification of recombinant proteins. Proteins with a known affinity are protein tagged in order to aid their purification. The protein may have been genetically modified so as to allow it to be selected for affinity binding, this is known as a fusion protein. Tags include glutathione-S-transferase (GST), hexahistidine (His，六聚组氨酸), and maltose binding protein (MBP). Histidine tags, have an affinity for nickel or cobalt ions which have been immobilized by forming coordinate covalent bonds with a chelator incorporated in the stationary phase. For elution, an excess amount of a compound able to act as a metal ion ligand, such as imidazole, is used. GST has an affinity for glutathione — commercially available, immobilized as glutathione agarose. During elution, excess glutathione is used to displace the tagged protein.

Lectins（凝集素）

Lectin affinity chromatography is a form of affinity chromatography where lectins are used to separate components within the sample. Lectins, such as concanavalin（伴刀豆球蛋白）are proteins which can bind specific carbohydrate (sugar) molecules. The most common application is to separate proteins based on their Glycosylation（糖基化）groups.

3.3.3 Refolding of denatured protein（变性蛋白的复性）

The Gram-negative bacterium *Escherichia coli* is one of the most attractive systems for heterologous protein expression, because of its ability to grow rapidly, its well-characterized genetics, high efficiency, low cost, and the availability of an increasingly large number of cloning vectors and mutant host strains. Recombinant protein yields of more than 50% of the total cellular protein can be obtained.

However, there is no guarantee of obtaining biologically active heterologous protein, as the high level expression of recombinant protein in *Escherichia coli* is often accompanied by misfolding, leading to protein aggregation and formation of inclusion bodies which are insoluble and inactive. In case of a eukaryotic target protein the product is often enriched in inclusion bodies. These aggregates usually contain the product in a non-native conformation, however in a high concentration.

Although the inclusion bodies are composed of inactive proteins, the formation of inclusion bodies also provides several advantages for the production of recombinant proteins. The Inclusion bodies are ready to be separated and purified due to their high density. The target recombinant protein, existing in the form of inclusion bodies, can effectively resist the degradation caused by the proteases in *Escherichia coli*. Furthermore, inclusion body formation is the best option for producing heterogenous proteins that are toxic to host cells when existing in their natural conformation.

Even though existing in the form of inclusion bodies has some advantages such as enriching target proteins, being protease-resistant, and being less toxic to the host, the greatest disadvantage of this is the problems encountered during attempted solubilization and renaturation of the target protein — the renaturation rate and renaturation yield of inclusion body proteins is generally low, and proteins often cannot be renatured at all, which greatly raise the cost of producing recombinant protein product. This is most common with mammalian proteins which are, in most cases, multidomain and/or disulphide-bonded proteins. The accumulation of newly synthesized polypeptide chains expressed from cloned genes as non-native aggregates has become an important factor in the recovery of such proteins.

In order to solve the problem of low renaturation rate of inclusion body protein, on the one hand, one can address the issue at the upstream level, by promoting the soluble expression of recombinant proteins in *E. coli*, changing growth condition of *E. coli*, fusion expressing or co-expressing the recombinant proteins with other proteins — expression in the cytoplasm using some fusion partners can greatly increase the solubility of passenger proteins that may otherwise accumulate as insoluble aggregates in the cytoplasm, or by using the strategy of secretory expression to direct recombinant protein towards bacteria periplasmic space. In doing so recombinant protein can be expressed in *E. coli* in a soluble form which remains active.

On the other hand, this problem can be solved by using bioengineering technology, optimizing the process of renaturation, and renaturating the inclusion bodies *in vitro* to obtain bioactive proteins. Since inclusion bodies are rich in recombinant proteins, which can be easily purified. As long as successfully refolded *in vitro*, the inclusion body formation and the recovery of aggregated proteins will be one of the most effective ways to mass produce a large number of recombinant proteins.

3.3.3.1   *Reasons for inclusion body formation*（包涵体形成的原因）

The main reason for inclusion body formation is high level expression of protein. The formation of inclusion bodies mainly depends on the kinetic competition between protein-specific folding and aggregation rates connected to the synthesis rate. When a protein or a peptide is expressed at a high level, inclusion body would form once the aggregation rate of nascent peptide chain exceeds the critical folding rate. Aggregation is a predominant feature in very strong expression systems, but also increases with high inducer concentration, with the use of complex growth media and at higher cultivation temperature. According to Rudolph, it can be concluded that the inclusion body formation depends on the specific folding behavior rather than on the general characteristics of a protein such as size, fusion partners, subunit structure and relative hydrophobicity.

The aggregation process in both homologous and heterologous cytoplasms may be driven by partial intracellular denaturation of intermediates. Studies of both the refolding of denatured proteins in *vitro*, and of *in vivo* folding and maturation pathways, indicate that aggregates derive from specific partially folded intermediates and not from mature native, or fully unfolded proteins. Folding-rate-limiting structural characteristics such as disulfide bonds and certain point mutations can significantly promote the formation of aggregates.

When recombinant protein is expressed in *Escherichia coli*, the absence of a critical factor — certain enzymes and cofactors necessary for protein folding, such as foldases and molecular chaperones, subunit, prosthetic group — during the maturation process, or high temperature, is another reason for the inclusion body formation.

All of these processes appear to be highly specific and subject to modification by genetic engineering of the intermediates, or alteration of their environment. This requires an appreciation of the properties of such intermediates as distinct from the native states.

3.3.3.2 *Separation and dissolution of inclusion bodies*（包涵体的分离和溶解）

Some detergents have been shown to increase the solubility of recombinant proteins.

Traditionally, proteins refolded from inclusion bodies are solubilized in urea or a similar denaturant, which disrupts protein structure. The basic strategy involves reducing the concentration of denaturant, so that intramolecular interactions can occur, followed by folding in the presence of an oxidizing agent. During the process, the protein concentration must be kept to a minimum to avoid intermolecular aggregation. Several methods can be employed to remove or reduce excess denaturing agents, including dilution, dialysis, diafiltration（渗滤）, gel permeation chromatography, and immobilization onto a solid support.

1. Separation of inclusion bodies

The first step of separating inclusion bodies is to crush the cultured microbes collected. The crushing technology includes high pressure slurry, ultrasonic broken, *etc*. To increase the broken rate, a certain amount of lysozyme can be added. Inclusion bodies contain high shear stability. After using the above-mentioned cell disruption method, they can still keep their structures intact.

After centrifugation, discard the supernatant and wash the precipitation pellet with low concentration of denaturant (such as urea and guanidine hydrochloride), detergent (such as Triton X-100), or sodium deoxycholic acid（脱氧胆酸钠）. If further purification is needed, sucrose density gradient centrifugation is mostly considered.

2. Dissolution of inclusion bodies

The inclusion bodies are usually dissolved with strong denaturants such as urea, guanidine hydrochloride or thiocyanate, or detergents such as SDS, n-hexadecyl trimethylammonium chloride, *etc*. For proteins containing cysteine, reductants such as mercaptoethanol, dithiothreitol and cysteine should be added. 30℃ is generally chosen to be the temperature to promote dissolution. In addition, since those proteins are prone to oxidation catalysis in the presence of metal ions, it is often necessary to add metal chelators such as EDTA to remove metal ions.

Dissolution of inclusion bodies needs to break various chemical bonds intra-molecules and inter-molecules, so as to isolate the polypeptide chains from each other. Each dissolution method has its own strengths and shortcomings. Generally speaking, among them, guanidine hydrochloride is better than urea, in that the guanidine hydrochloride is a stronger denaturant than urea, and isocyanates, which usually contained in urea preparations, would irreversibly modify amino groups or sulhydryl groups of proteins.

3.3.3.3 *Inclusion body protein renaturation method*（包涵体蛋白复性方法）

An effective and ideal refolding method should have the following characteristics: ① Higher rate of recovery of bioactive protein. ② The properly refolded products could be easily separated from the misfolded protein species. ③ A higher concentration of protein products should be obtained after refolding. ④ The refolding method chosen is easy to scale-up. ⑤ Less time would be spent in the renaturation process.

Various process parameters (*e.g.*, protein concentration, temperature, pH, and ion strength) should be optimized in the process of protein renaturation according to the different physicochemical properties of each protein. In the cases of proteins containing disulfide bonds, the process of renaturation should be able to facilitate disulfide bond formation.

1. Dilution and dialysis approach

In order to obtain the active protein correctly folded, the denaturants and reductants should be removed by dilution, dialysis, filtration and gel filtration chromatography before the recovery, so as to promote protein renaturation.

Being in strict control of temperature, pH, and ionic strength conditions, the concentration of a recombinant protein can be simply reduced, hence reducing protein aggregation. However, the dilution of the recombinant protein would bring about issues such as the need for enlarged renaturation containers, production would therefore be affected. To solve those problems, the recombinant protein should be refolded at high concentration, by adding the denatured protein to the renaturation buffer slowly and continuously, or intermittently. This requires enough time to avoid aggregation; Renaturation via dialysis can gradually reduce the concentration of denaturant in dialysis buffer. Another approach is to use the renaturation buffer to dilute the denaturant to make its concentration decrease. In the process of renaturation *in vitro*, denatured protein would undergo a series of folding intermediates, eventually completing its conversion to the natural conformation of the protein. In the process of protein folding, hydrophobic bonds of the partially folded intermediates would expose, and the intermolecular hydrophobic interactions would cause protein aggregation. Since aggregation is an intermolecular reaction, hence is a secondary order (or advanced) reaction, while correctly folding is a first order reaction, aggregation is more dependent on a high protein concentration. Therefore, the most direct way to prevent aggregation is to reduce the protein concentration. A higher refolding rate can be obtained in a protein concentration between 10 to 50 μg/ml.

2. Renaturation of proteins containing disulfide bonds

In the case of disulfide bond-containing proteins, there are disulfide bonds in the inclusion bodies that are mostly mismatched (intramolecular or intermolecular), hence renaturation of these inclusion body proteins also involves the reconstruction of those disulfide bonds. The correct methods for disulfide bond formation basically include the following: (1) Air oxidation method, generally speaking, is the use of oxygen in the air to oxidize sulfhydryl group during refolding process. The presence of trace metal ions, such as Cu^{2+} may have catalytic effect. This method is simple and cost effective, but the renaturation rate is low and it is difficult to accurately control oxidation process. (2) REDOX reagents such as reduced glutathione/oxidized glutathione are added to the refolding system. (3) Addition of oxidized glutathione before the protein renaturation, make the oxidized glutathione and the protein with reduced cysteine form disulfide complexes. While during renaturation, gradually remove GSH and the denaturants, and then add a low concentration of cysteine to replace glutathione in the protein — S — S — glutathione complex and make disulfide bond form correctly. (4) Application of reducing reagent or sodium sulfite/sodium tetrathionate (by S-sulfonation of cysteine residues) to protect sulfhydryl group of the denatured protein. During renaturation, a small amount of reducing reagent can remove those protection groups and offer opportunity for the disulfide bond to match correctly. (5) Application with some reducing agents such as dithiothreitol（二硫苏糖醇）.

3. Blocking the hydrophobic clusters of a protein to facilitate *in vitro* protein renaturation

The hydrophobic clusters that may cause molecular interactions among proteins can be determined through analysis of protein structures and sequences. Some designed amino acid site-specific mutation that can change or destroy those hydrophobic clusters, may reduce such kinds of aggregation. Monoclonal antibodies specific to those hydrophobic clusters are used to block those clusters and reduce the aggregation caused by intermolecular binding.

4. Renaturation via gel filtration chromatography

To reduce aggregation reactions caused by high concentrations of proteins, gel filtration chromatography technology has also been used for refolding the denatured proteins *in vitro*. Chromatography medium has some isolation effect, and reduces the aggregation caused by interaction between proteins. Therefore the protein concentration for renaturation can be elevated, and the renaturation rate can be greatly improved. Meanwhile, the protein itself can be purified via gel filtration chromatography.

5. Small molecule additives promote renaturation

A simple and effective strategy for reducing protein aggregation is to use some small molecule additives. A series of additives are proven to be able to prevent protein aggregation, they may have some role in stabilizing the active state of some target proteins, reducing the stability of the incorrectly folded molecules, increasing the stability of the folding intermediates, increasing the stability of the conformation of the unfolded state. Additives do not speed up the folding process, but only inhibit the occurrence of molecular aggregation.

6. Molecular chaperones or foldases promote renaturation

The use of molecular chaperones and foldases *in vitro* help proteins refold, they can also improve the refolding yield. However, the removal of molecular chaperones and foldases after renaturation is a complicated and tedious process. If the molecular chaperones and foldase enzymes could not be reused, the cost would be increased.

7. Artificial molecular chaperones promote refolding

Denatured protein can be captured by some kind of detergent in refolding buffer, forming protein-detergent complex. The formation of the complex inhibits protein aggregation, and then the cyclodextrin （环糊精）should be added to strip （除去）the detergent molecule from the complex to prompt protein refolding.

3.3.4 Basis for selecting separation and purification methods （选择分离纯化方法的依据）

Sample extraction procedures and the selection of buffers, additives, and detergents hinge largely on the source of the material, the stability of the target molecule, the chromatographic techniques that will be employed, and the intended use of the product.

3.3.4.1 *Choose the appropriate separation and purification strategy according to the expression pattern of products* （根据产物表达形式选择）

Secretion expression has three major potential advantages over intracellular accumulation: the secreted target protein is usually naturally folded; yields can be as high as or higher than that obtained from intracellular *E. coli* host/vector systems; there is a reduced requirement for extraction and purification procedures which are expensive, and reduced risks of contamination with host proteins and nucleic acids; and contamination with endotoxin is avoided, when the host is not Gram-negative.

Secretory products are usually contained in a large volume of fermentation broth at low concentrations, so they must be concentrated before purification to reduce the sample volume as soon as possible. The method for the concentration of the sample includes precipitation and ultrafiltration.

Affinity chromatography was the first choice of approach to be employed for the isolation of the expressed product, which has been accumulated in a soluble form in *E. coli* lysate after cell disruption. If there is no monoclonal antibody or affinity ligand with relative specificity available, ion exchange chromatography is generally used. Proteins with an extreme isoelectric point can be separated using ion exchange chromatography to obtain a satisfactory purification effect with most impurities or contaminants removed.

Periplasmic expression is an expression pattern in-between the intracellularly soluble expression and secretory expression. It is a way to keep the target protein away from other soluble proteins in the *E. coli* and protein impurities in culture media, which is to some extent in favor of separation and purification afterward. In order to obtain a recombinant periplasmic protein, *E. coli* is generally treated with a low concentration of lysozyme, then subject to osmotic shock. Because in the periplasmic space there are only a few secreted proteins, hence no problems with protease contamination, high-quality products are usually harvested.

The formation of insoluble intracellular expression products — inclusion bodies affect protein isolation and purification in two ways. On the one hand, it can be easily separated from soluble intracellular protein impurities, hence making it easy to accomplish the purification. On the other hand, it is supposed to undergo a process of denaturing and refolding, during which misfolded and/or aggregated products would form. The inclusion bodies can be separated from the crude extract by centrifuging at low speed, then redissolved in some dissolution enhancers, such as urea, guanidine hydrochloride, and sodium dodecyl sulfate, and finally refolded under appropriate conditions (pH, ionic strength and dilutability). Although the formation of inclusion bodies needs additional steps for extraction, it can also bring about some advantages, *e.g.*, the purity of the target protein in the inclusion bodies is relatively higher (up to 20%~80%). Meanwhile, inclusion bodies are resistant to proteolytic attack by intracellular proteases. If the presence of impurities or contaminants affects the refolding yield, the alternative way is doing so after purification.

3.3.4.2 Select the order of the separation and purification steps according to the means of connecting（根据分离单元之间的衔接选择）

Some separating units with different mechanisms should be selected to form a set of separation and purification process. Some efficient separation approaches should be adopted as early as possible to separate and remove the most abundant impurities or contaminants, while the most expensive and time-consuming separating units should be arranged in the final stage. In other words, operational units which are non-specific and with low-resolution, such as precipitation, ultrafiltration and adsorption, are usually applied first. The main purpose of this stage is to reduce sample volume as quickly as possible, increase the concentration of the desired protein and remove the most abundant impurities or contaminants (including non-protein impurities). High resolution operational units, such as ion exchange chromatography and affinity chromatography, which have the advantage of high selectivity, were then used. The operational units, such as gel-exclusion chromatography, with its small scale and low efficiency, are usually arranged as the final stage to improve the separation effect.

Specific sample preparation steps might be required if the crude sample is known to contain contaminants such as lipids, lipoproteins, or phenol red, which tend to accumulate on a column. Sample preparation might also be required if certain gross impurities, such as bulky protein, need be removed before any chromatographic step.

Fractional precipitation is occasionally used at laboratory scale to remove gross impurities but is generally not required in the purification of affinity-tagged proteins. In some cases, precipitation can be useful as a combined technique of protein concentration and purification.

The selection and order of chromatographic separation steps are also important. A reasonable order in a combination of different chromatographic methods can overcome some shortcomings, and the transition between the separation steps can be achieved without changing the conditions. When several methods are used successively, it would be better for each to be based on different separation mechanisms. Moreover, the fractions collected during the former stage should be able to be used directly as the feed liquid of a matching method in the latter stage. In this way, no desalting or concentration steps are needed, *e.g.*, if a crude product is obtained after salting out, it is not suitable to undergo ion exchange chromatography. The hydrophobic interaction chromatography (HIC) is often an excellent next purification step, as the fraction already contains a high salt concentration and can be applied directly to the HIC column with little or no additional preparation. The elevated salt level enhances the interaction between the hydrophobic components of the sample and the chromatography medium. Ion exchange, hydrophobic interaction and affinity chromatography usually have a protein concentrating effect, while gel filtration chromatography often dilutes the sample. It is appropriate to arrange hydrophobic chromatography after ion exchange chromatography without the need to replace buffer, because most proteins tend to bind strongly with hydrophobic medium under high ionic strength. Affinity chromatography is a separation method with the largest selectivity, but it is not suitable to be employed as the initial step. On the one hand, since too much impurities or contaminants are contained in the cell lysate at the initial phase, it is difficult to avoid the affinity chromatographic medium from being polluted, hence reducing service life. On the other hand, the sample volume is usually large in the initial phase, and a larger volume of sample solution requires a large amount of medium, while affinity chromatographic medium is generally more expensive. Therefore, affinity chromatography is often employed after the second step. Sometimes, a protective column — usually packed with a corresponding medium without any ligand — is added in front of an affinity column to prevent the poisoning of the latter medium. After affinity chromatography, the falling-off ligands may also exist in the fractions collected. Furthermore, some of the target proteins would aggregate to form dimers or oligomers in the process of separating and purifying them. It is more likely for those desired proteins to form oligomers, especially when the concentration is higher, or some degradation products are present in the solution. Therefore further purification is usually required afterward, and gel filtration chromatography is generally considered the method of choice. High-performance liquid chromatography (HPLC) is an alternative, but the cost is much higher. Furthermore, if gel filtration is used as the last step, the **eluent** can be directly transitioned to an appropriate buffer system to facilitate the moulding and preservation of the product.

3.3.4.3 *Select according to the requirements of separation and purification process* （根据分离纯化工艺的要求选择）

(1) The technical process （工艺流程） should have good stability and repeatability. The stability of the process includes that the quality of the product would not be affected by or less affected by some subtle changes in the fermentation techniques, conditions and sources of raw materials, it should be repeatable in

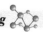

any environment to produce products of the same specification. In order to ensure the repeatability of the process, it is necessary to define the steps and techniques to be strictly controlled in the process, as well as the permissible variation range. The fewer the technical steps and techniques are to be strictly controlled, the wider the variation range of the technical conditions and the better the technical repeatability.

(2) The steps of the process should be minimized. The more steps there are, the lower the yield of the product after the final purification step — but the principle is that the quality of the product must be guaranteed. This requires that the techniques which compose the technology are highly efficient, and in general the technique with the same separation principle should not be used repeatedly in the process.

(3) The techniques or steps composing the technical process should be able to adapt and coordinate with each other, as well as the techniques and the equipments, to simplify the operation procedure, to reduce or omit the material handling needs and condition adjustment between steps.

(4) Reagents should be used as little as possible during the process to avoid additional separation and purification steps or disturbance of product quality.

(5) Process time should be as short as possible, because yield, especially the yield of the biologically active form would decline with increasing process time for the product with poor stability, hence the quality of the product .

(6) Make sure that the processes and techniques are easy to operate, with high efficiency, high yield, low equipment requirements and low energy consumption.

(7) High security. When selecting post-treatment techniques, processes and operating conditions, make sure the removal of dangerous impurities, the quality and safety of the product, and the safety of the production process. Drug production must be safe, sterile, pyrogen-free and pollution-free.

3.4 Analysis and determination of recombinant proteins（基因重组蛋白的分析和测定）

3.4.1 Protein content determination（蛋白质含量的测定）

3.4.1.1 Ultraviolet-visible spectroscopy [紫外（UV）吸收光谱法]

Ultraviolet-visible spectroscopy or **ultraviolet-visible spectrophotometry (UV-Vis or UV/Vis)** refers to absorption spectroscopy or reflectance spectroscopy（反射光谱法）in the ultraviolet-visible spectral region. This means it uses light in the visible and adjacent [near-UV and near-infrared（NIR）] ranges. The absorption or reflectance in the visible range directly affects the perceived color of the chemicals involved. In this region of the electromagnetic spectrum（电磁波谱）, molecules undergo electronic transitions（电子跃迁）. This technique is complementary to fluorescence spectroscopy, in that fluorescence deals with transitions from the excited state to the ground state（基态）, while absorption measures transitions from the ground state to the excited state.

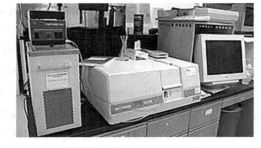

Beckman DU640 UV/Vis spectrophotometer.

Principle of ultraviolet-visible absorption

Molecules containing π-electrons or non-bonding electrons (n-electrons) can absorb the energy in the form of ultraviolet or visible light to excite these electrons to higher anti-bonding molecular orbitals. The more easily excited the electrons [*i.e.,* lower energy gap between the HOMO（最高已占轨道）and the LUMO（最低未占轨道）], the longer the wavelength of light it can absorb.

Applications

UV/Vis spectroscopy is routinely used in analytical chemistry for the quantitative determination of different analytes, such as transition metal（过渡金属）ions, highly conjugated organic compounds, and biological macromolecules. Spectroscopic analysis is commonly carried out in solutions but solids and gases may also be studied.

The Beer-Lambert law（比尔 — 朗伯定律）states that the absorbance of a solution is directly proportional to the concentration of the absorbing species in the solution and the path length. Thus, for a fixed path length, UV/Vis spectroscopy can be used to determine the concentration of the absorber（吸收体）in a solution. It is necessary to know how quickly the absorbance changes with concentration. This can be taken from references [tables of molar extinction coefficients（摩尔消光系数）], or more accurately, determined from a calibration curve（校正曲线）.

A UV/Vis spectrophotometer may be used as a detector for HPLC. The presence of an analyte（分析物，被分析物）gives a response assumed to be proportional to the concentration. For accurate results, the instrument's response to the analyte in the unknown should be compared with the response to a standard; this is very similar to the use of calibration curves. The response (*e.g.,* peak height) for a particular concentration is known as the response factor（响应因子）.

The wavelengths of absorption peaks can be correlated with（与…有关）the types of bonds in a given molecule and are valuable in determining the functional groups within a molecule. The Woodward-Fieser rules, for instance, are a set of empirical observations used to predict λ_{max}, the wavelength of the most intense UV/Vis absorption, for conjugated organic compounds such as dienes（二烯烃，双烯）and ketones（酮类）. The spectrum alone is not, however, a specific test for any given sample. The nature of the solvent, the pH of the solution, temperature, high electrolyte concentrations, and the presence of interfering substances can influence the absorption spectrum. Experimental variations such as the slit width（狭缝宽度）[effective bandwidth（带宽）] of the spectrophotometer will also alter the spectrum. To apply UV/Vis spectroscopy（光谱）to analysis, these variables must be controlled or accounted for（解释）in order to identify the substances present.

The method is most often used in a quantitative way to determine concentrations of an absorbing species in solution, using the Beer-Lambert law:

$$A = \log_{10}(I_0/I) = \varepsilon cL,$$

where A is the measured absorbance, in **Absorbance Units (AU)**, I_0 is the intensity of the incident light at a given wavelength, I is the transmitted intensity, L the path length through the sample, and c the concentration of the absorbing species. For each species and wavelength, ε is a constant known as the molar absorptivity（摩尔吸光系数）or extinction coefficient. This constant is a fundamental molecular property in a given solvent, at a particular temperature and pressure, and has units of $1/M * cm$ or often $AU/M * cm$.

The absorbance and extinction ε are sometimes defined in terms of the natural logarithm（自然对数）

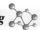

instead of the base-10 logarithm（以 10 为底的对数）.

The Beer-Lambert Law is useful for characterizing many compounds but does not hold as a universal relationship for the concentration and absorption of all substances. A 2nd order polynomial relationship （二阶多项式）between absorption and concentration is sometimes encountered for very large, complex molecules such as organic dyes [Xylenol Orange（二甲酚橙）or Neutral Red（中性红）, for example].

Quantitative determination of proteins

Near UV Absorbance (280 nm)

Quantitation of the amount of protein in a solution is possible in a simple spectrometer. Absorption of radiation in the near UV by proteins depends on the Tyr and Trp content (and to a very small extent on the amount of Phe and disulfide bonds). Therefore the A_{280} varies greatly between different proteins [for a 1 mg/ml solution, from 0 up to 4（for some tyrosine-rich wool proteins）, although most values are in the range 0.5~1.5]. The advantages of this method are that it is simple, and the sample is recoverable. The method has some disadvantages, including interference from other chromophores（发色团）, and the specific absorption value for a given protein must be determined. The extinction of nucleic acid in the 280-nm region may be as much as 10 times that of protein at their same wavelength, and hence, a few percent of nucleic acid can greatly influence the absorption.

Far UV Absorbance

The peptide bond absorbs strongly in the far UV with a maximum at about 190 nm. This very strong absorption of proteins at these wavelengths has been used in protein determination. Because of the difficulties caused by absorption by oxygen and the low output（输出）of conventional spectrophotometers at this wavelength, measurements are more conveniently made at 205 nm, where the absorbance is about half that at 190 nm. Most proteins have extinction coefficients at 205 nm for a 1 mg/ml solution of 30~35 and between 20 and 24 at 210 nm.

Various side chains, including those of Trp, Phe, Tyr, His, Cys, Met, and Arg (in that descending order), make contributions to the A_{205}.

The advantages of this method include simplicity and sensitivity. The sample is recoverable and in addition there is little variation in response between different proteins, permitting near absolute determination of protein.

Disadvantages of this method include the necessity for accurate calibration of the spectrophotometer （分光光度计）in the far UV. Many buffers and other components, such as heme（血红素）or pyridoxal groups（吡哆醛）, absorb strongly in this region.

Practical considerations

The Beer-Lambert law has implicit（未言明的）assumptions that must be met experimentally for it to apply, otherwise there is a possibility of deviations from the law to be observed. For instance, the chemical makeup and physical environment of the sample can alter its extinction coefficient. The chemical and physical conditions of a test sample therefore must match reference measurements for conclusions to be valid.

3.4.1.2 Lowry protein assay（Lowry 法）

The **Lowry protein assay** is a biochemical assay for determining the total level of protein in a solution. The total protein concentration is exhibited by a color change of the sample solution in proportion to protein concentration, which can then be measured using colorimetric techniques. It is named for the biochemist Oliver H. Lowry who developed the reagent in the 1940s. His 1951 paper describing the technique is the most-highly cited paper ever in the scientific literature, cited over 300 000 times.

Mechanism

The method combines the reactions of copper ions with the peptide bonds under alkaline conditions (the Biuret test) with the oxidation of aromatic protein residues. The Lowry method is best used with protein concentrations of 0.01~1.0 mg/ml and is based on the reaction of Cu^+, produced by the oxidation of peptide bonds, with Folin-Ciocalteu reagent [a mixture of phosphotungstic acid（磷钨酸）and phosphomolybdic acid（磷钼酸）in the Folin-Ciocalteu reaction]. The reaction mechanism is not well understood, but involves reduction of the Folin-Ciocalteu reagent and oxidation of aromatic residues (mainly tryptophan, also tyrosine). Experiments have shown that cysteine is also reactive to the reagent. Therefore, cysteine residues in protein probably also contribute to the absorbance seen in the Lowry Assay. The concentration of the reduced Folin reagent is measured by absorbance at 750 nm. As a result, the total concentration of protein in the sample can be deduced from the concentration of Trp and Tyr residues that reduce the Folin-Ciocalteu reagent.

The method was first proposed by Lowry in 1951. The Bicinchoninic acid assay（二喹啉甲酸）and the Hartree-Lowry assay are subsequent modifications of the original Lowry procedure.

3.4.1.3 *Bradford protein assay*（考马斯亮蓝法）

The **Bradford protein assay** is a spectroscopic analytical procedure used to measure the concentration of protein in a solution. It is subjective, *i.e.*, dependent on the amino acid composition of the measured protein. The Bradford protein assay was developed by Marion M. Bradford.

The Bradford assay, a colorimetric（比色的，色度的）protein assay, is based on an absorbance shift of the dye Coomassie Brilliant Blue G-250. Under acidic conditions the red form of the dye is converted into its bluer form, binding to the protein being assayed. During the formation of this complex, two types of bond interaction take place: the red form of Coomassie dye first donates its free electron to the ionizable groups on the protein, which causes a disruption of the protein's native state, consequently exposing its hydrophobic pockets. These pockets in the protein's tertiary structure bind non-covalently to the non-polar region of the dye via van der Waals forces, positioning the positive amine groups in proximity with the negative charge of the dye. The bond is further strengthened by the ionic interaction between the two. The binding of the protein stabilizes the blue form of the Coomassie dye; thus the amount of the complex present in solution is a measure for the protein concentration, and can be estimated by use of an absorbance reading.

The **bound** form of the dye has an absorption spectrum maximum historically held to be at 595 nm. The cationic (**unbound**) forms are green or red. The binding of the dye to the protein stabilizes the blue anionic form. The increase of absorbance at 595 nm is proportional to the amount of bound dye, and thus to the amount (concentration) of protein present in the sample.

Unlike other protein assays, the Bradford protein assay is less susceptible to interference by various chemicals that may be present in protein samples. An exception of note is elevated concentrations of detergent. Sodium dodecyl sulfate (SDS), a common detergent, may be found in protein extracts because it is used to lyse cells by disrupting the membrane lipid bilayer. While other detergents interfere with the

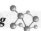

assay at high concentration, the interference caused by SDS is of two different modes, and each occurs at a different concentration. When SDS concentrations are below critical micelle concentration（临界胶束浓度）(known as CMC, 0.00333 %W/V to 0.0667 %) in a Coomassie dye solution, the detergent tends to bind strongly with the protein, inhibiting the protein binding sites for the dye reagent. This can cause underestimations of protein concentration in solution. When SDS concentrations are above CMC, the detergent associates strongly with the green form of the Coomassie dye, causing the equilibrium to shift, thereby producing more of the blue form. This causes an increase in the absorbance at 595 nm independent of protein presence.

Other interference may come from the buffer used when preparing the protein sample. A high concentration of buffer will cause an overestimated protein concentration due to depletion of free protons from the solution by conjugate base from the buffer. This will not be a problem if a low concentration of protein (subsequently the buffer) is used.

Advantages

The procedure for Bradford protein assay is very easy and simple to follow. It is done in one step where the Bradford reagent is added to a test tube along with the sample. After mixing well, the mixture almost immediately changes to a blue color and the absorbance can be read at 595 nm using a spectrophotometer — an easily accessible machine.

This assay is one of the fastest assays performed on proteins. The total time it takes to set up and complete the assay is under 30 minutes. The entire experiment is done at room temperature.

Also, the Bradford protein assay can measure protein concentration ranging from 1 to 20 μg. It is an extremely sensitive technique.

The dye reagent is a stable ready to use product prepared in phosphoric acid（磷酸）. It can remain at room temperature for up to 2 weeks before it starts to degrade.

Protein samples usually contains salts, solvents, buffers, preservatives, and metal chelating agents. Using Bradford can be advantageous against these molecules because they are compatible with each other and will not interfere.

The linear graph acquired from the assay (absorbance versus protein concentration in μg/ml) can be easily extrapolated to determine the concentration of proteins by using the slope of the line.

Disadvantages

The Bradford assay is linear over a short range, typically from 0 μg/ml to 2 000 μg/ml, often making dilutions of a sample necessary before analysis.

It is also inhibited by the presence of detergents.

Much of the non-linearity stems from the equilibrium between two different forms of the dye which is perturbed by adding the protein. The Bradford assay linearizes by measuring the ratio of the absorbances, 595 over 450 nm. This modified Bradford assay is approximately 10 times more sensitive than the conventional one.

Sample Bradford procedure
Materials

➢ Lyophilized bovine plasma gamma globulin

➢ Coomassie Brilliant Blue 1

➢ 0.15 M NaCl

➢ Spectrophotometer and tubes

➢ Micropipettes

Procedure (Standard Assay, 20~150 μg protein; 200~1500 μg/ml)

1. Prepare a series of protein standards diluted with 0.15 M NaCl to final concentrations of 0 (blank = NaCl only), 250, 500, 750 and 1 500 μg/ml. Also prepare serial dilutions of the unknown sample to be measured.

2. Add 100 μl of each of the above to a separate test tube (or spectrophotometer tube if using a Spec 20).

3. Add 5.0 ml of Coomassie Blue to each tube and mix by vortex, or inversion.

4. Adjust the spectrophotometer to a wavelength of 595 nm, and blank using the tube which contains no protein.

5. Wait 5 minutes and read each of the standards and each of the samples at 595 nm wavelength.

6. Plot the absorbance of the standards vs. their concentration. Compute the extinction coefficient and calculate the concentrations of the unknown samples.

Procedure (Micro Assay, 1~10 μg protein/ml)

1. Prepare standard concentrations of protein of 1, 5, 7.5 and 10 μg/ml. Prepare a blank of NaCl only. Prepare a series of sample dilutions.

2. Add 100 μl of each of the above to separate tubes (use microcentrifuge tubes) and add 1.0 ml of Coomassie Blue to each tube.

3. Turn on and adjust a spectrophotometer to a wavelength of 595 nm, and blank the spectrophotometer using 1.5 ml cuvettes.

4. Wait 2 minutes and read the absorbance of each standard and sample at 595 nm.

5. Plot the absorbance of the standards vs. their concentration. Compute the extinction coefficient and calculate the concentrations of the unknown samples.

3.4.1.4 *Bicinchoninic acid*（二喹啉甲酸）*assay (BCA protein assay)*（BCA 法）

The **bicinchoninic acid assay (BCA assay)**, also known as the **Smith assay**, after its inventor, Paul K. Smith at the Pierce Chemical Company, is a biochemical assay for determining the total concentration of protein in a solution (0.5 μg/ml to 1.5 mg/ml), similar to Lowry protein assay, Bradford protein assay or biuret reagent（双缩脲试剂）. The total protein concentration is exhibited by a color change of the sample solution from green to purple in proportion to protein concentration, which can then be measured using colorimetric techniques.

Mechanism

A stock BCA solution contains the following ingredients in a highly alkaline solution with a pH 11.25:

● Bicinchoninic acid

● Sodium carbonate

● Sodium bicarbonate（碳酸氢钠）

● Sodium tartrate（酒石酸钠）

● Copper (II) sulfate pentahydrate（五水合硫酸铜）

The BCA assay primarily relies on two reactions.

First, the peptide bonds in protein reduce Cu^{2+} ions from the copper (II) sulfate to Cu^+ (a temperature

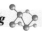

dependent reaction). The amount of Cu^{2+} reduced is proportional to the amount of protein present in the solution. Next, two molecules of bicinchoninic acid chelate with each Cu^+ ion, forming a purple-colored complex that strongly absorbs light at a wavelength of 562 nm.

The bicinchoninic acid Cu^+ complex is influenced in protein samples by the presence of cysteine/cystine, tyrosine, and tryptophan side chains. At higher temperatures (37℃ to 60℃), peptide bonds assist in the formation of the reaction complex. Incubating the BCA assay at higher temperatures is recommended as a way to increase assay sensitivity while minimizing the variances caused by unequal amino acid composition.

The amount of protein present in a solution can be quantified by measuring the absorption spectra and comparing with protein solutions of known concentration.

3.4.1.5 *Quantitative SDS gel staining and scanning*（SDS- 凝胶染色与扫描分析法）

Nonradioactive

Methods described for estimation of the amount of protein present in a sample, such as amino acid analysis and the bicinchoninic acid (BCA) method, quantify total protein present but not of one protein in a mixture of several. For this, the mixture must be resolved. Liquid chromatography achieves this, and the various proteins may be quantified by their absorbancy at 220 nm or 280 nm. Microgram to submicrogram amounts of protein can be analyzed in this way, using microbore（微内径，微径柱）high-performance liquid chromatography (HPLC).

An alternative is polyacrylamide gel electrophoresis (as the mixture-resolving step) followed by protein staining and densitometry. Exceptions are small peptides that are not successfully resolved and stained in gels, and which are more suited to chromatography. Microgram to submicrogram amounts of protein (of more than a few kilodaltons in size) may be quantified in this way.

Quantitation of proteins on SDS-polyacrylamide gels began at least from 1975, with peak areas corresponding to individual proteins determined and the area ratios of proteins to lysozyme (used as internal standard) were calculated. Whereas in a 1982 report quantitative analysis of individual protein spots was accomplished by computer-assisted densitometry (a PDP-ll/60 computer). Each gel was first photographed next to a calibrated density standard using 120-mm Tri-X Kodak film — for computerized densitometry.

Coomassie Brilliant Blue and silver stain are two commonly used stain methods for qualitative analysis via SDS-PAGE.

Staining by Coomassie dye is difficult to control — it may not fully penetrate and stain dense bands of protein, it may demonstrate a metachromatic（异染色的）effect (whereby the protein-dye complex may show any of a range of colors from blue through purple to red), and it may be variably or even completely decolorized by excessive destaining procedures (because the dye does not bind covalently). As a consequence, stoichiometric binding of Coomassie dye to protein is commonly not achieved. While silver stain methods have great sensitivity, they are problematical for quantification purposes. For various reasons, proteins vary widely in their stainability by silver — some do not stain at all, others may show a metachromatic effect, and it is difficult in obtaining staining throughout the gel, not just at the surface.

Procion navy MXRB. Various factors may influence the choice of dye to be used. Procion navy MXRB was used for quantitative staining suitable for proteins on acid/urea or SDS polyacrylamide gels.

By comparing with Coomassie Brilliant, Blue R250 (BBR250) Procion Navy MXRB has the following strengths ——

Firstly, given time, Procion Navy can penetrate dense bands of protein and stain them. Secondly, Procion Navy gives the same color with every protein, with no metachromatic effect. Thirdly, results are more consistent with Procion Navy, which binds covalently to proteins so that prolonged destaining does not remove it. Fourthly, the efficacy of Procion Navy MXRB doesn't vary from batch to batch. Furthermore, standard curves of Procion Navy MXRB binding to various proteins are straight lines passing through the origin, although they do plateau at higher protein quantities. On such gels, a loading of less than 0.5 μg is detectable and 1 μg is sufficient for quantification. Therefore, Procion Navy MXRB (and probably other members of the Procion dye family) is potentially the better choice for quantification purposes.

Colloidal Coomassie Brilliant Blue G Method. Colloidal stain does not stain the background in a gel and so washing can give crystal-clear backgrounds. A method used 0.4% (w/v) Brilliant Blue G250 in 3.5% (w/v) perchloric acid (高氯酸) has proven useful for quantification of proteins on gels.

(1) At the end of electrophoresis, wash the gel for a few minutes with several changes of water, then immerse the gel (with gentle shaking) in the colloidal Coomassie Brilliant Blue G protein stain — 0.4% (w/v) Coomassie Brilliant Blue G (C.I. 42 655; Sigma, code B0770)* in 3.5% (w/v) perchloric acid. This time varies with the gel type [*e.g.*, 1.0~1.5 h for a 1~1.5 mm thick sodium dodecyl sulfate (SDS) polyacrylamide gel slab], but cannot really be overdone. Discard the stain after use, for its efficacy declines with use.

*A commercially-available alternative is the GelCode blue stain reagent from Pierce.

Because performance of the Coomassie Brilliant Blue G stain is variable it is essential to run and stain standards and samples on the same gel, and to do so in duplicate.

(2) At the end of the staining period, decolorize the background by immersion in distilled water, with agitation, and a change of water whenever it becomes colored. Background destaining is fairly rapid, giving a clear background after a few hours.

(3) Measure the extent of blue dye bound by each band by scanning densitometry. The Coomassie Brilliant Blue G-stained gel may be dried between transparent sheets of dialysis membrane or cellophane for storage and later scanning. Beware that bubbles or marks in the membrane may add to the background noise upon scanning. A suitable scanning densitometer, for example, the Molecular Dynamics Personal Densitometer SI with Image Quant software or the Bio-Rad Fluor S MultiImager with Multi Analyst software. Such equipment can scan transparent objects such as wet gels, gels dried between transparent films, and photographic film, and digitize the image that may then be analyzed. Compare the dye bound by a sample with those for standard proteins run and stained in parallel with the sample, on the same gel.

When analyzing the results of scanning, construct a curve of absorbency vs protein concentration from standard samples and compare the experimental sample(s) with this. Construct a standard curve for each experiment.

The staining by Coomassie Brilliant Blue G may be quantitative, or nearly so, from about 10 to 20 ng/mm^2 up to large loadings of 1~5 μg/mm^2. Whatever method is used for quantification, it should be checked with the protein of interest, to confirm that staining is linear (quantitative) over the range of sample size being used. The stoichiometry of dye binding is subject to some variation, such that standard curves may be either linear or slightly curved, but even the latter case is acceptable provided standards are run on the same gel as samples.

Sypro Ruby Method. Better luminescent stains have been developed by Molecular Probes — the Sypro family of dyes. The Sypro Ruby stain is possibly the most sensitive of these, approaching the sensitivity of silver stains. The method for use of this stain is given below.

(1) At the end of electrophoresis, rinse the gel in water briefly, put it into a clean dish and then cover it with Sypro Ruby gel stain (Molecular Probes, product number S-12 000 or S-12 001) solution. Use fresh, undiluted stain only. Gently agitate until staining is completed, which may take up to 24 h or longer. Overstaining will not occur during prolonged stained. Do not let the stain dry up on the gel during long staining procedures. Discard the stain after use, for it becomes less efficacious with use. During the staining procedure the gel may be removed from the stain and inspected under UV light to monitor progress. If the staining is insufficient, the gel may be replaced in the stain for further incubation. A Sypro dye blot stain equivalent to the method described above for gels is available from Molecular Probes.

(2) Destain the background by washing the gel in a few changes of water for 15~30 min.

(3) Measure the extent of dye bound, that is, the luminescence. Although more sensitive than the blue stain, it does require UV irradiation for detection, by each band by scanning. Compare the dye bound by a sample with that for standard proteins run and stained in parallel with the sample, on the same gel.

Methods have been described for quantification of sub-microgram amounts of proteins that have been transferred from gels to polyvinylidene difluoride (聚偏氟乙烯) or similar membrane.

Equipment for scanning fluorescent bands on gels, for example, the Bio-Rad Fluor S MultiImager with Multi Analyst software, which can be used to photographically record or scan wet gels, allowing repeated scanning procedures (as staining or destaining proceeds). Simple viewing of stained bands may be done under a hand-held 300-nm UV lamp or on a transilluminator. Protect eyes with UV-opaque glasses. The Sypro dye may be excited at 280 or 450 nm and emits at 610 nm.

Other approaches and progress

"Scanplot". Area integration of protein bands from single line scans is relatively inaccurate when quantifying load. The software "Scanplot", allows volume integration of the complete protein band. Volume integration allows a more robust analysis of protein bands that may have irregular shapes and intensities and would perform equally well for the analysis of 1-D and 2-D gels. Scanplot also allows the user to select a region of interest (ROI) to provide background values which are then subtracted from values measured within the protein band ROI. The HP ScanJet Plus scanner and Scanplot software analyses demonstrated a linear relationship between protein load and densitometric volume for three different proteins. The HP ScanJet Plus offers both an affordable alternative to laser densitometry as well as an accurate tool in the quantification of CBB-stained proteins for loads ranging from 0.125 to 10.0 pg. Reliability may be improved by the use of standardized gel formation and staining/destaining protocols.

Zn^{2+} reverse staining. Zn^{2+} reverse staining method is a quantitative staining method which generates negatively stained bands. The technique generates a white background of precipitated zinc salt — imidazole-zinc complex, against which clear bands of protein (where precipitation is inhibited). This may be viewed by dark field illumination. The gel may be scanned at this stage, the negative staining being approximately quantitative (for horse myoglobin) in a range from about 100 ng/mm^2 to 2 μg/mm^2 or more. Sensitivity may be improved by staining of the background by incubation with tolidine (联甲

苯胺）. The method was described for 12% and 15% T gels, but the degree of zinc salt precipitation and subsequent toning — a "toning precedure" which turns the formerly white background into a deep blue, leaving the protein bands transparent and colorless — is dependent upon %T and at closer to 20%T the toning procedure may completely destain the gel, restricting the usefulness of the method.

Radioactive

Autoradiography is often used to detect and quantify radiolabeled proteins present after separation by polyacrylamide gel electrophoresis (PAGE). The use of a cleavable crosslinking agent in the polyacrylamide gels that allows the solubilization of the protein for quantification by scintillation counting. Although developed for tritium, the method works well with any covalently bound label. Resolution is as good as or better than autoradiography (Fig. 3-21), turnaround time（周转时间）can be greatly reduced, and quantification is more easily accomplished.

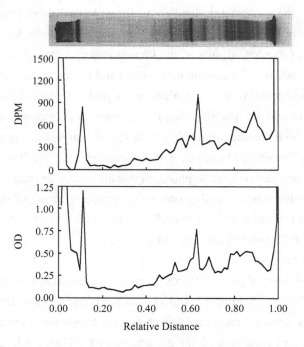

Fig. 3-21 Comparison of an autoradiogram, densitometry scan, and radioactivity in gel slices from a mixture of labeled proteins separated by PAGE. Identical aliquots of ^{35}S-methionine labeled proteins from the membranes of the cellular slime mold, *D. purpureum*, were separated using the methods described above in **SDS-Polyacrylamide Gels** section. One lane was fixed, soaked in Fluoro-Hance (Research Products International Corp., Mount Prospect, IL), dried, and autoradiographed (photograph). Another lane was cut from the gel, sliced into 1-mm pieces, solubilized, and counted using a Tracor Mark III liquid scintillation counter with automatic quench correction (TM Analytic, Elk Grove Village, IL) as described in **Slicing and Counting of Gel Slices** section. The resultant disintegrations per minute (DPM) were plotted vs the relative distance from the top of the running gel (**top figure**). The autoradiogram (photograph) was scanned relative to the top of the running gel using white light on a Transidyne RFT densitometer (**bottom figure**).

Reagents should be of high quality, particularly the sodium dodecyl sulfate (SDS) to obtain the best resolution, glycerol to eliminate extraneous bands, and ammonium persulfate to obtain proper polymerization.

The general requirements to construct, prepare, and run SDS-PAGE gels as described by Laemmli. For most of the methods described a preferred preparation of a standard gel can be substituted, except for the requirement of the replacement of DATD for bis at a ratio of 1 ：10 DATD ：acrylamide in the original

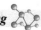

formulation.

SDS-Polyacrylamide Gels

Sufficient medium for one $8 \times 10 \times 0.75$ to 1.0-cm gel can be made by combining stock solutions and various amounts of acrylamide-DATD and water to achieve the required percentage of acrylamide by using the quantities listed in **Table 3-6**. The stacking gel is that described by Laemmli and is formed by combining 0.55 ml of acrylamide-*bis* with 1.25 ml of Tris III, 3.2 ml of water, 0.015 ml of fresh 10% APS, and 0.005 ml of TEMED.

Table 3-6   Recipe for Various Percentages of SDS-PAGE Gels

Stock Solution	Percentage of Acrylamide		
	7.5%	10%	12.5%
Acrylamide-DATD	0.96 ml	1.33 ml	1.66 ml
Tris II	1.50 ml	1.50 ml	1.50 ml
Water	3.50 ml	3.13 ml	2.80 ml
APS	0.03 ml	0.03 ml	0.03 ml
TEMED	0.003 ml	0.003 ml	0.003 ml

(1) For both the running and the stacking gel, degas the solutions by applying a vacuum for approx 30 s before adding the TEMED.

(2) After the addition of the TEMED, pour the gels, insert the comb in the case of the stacking gel, and overlay quickly with 0.1% SDS to provide good polymerization.

(3) Prepare protein samples by dissolving two parts of the protein sample in one part of sample buffer and heating to 100℃ for 2 min.

(4) Run gels at 200 V constant voltage for 45 min to 1 h or until the dye front reaches the bottom of the plate.

Special Reagent preparation

(1) Acrylamide-DATD: Acrylamide (45 g) and *N,N'*-diallyltartardiamide (DATD 4.5 g) are dissolved in water to a final volume of 100 ml. Water should be added slowly and time allowed for the crystals to dissolve.

(2) Acrylamide-*bis*: Acrylamide (45 g) and *N,N'*-methylenebis (acrylamide) (*bis*-acrylamide, 1.8 g), are dissolved as in item 1 in water to a final volume of 100 ml.

(3) Tris I: 0.285 *M* Tris-HCl, pH 6.8.

(4) Tris II: 1.5 *M* Tris-HCl, pH 8.8, 0.4% SDS.

(5) Tris III: 0.5 *M* Tris-HCl pH 6.8, 0.4% SDS.

(6) $10 \times$ Running buffer: Tris base (30.2 g), glycine (144.1 g), and SDS (10.00 g) are made up to 1 L with distilled water.

(7) Sample buffer: The following are mixed together and stored at 4℃: 1.5 ml 20% (w/v) SDS, 1.5 ml glycerol, 0.75 ml 2-mercaptoethanol, 0.15 ml 0.2% (w/v) Bromophenol blue, and 1.1 ml Tris I.

Silver Staining of Gels

The method used is that of Morrissey J.X. (1981)

(1) Remove gels from the plates, and immerse in solution A for 15 min.

(2) Transfer to solution B for 15 min and then solution C for 15 min, all while gently shaking.

(3) At this point, the gel can be rinsed in glass-distilled water for 2 h to overnight.

(4) After the water rinse, add fresh water and enough crystalline dithiotreitol (DTT) to make the solution 5 μg/ml.

(5) After 15 min, remove the DTT, and add 0.1% silver nitrate made fresh from the 1% stock solution. Shake for 15 min.

(6) Rapidly rinse the gel with a small amount of water followed by two 5~10 ml rinses with developer followed by the remainder of the developer.

(7) Watch the gel carefully, and add stop bath to the gel and developer when the desired darkness of the bands is reached.

(8) Store the stopped gel in water until the next step.

Reagent preparation

All solutions must be made with good-quality water.

(1) Solution A : methanol : acetic acid : water (50：10：40).

(2) Solution B : methanol:acetic acid : water (5：7：88).

(3) Solution C : 10% (*V/V*) glutaraldehyde（戊二醛）.

(4) 10× Silver nitrate: 1% (*W/V*) silver nitrate stored in brown glass bottle.

(5) Developer: Just before use, 25 μl of 37% formaldehyde is added to freshly made 3% (*W/V*) sodium carbonate.

(6) Stop bath: 2.3 *M* Citric acid (48.3 g/100 ml).

Slicing and Counting of Gel Slices

1. Remove individual lanes from the gel for slicing by cutting with a knife or spatula.

2. Cut each lane into uniform slices, or cut identified bands in the gel.

3. Place each slice into a glass scintillation vial, and add 0.5 ml of 2% sodium metaperiodate（偏过碘酸钠）(Solubilizer) solution.

4. Shake the vials for 30 min to dissolve the gel.

5. Add a 10-ml aliquot of scintillation fluid — Ecolume (+) (ICN Biomedical, Inc., Irvine, CA) or other scintillants to the vial, cool the vial, and count in a refrigerated scintillation counter.

Fig. 3-21 shows the results of a typical experiment using ^{35}S-methionine to label proteins metabolically from the cellular slime mold, *Dictyostelium purpureum*（盘基网柄菌）, and quantify them using the method described or by autoradiography. If one were interested in a particular protein, it would be fairly easy to isolate the slice of gel containing that protein for quantification. This makes this method extremely useful for comparing incorporation into a single protein over time as in pulse/chase experiments（脉冲追踪实验）.

It was found that as little as 400 dpm（每分钟衰变数）of tritium（氚）associated with a protein could be detected, which makes this method particularly useful for scarce proteins or small samples.

3.4.2 Assessment of protein purity（蛋白质纯度的评价）

3.4.2.1 SDS-PAGE（SDS-聚丙烯酰胺凝胶电泳法）

Introduction to SDS-PAGE

This material is accompanied by a presentation on protein structure and principles behind denaturing samples and discontinuous gel electrophoresis.

The separation of macromolecules in an electric field is called *electrophoresis*. A very common method for separating proteins by electrophoresis uses a discontinuous polyacrylamide gel as a support medium and sodium dodecyl sulfate (SDS) to denature the proteins. The method is called **sodium dodecyl sulfate polyacrylamide gel electrophoresis** (SDS-PAGE). The most commonly used system is also called the Laemmli method after U.K. Laemmli, who was the first to publish a paper employing SDS-PAGE in a scientific study.

SDS (also called lauryl sulfate) is an anionic detergent, meaning that when dissolved its molecules have a net negative charge within a wide pH range. A polypeptide chain binds certain amounts of SDS in proportion to its relative molecular mass. The negative charges on SDS destroy most of the complex structure of proteins, and are strongly attracted toward an anode (positively-charged electrode) in an electric field.

Polyacrylamide gels restrain larger molecules from migrating as fast as smaller molecules. Because the charge-to-mass ratio is nearly the same among SDS-denatured polypeptides, the final separation of proteins is dependent almost entirely on the differences in relative molecular mass of polypeptides. In a gel of uniform density the relative migration distance of a protein (Rf, the f as a subscript) is negatively proportional to the log of its mass (Fig. 3-22). If proteins of known mass are run simultaneously with the unknowns, the relationship between Rf and mass can be plotted, and the masses of unknown proteins estimated.

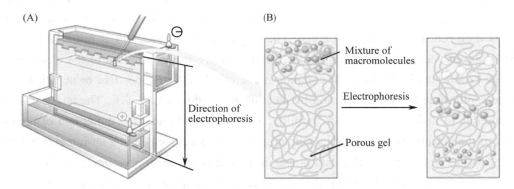

Fig. 3-22   Illustration of the equipment and operation of SDS-PAGE and its separation principle.

Protein separation by SDS-PAGE can be used to estimate relative molecular mass, to determine the relative abundance of major proteins in a sample, and to determine the distribution of proteins among fractions. The purity of protein samples can be assessed and the progress of a fractionation or purification procedure can be followed. Different staining methods can be used to detect rare proteins and to learn something about their biochemical properties. Specialized techniques such as Western blotting, two-dimensional electrophoresis, and peptide mapping can be used to detect extremely scarce gene products, to find similarities among them, and to detect and separate isoenzymes of proteins.

Polyacrylamide gels for SDS-PAGE

Regardless of the system, preparation requires casting two different layers of acrylamide between glass plates. The lower layer (separating, or resolving, gel) is responsible for actually separating polypeptides by size. The upper layer (stacking gel) includes the sample wells. It is designed to sweep up proteins in a sample between two moving boundaries so that they are compressed (stacked) into micrometer thin layers when they reach the separating gel.

3.4.2.2 *Capillary electrophoresis*（毛细管电泳法）

Capillary electrophoresis (CE) is a family of electrokinetic separation methods performed in submillimeter（亚毫米）diameter capillaries and in micro- and nanofluidic（纳流控的）channels. Very often, CE refers to capillary zone electrophoresis (CZE，毛细管区带电泳), but other electrophoretic techniques including capillary gel electrophoresis (CGE), capillary isoelectric focusing (CIEF), capillary isotachophoresis（等速电泳）and micellar electrokinetic chromatography (MEKC，毛细管胶束电动力学色谱) belong also to this class of methods. In CE methods, analytes migrate through electrolyte（电解质）solutions under the influence of an electric field. Analytes can be separated according to ionic mobility（离子迁移率）and/or partitioning into an alternate phase via Non-covalent interactions. Additionally, analytes may be concentrated or "focused" by means of gradients in conductivity and pH.

Instrumentation

The instrumentation（仪器）needed to perform capillary electrophoresis is relatively simple. A basic schematic of a capillary electrophoresis system is shown in Fig. 3-23. The system's main components are a sample vial（小瓶）, source and destination vials, a capillary, electrodes, a high-voltage power supply, a detector, and a data output and handling device. The source vial, destination vial and capillary are filled with an electrolyte such as an aqueous buffer solution. To introduce the sample, the capillary inlet is placed into a vial containing the sample. Sample is introduced into the capillary via capillary action, pressure, siphoning（虹吸，用虹吸管输送）, or electrokinetically（电动力地）, and the capillary is then returned to the source vial. The migration of the analytes is initiated by an electric field that is applied between the source and destination vials and is supplied to the electrodes by the high-voltage power supply. In the most common mode of CE, all ions, positive or negative, are pulled through the capillary in the same direction by electroosmotic flow（电渗流）. The analytes separate as they migrate due to their electrophoretic mobility, and are detected near the outlet end of the capillary. The output of the detector is sent to a data output and handling device such as an integrator（积分仪，积分器，集成器）or computer. The data is then displayed as an electropherogram（电泳图谱）, which reports detector response as a function of time. Separated chemical compounds appear as peaks with different retention times in an electropherogram. Capillary electrophoresis was first combined with mass spectrometry by Richard D. Smith and coworkers, and provides extremely high sensitivity for the analysis of very small sample sizes. Despite the very small sample sizes (typically only a few nanoliters

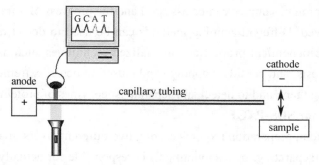

Fig. 3-23 Schematic of capillary electrophoresis system. Samples enter the tube from the right and travel to the left to the detection system which records the chromatogram output on a computer.

of liquid are introduced into the capillary), high sensitivity and sharp peaks are achieved in part due to injection strategies that result in concentration of analytes into a narrow zone near the inlet of the capillary. This is achieved in either pressure or electrokinetic injections simply by suspending the sample in a buffer of lower conductivity (*e.g.*, lower salt concentration) than the running buffer（运行缓冲液）. A process called field-amplified sample stacking（场放大样品电堆积，场放大样品富积）(a form of isotachophoresis) results in concentration of analyte in a narrow zone at the boundary between the low-conductivity sample and the higher-conductivity running buffer.

To achieve greater sample throughput（通量，流量，通过量，总处理能力）, instruments with arrays of capillaries are used to analyze many samples simultaneously. Such capillary array electrophoresis (CAE) instruments with 16 or 96 capillaries are used for medium- to high-throughput capillary DNA sequencing, and the inlet ends of the capillaries are arrayed（排列）spatially to accept samples directly from SBS-standard footprint 96-well plates. Certain aspects of the instrumentation (such as detection) are necessarily more complex than for a single-capillary system, but the fundamental principles of design and operation are similar to those shown in Fig. 3-24.

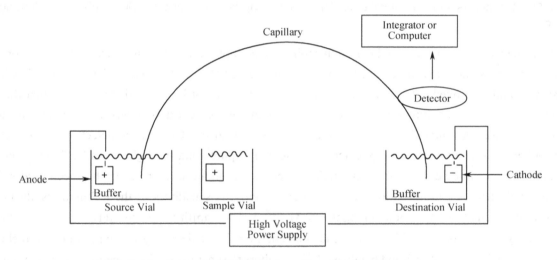

Fig. 3-24　Schematic diagram of capillary electrophoresis system.

Detection

Separation by capillary electrophoresis can be detected by several detection devices. The majority of commercial systems use UV or UV-Vis absorbance as their primary mode of detection. In these systems, a section of the capillary itself is used as the detection cell. The use of on-tube detection enables detection of separated analytes with no loss of resolution. In general, capillaries used in capillary electrophoresis are coated with a polymer [frequently polyimide（聚酰亚胺）or Teflon（特氟龙，聚四氟乙烯）] for increased flexibility. The portion of the capillary used for UV detection, however, must be optically transparent. For polyimide-coated capillaries, a segment of the coating is typically burned or scraped off （刮掉，擦去）to provide a bare window several millimeters long. This bare section of capillary can break easily, and capillaries with transparent coatings are available to increase the stability of the cell window. The path length of the detection cell in capillary electrophoresis (~ 50 micrometers) is far less than that of a traditional UV cell (~ 1 cm). According to the Beer-Lambert law, the sensitivity of the detector is proportional to the path length of the cell. To improve the sensitivity, the path length can be increased, though this results in a loss of resolution. The capillary tube itself can be expanded at the detection point, creating a "bubble cell" with a longer path length or additional tubing (管，管子) can be added at the detection point as shown in Fig. 3-25. Both of these methods, however, will decrease the resolution of the separation. Post-column detection utilizing a sheath flow (鞘流，包层液) configuration has also been described.

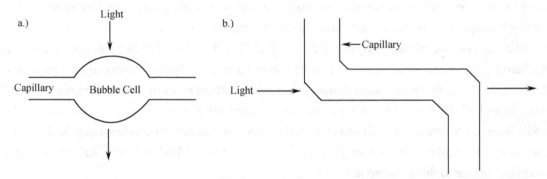

Fig. 3-25 Techniques for increasing the pathlength of the capillary: a.) a bubble cell and b.) a z-cell (additional tubing).

Fluorescence detection can also be used in capillary electrophoresis for samples that naturally fluoresce or are chemically modified to contain fluorescent tags (荧光标签). This mode of detection offers high sensitivity and improved selectivity for these samples, but cannot be utilized for samples that do not fluoresce. Numerous labeling strategies are used to create fluorescent derivatives or conjugates of non-fluorescent molecules, including proteins and DNA. The set-up for fluorescence detection in a capillary electrophoresis system can be complicated. The method requires that the light beam be focused on the capillary, which can be difficult for many light sources. Laser-induced fluorescence has been used in CE systems with detection limits as low as 10^{-18} to 10^{-21} mol. The sensitivity of the technique is attributed to the high intensity of the incident light (入射光) and the ability to accurately focus the light on the capillary. Multi-color (多彩) fluorescence detection can be achieved by including multiple dichroic mirrors (二向色镜，二色镜) and bandpass (带通) filters to separate the fluorescence emission amongst multiple detectors [*e.g.*, photomultiplier tubes (光电倍增管)], or by using a prism (棱镜) or grating (格栅) to project spectrally resolved (光谱分辨的) fluorescence emission onto a position-sensitive detector such as a CCD array (电荷耦合元件阵列). CE systems with 4- and 5-color LIF (激光诱导荧光检测器) detection systems are used routinely for capillary DNA sequencing and genotyping (基因型分型) ("DNA fingerprinting") applications.

In order to obtain the identity of sample components, capillary electrophoresis can be directly coupled with mass spectrometers or Surface Enhanced Raman Spectroscopy (SERS，表面增强拉曼光谱). In most systems, the capillary outlet is introduced into an ion source that utilizes electrospray ionization (ESI，电喷雾电离). The resulting ions are then analyzed by the mass spectrometer. This set-up requires volatile buffer solutions, which will affect the range of separation modes that can be employed and the degree of resolution that can be achieved. The measurement and analysis are mostly done with a specialized gel analysis software.

For CE-SERS, capillary electrophoresis eluants (洗脱剂，洗提液) can be deposited onto (沉淀于) a SERS-active substrate. Analyte retention times can be translated into spatial distance by moving the

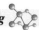

SERS-active substrate at a constant rate during capillary electrophoresis. This allows the subsequent spectroscopic technique（光谱技术）to be applied to specific eluants for identification with high sensitivity. SERS-active substrates can be chosen that do not interfere with the spectrum of the analytes.

Modes of separation

The separation of compounds by capillary electrophoresis is dependent on the differential migration（差速迁移）of analytes in an applied electric field. The electrophoretic migration velocity (u_p) of an analyte toward the electrode of opposite charge is:

$$u_p = \mu_p E$$

The electrophoretic mobility（电泳迁移率，电泳速率）can be determined experimentally from the migration time and the field strength:

$$\mu_p = \left(\frac{L}{t_r}\right)\left(\frac{L_t}{V}\right)$$

where L is the distance from the inlet to the detection point, t_r is the time required for the analyte to reach the detection point (migration time), V is the applied voltage (field strength), and L_t is the total length of the capillary. Since only charged ions are affected by the electric field, neutral analytes are poorly separated by capillary electrophoresis.

The velocity of migration of an analyte in capillary electrophoresis will also depend upon the rate of electroosmotic flow (EOF, 电渗流) of the buffer solution. In a typical system, the electroosmotic flow is directed toward the negatively charged cathode so that the buffer flows through the capillary from the source vial to the destination vial. Separated by differing electrophoretic mobilities, analytes migrate toward the electrode of opposite charge. As a result, negatively charged analytes are attracted to the positively charged anode, counter to the EOF, while positively charged analytes are attracted to the cathode, in agreement with the EOF as depicted in Fig. 3-26.

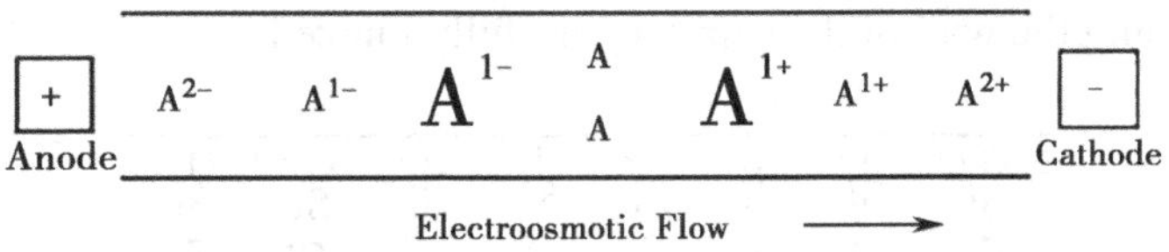

| + | A^{2-} | A^{1-} | $\mathbf{A}^{1-}$ | A A A | $\mathbf{A}^{1+}$ | A^{1+} | A^{2+} | − |

Anode ————————————————————— Cathode

Electroosmotic Flow ⟶

Fig. 3-26   Diagram of the separation of charged and neutral analytes (A) according to their respective electrophoretic and electroosmotic flow mobilities.

The velocity of the electroosmotic flow, u_o can be written as:

$$u_o = \mu_o E$$

where μ_o is the electroosmotic mobility（电渗迁移率）, which is defined as:

$$\mu_o = \frac{\epsilon\zeta}{\eta}$$

where ζ is the zeta potential of the capillary wall, and ϵ is the relative permittivity（相对介电常数）of the buffer solution. Experimentally, the electroosmotic mobility can be determined by measuring the retention time of a neutral analyte. The velocity (u) of an analyte in an electric field can then be defined as:

$$u_p + u_o = (\mu_p + \mu_o)E$$

Since the electroosmotic flow of the buffer solution is generally greater than that of the electrophoretic mobility of the analytes, all analytes are carried along with the buffer solution toward the cathode. Even small, triply charged anions can be redirected to the cathode by the relatively powerful EOF of the buffer solution. Negatively charged analytes are retained longer in the capillary due to their conflicting （冲突的，相矛盾的）electrophoretic mobilities. The order of migration seen by the detector is shown in Fig. 3-26: small multiply charged cations migrate quickly and small multiply charged anions are retained strongly.

Electroosmotic flow is observed when an electric field is applied to a solution in a capillary that has fixed charges on its interior wall. Charge is accumulated on the inner surface of a capillary when a buffer solution is placed inside the capillary. In a fused-silica capillary （熔融石英毛细管）, silanol (Si-OH) groups （硅羟基，硅烷醇基）attached to the interior wall of the capillary are ionized to negatively charged silanoate (Si-O⁻) groups at pH values greater than three. The ionization of the capillary wall can be enhanced by first running a basic solution, such as NaOH or KOH through the capillary prior to introducing the buffer solution. Attracted to the negatively charged silanoate groups, the positively charged cations of the buffer solution will form two inner layers of cations (called the diffuse double layer or the electrical double layer) on the capillary wall as shown in Fig. 3-27. The first layer is referred to as the fixed layer because it is held tightly to the silanoate groups. The outer layer, called the mobile layer, is farther from the silanoate groups. The mobile cation layer is pulled in the direction of the negatively charged cathode when an electric field is applied. Since these cations are solvated, the bulk buffer solution migrates with the mobile layer, causing the electroosmotic flow of the buffer solution. Other capillaries including Teflon capillaries also exhibit electroosmotic flow. The EOF of these capillaries is probably the result of adsorption of the electrically charged ions of the buffer onto the capillary walls. The rate of EOF is dependent on the field strength and the charge density of the capillary wall. The wall's charge density is proportional to the pH of the buffer solution. The electroosmotic flow will increase with pH until all of the available silanols lining the wall of the capillary are fully ionized.

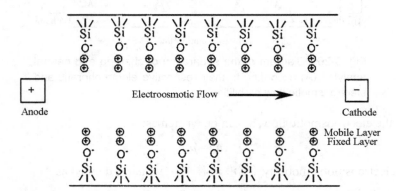

Fig. 3-27　Depiction of the interior of a fused-silica gel capillary in the presence of a buffer solution.

In certain situations where strong electroosmotic flow toward the cathode is undesirable, the inner surface of the capillary can be coated with polymers, surfactants, or small molecules to reduce electroosmosis to very low levels, restoring the normal direction of migration (anions toward the anode, cations toward the cathode). CE instrumentation typically includes power supplies with reversible （可

反转的）polarity（极性）, allowing the same instrument to be used in "normal" mode (with EOF and detection near the cathodic end of the capillary) and "reverse" mode (with EOF suppressed or reversed, and detection near the anodic end of the capillary). One of the most common approaches to suppressing EOF, reported by Stellan Hjertén in 1985, is to create a covalently attached layer of linear polyacrylamide. The silica surface of the capillary is first modified with a silane reagent bearing a polymerizable vinyl group（乙烯基）(*e.g.,* 3-methacryloxypropyltrimethoxysilane [3-（甲基丙基酰氧基）丙基三甲氧基硅烷）], followed by introduction of acrylamide monomer and a free radical initiator（自由基引发剂）. The acrylamide is polymerized *in situ*, forming long linear chains, some of which are covalently attached to the wall-bound silane reagent. Numerous other strategies for covalent modification of capillary surfaces exist. Dynamic or adsorbed coatings (which can include polymers or small molecules) are also common. For example, in capillary sequencing of DNA, the sieving polymer（筛分介质，筛分聚合物）(typically polydimethylacrylamide) suppresses electroosmotic flow to very low levels. A variety of dynamic capillary coating agents are commercially available to modify, suppress, or reverse the direction of electroosmotic flow. Besides modulating electroosmotic flow, capillary wall coatings can also serve the purpose of reducing interactions between "sticky" analytes (such as proteins) and the capillary wall. Such wall-analyte interactions, if severe, manifest as reduced peak efficiency, asymmetric (tailing) peaks, or even complete loss of analyte to the capillary wall.

Efficiency and resolution

The number of theoretical plates, or separation efficiency, in capillary electrophoresis is given by:

$$N = \frac{\mu V}{2Dm}$$

where N is the number of theoretical plates, μ is the apparent mobility（表观迁移率）in the separation medium and D_m is the diffusion coefficient of the analyte. According to this equation, the efficiency of separation is only limited by diffusion and is proportional to the strength of the electric field, although practical considerations limit the strength of the electric field to several hundred volts per centimeter. Application of very high potentials (>20~30 kV) may lead to arcing or breakdown of the capillary. Further, application of strong electric fields leads to resistive heating（电阻热）(Joule heating) of the buffer in the capillary. At sufficiently high field strengths, this heating is strong enough that radial temperature gradients can develop within the capillary. Since electrophoretic mobility of ions is generally temperature-dependent (due to both temperature-dependent ionization and solvent viscosity effects), a non-uniform temperature profile results in variation of electrophoretic mobility across the capillary, and a loss of resolution. The onset of significant Joule heating can be determined by constructing an "Ohm's Law plot", wherein the current through the capillary is measured as a function of applied potential. At low fields, the current is proportional to the applied potential [Ohm's Law（欧姆定律）], whereas at higher fields the current deviates from the straight line as heating results in decreased resistance of the buffer. The best resolution is typically obtained at the maximum field strength for which Joule heating is insignificant [*i.e.,* near the boundary between the linear and nonlinear regimes（状况，态，动态）of the Ohm's Law plot]. Generally capillaries of smaller inner diameter support use of higher field strengths, due to improved heat dissipation and smaller thermal gradients relative to larger capillaries, but with the drawbacks of lower sensitivity in absorbance detection due to shorter path length, and greater difficulty in introducing buffer and sample into the capillary (small capillaries require greater pressure and/or longer times to force fluids through the capillary).

The efficiency of capillary electrophoresis separations is typically much higher than the efficiency of other separation techniques like HPLC. Unlike HPLC, in capillary electrophoresis there is no mass transfer (传质, 质量传递) between phases. In addition, the flow profile in EOF-driven systems is flat, rather than the rounded laminar flow (层流) profile characteristic of the pressure-driven flow in chromatography columns as shown in Fig. 3-28. As a result, EOF does not significantly contribute to band broadening as in pressure-driven chromatography. Capillary electrophoresis separations can have several hundred thousand theoretical plates.

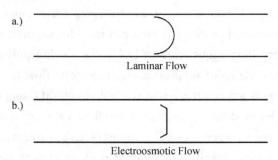

Fig. 3-28   Flow profiles of laminar and electroosmotic flow.

The resolution (R_s) of capillary electrophoresis separations can be written as:

$$R_s = \frac{1}{4} \left(\frac{\triangle \mu_p \sqrt{N}}{\mu_p + \mu_o} \right)$$

According to this equation, maximum resolution is reached when the electrophoretic and electroosmotic mobilities are similar in magnitude and opposite in sign. In addition, it can be seen that high resolution requires lower velocity and, correspondingly, increased analysis time.

Besides diffusion and Joule heating (discussed above), factors that may decrease the resolution in capillary electrophoresis from the theoretical limits in the above equation include, but are not limited to, the finite widths (有限宽度) of the injection plug and detection window; interactions between the analyte and the capillary wall; instrumental non-idealities (非理想特性) such as a slight difference in height of the fluid reservoirs (储液罐, 储液室) leading to siphoning (虹吸作用); irregularities in the electric field due to, *e.g.,* imperfectly cut capillary ends; depletion (消耗, 损耗, 耗竭) of buffering capacity (缓冲能力, 缓冲量) in the reservoirs; and electrodispersion (电分散, 电分解作用, 电分散作用) (when an analyte has higher conductivity than the background electrolyte). Identifying and minimizing the numerous sources of band broadening is key to successful method development in capillary electrophoresis, with the objective of approaching as close as possible to the ideal of diffusion-limited resolution.

3.4.3 Western blotting (蛋白质印迹)

Blotting includes various methods for transferring biological molecules (*e.g.,* proteins, nucleic acid fragments) from a gel matrix to a membrane support for the subsequent detection of those molecules, and Western blotting is the method used for immunodetection of detect proteins.

Overview

Western blotting, also called protein blotting or immunoblotting, is a widely used analytical technique used to detect specific proteins in a sample of tissue homogenate (匀浆) or extract. It uses gel electrophoresis to separate native proteins by 3-D structure or denatured proteins by the length of the polypeptide. The proteins are then transferred to a membrane [typically nitrocellulose or PVDF (Polyvinylidene Fluoride 聚偏氟乙稀)], where they are stained with antibodies specific to the target protein. The gel electrophoresis step is included in Western blot analysis to resolve the issue of (解决······ 问题) the cross-reactivity of antibodies. Then antibodies are used to identify specific protein targets bound to a membrane — the specificity of the antibody-antigen interaction enables a target protein to be identified in the midst of a complex protein mixture. Western blotting can produce qualitative and semi-quantitative data on a protein of interest.

The first step in a Western blotting procedure is to separate the proteins in a sample by size using denaturing gel electrophoresis (*i.e.*, SDS-PAGE). Alternatively, proteins can be separated by their isoelectric point (pI) using isoelectric focusing (IEF). After electrophoresis, the separated proteins are transferred, or "blotted", onto a solid support matrix, which is generally a nitrocellulose or polyvinylidene difluoride (PVDF) membrane. In procedures where protein separation is not required, the proteins may be directly applied to the solid support by spotting the sample on the membrane using an approach called dot blotting (the dot blot analysis) .

In most cases, the membrane must be blocked (封闭) to prevent nonspecific binding of the antibody probes to the membrane surface, and the transferred protein is then complexed with an antibody and detection probe (*e.g.*, enzyme, fluorophore, isotope). An appropriate method is then used to detect the localized probe to document the position and relative abundance of the target protein.

In addition to the challenges of immunodetection in the protein blotting workflow (工作流程), the transfer of proteins from a gel matrix to a membrane is a potential hurdle. The best results depend on the nature of the gel, the molecular weight of the proteins being transferred, the type of membrane and transfer buffers used and the transfer method.

There are many reagent companies that specialize in providing antibodies (both monoclonal and polyclonal antibodies) against tens of thousands of different proteins. Commercial antibodies can be expensive, although the unbound antibodies can be reused between experiments. This method is used in the fields of molecular biology, immunogenetics (免疫遗传学) and other molecular biology disciplines. A number of search engines, such as CiteAb, Antibodypedia, and SeekProducts, are available that can help researchers find suitable antibodies for use in Western blotting.

Other related techniques include immunohistochemistry and immunocytochemistry where antibodies are used to detect proteins in tissues and cells by immunostaining, and enzyme-linked immunosorbent assay (ELISA).

Western blotting was introduced by Towbin *et al.* in 1979 and is now a routine technique for protein analysis. Since the method originated in the laboratory of Harry Towbin at the Friedrich Miescher Institute, the name *Western blot* was given to the technique by W. Neal Burnette and is a play on the name Southern blot, a technique for DNA detection developed earlier by Edwin Southern. Detection of RNA is termed Northern blot and was developed by George Stark at Stanford.

Blotting Membranes

Blotting membranes may be available in either sheets or rolls and commonly have a thickness of 100 μm with typical pore sizes of 0.1, 0.2 or 0.45 μm. Most proteins can be successfully blotted using a 0.45

μm pore size membrane, while a 0.1 or 0.2 μm pore size membrane is recommended for low molecular weight proteins or peptides (<20 kDa).

Following gel electrophoresis, there are a number of supports for protein transfer [including glass, plastic, latex （乳胶，乳液） and cellulose]. The most common immobilization membranes are nitrocellulose, polyvinylidene difluoride (PVDF) and nylon. These membranes have the following characteristics:

- A large surface area-to-volume area ratio
- A high binding capacity
- Provide the extended storage of immobilized macromolecules
- Are easy to use
- Can be optimized for low background signal and reproducibility

Nitrocellulose Membranes

Nitrocellulose membranes are a popular matrix used in protein blotting because of their high protein-binding affinity, compatibility with a variety of detection methods, and the ability to immobilize proteins, glycoproteins or nucleic acids. Protein immobilization is thought to occur by hydrophobic interactions, and high salt and low methanol concentrations improve protein immobilization to the membrane during electrophoretic transfer, especially proteins with higher molecular weights. Nitrocellulose membranes are not optimal for electrophoretic transfer of nucleic acids, as the high salt concentrations that are required for efficient binding will effectively elute some or all of the charged nucleic acid fragments.

PVDF Membranes

PVDF membranes are highly hydrophobic and must be pre-wetted with methanol or ethanol prior to submersion （浸没） in transfer buffer. PVDF membranes have a high binding affinity for proteins and nucleic acids and may be used for applications such as Western, Southern, Northern and dot blots; binding likely occurs via dipole and hydrophobic interactions. PVDF membranes offer better retention of adsorbed proteins than other supports because of the greater hydrophobicity. PVDF is also less brittle than nitrocellulose.

Nylon Membranes

Charged nylon (polyamide，聚酰胺) membranes bind by ionic, electrostatic and hydrophobic interactions, and many of the charged nylons contain quaternary amines that form stable linkages with nucleic acids under alkaline conditions. While not always required, nucleic acids are typically fixed to the membrane by UV-crosslinking, while uncharged nylon membranes rely on hydrophobic interactions that are formed when nucleic acids are dried on to the membrane surface. A significant drawback to using nylon membranes for blotting applications is the possibility for nonspecific binding and strong binding to anions like SDS and Ponceau S （丽春红 S）. Membranes with a positive zeta charge are recommended for blotting applications with negatively-charged nucleic acids, such as electrophoretic mobility shift assays (EMSA).

Transfer Buffers

Common buffers used for Western blotting are:

- Towbin system buffer [25 mM Tris-HCl pH 8.3, 192 mM glycine, 20% ($V : V$) methanol]
- CAPS buffer system [10 mM CAPS pH 10.5, 10% ($V : V$) methanol]

In most experiments, SDS should be omitted from the Western transfer buffer because the negative charge imparted to proteins can cause them to pass through the membrane. Typically, there is enough SDS associated with the proteins in SDS-PAGE gels to effectively carry them out of the gel and onto the membrane support. For proteins that tend to precipitate, the addition of low concentrations of SDS (<0.01%) may be necessary. It should be noted that adding SDS to the transfer buffer may require optimization of other transfer parameters (*e.g.*, time, current) to prevent "over-transfer" of proteins through the membrane [also known as "blowout" (喷出，井喷)].

Methanol in the transfer buffer aids in stripping the SDS from proteins in SDS-PAGE gels, increasing their ability to bind to support membranes. However, methanol can inactivate enzymes required for downstream analyses and shrinks the gel and membrane, which may increase the transfer time of large molecular weight proteins (150 000 Da) with poor solubility in methanol. In the absence of methanol, though, protein gels may swell in low ionic strength buffers, and therefore it is recommended to pre-swell gels for 30 minutes to 1 hour to prevent band distortion.

Transfer Methods

There are four major ways to transfer macromolecules from SDS-PAGE or native gels to nitrocellulose, PVDF or nylon membranes: Diffusion blotting, Vacuum blotting, Tank (Wet) electrotransfer (湿转) and Semi-dry electrotransfer (半干转).

Diffusion Blotting

Diffusion blotting relies on the thermal motion of molecules, which causes them to move from an area of high concentration to an area of low concentration. In blotting methods, the transfer of molecules is dependent upon the diffusion of proteins out of the gel matrix and absorption to the transfer membrane. As the absorbed proteins are "removed" from solution, it helps maintain the concentration gradient that drives proteins towards the membrane. Originally developed for transferring proteins from isoelectric focusing (IEF) gels, diffusion blotting is also useful for other macromolecules, especially nucleic acids. Diffusion blotting is most useful when preparing multiple immunoblots from a single gel. Blots obtained by this method can also be used to identify proteins by mass spectrometry and analyze proteins by zymography (酶谱法). Protein recoveries are typically 25%~50% of the total transferrable protein, which is lower than other transfer methods. Additionally, protein transfer is not quantitative. Diffusion blotting may be difficult for very large proteins in SDS-PAGE gels, but smaller proteins are typically easily transferred.

Vacuum Blotting (Vacuum Capillary Blotting)

Vacuum blotting is a variant of capillary blotting, where buffer from a reservoir is drawn through a gel and blotting membrane into dry tissue paper or other absorbent material. Vacuum blotting uses a slab (平板) gel dryer system or other suitable gel drying equipment to draw polypeptides from a gel to membrane, such as nitrocellulose. Strong pumps cannot be used because the high vacuum will shatter (粉碎，损坏) the gel or transfer membrane. Gels may dry out (变干，干透) after 45 minutes under vacuum, requiring plenty of reserve buffer. Gels also have a tendency to adhere to the membrane after transfer, but rehydration of the gel can help facilitate separation.

The transfer efficiency of vacuum blotting varies within a range of 30%~65%, with low molecular weight proteins (14.3 kDa) at the high end of this efficiency range and high molecular weight proteins (200 kDa) at the low end. Like diffusion blotting, vacuum blotting allows only a qualitative transfer.

Wet Electroblotting (Tank Transfer) (电转移法 - 湿转)

When performing a wet transfer, the gel is first equilibrated in transfer buffer. The gels is then placed in the 'transfer sandwich' (filter paper-gel-membrane-filter paper), cushioned by pads (安置在垫子上)

and pressed together by a support grid（网格，格子，格网）. The supported gel "sandwich" is placed vertically in a tank between stainless steel/platinum（铂）wire electrodes and filled with transfer buffer (Fig. 3-29).

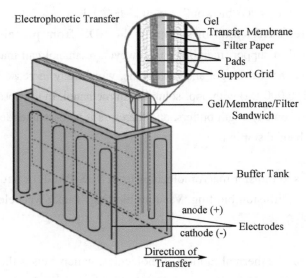

Fig. 3-29　Tank transfer apparatus for Western blotting. Schematic showing the assembly of a typical Western blot apparatus with the position of the gel, transfer membrane and direction of protein in relation to the electrode position.

Multiple gels may be electrotransferred in the standard field option, which is performed either at constant current (0.1 to 1 A) or voltage (5 to 30 V) from as little as 1 hour to overnight. Transfers are typically performed with an ice pack（冰袋）and at 4℃ to mitigate the heat produced. A high-field option exists for a single gel, which may bring transfer time down to as little as 30 minutes, but it requires the use of high voltage (up to 200 V) or high current (up to 1.6 A) and a cooling system to dissipate the tremendous heat produced.

Transfer efficiencies of 80%~100% are achievable for proteins between 14~116 kDa. The transfer efficiency improves with increased transfer time and is better, in general, for lower molecular weight proteins than higher molecular weight proteins. With increasing time, however, there is a risk of over-transfer (stripping, blowout) of the proteins through the membrane, especially for lower molecular weight (<30 kDa) proteins when using membranes with a larger pore size (0.45 μm).

Semi-dry Electroblotting (Semi-dry Transfer)（电转移法 - 半干转）

For semi-dry protein transfer, the transfer sandwich is placed horizontally between two plate electrodes in a semi-dry transfer apparatus. For this semi-dry transfer, it is very important that the gel is pre-equilibrated in transfer buffer. To maximize the current passing through the gel instead of around the gel, the amount of buffer available during transfer is limited to that contained in the sandwich, so it is helpful if the extra-thick filter paper (~3 mm thickness) and membrane are also sufficiently soaked in buffer. Likewise, it is key that the filter paper sheets and membrane are cut to the size of the gel.

One to four gels may be rapidly electroblotted to membranes. Methanol may be included in the transfer buffer, but other organic solvents, including aromatic hydrocarbons（芳烃）, chlorinated hydrocarbons（氯化烃）and acetone, should not be used to avoid damage to the semi-dry blotter. Electrotransfer is performed either at constant current (0.1 up to ~0.4 A) or voltage (10 to 25 V) for 10 to 60 minutes.

Methanol-free transfer buffers are recommended to reduce transfer time to 7 to 10 minutes. Transfer efficiencies of 60%~80% may be achievable for proteins between 14 and 116 kDa.

Steps

Tissue preparation

Samples can be taken from whole tissue or from cell culture. Solid tissues are first broken down mechanically using a blender (for larger sample volumes), using a homogenizer (smaller volumes), or by sonication. Cells may also be broken open by one of the above mechanical methods. However, virus or environmental samples can be the source of protein and thus Western blotting is not restricted to cellular studies only.

Assorted detergents, salts, and buffers may be employed to encourage lysis of cells and to solubilize proteins. Protease and phosphatase inhibitors are often added to prevent the digestion of the sample by its own enzymes. Tissue preparation is often done at cold temperatures to avoid protein denaturing and degradation.

A combination of biochemical and mechanical techniques — comprising various types of filtration and centrifugation — can be used to separate different cell compartments and organelles.

Gel electrophoresis

The proteins of the sample are separated using gel electrophoresis. Separation of proteins may be by isoelectric point (pI), molecular weight, electric charge, or a combination of these factors. The nature of the separation depends on the treatment of the sample and the nature of the gel. This is a very useful way to identify a protein.

By far the most common type of gel electrophoresis employs polyacrylamide gels and buffers loaded with sodium dodecyl sulfate (SDS). SDS-PAGE maintains polypeptides in a denatured state once they have been treated with strong reducing agents to remove secondary and tertiary structure (*e.g.*, disulfide bonds [S — S] to sulfhydryl groups [SH and SH]) and thus allows separation of proteins by their molecular weight. Sampled proteins become covered in the negatively charged SDS and move to the positively charged electrode through the acrylamide mesh (网眼, 网格) of the gel. Smaller proteins migrate faster through this mesh and the proteins are thus separated according to size (usually measured in kilodaltons, kDa). The concentration of acrylamide determines the resolution of the gel — the greater the acrylamide concentration, the better the resolution of lower molecular weight proteins. The lower the acrylamide concentration, the better the resolution of higher molecular weight proteins. Proteins travel only in one dimension along the gel for most blots.

Samples are loaded into *wells* in the gel. One lane is usually reserved for a *marker* or *ladder*, a commercially available mixture of proteins having defined molecular weights, typically stained so as to form visible, colored bands. When voltage is applied along the gel, proteins migrate through it at different speeds dependent on their size. These different rates of advancement (前进) (different *electrophoretic mobilities*) separate into *bands* within each *lane*.

It is also possible to use a two-dimensional (2-D) gel which spreads the proteins from a single sample out in two dimensions. Proteins are separated according to isoelectric point (pH at which they have neutral net charge) in the first dimension, and according to their molecular weight in the second dimension.

Transfer

In order to make the proteins accessible to antibody detection, they are moved from within the gel onto a membrane made of *nitrocellulose or polyvinylidene difluoride (PVDF)*. The primary method for transferring the proteins is called electroblotting（电印迹）and uses an electric current to pull proteins from the gel into the PVDF or nitrocellulose membrane (Fig. 3-30). The proteins move from within the gel onto the membrane while maintaining the organization they had within the gel. An older method of transfer involves placing a membrane on top of the gel, and a stack of filter papers on top of that. The entire stack is placed in a buffer solution that moves up the paper by capillary action, bringing the proteins with it. In practice this method is not used as it takes too much time; electroblotting is preferred. As a result of either "blotting" process, the proteins are exposed on a thin surface layer for detection. Both varieties of membrane are chosen for their non-specific protein binding properties (*i.e.,* binds all proteins equally well). Protein binding is based upon hydrophobic interactions, as well as charged interactions between the membrane and protein. Nitrocellulose membranes are cheaper than PVDF, but are far more fragile and do not stand up well to repeated probings.

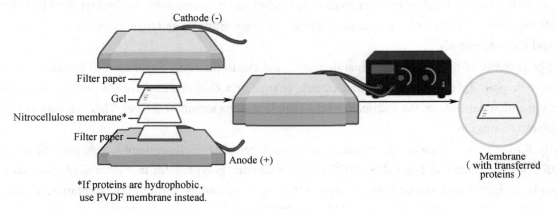

Fig. 3-30 Diagram of electroblotting.

The uniformity and overall effectiveness of transfer of protein from the gel to the membrane can be checked by staining the membrane with Coomassie Brilliant Blue or Ponceau S dyes. Ponceau S is the more common of the two, due to its higher sensitivity and water solubility, the latter making it easier to subsequently destain and probe the membrane.

Blocking

Since the membrane has been chosen for its ability to bind protein and as both antibodies and the target are proteins, steps must be taken to prevent the interactions between the membrane and the antibody used for detection of the target protein. Blocking of non-specific binding is achieved by placing the membrane in a dilute solution of protein — typically 3%~5% Bovine serum albumin (BSA) or non-fat dry milk（脱脂奶粉）(both are inexpensive) in Tris-Buffered Saline (TBS) or I-Block, with a minute percentage (0.1%) of detergent such as Tween 20 or Triton X-100. The protein in the dilute solution attaches to the membrane in all places where the target proteins have not attached. Thus, when the antibody is added, there is no room on the membrane for it to attach other than on the binding sites of the specific target protein. This reduces background in the final product of the Western blot, leading to clearer results, and eliminates false positives.

Incubation

During the detection process the membrane is "probed" for the protein of interest with a modified antibody which is linked to a reporter enzyme; when exposed to an appropriate substrate, this enzyme drives a colorimetric reaction and produces a color. For a variety of reasons, this traditionally takes place in a two-step process, although there are now one-step detection methods available for certain applications.

Two steps

1. *Primary antibody*

The primary antibodies are generated when a host species or immune cell culture is exposed to protein of interest [or a part thereof (它的)]. Normally, this is part of the immune response, whereas here they are harvested and used as sensitive and specific detection tools that bind the protein directly.

After blocking, a dilute solution of primary antibody (generally between 0.5 and 5 micrograms/ml) is incubated with the membrane under gentle agitation. Typically, the solution is composed of buffered saline solution with a small percentage of detergent, and sometimes with powdered milk or BSA(牛血清白蛋白). The antibody solution and the membrane can be sealed and incubated together for anywhere from 30 minutes to overnight. It can also be incubated at different temperatures, with lesser temperatures being associated with more binding, both specific (to the target protein, the "signal") and non-specific ("noise").

2. *Secondary antibody*

After rinsing the membrane to remove unbound primary antibody, the membrane is exposed to another antibody, directed at a species-specific portion of the primary antibody. Antibodies come from animal sources (or animal sourced hybridoma cultures); an anti-mouse secondary will bind to almost any mouse-sourced primary antibody, which allows some cost savings by allowing an entire lab to share a single source of mass-produced antibody, and provides far more consistent results. This is known as a secondary antibody, and due to its targeting properties, tends to be referred to as "anti-mouse", "anti-goat", *etc*. The secondary antibody is usually linked to biotin or to a reporter enzyme such as alkaline phosphatase or horseradish peroxidase (辣根过氧化物酶). This means that several secondary antibodies will bind to one primary antibody and enhance the signal.

Most commonly, a horseradish peroxidase-linked secondary antibody is used to cleave a chemiluminescent agent, and the reaction product produces luminescence in proportion to the amount of protein. A sensitive sheet of photographic film (感光胶片，胶卷) is placed against the membrane, and exposure to the light from the reaction creates an image of the antibodies bound to the blot. A cheaper but less sensitive approach utilizes a 4-chloronaphthol stain with 1% hydrogen peroxide; the reaction of peroxide radicals with 4-chloronaphthol produces a dark purple stain that can be photographed without using specialized photographic film.

As with the ELISPOT (酶联免疫斑点测定法) and ELISA procedures, the enzyme can be provided with a substrate molecule that will be converted by the enzyme to a colored reaction product that will be visible on the membrane.

Another method of secondary antibody detection utilizes a near-infrared (NIR) fluorophore-linked antibody. Light produced from the excitation of a fluorescent dye is static, making fluorescent detection a more precise and accurate measure of the difference in signal produced by labeled antibodies bound to proteins on a Western blot. Proteins can be accurately quantified because the signal generated by the different amounts of proteins on the membranes is measured in a static state, as compared to chemiluminescence (化学发光), in which light is measured in a dynamic state (动态).

A third alternative is to use a radioactive label rather than an enzyme coupled to the secondary antibody, such as labeling an antibody-binding protein like *Staphylococcus* Protein A or Streptavidin (链霉亲和素) with a radioactive isotope of iodine. Since other methods are safer, quicker, and cheaper, this method is now rarely used; however, an advantage of this approach is the sensitivity of auto-radiography-based imaging, which enables highly accurate protein quantification when combined with optical software (*e.g.*, Optiquant).

One step

Historically, the probing process was performed in two steps because of the relative ease of producing primary and secondary antibodies in separate processes. This gives researchers and corporations huge advantages in terms of flexibility, and adds an amplification step to the detection process. Given the advent (出现) of high-throughput protein analysis and lower limits of detection, however, there has been interest in developing one-step probing systems that would allow the process to occur faster and with fewer consumables (消耗品，耗材). This requires a probe antibody which both recognizes the protein of interest and contains a detectable label, probes which are often available for known protein tags. The primary probe is incubated with the membrane in a manner similar to that for the primary antibody in a two-step process, and then is ready for direct detection after a series of wash steps.

Detection/Visualization

After the unbound probes are washed away, the Western blot is ready for detection of the probes that are labeled and bound to the protein of interest. In practical terms, not all Westerns reveal protein only at one band in a membrane. Size approximations are taken by comparing the stained bands to that of the marker or ladder loaded during electrophoresis. The process is commonly repeated for a structural protein, such as actin (肌动蛋白) or tubulin (微管蛋白), that should not change between samples. The amount of target protein is normalized (归一化) to the structural protein to control between groups. A superior strategy is the normalization to the total protein visualized with trichloroethanol (三氯乙醇) or epicocconone. This practice ensures correction for the amount of total protein on the membrane in case of errors or incomplete transfers.

Colorimetric detection

The colorimetric (比色的) detection method depends on incubation of the Western blot with a substrate that reacts with the reporter enzyme (such as peroxidase) that is bound to the secondary antibody. This converts the soluble dye into an insoluble form of a different color that precipitates next to the enzyme and thereby stains the membrane. Development (显影) of the blot is then stopped by washing away the soluble dye. Protein levels are evaluated through densitometry (光密度测定法，显微测密术) (how intense the stain is) or spectrophotometry (分光光度测定法).

Chemiluminescent detection

Chemiluminescent (化学发光的) detection methods depend on incubation of the Western blot with a substrate that will luminesce when exposed to the reporter on the secondary antibody. The light is then detected by CCD cameras (电荷耦合摄像机) which capture a digital image of the Western blot or photographic film. The use of film for Western blot detection is slowly disappearing because of non linearity of the image (non-accurate quantification). The image is analyzed by densitometry, which evaluates the relative amount of protein staining and quantifies the results in terms of optical density（光密度）. Newer software allows further data analysis such as molecular weight analysis if appropriate standards are used.

The main companies offering Chemiluminescence imaging systems are Analytik Jena, Syngene, UVP, Azure Biosystems, UVITEC, GE, Biorad and Vilber Lourmat.

Radioactive detection

Radioactive labels do not require enzyme substrates, but rather, allow the placement of medical X-ray film directly against the Western blot, which develops as it is exposed to the label and creates dark regions which correspond to the protein bands of interest. The importance of radioactive detections methods is declining due to its hazardous radiation, because it is very expensive, health and safety risks are high, and ECL (enhanced chemiluminescence) provides a useful alternative.

Fluorescent detection

The fluorescently labeled probe is excited by light and the emission of the excitation is then detected by a photosensor such as a CCD camera equipped with appropriate emission filters which captures a digital image of the Western blot and allows further data analysis such as molecular weight analysis and a quantitative Western blot analysis. Fluorescence is considered to be one of the best methods for quantification but is less sensitive than chemiluminescence.

Secondary probing

One major difference between nitrocellulose and PVDF membranes relates to the ability of each to support "stripping"（剥离，剥脱）antibodies off and reusing the membrane for subsequent antibody probes. While there are well-established protocols available for stripping nitrocellulose membranes, the sturdier（更结实的，更坚固的）PVDF allows for easier stripping, and for more reuse before background noise limits experiments. Another difference is that, unlike nitrocellulose, PVDF must be soaked in 95% ethanol, isopropanol or methanol before use. PVDF membranes also tend to be thicker and more resistant to damage during use.

2-D gel electrophoresis

2-dimensional SDS-PAGE uses the principles and techniques outlined above. 2-D SDS-PAGE, as the name suggests, involves the migration of polypeptides in 2 dimensions. For example, in the first dimension, polypeptides are separated according to isoelectric point, while in the second dimension, polypeptides are separated according to their molecular weight. The isoelectric point of a given protein is determined by the relative number of positively (*e.g.*, lysine, arginine) and negatively (*e.g.*, glutamate, aspartate) charged amino acids, with negatively charged amino acids contributing to a low isoelectric point and positively charged amino acids contributing to a high isoelectric point. Samples could also be separated first under nonreducing conditions using SDS-PAGE, and under reducing conditions in the second dimension, which breaks apart disulfide bonds that hold subunits together. SDS-PAGE might also be coupled with urea-PAGE for a 2-dimensional gel.

In principle, this method allows for the separation of all cellular proteins on a single large gel. A major advantage of this method is that it often distinguishes between different isoforms（亚型，同工型，蛋白质异形体）of a particular protein — *e.g.*, a protein that has been phosphorylated (by addition of a negatively charged group). Proteins that have been separated can be cut out of the gel and then analyzed by mass spectrometry, which identifies the protein.

Medical diagnostic applications

● The confirmatory（证实的，确定的）HIV test employs a Western blot to detect anti-HIV antibody in a human serum sample. Proteins from known HIV-infected cells are separated and blotted on a membrane as above. Then, the serum to be tested is applied in the primary antibody incubation step; free antibody is washed away, and a secondary anti-human antibody linked to an enzyme signal is added. The stained bands then indicate the proteins to which the patient's serum contains antibodies.

● A Western blot is also used as the definitive（决定性的，最后的）test for bovine spongiform encephalopathy（疯牛病，牛绵状脑病）(BSE, commonly referred to as 'mad cow disease').

● Some forms of Lyme disease（莱姆病）testing employ Western blotting.

● A Western blot can also be used as a confirmatory test for Hepatitis B infection and HSV-2 (Herpes simplex virus type 2，II 型单纯疱疹病毒) infection.

● In veterinary medicine, a Western blot is sometimes used to confirm FIV$^+$（猫免疫缺陷病毒，猫艾滋）status in cats.

3.4.4　Isoelectric point determination of proteins（蛋白质等电点的测定）

Isoelectric focusing

Isoelectric focusing (IEF), also known as **electrofocusing**, is a technique for separating different molecules by differences in their isoelectric point (pI). It is a type of zone electrophoresis, usually performed on proteins in a gel, that takes advantage of the fact that overall charge on the molecule of interest is a function of the pH of its surroundings.

Isoelectric focusing in laboratory

IEF involves adding an ampholyte（两性电解质）solution into **immobilized pH gradient** (IPG) gels. IPGs are the acrylamide gel matrix copolymerized with the pH gradient, which results in completely stable gradients except the most alkaline (>12) pH values. The immobilized pH gradient is obtained by the continuous change in the ratio of *Immobilines*（固定化电解质）. An Immobiline is a weak acid or base defined by its pK value.

A protein that is in a pH region below its isoelectric point (pI) will be positively charged and so will migrate towards the cathode (negatively charged electrode，阴极). As it migrates through a gradient of increasing pH, however, the protein's overall charge will decrease until the protein reaches the pH region that corresponds to its pI. At this point it has no net charge and so migration ceases (as there is no electrical attraction towards either electrode). As a result, the proteins become focused into sharp stationary bands with each protein positioned at a point in the pH gradient corresponding to its pI. The technique is capable of extremely high resolution with proteins differing by a single charge being fractionated into separate bands.

Molecules to be focused are distributed over a medium that has a pH gradient (usually created by aliphatic ampholytes). An electric current is passed through the medium, creating a "positive" anode and "negative" cathode end. Negatively charged molecules migrate through the pH gradient in the medium toward the "positive" end while positively charged molecules move toward the "negative" end. As a particle moves towards the pole opposite of its charge it moves through the changing pH gradient until it reaches a point in which the pH of that molecules isoelectric point is reached. At this point the molecule no longer has a net electric charge (due to the protonation or deprotonation of the associated functional groups) and as such will not proceed any further within the gel. The gradient is established before adding the particles of interest by first subjecting a solution of small molecules such as polyampholytes (聚两性电解质) with varying pI values to electrophoresis (Fig. 3-31).

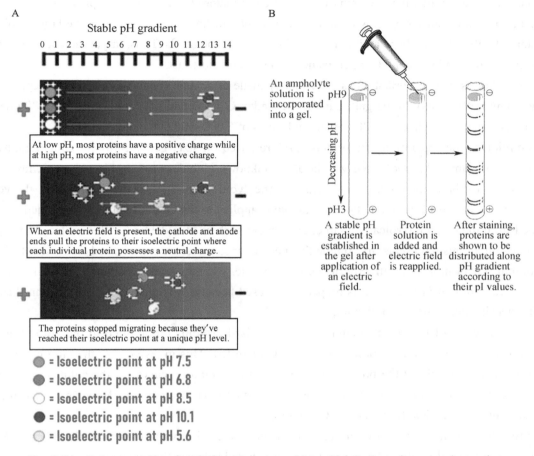

Fig. 3-31   Schemes of Isoelectric focusing. A. working principle. B. equipment and operation.

The method is applied particularly often in the study of proteins, which separate based on their relative content of acidic and basic residues, whose value is represented by the pI. Proteins are introduced into an immobilized pH gradient gel composed of polyacrylamide (聚丙烯酰胺), starch, or agarose where a pH gradient has been established. Gels with large pores are usually used in this process to eliminate any "sieving" effects, or artifacts (假象) in the pI caused by differing migration rates for proteins of differing sizes. Isoelectric focusing can resolve proteins that differ in pI value by as little as 0.01. Isoelectric focusing is the first step in two-dimensional gel electrophoresis, in which proteins are first separated by their pI and then further separated by molecular weight through SDS-PAGE.

3.4.5 Molecular weight determination of proteins (蛋白质分子量的测定)

3.4.5.1 *Gel filtration chromatography* (凝胶色谱法)

Size Exclusion Chromatography (Gel Filtration Chromatography)

SEC is a preparative, non-destructive analytical technique that permits the separation of molecules by their size. This is especially useful in protein purification because while there may be many proteins in a sample, their molecular weights can vary widely. This allows one to separate a mixture of proteins based on this wide size distribution. It also provides a simple procedure for removing salt (desalting) from a protein sample.

Molecules smaller than the exclusion limit of the gel material will become trapped in the gel beads. Those of larger molecular weight will not be trapped but will flow through the gel. The larger molecules are retarded only by their shape and their ease of passing by the beads. Thus, larger molecules elute first, while smaller molecules are held longer inside the beads and elute last.

Gel selection is very important. Gels are typically made of dextran (Sephadex), agarose (Sepharose) or polyacrylamide (Bio-Gel). Some gels, such as Sephadex G-10, retain only molecules of 0~700 daltons, while others, such as Sephadex G-200 retain molecules of 5 000~600 000 daltons.

In addition to the separation of a protein mixture based on size, gel filtration chromatography also allows one to estimate the molecular weight of an unknown globular protein. First, the column must be calibrated. To calibrate the column, one measures the "void volume" V_o of the column, *i.e.*, the volume of liquid collected from the minute that the sample is applied to the column until an unretained molecule is eluted from the column (typically a large, dyed sugar such as blue dextran with a molecular weight of 2×10^6 daltons). This represents the volume that non-retained molecule experienced on its travels through the column. Each molecule will experience this volume, whether retained or not. This value must be measured each time a SEC column is prepared and used because it is unique to each column (based on packing density, gel composition, length, *etc.*).

Second, a series of known molecular weight standard proteins are applied to the column and the volume at which each standard protein is eluted is recorded. This gives you V_r, the elution volume. A plot of molecular weight of the protein vs. V_r/V_o gives a calibration curve for the column. This is time consuming and the data for the calibration curve is unique to that column only. However, this is the most accurate way to obtain data from your SEC column.

In order to compare data between columns, a relative elution volume is used. Recall that K_d, the distribution constant describes how the protein is distributed between the two phases:

$$K_d = \frac{[Concentration\ in\ Mobile\ phase]}{[Concentration\ in\ Stationary\ phase]}$$

In SEC, this ratio can be expressed as a ratio of retention times or retention volumes.

$$K_d = \frac{V_r - V_o}{V_s}$$

Where V_r is the retention volume of the protein, V_o is the void volume and V_s is the volume of the stationary phase. The volume of the stationary phase is difficult to calculate accurately since the gel particles vary in size and volume in each batch and column. Instead, the average distribution constant is used:

$$K_{avg} = \frac{[V_r - V_o]}{[V_t - V_o]}$$

where V_t is the maximum retention volume experienced by a small molecule such as a dye labeled amino acid. This is a close approximation of the stationary phase volume in the column. K_{avg} values have been determined for a number of gels and for a number of proteins. This allows one to compare K_{avg} values across different columns and different experiments. One can also plot log MW vs. K_d to get an estimate of the molecular weight of a protein. Remember, this is not as accurate as doing a full column calibration. One must be careful in interpreting these results. SEC separations are influenced by protein shape as well as ionic strength.

Concerning how do we know when a protein is eluting from the column — in the case of blue dextran and the dye-labeled amino acid (any DNP amino acid), the molecules are colored blue or yellow respectively and one can see them elute from the column visually. While for most proteins, they do not exhibit a visual color (proteins containing hemes, like cytochrome c or myoglobin will be red). Instead, they absorb at 280 nm with an extinction coefficient that is related to the number of aromatic amino acids in the protein. As we collect fractions, we need to monitor each fraction on the UV-VIS at 280 nm in order to plot Abs. vs. Volume to determine where the proteins elute, based on an increase in absorbance at 280 nm.

3.4.5.2　SDS-PAGE（SDS-聚丙烯酰胺凝胶电泳法）

Determining Protein Molecular Weight with SDS-PAGE: An Overview of the Process

The molecular weight of an unknown protein can be estimated by using the SDS-PAGE method. Although there are some other methods (*i.e.*, analytical ultracentrifugation and light scattering) for calculating the size or molecular weight (MW) of an unknown protein, they are not commonly used for this purpose since they use large amounts of highly purified proteins and require costly equipment.

SDS-PAGE for Molecular Weight Determination: An Overview of the Process

To determine the molecular weight of an unknown protein, you should separate the sample on the same gel with a set of molecular weight standards. After running the standards and the unknown protein sample, the gel is processed with the desired stain and then destained for about 12 to 14 hours to visualize the protein bands.

After running the gel, you should then determine the relative migration distance (*Rf*) of the protein standards and the unknown protein. The migration distance can be determined using the following equation:

Rf = Migration distance of the protein/Migration distance of the dye front

Note: You can use a ruler to measure the migration distance (in centimeters) from the top of the gel to every major band in the gel. Alternatively, an appropriate software may also be used to determine the *Rf* values of the resulting bands.

Based on the values obtained for the bands in the standard, the logarithm of the molecular weight of an SDS-denatured polypeptide and its relative migration distance (*Rf*) is plotted into a graph. Please take note that you will generate a linear plot for most proteins if your samples are fully denatured and the gel percentage is appropriate for the molecular weight range of the sample. If you get a sigmoidal curve（S 形曲线）, it means that the sieving effect of your matrix is either too large that it restricts the penetration of the molecules into the gel or is nearly negligible that it allows protein molecules to migrate almost at their free mobility.

Interpolating（插入，补充）the value from this graph will then give you the molecular weight of the unknown protein band. Please note that the accuracy of this method in determining the molecular weight of an unknown protein typically ranges from 5% to 10%. The presence of polypeptides such as glycol- and lipoproteins usually leads to erroneous results since they are not fully coated with SDS and thus, would not behave as expected.

For instance, the unknown protein has an Rf of 0.7084. Using the equation for the linear plot we can calculate the Log (MW):

$$(-2.0742 \times 0.7084) + 2.8 = 1.3305$$

So the inverse log（反对数）is $10^{1.3305}$ = 21.4 kDa for the molecular weight of the unknown protein.

Creating Ideal Separation Conditions: Some Factors to Consider

Given its importance in determining the molecular weight of an unknown protein sample, you need to select the appropriate separation conditions when doing your experiment. To do this, you need to take the following factors into consideration:

- The standard protein and the unknown protein should be electrophoresed on the same gel under identical conditions.

- Multiple data points should be generated to make sure that the data carries a statistical significance. For best results, try using at least **three** gels.

- In solubilizing the proteins, the sample buffer should contain reducing agents such as dithiothreitol （二硫苏糖醇）or β-mercaptoethanol（β- 巯基乙醇）to ensure that the disulfide bonds will be broken. As you may already know, disulfide bonds reduce the effect of secondary structure on migration.

- The sample buffer should also contain SDS. SDS binds to hydrophobic protein regions to denature secondary, tertiary and quaternary structures and give a net negative charge on the proteins. SDS causes proteins to unfold to random, rod-like chains without breaking any covalent bonds in the process. This causes proteins to lose their biological functions without damaging their primary structures.

Keep in mind that the unknown protein should be within the linear range of the standard curve to allow for the accurate determination of its molecular weight. In addition, the amount of the unknown protein should match the corresponding standard to increase the accuracy of the results.

3.4.5.3 *Mass spectrum* （质谱法）

1. Electrospray ionization （ESI，电喷雾离子化）

Electrospray ionization (ESI) is a technique used in mass spectrometry to produce ions using an electrospray in which a high voltage is applied to a liquid to create an aerosol（气溶胶，气雾剂）. It is especially useful in producing ions from macromolecules because it overcomes the propensity（倾向）of these molecules to fragment when ionized. ESI is different from other atmospheric pressure ionization processes (*e.g.*, MALDI) since it may produce multiple charged ions, effectively extending the mass range of the analyzer to accommodate the kDa-MDa orders of magnitude observed in proteins and their associated polypeptide fragments.

Mass spectrometry using ESI is called electrospray ionization mass spectrometry (ESI-MS) or, less commonly, electrospray mass spectrometry (ES-MS). ESI is a so-called "soft ionization" technique, since there is very little fragmentation. This can be advantageous in the sense that the molecular ion (or more accurately a pseudo molecular ion) is always observed, however very little structural information can be gained from the simple mass spectrum obtained. This disadvantage can be overcome by coupling ESI with tandem mass spectrometry (ESI-MS/MS，串联质谱). Another important advantage of ESI is that solution-phase information can be retained（保留）into the gas-phase.

The electrospray ionization technique was first reported by Masamichi Yamashita and John Fenn in

1984. The development of electrospray ionization for the analysis of biological macromolecules was rewarded with the attribution（归因）of the Nobel Prize in Chemistry to John Bennett Fenn in 2002. One of the original instruments used by Dr. Fenn is on display（陈列，展出，展览）at the Chemical Heritage Foundation in Philadelphia, Pennsylvania.

History

In 1882, Lord Rayleigh theoretically estimated the maximum amount of charge a liquid droplet could carry before throwing out fine jets（细喷射流）of liquid. This is now known as the Rayleigh limit.

In 1914, John Zeleny published work on the behavior of fluid droplets at the end of glass capillaries and presented evidence for different electrospray modes. Wilson and Taylor and Nolan investigated electrospray in the 1920s and Macky in 1931. The electrospray cone (now known as the Taylor cone) was described by Sir Geoffrey Ingram Taylor (Fig. 3-32).

A.

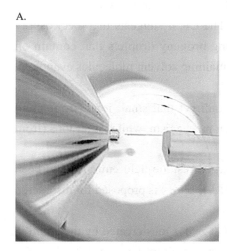

B.

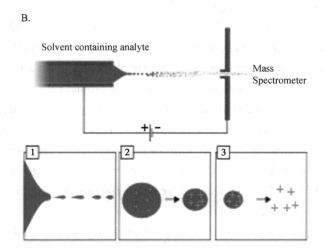

Fig. 3-32A   Electrospray (nanoSpray) ionization source

Fig. 3-32B   Diagram of Electrospray Ionization. (1) Under high voltage, the Taylor Cone （泰勒锥，泰勒圆锥）emits a jet of liquid drops; (2) The solvent from the droplets progressively evaporates, leaving them more and more charged; (3) When the charge exceeds the Rayleigh limit（瑞利限度，瑞利极限）the droplet explosively dissociates, leaving a stream of charged ions.

The first use of electrospray ionization with mass spectrometry was reported by Malcolm Dole in 1968. John Bennett Fenn was awarded the 2002 Nobel Prize in Chemistry for the development of electrospray ionization mass spectrometry in the late 1980s.

Ionization mechanism

The liquid containing the analyte(s) of interest is dispersed（扩散，使分散）by electrospray, into a fine aerosol. Because the ion formation involves extensive solvent evaporation [also termed desolvation （去溶剂化，脱溶，退溶）], the typical solvents for electrospray ionization are prepared by mixing water with volatile organic compounds (*e.g.*, methanol, acetonitrile). To decrease the initial droplet size, compounds that increase the conductivity (*e.g.*, acetic acid) are customarily（通常）added to the solution. These species also act to provide a source of protons to facilitate the ionization process. Large-flow electrosprays can benefit from nebulization（雾化）— a heated inert gas such as nitrogen or carbon dioxide in addition to the high temperature of the ESI source. The aerosol is sampled into the first vacuum stage of a mass spectrometer through a capillary carrying a potential difference of approximately 3 000 V, which can be heated to aid further solvent evaporation from the charged droplets. The solvent evaporates from a charged droplet until it becomes unstable upon reaching its Rayleigh limit. At this point, the droplet deforms as the electrostatic repulsion of like charges, in an ever-decreasing (逐渐下降) droplet size, becomes more powerful than the surface tension holding the droplet together. At this point the droplet undergoes Coulomb fission (库伦裂变), whereby the original droplet "explodes" creating many smaller, more stable droplets. The new droplets undergo desolvation and subsequently further Coulomb fissions. During the fission, the droplet loses a small percentage of its mass (1.0%~2.3%) along with a relatively large percentage of its charge (10%~18%).

There are two major theories that explain the final production of gas-phase ions: the ion evaporation model (IEM) and the charge residue model (CRM, 电荷残留模式). The IEM suggests that as the droplet reaches a certain radius, the field strength at the surface of the droplet becomes large enough to assist the field desorption (场解析, 场致退吸, 场脱附) of solvated ions. The CRM suggests that electrospray droplets undergo evaporation and fission cycles, eventually leading progeny droplets that contain on average one analyte ion or less. The gas-phase ions form after the remaining solvent molecules evaporate, leaving the analyte with the charges that the droplet carried.

A large body of evidence, which is considered either direct or indirect that small ions (from small molecules) are liberated into the gas phase through the ion evaporation mechanism, while larger ions (from folded proteins for instance) form by charged residue mechanism.

A third model invoking (援引, 受……启发) combined charged residue-field emission has been proposed. Another model called the **chain ejection model** (CEM, 链弹射理论) is proposed for disordered polymers (unfolded proteins).

The ions observed by mass spectrometry may be quasimolecular (准分子) ions created by the addition of a hydrogen cation and denoted $[M + H]^+$, or of another cation such as sodium ion, $[M + Na]^+$, or the removal of a hydrogen nucleus, $[M-H]^-$. Multiply charged ions such as $[M + nH]^{n+}$ are often observed. For large macromolecules, there can be many charge states, resulting in a characteristic charge state envelope (外表, 外层). All these are even-electron ion species: electrons (alone) are not added or removed, unlike in some other ionization sources. The analytes are sometimes involved in electrochemical processes, leading to shifts of the corresponding peaks in the mass spectrum. This effect is demonstrated in the direct ionization of noble metals (贵金属) such as copper, silver and gold using electrospray.

Variants

The electrosprays operated at low flow rates generate much smaller initial droplets, which ensure improved ionization efficiency. In 1993 Gale and Richard D. Smith reported significant sensitivity increases could be achieved using lower flow rates, and down to 200 nl/min. In 1994, two research groups coined the name micro-electrospray (microspray) for electrosprays working at low flow rates. Emmett and Caprioli demonstrated improved performance for HPLC-MS analyses when the electrospray was operated at 300~800 nl/min. Wilm and Mann demonstrated that a capillary flow of ~ 25 nl/min can sustain an electrospray at the tip of emitters (发射器) fabricated by pulling glass capillaries to a few micrometers. The latter was renamed nano-electrospray (nanospray) in 1996. Currently the name nanospray is also in use for electrosprays fed (供应) by pumps at low flow rates, not only for self-fed electrosprays. Although there may not be a well-defined flow rate range for electrospray, microspray, and nano-electrospray, the effect of flow rate on ion signals was studied systematically using mixtures of compounds with different physicochemical properties (*i.e.*, detergent/oligosaccharide and oligosaccharide/peptide). For these model systems, the functional dependence of certain analyte-ion ratios upon the flow rate can be correlated to "changes in analyte partition during droplet fission prior to ion release".

Cold spray ionization is a form of electrospray in which the solution containing the sample is forced through a small cold capillary (10~80℃) into an electric field to create a fine mist of cold charged droplets. Applications of this method include the analysis of fragile molecules and guest-host interactions that cannot be studied using regular electrospray ionization.

Electrospray ionization has also been achieved at pressures as low as 25 torr and termed sub-ambient pressure (低压) ionization with nanoelectrospray (SPIN) based upon a two-stage ion funnel (离子漏子) interface developed by Richard D. Smith and coworkers. The SPIN implementation provided increased sensitivity due to the use of ion funnels that helped confine and transfer ions to the lower-pressure region of the mass spectrometer. Operation at low pressure was particularly effective for low flow rates where the smaller electrospray droplet size allowed effective desolvation and ion formation to be achieved. As a result, later the researchers were able to demonstrate achieving in excess of 50% overall ionization utilization efficiency for transfer of ions from the liquid phase, into the gas phase as ions, and through the dual ion funnel interface to the mass spectrometer.

Ambient ionization (常压电离)

In ambient ionization, the formation of ions occurs outside the mass spectrometer without sample preparation. Electrospray is used for ion formation in a number of ambient ion sources.

Desorption electrospray ionization (DESI, 解吸附电喷雾离子化) is an ambient ionization technique in which a solvent electrospray is directed at a sample. The electrospray is attracted to the surface by applying a voltage (电压) to the sample. Sample compounds are extracted (提取) into the solvent which is again aerosolized as highly charged droplets that evaporate to form highly charged ions (Fig. 3-33). After ionization, the ions enter the atmospheric pressure interface of the mass spectrometer. DESI allows for ambient ionization of samples at atmospheric pressure, with little sample preparation.

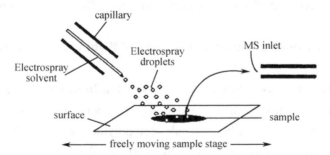

Fig. 3-33　Diagram of a DESI ambient ionization source.

Extractive electrospray ionization (电喷雾萃取电离，电喷雾萃取离子化) is a spray-type, ambient ionization method that uses two merged sprays, one of which is generated by electrospray.

Laser-based electrospray-based ambient ionization is a two-step process in which a pulsed laser is used to desorb (解除吸附，脱附) or ablate (使……脱落，融化，激光烧蚀) material from a sample and the plume (一缕) of material interacts with an electrospray to create ions. For ambient ionization, the sample material is deposited on (把……放在……上) a target near the electrospray. The laser desorbs or ablates material from the sample which is ejected from the surface and into the electrospray which produces highly charged ions. Examples are electrospray laser desorption ionization, matrix-assisted laser desorption electrospray ionization, and laser ablation electrospray ionization.

Applications

Electrospray is used to study protein folding. Additionally, ESI-MS is used to test for the presence of nano clusters, for example U-60.

Liquid chromatography-mass spectrometry (LC-MS)

Electrospray ionization is the ion source of choice to couple liquid chromatography with mass spectrometry. The analysis can be performed online, by feeding the liquid eluting from the LC column directly to an electrospray, or offline, by collecting fractions to be later analyzed in a classical nanoelectrospray-mass spectrometry setup. Among the numerous operating parameters in ESI-MS, the electrospray voltage has been identified as an important parameter to consider in ESI LC/MS gradient elution. The effect of various solvent compositions [such as TFA or ammonium acetate, or supercharging (增压) reagents, or derivatizing (衍生) groups] or spraying conditions on Electrospray-LCMS spectra and/or nanoESI-MS spectra have been studied.

Capillary electrophoresis-mass spectrometry (CE-MS)

Capillary electrophoresis-mass spectrometry was enabled by an ESI interface that was developed and patented by Richard D. Smith and coworkers at Pacific Northwest National Laboratory, and shown to have broad utility for the analysis of very small biological and chemical compound mixtures, and even extending to a single biological cell.

Noncovalent gas phase interactions

Electrospray ionization is also utilized in studying noncovalent gas phase interactions. The electrospray process is thought to be capable of transferring liquid-phase noncovalent complexes into the gas phase without disrupting the noncovalent interaction. Problems such as non-specific interactions have been identified when studying ligand substrate complexes by ESI-MS or nanoESI-MS. An interesting example of this is studying the interactions between enzymes and drugs which are inhibitors of the enzyme. Competition studies between STAT6 and inhibitors have used ESI as a way to screen for potential new drug candidates.

2. Matrix-assisted laser desorption/ionization-Time of flight (MALDI-TOF, 基质辅助激光解析离子化 - 飞行时间)

In mass spectrometry **matrix-assisted laser desorption/ionization (MALDI)** is an ionization technique that uses a laser energy absorbing matrix to create ions from large molecules with minimal fragmentation, allowing the analysis of biomolecules (biopolymers such as DNA, proteins, peptides and carbohydrates) and large organic molecules [such as polymers, dendrimers (树枝状大分子) and other macromolecules], which tend to be fragile and fragment when ionized by more conventional ionization methods. It is similar in character to electrospray ionization (ESI) in that both techniques are relatively soft (low fragmentation) ways of obtaining ions of large molecules in the gas phase, though MALDI typically produces far fewer multiply charged ions.

MALDI methodology is a three-step process. First, the sample is mixed with a suitable matrix material and applied to a metal plate. Second, a pulsed laser irradiates (照射) the sample, triggering ablation and desorption of the sample and matrix material. Finally, the analyte molecules are ionized by being

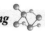

protonated or deprotonated in the hot plume（飘升之物，一缕，羽状烟柱，羽流）of ablated（烧蚀）gases, and then they can be accelerated into whichever mass spectrometer is used to analyze them.

History

The term matrix-assisted laser desorption ionization (MALDI) was coined in 1985 by Franz Hillenkamp, Michael Karas and their colleagues. These researchers found that the amino acid alanine could be ionized more easily if it was mixed with the amino acid tryptophan and irradiated with a pulsed 266 nm laser. The tryptophan was absorbing the laser energy and helping to ionize the non-absorbing alanine. Peptides up to the 2 843 Da peptide melittin（蜂毒肽）could be ionized when mixed with this kind of "matrix". The breakthrough for large molecule laser desorption ionization came in 1987 when Koichi Tanaka of Shimadzu Corporation and his co-workers used what they called the "ultra fine metal plus liquid matrix method" that combined 30 nm cobalt particles in glycerol with a 337 nm nitrogen laser for ionization. Using this laser and matrix combination, Tanaka was able to ionize biomolecules as large as the 34 472 Da protein carboxypeptidase A（羧肽酶 A）. Tanaka received one-quarter of the 2002 Nobel Prize in Chemistry for demonstrating that, with the proper combination of laser wavelength and matrix, a protein can be ionized. Karas and Hillenkamp were subsequently able to ionize the 67 kDa protein albumin（白蛋白）using a nicotinic acid（烟酸，尼克酸）matrix and a 266 nm laser. Further improvements were realized through the use of a 355 nm laser and the cinnamic acid（肉桂酸，苯丙烯酸）derivatives ferulic acid（阿魏酸），caffeic acid（咖啡酸，二羟基桂皮酸）and sinapinic acid（芥子酸）as the matrix. The availability of small and relatively inexpensive nitrogen lasers operating at 337 nm wavelength and the first commercial instruments introduced in the early 1990s brought MALDI to an increasing number of researchers. Today, mostly organic matrices are used for MALDI mass spectrometry.

Matrix and sample preparation

The matrix consists of crystallized molecules, of which the three most commonly used are sinapinic acid, α-cyano-4-hydroxycinnamic acid (α-CHCA, alpha-cyano or alpha-matrix) and 2,5-dihydroxybenzoic acid (DHB) (Table 3-7). A solution of one of these molecules is made, often in a mixture of highly

Table 3-7   UV MALDI Matrix List

Compound	Other Names	Solvent	Wavelength (nm)	Applications
2,5-dihydroxybenzoic acid (gentisic acid)	DHB, gentisic acid（龙胆酸）	acetonitrile, water, methanol, acetone, chloroform	337, 355, 266	peptides, nucleotides, oligonucleotides, oligosaccharides
3,5-dimethoxy-4-hydroxycinnamic acid（3,5- 二甲氧基 -4- 羟基肉桂酸）	sinapic acid（芥子酸）；sinapinic acid（芥子酸）；SA	acetonitrile, water, acetone, chloroform	337, 355, 266	peptides, proteins, lipids
4-hydroxy-3-methoxycinnamic acid	ferulic acid（阿魏酸）	acetonitrile, water, propanol	337, 355, 266	proteins
α-cyano-4-hydroxycinnamic acid	CHCA	acetonitrile, water, ethanol, acetone	337, 355	peptides, lipids, nucleotides
picolinic acid（皮考啉酸，吡啶甲酸）	PA	ethanol	266	oligonucleotides
3-hydroxy picolinic acid	HPA	ethanol	337, 355	oligonucleotides

purified water and an organic solvent such as acetonitrile (ACN) or ethanol. A counter-ion source such as trifluoroacetic acid (TFA) is usually added to generate the $[M^+H]$ ions. A good example of a matrix-solution would be 20 mg/ml sinapinic acid in ACN : water : TFA (50 : 50 : 0.1).

Notation（编号）for cinnamic acid substitutions.

The identification of suitable matrix compounds is determined to some extent by trial and error, but they are based on some specific molecular design considerations:

- They are of a fairly low molecular weight (to allow easy vaporization), but are large enough (with a low enough vapor pressure) not to evaporate during sample preparation or while standing in the mass spectrometer.

- They are often acidic, therefore act as a proton source to encourage ionization of the analyte. Basic matrices have also been reported.

- They have a strong optical absorption in either the UV or IR range, so that they rapidly and efficiently absorb the laser irradiation. This efficiency is commonly associated with chemical structures incorporating several conjugated double bonds, as seen in the structure of cinnamic acid.

- They are functionalized with polar groups, allowing their use in aqueous solutions.

- They typically contain a chromophore.

The matrix solution is mixed with the analyte (*e.g.*, protein sample). A mixture of water and organic solvent allows both hydrophobic and water-soluble (hydrophilic) molecules to dissolve into the solution. This solution is spotted onto a MALDI plate (usually a metal plate designed for this purpose). The solvents vaporize, leaving only the recrystallized （融化并再结晶）matrix, but now with analyte molecules embedded into MALDI crystals. The matrix and the analyte are said to be co-

Naphthalene and naphthalene-like compounds can also be used as a matrix to ionize a sample.

crystallized. Co-crystallization is a key issue in selecting a proper matrix to obtain a good quality mass spectrum of the analyte of interest.

The matrix can be used to tune the instrument to ionize the sample in different ways. As mentioned above, acid-base like reactions are often utilized to ionize the sample, however, molecules with conjugated π systems, such as naphthalene like compounds, can also serve as an electron acceptor and thus a matrix for MALDI/TOF. This is particularly useful in studying molecules that also possess conjugated π systems. The most widely used application for these matrices is studying porphyrin（卟啉）-like compounds such as chlorophyll（叶绿素）. These matrices have been shown to have better ionization patterns that do not result in odd fragmentation patterns or complete loss of side chains. It has also been suggested that conjugated porphyrin-like molecules can serve as a matrix and cleave themselves eliminating the need for a separate matrix compound.

Ionization mechanism

The laser is fired at the matrix crystals in the dried-droplet spot. The matrix absorbs the laser energy and it is thought that primarily the matrix is desorbed（释出被吸收之物，使解除吸附，解吸）and ionized (by addition of a proton) by this event. The hot plume produced during ablation contains many species: neutral and ionized matrix molecules, protonated and deprotonated matrix molecules, matrix clusters and nanodroplets（纳米液滴）. Ablated species may participate in the ionization of analyte molecules, though the mechanism of MALDI is still debated. The matrix is then thought to transfer protons to the analyte molecules (*e.g.*, protein molecules), thus charging the analyte. An ion observed after this process will consist of the initial neutral molecule [M] with ions added or removed. This is called a quasimolecular ion（准分子离子）, for example $[M+H]^+$ in the case of an added proton, $[M+Na]^+$ in the case of an added sodium ion, or $[M-H]^-$ in the case of a removed proton. MALDI is capable of creating singly charged ions or multiply charged ions ($[M+nH]^{n+}$) depending on the nature of the matrix, the laser intensity, and/or the voltage used. Note that these are all even-electron species. Ion signals of radical cations (photoionized molecules) can be observed, *e.g.*, in the case of matrix molecules and other organic molecules.

The matrix-assisted ionization [MAI] method uses matrix preparation identical to MALDI but does not require laser ablation to produce analyte ions of volatile or nonvolatile compounds. Simply exposing the matrix [*e.g.*, 3-nitrobenzonitrile（3-硝基苯腈，3-硝基苯甲腈）] with analyte to the vacuum of the mass spectrometer creates ions with nearly identical charge states to electrospray ionization. It is suggested that there are likely mechanistic（机械论的）commonality（共性，共同点，共同之处）between this process and MALDI.

Technology and instrumentation（仪器）

There are several variations of the MALDI technology and comparable instruments are today produced for very different purposes. From more academic and analytical, to more industrial and high throughput. The mass spectrometry field has expanded into requiring ultrahigh resolution mass spectrometry such as the FT-ICR instruments as well as more high-throughput instruments. As many MALDI MS instruments can be bought with an interchangeable ionization source (Electrospray ionization, MALDI, Atmospheric pressure ionization, *etc.*), the technologies often overlap and many times any soft ionization method could potentially be used.

Laser

MALDI techniques typically employ the use of UV lasers such as nitrogen lasers (337 nm) and frequency-tripled and quadrupled Nd:YAG lasers (355 nm and 266 nm respectively). Infrared laser wavelengths used for infrared MALDI include the 2.94 μm Er : YAG laser, mid-IR optical parametric oscillator, and 10.6 μm carbon dioxide laser. Although not as common, infrared lasers are used due to their softer mode of ionization. IR-MALDI also has the advantage of greater material removal (useful for biological samples), less low-mass（低质量）interferences, and compatibility with other matrix-free laser desorption mass spectrometry methods.

Time of Flight

The type of a mass spectrometer most widely used with MALDI is the (time-of-flight mass spectrometer) TOF, mainly due to its large mass range. The TOF measurement procedure is also ideally suited to the MALDI ionization process since the pulsed laser takes individual "shots"（发射）rather than working in continuous operation. MALDI-TOF instruments are often equipped with a reflectron

（反射器）(an "ion mirror") that reflects ions using an electric field, thereby doubling the ion flight path,thereby increasing time of flight between ions of different m/z and increasing resolution. Modern, commercial reflectron TOF instruments reach a resolving power m/Δm of 50 000 FWHM (full-width half-maximum, Δm defined as the peak width at 50% of peak height) or more.

MALDI has been coupled with IMS-TOF MS to identify phosphorylated and non-phosphorylated peptides.

MALDI-FT-ICR MS has been demonstrated to be a useful technique where high-resolution MALDI-MS measurements are desired.

Atmospheric pressure matrix-assisted laser desorption/ionization

Atmospheric pressure (AP) matrix-assisted laser desorption/ionization (MALDI) is an ionization technique (ion source) that in contrast to vacuum MALDI operates at normal atmospheric environment. The main difference between vacuum MALDI and AP-MALDI is the pressure in which the ions are created. In vacuum MALDI, ions are typically produced at 10 mTorr or less while in AP-MALDI ions are formed in atmospheric pressure. In the past the main disadvantage of AP MALDI technique compared to the conventional vacuum MALDI has been its limited sensitivity; however, ions can be transferred into the mass spectrometer with high efficiency and attomole（阿摩尔）detection limits have been reported. AP-MALDI is used in mass spectrometry (MS) in a variety of applications ranging from proteomics to drug discovery. Popular topics that are addressed by AP-MALDI mass spectrometry include: proteomics; mass analysis of DNA, RNA, PNA, lipids, oligosaccharides, phosphopeptides, bacteria, small molecules and synthetic polymers, similar applications are also available for vacuum MALDI instruments. The AP-MALDI ion source is easily coupled to an ion trap mass spectrometer or any other MS system equipped with (electrospray ionization) ESI or nanoESI source.

Aerosol mass spectrometry

In aerosol mass spectrometry, one of the ionization techniques consists in firing a laser to individual droplets. These systems are called single particle mass spectrometers (SPMS). The sample may optionally be mixed with a MALDI prior to aerosolization.

Applications in biomedicine

Biochemistry

In proteomics, MALDI is used for the rapid identification of proteins isolated by using gel electrophoresis: SDS-PAGE, size exclusion chromatography, affinity chromatography, strong/weak ion exchange, isotope coded protein labeling (ICPL，同位素编码的标签蛋白), and two-dimensional gel electrophoresis. Peptide mass fingerprinting（肽质量指纹图谱）is the most popular analytical application of MALDI-TOF mass spectrometers. MALDI TOF/TOF mass spectrometers are used to reveal amino acid sequence of peptides using post-source decay（源后衰变，源后降解）or high-energy collision-induced dissociation（分解，分离）.

Loss of sialic acid has been identified in papers when DHB has been used as a matrix for MALDI MS analysis of glycosylated peptides. Using sinapinic acid, 4-HCCA and DHB as matrices, S. Martin studied loss of sialic acid in glycosylated peptides by metastable decay（亚稳衰变）in MALDI/TOF in linear mode and reflector（反射物，反射镜）mode. A group at Shimadzu Corporation derivatized the sialic acid by an amidation（酰胺化）reaction as a way to improve detection sensitivity and also demonstrated that ionic liquid matrix reduces a loss of sialic acid during MALDI/TOF MS analysis of sialylated oligosaccharides. THAP, DHAP, and a mixture of 2-aza-2-thiothymine（2- 氮杂 -2- 硫代胸腺嘧啶）and phenylhydrazine（苯肼）have been identified as matrices that could be used to minimize loss of sialic acid during MALDI MS analysis of glycosylated peptides.

MALDI-TOF has been used to characterize post-translational modification. It has been reported that a reduction in loss of some post-translational modifications can be accomplished if IR MALDI is used instead of UV MALDI.

Oligonucleotides have been characterized by MALDI-TOF e.g., in molecular biology, a mixture of 5-methoxysalicylic acid（5- 甲氧基水杨酸）and spermine（精胺，精素）can be used as a matrix for oligonucleotides analysis in MALDI mass spectrometry, for instance after oligonucleotide synthesis.

Medicine

MALDI/TOF spectra are often utilized in tandem with other analysis and spectroscopy techniques in the diagnosis of diseases. MALDI/TOF is a diagnostic tool with much potential because it allows for the rapid identification of proteins and changes to proteins without the cost or computing power of sequencing and the skill or time needed to solve a crystal structure in X-ray crystallography.

One example of this is **necrotizing enterocolitis（NEC，坏死性小肠结肠炎）**, which is a devastating （毁灭性的）disease that affects the bowels of premature infants. The symptoms of NEC are very similar to those of sepsis（败血症）, and many infants die awaiting diagnosis and treatment. MALDI/TOF was used to identify bacteria presentin the fecal（排泄物的）matter of NEC positive infants. There is hope that a similar technique could be used as a quick, diagnostic tool that would not require sequencing.

Another example of the diagnostic power of MALDI/TOF is in the area of cancer. Pancreatic cancer remains one of the most deadly and difficult to diagnose cancers. Impaired cellular signaling due to mutations in membrane proteins has been long suspected to contribute to pancreatic cancer. MALDI/TOF has been used to identify a membrane protein associated with pancreatic cancer and at one point（一度，在某一时刻）may even serve as an early detection technique.

MALDI/TOF can also potentially be used to dictate（指示，导致，影响）treatment as well as diagnosis. MALDI/TOF serves as a method for determining the drug resistance of bacteria, especially to β-lactams (Penicillin family). The MALDI/TOF detects the presence of carbapenemases（碳青霉烯酶）, which indicates drug resistance to standard antibiotics. It is predicted that this could serve as a method for identifying a bacterium as drug resistant in as little as three hours. This technique could help physicians decide whether to prescribe more aggressive antibiotics initially.

Details that need attention

In analysis of biological systems, inorganic salts, which are also part of protein extracts, interfere with the ionization process. The salts can be removed by solid phase extraction or by washing the dried-droplet MALDI spots with cold water. Both methods can also remove other substances from the sample. The matrix-protein mixture is not homogenous because the polarity difference leads to a separation of the two substances during co-crystallization. The spot diameter of the target is much larger than that of the laser, which makes it necessary to make many laser shots at different places of the target, to get the statistical average of the substance concentration within the target spot. The matrix chemical composition, the addition of trifluoroacetic acid, formic acid（甲酸，蚁酸）, fructose, delay time between the end of laser pulse and start of ion acceleration in the ion source (in vacuum MALDI sources), laser wavelength, UV energy (as well as its density and homogeneity) in a focused light spot produced by a pulsed laser, and the impact angle of the laser on the target are among critical parameters for the quality and reproducibility of the MALDI-TOF MS method.

Additionally, the thickness of the MALDI plate can affect the TOF measurements. The smaller plates (less thick) will have longer TOF measurements. This can potentially shift peaks in the spectra and make it difficult to compare to other published results.

3.4.6 Assignment of disulfide bonds in proteins（蛋白质中二硫键的鉴定）

Among the 20 natural amino acids, cysteine is unique because it is involved in many biological activities through oxidation and reduction to form disulfide bonds and sulfhydryls. These modifications play an important role in the protein's structure and biological function. Disulfide bonds are important for the stabilization of the native structures of proteins. The identification and characterization of protein disulfide bonds is an essential step to thoroughly understand their biological function, provide insights into their folds and information to guide structural determination and assess the folding of recombinant proteins. However, the determination of disulfide linkages can be a challenging task.

Several methods are used to determine the pattern of disulfide bond linkage. Among them, crystallography and NMR are excellent tools that can identify disulfide bond linkages with minimal disulfide bond interexchange. However, the application of both techniques is limited by large sample requirements and protein size.

The basic strategy for obtaining this information by using methods other than the above-described involves the identification of disulfide-linked peptides in digests of proteins and the characterization of their cysteinyl peptide constituents. Edman degradation can be used for the identification of disulfide bonds. But this technique requires ultra pure samples, digestion, and further purification of the peptides for protein sequencing. Mass spectrometry has also been successfully applied to identify disulfide bonds in solution and from gels. Researchers have successfully demonstrated that disulfide bridge patterns can be identified by mass spectrometry (MS) analysis, following protein digestion either under partial reduction or nonreduction conditions (Fig. 3-34).

Partial reduction is a widely accepted approach for the determination of disulfide bonds. In this approach, the protein is digested under controlled conditions such that disulfide bonds with different reduction kinetics are reduced and alkylated gradually. Peptide containing modified cysteines are further separated and analyzed by MS and/or tandem MS. However, when a protein is highly bridged, multiple reductions and separations are necessary for complete disulfide mapping. The approach requires relatively large sample amounts compared with direct tandem MS and can provide ambiguous results when disulfide bonds have the same or similar reduction rates. Tandem MS analysis of protein digests under nonreducing condition has also been used frequently for the investigation of disulfide bond patterns. With appropriate enzyme(s) digestion, disulfide bonds pattern can be identified in a single run. However, data processing may be extremely complicated and time/labor-consuming for proteins with multiple unknown disulfide bonds. Also, when the sample contains a large number of cysteines or multiple disulfide bonds exist in the sample, some disulfide bond linkages might go unidentified. Tools that can effectively search tandem MS data for the presence of disulfide bonds will facilitate disulfide analysis.

The objective of determining the disulfide arrangement of a protein accompanied the very first determination of the amino acid sequence of a protein. Knowledge of the disulfide arrangement

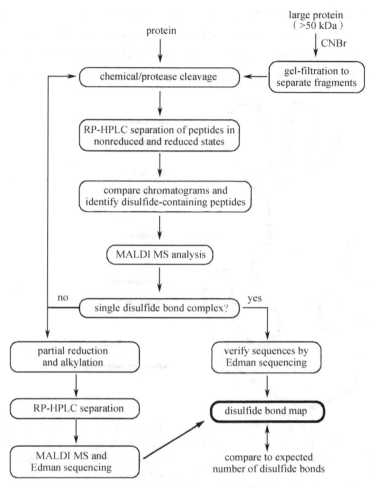

Fig. 3-34　Overall strategy for location of disulfide bond in proteins.

was sought to complete the description of the primary chemical structure of the protein in question. Characterization of the disulfides of ribonuclease was another informative study into the determination of protein disulfides. These studies established the basic strategy that still applies today for the determination of disulfide bond arrangements (Fig. 3-35). The steps involved in this strategy are: (1) fragmentation of the non-reduced protein of interest into disulfide-linked peptides with cleavages between all cysteine residues, if possible, and under conditions that avoid rearrangement (interchange) of disulfide bonds; (2) separation of disulfide-linked peptides from one another; (3) location/ identification of disulfide-linked peptides in various separated fractions; (4) fragmentation of the disulfide linked peptides at the disulfide bond; and (5) isolation and characterization of the cysteinyl products of the disulfide cleavage reaction.

These early studies also provided insights into the experimental conditions required for disulfide bond determination. It was observed that disulfide bond rearrangement could be promoted by strong acids, by the presence of thiols（巯基）at neutral pH, and by thiols produced by hydrolytic cleavage of disulfide bonds at neutral and alkaline pH. Disulfide interchange was noted under the conditions of enzymatic cleavage at slightly alkaline pH. Thus, conditions of the cleavage of the peptide backbone between cysteines must be carefully controlled. The concern regarding disulfide bond interchange at alkaline pH has been reinforced in a variety of subsequent reports. Consequently, protein cleavage methods that are performed in aqueous solvents at acid pH are preferred. Accordingly, dilute acids and/or cyanogen bromide（溴化氰）and pepsin（胃蛋白酶）are favored chemical and enzymatic cleavage agents. Acidic conditions also tend to disrupt protein conformation and enable optimal access to and requisite cleavage between cysteine residues. The broad substrate specificity of pepsin also potentiates（加强）cleavage between cysteines.

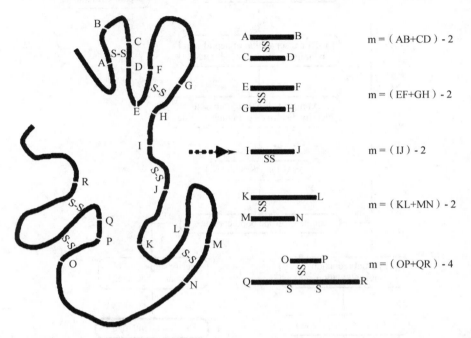

Fig. 3-35 Strategy for determination of disulfide bond arrangements of a protein. A protein of interest is cleaved in its non-reduced state, using methods to cleave between as many of the cysteine residues as possible. The resultant disulfide-linked peptides are separated, identified, and characterized. In principle, mass spectrometry may be used for separation, identification, and characterization. Mass spectrometric identification and characterization may be based on the computation of combinations of masses of cysteinyl sequences that would give rise to masses observed for disulfide-linked peptides. The computational process may be facilitated by measuring the masses of peptides that arise from the reduction of disulfide linked peptides and/or by performing MS/MS of disulfide-linked peptides.

Analytical technologies that require disulfide-linked fragments to be analyzed as pure components to define linkages, for example amino acid analysis or Edman degradation are highly dependent on purification strategies. Purification conditions must also avoid disulfide-bond rearrangements, and protocols have been devised for this purpose. Cation-exchange HPLC has been used to isolate disulfide-linked peptides due to the greater retention on cation-exchange media than single-chain peptides due to relative differences in cationic properties of these classes of peptides at acid pH. An elegant（简洁的）method for identification of disulfide-linked peptides and isolation of the component cysteinyl peptides for analysis involved diagonal（对角线的）peptide mapping by paper electrophoresis. This technique involved: (1) cleavage of the non-reduced protein with pepsin; (2) separation of the disulfide-linked peptides by one dimension of paper electrophoresis at acid pH; (3) exposure of the original electrophoretogram（电泳图）to performic acid（过甲酸）vapor; and (4) a second dimension of separation by paper electrophoresis at right angles to the initial direction of separation. Performic acid cleaves disulfide bonds, and converts the cysteine residues into highly negatively charged cysteic acids（磺基丙氨酸）. Thus, peptides not affected by performic acid migrated in a diagonal fashion after the combined electrophoretic steps, and peptides with disulfides prior to performic acid oxidation migrated off the diagonal. Peptides that were paired by inter-chain disulfide linkages prior to oxidative cleavage migrated with a vertical orientation to each other. The off-diagonal peptides were detected by minimal staining, eluted from the electrophoretograms, and characterized by amino acid analysis and/or amino acid sequence analysis.

The original diagonal electrophoretic concept has subsequently been adapted to create other two-dimensional methodologies for identification, isolation, and characterization of disulfide-linked peptides. For example, digests have been subjected to HPLC separations in non-reduced and reduced states. Alterations in HPLC mobility as a consequence of reduction are used as the equivalent of off-diagonal electrophoretic mobility. Likewise, mass spectrometric (MS) analysis of unfractionated digests in non-reduced and reduced states may also provide information on disulfide linkages.

Mass spectrometry and disulfide bond determination

Tools for disulfide bond analysis have improved dramatically in the recent decades, especially in terms of speed and sensitivity. This improvement is largely due to the development of matrix-assisted laser desorption/ionization (MALDI) and electrospray ionization (ESI), and complementary analyzers with high resolution and accuracy. The process of pairing cysteinyl peptides is now generally achieved by comparing masses of non-reduced and reduced aliquots of a digest of a protein that was proteolyzed with intact disulfide bonds. Pepsin has favorable properties for generating disulfide-linked peptides, including its acidic pH optimum, at which disulfide bond rearrangement is precluded and protein conformations are likely to be unfolded and accessible to cleavage, and broad substrate specificity. These properties potentiate cleavage between all cysteine residues of the substrate protein. However, pepsin produces complex digests that contain overlapping peptides due to ragged cleavage. This complexity can produce very complex spectra and/or hamper the ionization of some constituent peptides. It may also be more difficult to compute which cysteinyl sequences of the protein of interest are disulfide-linked in non-reduced peptic (胃蛋白酶的) digests. This ambiguity is offset (抵消，补偿，弥补) to some extent by sequence tags that may arise from ragged cleavages and aid sequence assignments. Problems associated with pepsin cleavage can be minimized by digestion in solvents that contain 50% $H_2^{18}O$. Resultant disulfide-linked peptides have distinct isotope profiles (combinations of isotope ratios and average mass increases) compared to the same peptides with only ^{16}O in their terminal carboxylates. Thus, it is possible to identify disulfide-linked peptides in digests and chromatographic fractions, using these mass-specific markers, and to rationalize (使······合理化) mass changes upon reduction in terms of cysteinyl sequences of the protein of interest. Some peptides may require additional cleavages due to their multiple disulfide bond contents and/or tandem mass spectrometry (MS/MS) to determine linkages. Interpretation of the MS/MS spectra of peptides with multiple disulfides in supplementary digests is also facilitated by the presence of ^{18}O in their terminal carboxylates.

Peptide Mass Analysis

The potential for mass spectrometry to facilitate the determination of disulfide bond linkages in proteins was realized with the advent of reliable methods, such as fast atom bombardment (FAB) and plasma desorption (PD, 等离子体解吸), for ionization of peptides and proteins. Development of instruments suitable for analysis of relatively small quantities of proteins and peptides, with reasonable mass range, resolution, and accuracy, was another contributory factor. One of the first reports on the use of mass spectrometry for disulfide bond analysis was very similar in principal to diagonal peptide mapping by paper electrophoresis. For instance, peptic digestion at acid pH was used to preclude disulfide interchange. The major difference was that separation and analysis were done simultaneously in the mass spectrometer. Disulfide bond-containing peptides in digests of non-reduced proteins were identified by comparison of spectra obtained with aliquots of the digests before and after reduction. Linkage arrangements were proposed on the basis of computations of combinations of masses of potentially linked cysteinyl sequences (Fig. 3-35). These assignments were confirmed by one cycle of manual Edman degradation. Ragged peptic cleavage produced sequence tags at the termini of the chains of some of the interchain disulfide-linked peptides. Although not specifically mentioned, the resultant sequence tags could have also been used to facilitate identification of the sequence partnerships within some of the interchain disulfide-linked peptides. Peptides with intrachain disulfides were identified by virtue of 2 U mass increases associated with reduction of their constituent cysteines.

Other groups made similar observations with FAB-MS. They observed that disulfide bonds were labile when bombarded in the ion source with high-energy xenon（氙）atoms, and that this effect was dependent upon the duration of bombardment prior to ion acceleration. Thus, mass changes were observed that were associated with the reduction of intrachain and interchain disulfide-linked peptides. Concomitantly, the products of reduction were observed at the masses of the constituent cysteinyl peptides of interchain disulfide linked peptides and at masses 2 U higher than non-reduced intrachain disulfide-linked peptides. Chemical reduction in solution was also used to produce the same changes in the masses of disulfide-linked peptides. A combination of dilute acid and/or cyanogen bromide cleavage at acid pH, followed by proteolysis with enzymes of well-defined substrate specificities at alkaline pH was used to produce disulfide-linked peptides. Variations on this approach have now been used to define the disulfide bond configurations of many complex disulfide linked proteins (Table 3-8). Many of these studies have been conducted（进行，实施）, using the more sensitive ionization methods of matrix-assisted laser desorption/ionization (MALDI) and electrospray ionization (ESI) in conjunction with improved mass analyzers, such as TOF（飞行时间）analyzers with delayed extraction (DE) ion sources and ion mirrors.

Table 3-8   Representative examples of protein disulfide bond arrangements determined by mass spectrometry

Protein	Methodology	Reference
Insulin	FAB-MS of peptic digest peptides	Morris & Pucci (1985)
Hen and duck egg-white lysozymes	FAB-MS of combined CNBr/peptic digest peptides	Takao *et al.*(1984)
Hen egg-white lysozyme and bovine ribonuclease A (RNaseA)	FAB-MS of peptides from various digests involving CNBr/trypsin/dilute acid/chymotrypsin/endoproteinase Glu-C	Yazdanparast *et al.* (1987)
RNase A	FAB-MS of combined CNBr/tryptic digest peptides	Smith & Zhou (1990)
Antithrombin III	FAB-MS of combined endoproteinase Glu-C/tryptic or peptic digest peptides	Zhou & Smith (1990b)
Paim 1, α-amylase inhibitor	FAB-MS of endoproteinase Glu-C digest peptides	Akashi *et al.* (1988)
Wheat kernel α-amylase inhibitor	FAB-MS of different combinations of elastase/trypsin or elastase/trypsin/chymotrypsin or elastase/trypsin/pepsin and of some peptides shortened by manual Edman degradation	Poerio *et al.* (1991)

continued

Protein	Methodology	Reference
Protozoan Er-1 and Er-2	MALDI-TOF-MS and ESI-TOF-MS of thermolytic digest peptides	Stewart *et al.* (1992)
Echistatin	ESI-MS and ESI-MS/MS of peptides derived by oxalic acid hydrolysis	Bauer *et al.* (1993)
Bovine dopamine β-hydroxylase	ESI-MS and MALDI-TOF-MS of tryptic or endoproteinase Glu-C or peptic digest peptides	Robertson *et al.* (1994)
Saposin C and B	ESI-MS and FAB-MS of combined CNBr/ peptic/endoproteinase Glu-C or CNBr/tryptic/ endoproteinase Asp-N/chymotryptic peptides	Vaccaro *et al.* (1995)
Brassica napus seed storage protein, napin	MALDI-TOF-MS of combined endoproteinase Lys-C/thermolytic digest peptides	Gehrig & Biemann (1996)
Plasmodium apical membrane antigen-1	Ion Trap-MS of combined tryptic/thermolytic digest peptides	Hodder *et al.* (1996)
Bitis arietans bitistatin	MALDI-TOF-MS and ESI-MS/MS of tryptic and oxalic acid digest peptides	Calvete *et al.* (1997)
Human insulin receptor ectodomain	MALDI-TOF-MS of combined CNBr/tryptic digest peptides	Sparrow *et al.* (1997)
Human respiratory syncytial virus attachment glycoprotein	MALDI-TOF-MS and MALDI-TOF-PSD-MS of combined tryptic/peptic or tryptic/ thermolytic digest peptides	Gorman *et al.*(1997)
Newcastle disease virus (NDV) hemagglutinin-neuraminidase (HN)	MALDI-TOF-MS and ESI-MS/MS of peptic or peptic/CNBr or peptic/tryptic or peptic/ chymotryptic digest peptides	Pitt *et al.* (2000)
Human agouti-related protein	MALDI-TOF-MS of tryptic/peptic digest peptides of partially reduced and alkylated protein	Bures *et al.* (1998)
Human leptin receptor	MALDI-TOF-MS of combined peptic/tryptic/ thermolytic/CNBr digest peptides	Haniu *et al.* (1998)
Human interleukin-6 receptor	ESI-Ion Trap-MS/MS of tryptic peptides	Cole *et al.* (1999)
Human signal transducer gp130 ectodomain	ESI-Ion Trap-MS/MS and MALDI-TOF-MS of tryptic peptides	Moritz *et al.*(2001)

Tandem Mass Spectrometry (*MS/MS*，串联质谱)

Fragmentation of ions may be required to define the linkage patterns within some disulfide-linked peptides. This requirement applies where three chains are linked and are not susceptible to further proteolysis between cysteines, or where two chains are linked but one of the chains contains an intrachain disulfide and no further proteolysis is possible between cysteines (Fig. 3-36). If a peptide contains two overlapping intrachain disulfides, then it is necessary to form a two- or three-chain peptide by further cleavages within the disulfide loops (Fig. 3-36) because peptide bonds within disulfide loops of peptide ions are generally resistant to gas-phase fragmentation. This resistance may be overcome if some of the intrachain disulfide is cleaved during ionization. Although peptide bonds and interchain disulfide bonds may be induced to fragment in MALDI and ESI ion sources, such in-source fragmentation is only informative with relatively pure analytes. Tandem MS may be used to define linkage patterns of disulfide-containing peptides in more complex mixtures. A variety of ionization techniques and mass analyzers have been used for this purpose. Combinations used include, FAB with tandem sector (扇形) mass spectrometers, ESI in conjunction with triple quadrupole (三重四级杆) analyzers, and MALDI post-source decay (PSD, 源后衰变) on TOF analyzers fitted with an ion mirror. In some instances, MS/MS has been used to achieve fragmentation of the peptide backbone between two sequential cysteine residues to define the partnerships of these cysteines with cysteines in attached chains.

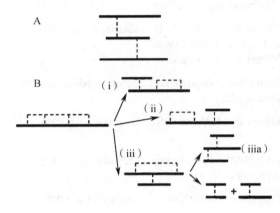

Fig. 3-36 Disulfide-linked peptide arrangements not directly amenable to solution by comparison of masses of non-reduced and reduced primary proteolysis products. Either MS/MS, additional enzymatic cleavage, and/or chemical cleavage would be required to determine linkages of a three-chain disulfide-linked peptide (A) or a single-chain peptide with multiple intrachain disulfide bonds (B). In the latter case, additional peptide bond cleavages would be required before MS/MS and (B (iii)) must be cleaved further to (B (iiia)) prior to MS/MS or into two chain disulfide linked peptides.

Ancillary methods and considerations

Isotope profiling (剖析研究) for disulfide-linked peptides, based on ^{18}O incorporation during proteolysis, adds an additional facility to the use of pepsin for the identification and characterization of disulfide-linked peptides.

It is necessary to use additional methods to characterize highly disulfide-linked peptic fragments. For example, where a two-chain peptide is produced in which one of the chains has an intrachain disulfide (Fig. 3-36). Even if peptides of this type can be converted to three-chain peptides, it may be that they are not amenable to (经得起检验) enzymatic cleavage between the two cysteines in the common chain or to MS/MS analysis. Adjacent cysteines (*i.e.*, -Cys-Cys-) in a chain of a multichain disulfide-linked peptide could pose particularly difficult challenges. Some methods that may be worth considering for use in these circumstances are discussed below.

Acid hydrolysis was used in the very early strategies to determine protein disulfides by mass spectrometry. The original work on insulin used acid hydrolysis for cleavage between cysteines. Oxalic acid (草酸) has been recommended as being a useful reagent for acid hydrolysis, particularly when disulfide interchange is observed under conditions of enzymatic cleavage.

Edman degradation can be a powerful complement to mass analysis for defining disulfide linkages. Manual Edman degradation may be used to cleave cysteines from chains that contain multiple cysteines. These cysteine derivatives are released with their linkages to cysteines in partnering chains intact. Thus, mass analysis of the shortened chains can be used to differentiate between alternate disulfide linkage arrangements. A proviso (附带条件，限制性条款) applies to this approach that cysteine cleavage from the chain that bears multiple cysteines precedes potential cleavage of a cysteine from a partnering chain. This approach has been used to define the linkages of sequential cysteines in an α-amylase inhibitor.

Selective susceptibility of disulfides to reducing agents has been used to simplify extremely complex disulfide-linked networks. Sequential reduction of disulfides with tris (2-carboxyethyl)phosphine (TCEP, 三羧乙基膦) at acid pH, followed by rapid alkylation with iodoacetamide (碘乙酰胺) or cyanylation with 2-nitro-5-thiocyanobenzoic acid (NTCB, 2-硝基-5-硫氰苯甲酸) at alkaline pH, has been used for this purpose. 1-Cyano-4- (dimethylamino) pyridinium tetrafluoroborate (CDAP, 1-氰基-4-二甲基氨基吡啶四氟硼酸盐) was subsequently used in place of NTCB because CDAP is able to cyanylate cysteines of selectively reduced disulfides at acid pH, thus minimizing any potential interchange during the alkylation step. Cyanylated cysteinyl peptides are susceptible to cleavage of the peptide backbone at the modified cysteines at alkaline pH and this may be used to simplify complex disulfide-linked peptides for subsequent mass analysis or MS/MS. The utility of this procedure was applied to resolving the partnerships of three sequential cysteines of the highly knotted protein sillucin.

It may also be helpful to use reduction with TCEP *in situ* in MALDI matrices to selectively disrupt complex networks immediately after the step of mass analysis of the disulfide-linked complex. *In situ* reduction was initially described with sinapinic acid (芥子酸) as the MALDI matrix; however, sinapinic acid may induce prompt fragmentation of disulfides in the ion source during laser irradiation in the absence of reducing agent. Dihydroxyacetophenone (DHAP, 二羟基苯乙酮) may be a more appropriate matrix for selective *in situ* reduction because it has been shown to be effective in avoiding fragmentation of fragile peptides and post-translational substituents such as disulfide bonds, and it is compatible with TCEP. DHAP may be useful in conjunction with TCEP for producing non-reduced or partially reduced disulfide-linked peptide ions for linkage analysis by MS/MS.

Caution must be exercised in the choice of reducing agents for selective reduction. Traditional biochemical reducing agents such as β-mercaptoethanol and dithiothreitol (DTT) are effective at reducing disulfide linkages, but they may also form covalent adducts with peptides, and such adducts complicate the interpretation of MS data. Tributylphosphine (TBP, 三丁基膦) is highly effective, and is not prone to this effect. Its volatility also means that excess reagent can be easily removed for subsequent analysis. However, the insolubility, high toxicity, and reactivity of this reagent require special handling precautions. TCEP is readily soluble in aqueous solutions, and is less toxic and more easily handled than TBP. Other advantages of TCEP over TBP include a greater compatibility with biochemical reagents and activity over a wider range of pH. Although not volatile, the concentrations of TCEP required for disulfide reductions do not interfere with subsequent analysis by MALDI.

Prompt in-source fragmentation during the MALDI process may also be used to selectively or partially reduce disulfide-linked peptides and may be useful for gaining some linkage information. Likewise, selective disulfide fragmentation has been observed in MS/MS spectra and may assist in defining linkages.

Particular care must be taken during the handling of proteins with unequal numbers of cysteines due to the increased potential for disulfide interchange to be initiated by thiols of unpaired cysteines. N-ethylmaleimide (N-乙基马来酰亚胺) and p-chloromercuribenzoate (对氯汞苯甲酸) may be added to block thiols of unpaired cysteines. These reagents can also be used to scavenge the thiols that maybe generated by the hydrolytic cleavage of disulfides at neutral and alkaline pH. Thiols of unpaired cysteines have also been shown to participate in other reactions that may complicated at an interpretation. The thiol of an unpaired cysteine residue of an insulin receptor was found to have reacted with the indole (吲哚) side chain of a tryptophan residue under the conditions of cyanogen bromide cleavage to produce a reduction-resistant tryptathionine (氨基羧乙基硫色氨酸) crosslink between two tryptic peptides. This side reaction had the advantage of eliminating the thiol of the unpaired cysteine from participation in interchange reactions during tryptic digestions and HPLC steps that followed the primary cyanogen bromide cleavage, but it caused confusion in the initial data interpretation. Cysteinylation of unpaired cysteine thiols in recombinant receptor proteins probably also precluded the interchange of disulfides during tryptic digestion to produce disulfide linked peptides for subsequent analyses. The tryptic digestion was performed at slightly acidic pH presumably in order to minimize any interchange expected to be induced by unpaired cysteine thiols. This cysteinylation probably occurred as an artifact (人工制品，矫作物，假象) of the fermentation conditions used to produce the proteins.

The use of mass spectrometry is pivotal to meet the contemporary challenges in determining disulfide linkage arrangements of proteins. It is now possible to determine the disulfide linkages of proteins, using mass spectrometry as the sole analytical tool in conjunction with enzymatic and chemical digestion and minimal chromatographic fractionation of digests. Stable isotope-labels on terminal carboxylates of peptides generated by proteolysis in $H_2^{18}O$ greatly facilitate the identification and characterization of disulfide-linked peptides. Isotope profiles, a combination of isotope ratios, and average mass increases of peptides produced in 50% $H_2^{18}O$, enable disulfide-linked peptides to be identified in complex digests produced by peptic digestion or in chromatographic fractions of such digests. This procedure allows the production and isolation of disulfide-linked peptides to be performed at an acid pH so as to preclude disulfide rearrangement. Stable isotope labeling with ^{18}O may also be used to aid the interpretation of MS/MS spectra of peptides with multiple disulfide bonds and that require MS/MS to define their constituent linkages. Isotope profiles produced by proteolytically mediated incorporation of ^{18}O may also be useful for identifying and characterizing other post-translational or chemical protein crosslinks.

3.4.7 Amino acid analysis and sequencing of proteins（蛋白质氨基酸分析和测序）

3.4.7.1 Amino acid analysis (composition)（氨基酸分析）

At a low level of resolution, we can determine the amino acid composition of the protein by hydrolyzing the protein in 6 N HCl, 100℃, under vacuum for various time intervals. After removing the HCl, the hydrolyzate is applied to an ion-exchange or hydrophobic interaction column, and the amino acids eluted and quantitated (测数量，用数量表示) with respect to known standards. A non-naturally-occurring amino acid like norleucine (正亮氨酸) is added in known amounts as an internal standard to monitor quantitative recovery during the reactions. The separated amino acids are often derivatized (衍生) with ninhydrin or Phenyl isothiocyanate (异硫氰酸苯酯) to facilitate their detection. The reaction is usually allowed to proceed for 24, 36, and 48 hours, since amino acids with OH (like Ser) are destroyed. A time course allows the concentration of Ser at time t = 0 to be extrapolated (外推). Trp is also destroyed during the process. In addition, the amide links in the side chains of Gln and Asn are hydrolyzed to form Glu and Asp, respectively.

3.4.7.2 Amino acid sequence（蛋白质测序）

Two methods exist to determine the entire sequence of a protein. In one, the protein is sequenced; in the other, the DNA encoding the protein is sequenced, from which the amino acid sequence can be derived. The actual protein can be sequenced by automated, sequential Edman degradation (Fig. 3-37).

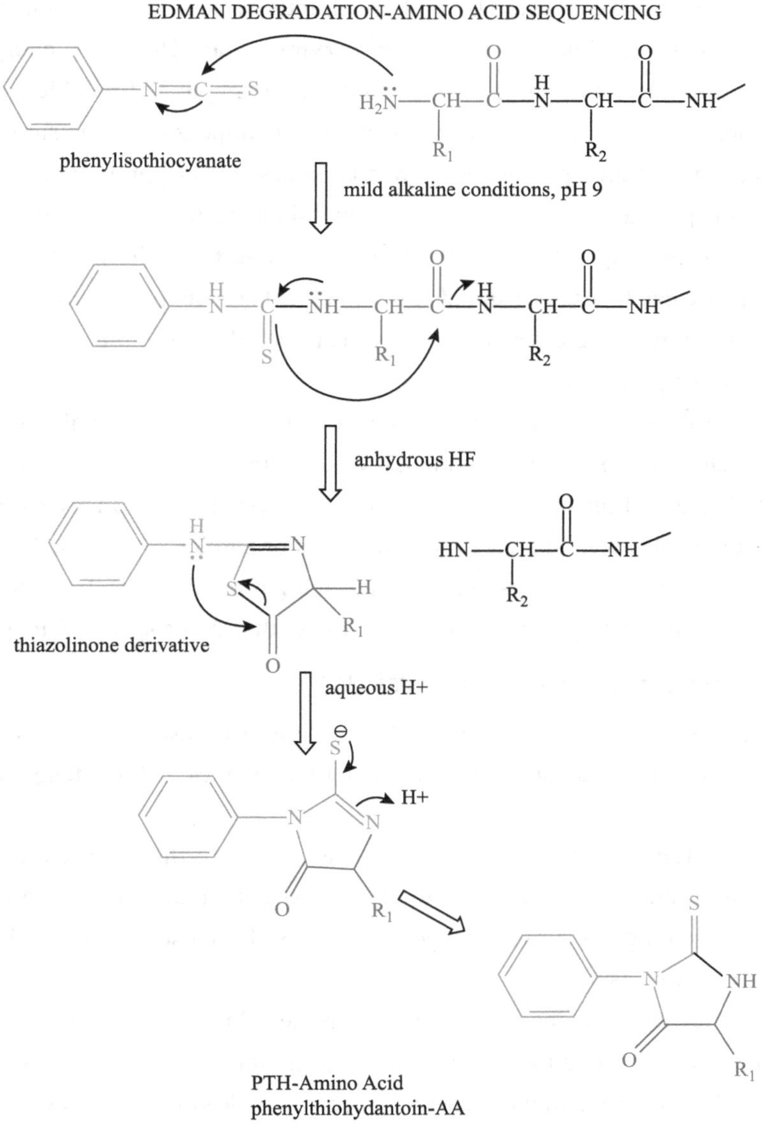

EDMAN DEGRADATION-AMINO ACID SEQUENCING

phenylisothiocyanate

mild alkaline conditions, pH 9

anhydrous HF

thiazolinone derivative

aqueous H+

PTH-Amino Acid
phenylthiohydantoin-AA

Fig. 3-37   Reaction steps of sequential Edman degradation used in amino acid sequencing.

3.4.8   Activity determination of recombinant proteins（基因重组蛋白活性的测定）

The production of a recombinant protein is a critical step in studying the function of proteins, while not all proteins produced by recombinant DNA technique possess biological activity, *i.e.*, some of the proteins produced in such ways lose biological activity partly or completely in the process of isolation and purification. Therefore, the most important qualitative criterion for a successful isolation and purification of a recombinant protein is hinged on whether biological activity of the protein still remains intact after the whole process for isolation and purification. Therefore, it is not surprising that protein activity determination is an indispensable segment to be arranged after isolation and purification.

However in many cases, there is no unified approach for the determination of the activity of recombinant proteins.

The first approach to determine the activity of recombinantly expressed protein is to directly assess the purified protein in a specific assay. The biological activity of a recombinantly expressed protein is routinely measured using a bioassay such as an **enzyme assay**. However, many proteins have no enzymatic activity and in many cases it is difficult to devise a simple and reliable approach to test their activities. And if a protein shows no activity in detection, it is impossible to be sure whether its activity was lost along with the purification process or the particular assay is inappropriate.

Some of the proteins play their biological roles through binding to another molecule, such as another protein, a nucleic acid, or a ligand, hence the **binding capacity** of the purified protein with those corresponding molecules, can be used as an index of biological activity of the protein to be tested.

Other approaches used in biological activity assessment include determining the impact of the protein on certain cell, tissue or organ system physiologies.

While only when all the determination approaches are established on a qualitative basis, can we get accurate bioactivity data. For instance, immunoassay is a commonly used method to assess biological activity. This method is based on specific antigen-antibody responses. In many cases, an antibody can bind to a variety of molecules with shared structural motifs or similar structures. And it is those specific structures either on antigens or on antibodies hence their mutual interactions that are the basis of immunodetection for recombinantly expressed protein, rather than some special functions.

3.4.8.1 Enzymatic activity（依据酶促活性检测）

Some substrates, substrate analogues, or a cofactor should be used to evaluate the activity of an enzyme. Various enzyme traits and parameters, including the kinetics, pH and temperature profile should also be determined.

The **Michaelis-Menten** equation is commonly used to study the kinetics of enzyme catalysis. Typically, the rate of reaction (or reaction velocity) is experimentally measured at several substrate concentration values. The range of substrate concentrations is chosen such that very low reaction rates as well as saturating rates are measured.

At low substrate concentrations, the reaction rate increases almost in a linear fashion with increasing substrate concentration. However, at higher substrate concentrations, the reaction rate no longer increases in a linear manner. Rather, increases in the substrate concentration lead to progressively smaller and smaller increases in the reaction rate. In fact, at very high substrate concentrations, the rate begins to approach asymptoticcally（渐进地）to a **steady-state** level, and additional increases in the substrate concentration do not lead to an increase in the reaction rate (see Fig. 3-38). This type of relationship is referred to as **hyperbolic**（双曲线的）and demonstrates **saturation** of the enzyme at high substrate concentrations.

A plot of the reaction rate versus the substrate concentration reveals two important kinetic parameters: V_{max} and K_m (see Fig. 3-38). V_{max} is the maximum reaction rate that is observed at saturating substrate concentrations. V_{max} is a function of the intrinsic rate of the enzyme as well as a function of the total number of enzyme molecules that give rise to the measured rate. K_m is referred to as the **Michaelis constant** and is the substrate concentration at which the reaction rate is exactly half of V_{max}. K_m is inversely related to the apparent affinity of the enzyme for its substrate. Therefore, a low numerical value of K_m refers to a very high affinity of interaction between the enzyme and its substrate. Conversely, a high numerical value of K_m is indicative of a low affinity of the enzyme for its substrate.

$$V = \frac{V_{max}[S]}{K_m + [S]}$$

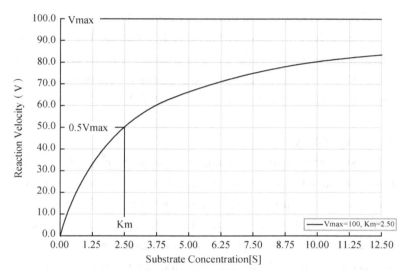

Fig. 3-38   A plot of the reaction velocity as a function of the substrate concentration as described by the Michaelis-Menten equation.

The activity of the enzyme was calculated from the linear part of the plot, *i.e.*, the initial specific activity of an enzyme was calculated as the change in the substrate amount in the time of the linear part according to the following equation:

$$a = (n_1 - n_2) / (t_1 - t_2)$$

If the enzyme under study has more than one (*i.e.*, two or more) substrate binding sites, and if there is cooperativity（协同性，协同作用）with respect to substrate binding to the enzyme, a plot of the reaction rate as a function of the substrate concentration is no longer hyperbolic and may assume a **sigmoidal**（S 形的）shape. In this case, the Michaelis-Menten equation is no longer the appropriate equation to use for studying the rate of reaction as a function of the substrate concentration. Instead, the **Hill equation** is the appropriate equation to use. Indeed, the Michaelis-Menten equation is a special case of the Hill equation where the enzyme under study has only one substrate binding site.

3.4.8.2   *Binding capacity*（依据结合能力检测）

In a biochemical reaction, a **ligand** forms a complex with a biomolecule to serve a biological purpose. In protein-ligand binding, the ligand is usually a molecule which produces a signal by binding to a site on a target protein. The binding typically results in a change in conformation of the target protein. In DNA-ligand binding studies, the ligand can be a small molecule, ion, or protein which binds to the DNA double helix. The relationship between ligand and binding partner is a function of charge, hydrophobicity, and molecular structure. The instance of binding occurs over an infinitesimal（无限小的）range of time and space, so the rate constant（速率常数，反应速度常数）is usually a very small number.

Binding occurs by intermolecular forces, such as ionic bonds, hydrogen bonds and Van der Waals forces. The association of docking is reversible through dissociation.

Ligand binding to a receptor protein alters the chemical conformation by affecting the three-dimensional shape, orientation. The conformation of a receptor protein composes the functional state. Ligands include substrates, inhibitors, activators, and neurotransmitters. The rate of binding is called affinity（亲和力），and this measurement typifies（代表，具有……特点）a tendency or strength of the effect. Binding

467

affinity is actualized (实现) not only by host-guest interactions, but also by solvent effects that can play a dominant, steric role that drives non-covalent binding in solution. The solvent provides a chemical environment for the ligand and receptor to adapt, and thus accept or reject each other as partners.

Radioligands (放射性配体) are radioisotope-labeled compounds used *in vivo* as tracers in PET (positron emission tomography, 正电子发射计算机断层显像, 正电子成像术) studies and for *in vitro* binding studies.

Receptor/ligand binding affinity

The interaction of most ligands with their binding sites can be characterized in terms of a binding affinity. In general, high-affinity ligand binding results from greater intermolecular force between the ligand and its receptor while low-affinity ligand binding involves less intermolecular force between the ligand and its receptor (Fig. 3-39). In general, high-affinity binding involves a longer residence time (滞留时间) for the ligand at its receptor binding site than is the case for low-affinity binding. High-affinity binding of ligands to receptors is often physiologically important when some of the binding energy can be used to cause a conformational change in the receptor, resulting in altered behavior of an associated ion channel or enzyme.

A ligand that can bind to a receptor, alter the function of the receptor, and trigger a physiological response is called an **agonist** for that receptor. Ligands that bind to a receptor but fail to activate the physiological response are receptor **antagonists**.

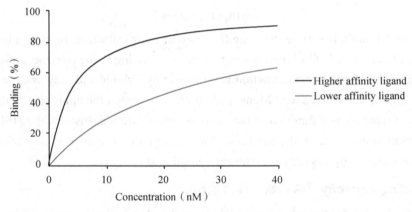

Fig. 3-39 Two ligands with different receptor binding affinity.

Binding affinity is most commonly determined using a radiolabeled ligand, known as a tagged ligand. *Homologous competitive binding experiments* (同源竞争结合实验) involve binding competition between a tagged ligand and an untagged ligand. Non-labeled methods such as surface plasmon resonance (表面等离子体共振, 表面等离激元共振), dual polarization interferometry (双偏振干涉测量, 双偏振/极化干涉测量技术) and Multi-Parametric Surface Plasmon Resonance (MP-SPR, 多参数表面等离子体共振) can not only quantify the affinity from concentration based assays; but also from the kinetics of association and dissociation, and in the later cases, the conformational change induced upon binding. MP-SPR also enables measurements in high saline dissociation buffers thanks to a unique optical setup. Microscale Thermophoresis (MST, 微量热泳, 微尺度热泳), an immobilization-free method was developed. This method allows the determination of the binding affinity without any limitation to the ligand's molecular weight.

When an immunoassay is used to test the intermolecular binding between an antigen and an antibody, it should be noted that sometimes the reaction is not the only one, cross reactions occur at the same time. One should make sure that a special determinant is chosen, lest cross reactions occur.

The **Western blot** (sometimes called the **protein immunoblot**) is an analytical technique widely used to detect specific proteins in a sample of tissue homogenate or extract. It uses gel electrophoresis to separate native proteins by 3-D structure or denatured proteins by the length of the polypeptide. The proteins are then transferred to a membrane (typically nitrocellulose or PVDF), where they are stained with antibodies specific to the target protein. The gel electrophoresis step is included in Western blot analysis to resolve the issue of the cross-reactivity of antibodies.

Drug potency and binding affinity

Binding affinity data alone does not determine the overall potency of a drug. Potency is a result of the complex interplay of both the binding affinity and the ligand efficacy. Ligand efficacy refers to the ability of the ligand to produce a biological response upon binding to the target receptor and the quantitative magnitude of this response. This response may be as an agonist, antagonist, or inverse agonist, depending on the physiological response produced.

Isothermal titration calorimeter

Isothermal titration calorimetry (ITC，等温滴定量热法) is a physical technique used to determine the thermodynamic（热力学的）parameters of interactions in solution. It is most often used to study the binding of small molecules (such as medicinal compounds) to larger macromolecules (proteins, DNA, *etc.*).

In an **isothermal titration calorimeter**（等温滴定量热仪）, the heat of reaction is used to follow a titration experiment. This permits determination of the midpoint (stoichiometry, 化学计量学) (N) of a reaction as well as its enthalpy (ΔH), entropy (ΔS) and of primary concern the binding affinity (Ka).

The technique is gaining in importance particularly in the field of biochemistry, because it facilitates determination of substrate binding to enzymes. The technique is commonly used in the pharmaceutical industry to characterize potential drug candidates.

Thermodynamic measurements

ITC is a quantitative technique that can determine the binding affinity (K_a), enthalpy changes (ΔH), and binding stoichiometry(n) of the interaction between two or more molecules in solution. From these initial measurements, Gibbs energy changes (ΔG) and entropy changes (ΔS) can be determined using the relationship:

$$\Delta G = -RT \ln K_a = \Delta H - T\Delta S$$

(where R is the gas constant（气体常数）and T is the absolute temperature).

The instrument

An isothermal titration calorimeter is composed of two identical cells made of a highly efficient thermally conducting and chemically inert material such as Hastelloy alloy（哈斯特洛伊耐蚀镍基合金）or gold, surrounded by an adiabatic（绝热的，隔热的）jacket (Fig. 3-40). Sensitive thermopile（热电堆）/thermocouple circuits（热电偶电路）are used to detect temperature differences between the reference cell (filled with buffer or water) and the sample cell containing the macromolecule. Prior to addition of ligand, a constant power（功率）（<1 mW）is applied to the reference cell. This directs a feedback circuit, activating a heater located on the sample cell. During the experiment, ligand is titrated into the sample cell in precisely known aliquots, causing heat to be either taken up or evolved（散发）(depending on the nature of the reaction). Measurements consist of the time-dependent input（输入）of power required to maintain equal temperatures between the sample and reference cells.

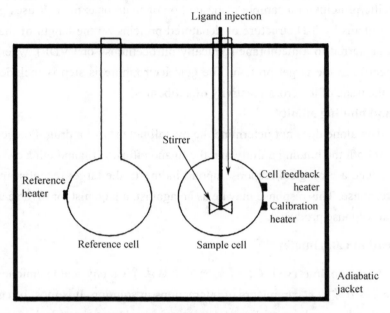

Fig. 3-40　Schematic of an ITC instrument.

In an exothermic（放热的）reaction, the temperature in the sample cell increases upon addition of ligand. This causes the feedback power to the sample cell to be decreased (remember: a reference power is applied to the reference cell) in order to maintain an equal temperature between the two cells. In an endothermic（吸热的）reaction, the opposite occurs; the feedback circuit increases the power in order to maintain a constant temperature (isothermic/isothermal operation).

Observations are plotted as the power needed to maintain the reference and the sample cell at an identical temperature against time. As a result, the experimental raw data consists of a series of spikes（尖脉冲）of heat flow (power), with every spike corresponding to one ligand injection. These heat flow spikes/pulses are integrated with respect to time, giving the total heat exchanged per injection. The pattern of these heat effects as a function of the molar ratio [ligand]/[macromolecule] can then be analyzed to give the thermodynamic parameters of the interaction under study. It should be noted that degassing （除气的，排气的）samples is often necessary in order to obtain good measurements as the presence of gas bubbles within the sample cell will lead to abnormal data plots in the recorded results. The entire experiment takes place under computer control.

Application in drug discovery

ITC is one of the latest techniques to be used in characterizing the binding affinity of ligands for proteins. It is typically used as a secondary screening technique in high throuput screening. ITC is particularly useful as it gives not only the binding affinity, but also the thermodynamics（热力学）of the binding. This thermodynamic characterization allows for further optimization of compounds.

3.4.8.3   *The impact of the protein on biological functions* （依据对生物功能的影响检测）

By exploiting some well-investigated and established findings, various bioassays have been designed and developed to determine the bioactivity of a recombinantly expressed protein. The assay may be based on the corresponding ligand-receptor interaction, which is associated with a cascade of events, an intracellular, inter-organelle, or intra-organelle signaling, in which a series of signaling molecules are involved.

For instance, the PTH receptor uses cyclic AMP as a second messenger. Almost all renal cyclic AMP production [Nephrogenic（肾发生的，肾源性的）cAMP] is in response to PTH, therefore **Nephrogenic cyclic AMP assay** is the "gold standard" against which PTH assays are judged. Urinary cAMP is measured by radioimmunoassay and corrected for the amount filtered from plasma (calculated from urine and plasma creatinine and plasma cAMP). This assay detects all bioactive PTH (including PTHrP). The stimulation of cAMP formation can also be performed in an isolated perfused rat femur preparation.

When it comes to measuring the impact of a protein on biological functions of certain cell types, for instance, the leakage of cytochrome *c* from mitochondria into the cytoplasm is known to activate caspases and initiate apoptosis. If a recombinantly expressed protein is able to induce apoptosis, and the apoptotic mechanism is supposed to associate with mitochondrial damage or mitochondrial swelling and release of intermembrane protein, including leakage of cytochrome *c*, then **Measurement of Cytochrome *c* Leakage from Mitochondria** is a nice choice since the cells can be assayed with the cytochrome *c*-releasing apoptosis kit (BioVision).

Chapter 4
The Genetic Engineering of Monoclonal Antibodies
第4章　单克隆抗体基因工程

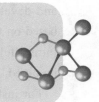

4.1　Introduction（简介）

The use of antibody-based therapeutics has grown exponentially in the past few decades, now representing a large component of therapeutic drugs that was dominated by small organic molecules up until the late 1990s. Antibodies have proven versatile in treating a variety of diseases including cancer, autoimmunity, infectious diseases, and even neurodegenerative disorders. As of 2020, 231 therapeutic antibodies have been approved by the FDA and around 2770 promising candidates are in different phases of clinical trials. They currently represent 28% of the top 100 selling drugs, up from just 1% in 2007. Actually, they represent 45% of the top 20 selling drugs and 50% of the top 10 selling drugs in 2020. However, major improvements and breakthroughs have been necessary to achieve these impressive results.

The 1970s were the start of great revolutions in the field: Gerald Edelman and Rodney porter were awarded the Nobel Prize for their work on the molecular structure of antibodies, the first atomic resolution structure of an antibody fragment was published, followed by the groundbreaking development of hybridoma technology by Georges J. F. Kohler and Cesar Milstein. This technology allowed antibodies to be produced and characterized as monoclonals, starting the modern era of antibody engineering.

Monoclonal antibody technology has yielded immunoglobulins with specificities to a wide range of antigens, including tumor-associated markers, viral coat proteins and lymphocyte cell surface glycoproteins. Such antibodies have great potential as agents in the diagnosis and treatment of human diseases. Clinical applications include the imaging of tumors with radiolabeled antibodies, passive immunotherapy in the treatment of viral infections and immunosuppression.

Despite the revolution mentioned above, the success of antibodies as therapeutic molecules was not immediate, and most clinical studies led to disappointments. For instance, the use of rodent antibodies in human diagnosis or therapy poses many problems, such as a short *in vivo* half-life, limited tumor penetration, inefficient recruitment of host effector functions, and most of all, the immune response from the patient against the injected antibody, also called "HAMA" response, referring to the production of neutralizing human anti-mouse antibodies, when the first murine antibody was used as treatment. Foremost（最重要的，居于首位的）amongst these is the immunogenic nature of the immunoglobulins.

Because mice are convenient for immunization and recognize most human antigens as foreign, mAbs against human targets with therapeutic potential have typically been of murine origin. However, murine mAbs have inherent disadvantages as human therapeutics.

When rodent antibodies are used for prolonged human therapy, antiglobulin response would appear, due to the sequence differences between rodent immunoglobulins and human immunoglobulins, hence precluding further treatment.

Many therapeutic applications for mAbs would require repeated administrations, especially for chronic diseases such as autoimmunity or cancer. Murine antibodies require more frequent dosing to maintain a therapeutic level of mAb because of a shorter circulating half-life in humans than human antibodies. More critically, repeated administration of murine immunoglobulin (Ig) creates the likelihood that the human immune system will recognize the mouse protein as foreign, repeated doses of rodent antibodies elicit an anti-immunoglobulin response, referred to as **human anti-mouse antibody (HAMA)**. At best, a HAMA response will result in rapid clearance of the murine antibody upon repeated administration, rendering the therapeutic useless. Worse, a HAMA response can cause a severe allergic reaction. This limits the use of repeated antibody administration essential for chronic treatments.

This possibility of reduced efficacy and increased safety risks has led to the development of a number of technologies for reducing the immunogenicity of murine mAbs.

The use of human monoclonal antibodies would greatly reduce the probability of occurrence of HAMA response, but such antibodies are generally restricted in their range of specificities. Intrinsic properties of immunoglobulins, whether rodent or human-derived, may also limit their effective clinical use. For example, for certain applications, the effector functions of the antibody may be required. However, the necessary isotype may not be readily obtained with the correct specificity. Further, human hybridomas are often unstable and/or poor producers preventing the production of large amounts of the human immunoglobulin.

For many years, researchers developed strategies to abrogate those problems — the journey toward antibody humanization began. Fully murine antibodies first progressed to chimeras, where variable regions from murine origin were assembled onto human constant domains, then to humanized antibodies by insertion of only the relevant CDRs onto human antibody scaffolds. Finally, fully human antibodies were generated, directly in genetically modified mice, selected from human synthetic antibody libraries or by sequencing of human plasma cells.

At the beginning of the 1990s, some of the limitations of monoclonal antibodies as therapeutic agents have been addressed (设法解决) by genetic engineering. Thus it is possible to replace much of the rodent-derived sequence of an antibody with sequences derived from human immunoglobulins without loss of function. This new generation of 'humanized' antibodies represents an alternative to human hybridoma derived antibodies and should be less immunogenic. Expression of the humanized antibody also offers the opportunity of tailoring the Fc of the antibody to best suit its application. Furthermore, genetically truncated versions of the antibody may be produced ranging in size from the smallest antigen-binding unit or Fv through Fab' to F (ab')$_2$ fragments. The expression technology can equally well be applied to human hybridoma derived antibodies. In this way unstable or poorly producing antibodies may be rescued and re-expressed in high-yielding mammalian or microbial systems. The genetic engineering of immunoglobulins may be extended to include non-clinical applications. In particular, the relatively low-cost production of antibody derivatives in microbial systems opens up the possibility of developing immune-purification agents.

An optimal technology for the generation of mAbs lacking immunogenicity in humans should have several characteristics. Ideally, the technology should produce mAbs that are fully human in sequence, lacking any murine amino acid components. It should generally be able to generate mAbs against human antigens. These mAbs should routinely be of high affinity and high specificity. The technology should easily generate a mAb with the desired effector function. Critically, the technology should be easy to use so that many users can generate mAbs without the need for sophisticated molecular biology techniques.

However, immunogenicity was not the only factor holding up the development of antibodies. Indeed, the classical architecture of immunoglobulin molecules bears some inherent limitations. The relatively large molecular size of immunoglobulins may mitigate against their effectiveness *in vivo*. Many innovative formats have been explored to overcome these major hurdles, such as reducing the antibody to its minimal functional size, modulating the valency, the (multi)specificity, increasing the half-life, and enhancing the recruitment of immune effector cells. Antibody fragments may be the reagents of choice for some clinical applications since they have much shorter half-lives *in vivo* compared with intact antibodies.

The following sections discuss the technology available for protein engineering and subsequent re-expression of antibodies.

4.2 Chimeric antibodies（嵌合抗体）

Immunoglobulin is a Y-shaped protein consisting of two heavy chains and two light chains connected by disulfide bonds, each chain can be divided into a variable region and a constant region.

The antigen-binding sites of an antibody are located in variable regions, and three loops within each variable region are hypervariable in amino acid sequences, which are called **Complementarity Determining Regions (CDR)**.

In a chimeric antibody a constant region of a human antibody is used to replace the homologous region in antibodies from non-human species (*i.e.*, mouse), which makes the immunogenicity decrease significantly.

In 1984, Morrion SL reported that they had created mouse-human antibody molecules of defined antigen-binding specificity by taking the variable region genes of a mouse antibody-producing myeloma cell line with known antigen-binding specificity and joining them to human immunoglobulin constant region genes using recombinant DNA techniques. Both chimeric mouse heavy chain V region exon (Vh)-human heavy chain C region genes and chimeric mouse light chain V region exon (V_K)-human K light chain gene constructs are expressed when transfected into mouse myeloma cell lines. When both chimeric heavy and light chain genes are transfected into the same myeloma cell, an intact tetrameric (H_2L_2) chimeric antibody is produced. The chimeric molecules were present in the ascitic fluids and sera of tumor-bearing mice. It is characterized by greatly reducing the immunogenicity of mouse monoclonal antibodies while preserving the specificity and affinity of parent antibodies. In addition, the effector function of antibodies is altered by linking different human homologous genes.

Although the issue of immunogenicity still exists in the chimeric antibodies, several kinds of chimeric antibodies have successfully passed the clinical trials. Chimeric antibody names contain a -*xi*- stem. Examples of chimeric antibodies approved for human therapy include abciximab（阿昔单抗）(ReoPro), basiliximab（巴利昔单抗）(Simulect), cetuximab（西妥昔单抗）(Erbitux), infliximab（英夫利昔单抗）

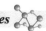

(Remicade) and rituximab（利妥昔单抗）(MabThera). There are also several examples of chimerics currently in clinical trials [*e.g.*, bavituximab（巴维昔单抗）].

The first generation of recombinant monoclonal antibodies consisted of the rodent derived variable regions fused genetically to human constant regions. The method of chimeric antibody construction is closely related to the method used to clone the variable domains and the two principal strategies for cloning and assembling chimeric antibody genes are summarized below.

4.2.1 Genomic vs. cDNA cloning to isolate variable region genes（基因组及 cDNA 克隆分离可变区基因）

Early work on the expression of recombinant antibodies relied on the isolation of the rearranged heavy and light chain variable region genes from genomic clones. This required the construction of genomic libraries from the hybridoma cell line using λ phage vectors and screening with either gene fragments or synthetic oligonucleotide probes. Although this was a relatively time-consuming process, the cloned immunoglobulin genes contained the necessary enhancer sequences for re-expression from immunoglobulin promoters (see sections on antibody expression). In addition, chimeric versions of the antibodies could be conveniently assembled using restriction sites present in the intron between the variable and constant gene segments.

Alternatively, V-region genes could be isolated from mRNA extracted from the hybridoma cell, via cDNA cloning. This appears to be a more rapid route than the genomic cloning approach but requires the use of site-directed mutagenesis to make chimeric constructs. The high levels of immunoglobulin mRNA in the hybridoma ensure that only small cDNA libraries (5 000~10 000 clones) are required to obtain full length heavy and light chain genes. Again the cDNA libraries are screened with synthetic oligonucleotide or gene fragment probes. It must be noted that many mouse hybridomas produce the mRNA for a non-functional light chain that is derived from the myeloma（骨髓瘤）fusion partner. The sequence of this light chain has been reported and can be distinguished from an authentic light chain by Cys^{23} to Tyr mutation in the first framework.

4.2.2 Use of polymerase chain reaction to isolate variable region genes（聚合酶链反应分离可变区基因）

Around 1990, the use of conventional gene cloning methods for isolating antibody genes has been superseded by strategies based on the polymerase chain reaction (PCR). The method depends upon the amplification of the required gene through repeated rounds of extension between two primers that hybridize to the 5′ and 3′ ends of the gene. The primers need not match the template sequence exactly, except at the very 3′ end, and often include restriction enzyme sites to permit the cloning of the amplified gene. The ability to isolate V-region genes by PCR has greatly reduced the time taken to produce genetically engineered antibodies. In addition, relatively few cells are required to produce sufficient mRNA for PCR cloning.

Two general PCR strategies have been reported for the cloning of both human and murine variable domains. The approaches differ only in the locations of the 5′ PCR primer, for both methods the 3′ primer is chosen to hybridize to the constant region. In the first method a set of upstream primers have been designed that hybridize to the DNA sequence encoding the signal peptide. Since there is a large number of potential leader sequences, a total of 61 heavy chain and 277 light chain primers are required to specify all known sequences for mouse antibodies. Rather fewer are required for human antibodies but this reflects the smaller database of known sequences. The major advantage of this strategy is that the cloned V-regions may be directly expressed without further engineering as either a murine or chimeric antibody (Fig. 4-1).

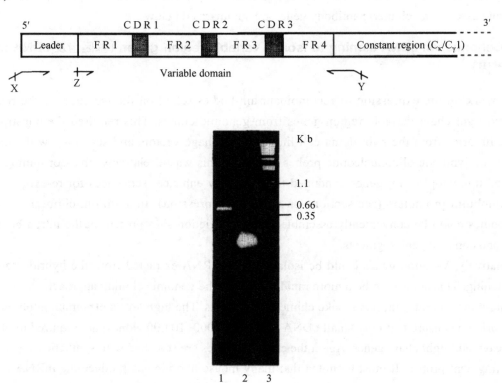

Fig. 4-1 Cloning antibody variable region genes by PCR amplification. The diagram shows the positions of oligonucleotide primers required to amplify variable region genes by the polymerase chain reaction (PCR). Two alternative locations of the 5′ end primers are illustrated. X, Y and Z represent restriction enzyme sites incorporated into the primer sequences to enable the PCR amplified gene to be cloned. The photograph shows the result of PCR amplification of a variable region gene analyzed on a 1.2% agarose gel stained with ethidium bromide and viewed under UV light. The variable region gene (track 1) was amplified from first strand cDNA, produced from total RNA by reverse transcriptase, using the conditions 94℃ 1 min, 55℃ 1 min; 72℃ 1 min for 30 cycles. A no DNA control (track 2) was run in the same experiment. DNA size markers are shown in track 3. Abbreviations: FR = framework region; CDR = complementarity determining region.

A potential weakness of this approach is the formal possibility that for any new antibody there may not be a primer that recognizes or is sufficiently similar to its leader to allow amplification. The second method avoids this since the 5′ primers bind to relatively conserved sequences in the first framework region of the heavy and light chain V domains. Again sets of primers for cloning both mouse and human V regions have been designed. Alternatively if the amino terminal sequence of either the light or heavy chain polypeptides can be determined by protein sequencing then a PCR primer can be synthesized that is specific to that sequence. Since the cloned V-regions lack signal sequences, these must be added to permit the expression of the antibody.

A potential problem with the framework primers is that the primer sequence becomes incorporated into the V-region sequence and may result in changes of amino-terminal residues. It was found that single amino acid changes in the first few amino terminal residues can drastically reduce the expression of the antibody. Nonetheless the framework primers have been used to clone a number of antibody specificities from both mouse splenocytes [*e.g.*, anti-(influenza hemagglutinin), 抗流感病毒血凝素] and the peripheral B lymphocytes of immunized human donors [*e.g.*, anti-(tetanus toxin)，抗破伤风毒素].

4.2.3   Choice of constant region（恒定区选择）

The construction of chimeric antibodies offers the opportunity of tailoring the constant region to the requirements of the antibody. Each immunoglobulin subclass differs in its ability to interact with Fc receptors and complement and thus to trigger cytolytic events. Thus human IgG1 would be the constant region of choice to retain or endow the chimeric antibody with the ability to mediate antigen-dependent cytotoxicity (ADCC) and complement-dependent cytotoxicity（CDC，补体依赖性细胞毒性反应）. For example mouse : human IgG1 chimeric antibodies have been shown to mediate the lysis of tumor cells and HIV-infected cells in the presence of human mononuclear cells. Alternatively if the antibody is required simply to activate or block a receptor then human IgG2 or IgG4 would be appropriate.

To avoid the unwanted side effects of a particular isotype it is possible to remove or modify effector functions by site-directed mutagenesis. It has recently been shown that the sites on IgG Fc involved in C1q and $Fc\gamma R'$ binding map to the CH2 of the heavy chain. Thus the ability of IgG to mediate complement-dependent lysis can be significantly reduced by point mutations at three positions, Glu^{318}, Lys^{320} and Lys^{322}. By constructing hybrids between human IgG1 and IgG4, Tao *et al* (1991) showed that other residues in the CH2 domain also contribute to C1q binding, the first step in the complement cascade. Similarly a number of reports have implicated（涉及）residues in the CH2 sequence 234-Leu-Leu-Gly-Gly-237 in their binding to both $Fc\gamma R'$ and $Fc\gamma R$ II cell surface receptors. Deviations from this sequence are suggested to account for the variable affinity of different IgG isotypes to these receptors. Thus the ability of an antibody to mediate ADCC can be removed by point mutations in the Leu-Leu-Gly-Gly motif.

However, it must be noted that creating unnatural constant region sequences may result in the production of novel antigenic sites. In this context, a further consideration in choosing the isotype of the recombinant antibody is the choice of allotype（同种异型）. Allotypes are known for three of the four human IgG heavy chains (IgG1, −2 and −3) in addition to IgA, IgE and κ type light chains. Combinations of allotypic（异型的）markers are not randomly distributed amongst different human populations being characteristic of particular racial groups.

4.3   Humanized antibody（人源化抗体）

Humanized antibodies (HAb), also called **CDR-grafted antibodies**（互补决定区移植抗体），**Reshaped antibodies**（RAb，改形抗体），are antibodies from non-human species whose protein sequences have been modified to reduce the heterology（异源性）of antibodies and increase their similarity to antibody variants produced naturally in humans.

To further reduce the mouse sequence content of the chimeric antibody the process of CDR grafting（嫁接法，移植法）has been developed. The CDR regions of an antibody are defined as that part of the variable domains that show hypervariability in sequence. From an analysis of a sequence database of antibody variable regions Wu and Kabat (1970) demonstrated that each variable domain contains three hypervariable sequences. They postulated that together these represented the antigen-binding site of the antibody. In general, the CDRs include the structural loops that connect the β-stranded framework at the top end of the variable region.

Since it was speculated that the transfer of rodent CDRs into human frameworks would transfer the ability to recognize the antigen seen by the rodent antibody, and the resultant reshaped humanized antibodies would possess both the specificity and the affinity of mouse-derived monoclonal antibodies. Humanization has been carried out by grafting the antigen-binding sites — substituting the CDR sequences of human antibody variable region (V) with CDR sequences of mouse monoclonal antibody by recombinant DNA technique. In this way, the exogenous (外源性) portion of the antibody would be minimized greatly, hence the immunogenicity of the antibody. RAb is also called "reconstituted antibody". Since the process of making it mainly involves CDR "grafting", it can be referred to as the "CDR grafting antibody" (CDR 移植抗体).

Work by Winter and colleagues showed that it was possible to transfer the CDR sequences from a mouse antibody and substitute them into a human antibody variable domain without significant loss of antigen-binding activity. In this way the hapten-binding of the antibody B1-8 was conferred (赋予) onto the human V_H of NEWM when co-expressed with the J5881 light chain.

Humanized antibodies are distinct from chimeric antibodies. The latter also have their protein sequences made more similar to human antibodies, but carry a larger stretch of non-human protein. Indeed immunogenicity of a chimeric antibody is drastically decreased when compared with that of a non-human monoclonal antibody, but the variable region still retains sequences of non-human origin. To further reduce the immunogenicity of antibodies, reshaped antibody (RAb) have been constructed in recent decades based on the chimeric antibody.

The main purpose for the preparation of humanized antibodies is to facilitate their clinical application. The process of "humanization" is usually applied to monoclonal antibodies developed for administration to humans (for example, antibodies developed as anti-cancer drugs). Humanization can be necessary when the process of developing a specific antibody involves generation in a non-human immune system (such as that in mice). The protein sequences of antibodies produced in this way are partially distinct from homologous antibodies occurring naturally in humans, and are therefore potentially immunogenic when administered to human patients.

The creation of "fully humanized" or "reshaped" variable region involves designing a variable region amino acid sequence that contains the rodent-derived CDRs and human-derived framework sequences. The rodent-derived CDRs from the monoclonal antibody of choice provide the specificity, so these residues are automatically included in the design of the reshaped variable region.

However, creating a reshaped antibody might require a more sophisticated approach than just splicing rodent CDRs into the most convenient human framework sequences. With only the sequences of the rodent CDR regions transplanted into the framework region sequences of a human antibody, the affinity of the antibody for antigen was usually unacceptable (low) until some residues in the human framework sequences were replaced with some corresponding residues in the rodent framework. Thus a dilemma arises between **immunogenicity and the affinity for antigen.** Through "saturation mutagenesis" or computer simulation analysis, the immunogenicity can be reduced as much as possible on the premise of retaining the original antigen-antibody specificity and affinity.

The generation and development of RAb make it possible to apply a variety of specific mouse monoclonal antibodies to clinical treatment, including specific anti-human antigen antibodies that are difficult to be induced to develop through the human immune system.

The Campath-1H antibody is the first humanized antibody clinically applied to treat non-hodgkin's lymphoma and rheumatoid arthritis. It represented the first "CDR grafted" or "fully shaped" antibody with the therapeutic potential. Although effective, more than half of the patients still have an immune response.

Other humanized antibodies, such as anti-CD33 antibody, a medicine used to treat myeloid leukemia （髓系白血病）, have negligible immune responsiveness.

There are other types of antibodies developed. The International Nonproprietary Names （国际非专利药名称） of humanized antibodies end in *-zumab*, as in *omalizumab*（奥马珠单抗）.

The best-fit strategy

The best-fit strategy holds that the human framework sequence used for antibody reshaping should be derived from the human variable region that is most homologous or similar to the rodent-derived variable region. This strategy is based upon the knowledge that the framework sequences serve to hold the CDRs in their correct spatial orientation for interaction with antigen, and the framework residues can sometimes even participate in antigen binding. Logic dictates （使人相信，导致） then, that if the selected human framework sequences are most similar to sequences of the rodent frameworks, this will maximize the likelihood that affinity will be retained in the reshaped antibody. In cases such as Campath-1H, the selection of a human variable region framework that is highly homologous to the rodent V region seems to be the best strategy for framework selection.

At its simplest level, the 'best fit' strategy involves comparing the donor rodent V-region with all known human V-region amino acid sequences, and then selecting the most homologous to provide the acceptor framework regions for the humanization exercises. In fact, comparing the chosen acceptor V regions with the database will help in identifying the discrepancies between their amino acid sequences.

As the process of humanization involves the joining of Fw (framework region) sequences from the acceptor V region to the CDR sequences of the donor, the important factor to consider is the homology between the framework region of the two V genes. If two possible acceptor V regions are identical having similar-homology scores to the donor, a choice can be made based on the number of framework region differences between them and the donor. The acceptor with the most homologous frameworks is the one of choices.

A variety of additional antibodies have been reshaped using a strategy similar to "best fit", in which acceptor frameworks are chosen on the basis of homology to the rodent monoclonal antibody, and then altered based on molecular modeling predictions prior to any experimental work in an attempt to maximize the affinity of the resultant reshaped antibody. Essentially, the goal of the computer modeling is to predict which key residues (if any) of the most homologous human framework should be left as in the rodent and which residues should be replaced with the corresponding rodent residues to optimize affinity in the reshaped antibody. These residues were chosen based on their possible influence on CDR conformation and/or binding to an antigen. Thus in such cases, modeling provided a potentially useful addition to the best-fit strategy. In fact, it is important to use computer molecular modeling or other strategies in helping to resolve problems that may arise.

Use of recombinant DNA in the humanization process

The humanization processe takes advantage of the fact that the production of monoclonal antibodies can be accomplished using recombinant DNA to create constructs (构成物，构建物) capable of expression in mammalian cell culture. That is, gene segments capable of producing antibodies are isolated and cloned into cells that can be grown in a bioreactor such that antibody proteins produced from the DNA of the cloned genes can be harvested *en masse* (全体地，一同地). The step involving recombinant DNA provides an intervention point (介入点，干预点，靶点) that can be readily exploited to alter the protein sequence of the expressed antibody. The alterations to antibody structure that are achieved in the humanization process are therefore all effectuated (完成，实行，招致) through techniques at the DNA level. Not all methods for deriving (获得) antibodies intended for human therapy require a humanization step (*e.g.*, phage display) but essentially all are dependent on techniques that similarly allow the "insertion" or "swapping-out" (交换，换出) of portions of the antibody molecule.

Distinction from "chimeric antibody"

Humanization is usually seen as distinct from the creation of a mouse-human antibody chimera (抗体嵌合体). So, although the creation of an antibody chimera is normally undertaken to achieve a more human-like antibody (by substituting the mouse Fc region of the antibody with that from human) simple chimeras of this type are not usually referred to as humanized. Rather, the protein sequence of a humanized antibody is essentially identical to that of a human variant, despite the non-human origin of some of its CDR segments responsible for the ability of the antibody to bind to its target antigen.

Humanizing via a chimeric intermediate

The humanization process may, however, include the creation of a mouse-human chimera in an initial step (mouse Fab spliced to human Fc). Thereafter the chimera might be further humanized by the selective alteration of the sequence of amino acids in the Fab portion of the molecule. The process must be "selective" to retain the specificity for which the antibody was originally developed. That is, since the CDR portions of the Fab are essential to the ability of the antibody to bind to its intended target, the amino acids in these portions cannot be altered without the risk of undermining (削弱…的基础，逐渐损毁) the purpose of the development. Aside from the CDR segments, the portions of the Fab sequence that differ from those in humans can be corrected by exchanging the appropriate individual amino acids. This is accomplished at the DNA level using mutagenesis (突变形成，变异发生).

The naming of humanized chimeras includes the stem for both designations (-*xi*- + -*zu*-). Otelixizumab is an example of a humanized chimera currently in clinical trials for the treatment of rheumatoid arthritis and diabetes mellitus.

Humanization by insertion of relevant CDRs into human antibody "scaffold"

It is possible to produce a humanized antibody without creating a chimeric intermediate. "Direct" creation of a humanized antibody can be accomplished by inserting the appropriate CDR coding segments (responsible for the desired binding properties) into a human antibody "scaffold". As discussed above, this is achieved through recombinant DNA methods using an appropriate vector and expression in mammalian cells. That is, after an antibody is developed to have the desired properties in a mouse (or other non-human), the DNA coding for that antibody can be isolated, cloned into a vector and sequenced. The DNA sequences corresponding to the antibody CDRs can then be determined. Once the precise sequences of the desired CDRs are known, a strategy can be devised for inserting these sequences appropriately into a construct containing the DNA for a human antibody variant. The strategy may also employ synthesis of linear DNA fragments based on the reading of CDR sequences.

Subsequently the construction of CDR-grafted antibodies to complex antigens has been reported [*e.g.*, cell surface receptors — Campath (一种抗肿瘤药, 含 alemtuzumab) and IL-2 receptor; viral antigens — respiratory syncytial virus (合胞体病毒, 融合后胞病毒) and hepatitis B]. In all cases, it has been shown that simply introducing the CDR sequences into the human antibody background is not sufficient to obtain full binding activity. Therefore the process of CDR grafting involves the manipulation of not only the CDR but also the framework sequences.

Alemtuzumab (阿仑单抗) is an early example of an antibody whose humanization did not include a chimeric intermediate. In this case, a monoclonal dubbed (授予称号, 被称为) "Campath-1" was developed to bind CD52 using a mouse system. The hypervariable loops of Campath-1 (that contain its CDRs and thereby impart its ability to bind CD52) were then extracted and inserted into a human antibody framework. Alemtuzumab is approved for treatment of B-cell chronic lymphocytic leukemia and is currently in clinical trials for a variety of other conditions including multiple sclerosis (多发性硬化).

Clinical experience around 1990 with chimeric antibodies indicates that though the immune response to these immunoglobulins is much reduced compared to murine antibodies, in some individuals a strong anti-idiotypic (抗个体基因型的) reaction is elicited. The results of two phase I studies using the anti-tumor antibodies 17-1A and B72.3 have been analyzed in detail. Both antibodies produced an immune response which has been mapped to the variable regions. No anti-(constant region) antibodies were detected. This contrasts with earlier work on the administration of the murine antibody OKT3 to renal transplant patients in which both an anti-isotype and anti-(idiotype) were elicited. However, it appears that not all variable regions will produce the same frequency of HAMA. It must be noted that these studies involved cancer patients with a variable history of immunosuppressive treatment.

A general approach to CDR grafting is outlined in Fig. 4-2.

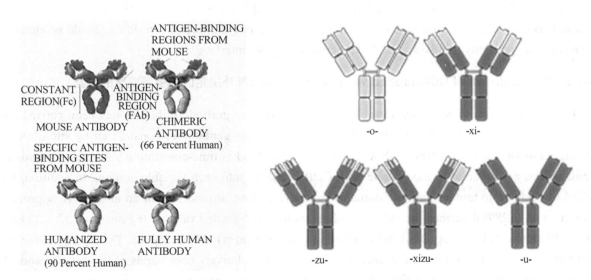

Fig. 4-2   Sketches of chimeric (top right), humanized (bottom left) and chimeric/humanized (bottom middle) monoclonal antibodies. Human parts are shown in brown, non-human parts in blue.

4.3.1 Design of CDR-grafted variable domains（互补决定区移植可变区的设计）

Starting with the sequence of the murine light and heavy chain variable regions, the first step in the design of a CDR-grafted variable region is to identify the boundaries of the CDRs. Most commonly these are defined according to Kabat *et al.* (1987). With the exception of CDR2 on the heavy chain (H2) the CDRs include all the sequences required to determine the local conformation of the apical（顶点的，顶上的）loops. In the case of H2, Cothia and Lesk showed from an examination of the resolved structures of antibodies, that residues adjacent to the Kabat CDR are important in determining the conformation of the loop.

Framework residues not contiguous（邻近的，接触的）to the CDRs have also been implicated in the positioning of the CDR loops. Thus Tramontano *et al.* argued again on structural grounds that residue 71 in framework 4 of the heavy chain is the major determinant of the position of the H2 loop. This position is one of a subset of framework residues that directly or indirectly interact with the CDR loops and determine their packing（包装）. Inclusion of some or all of these residues from the donor mouse antibody if they differ in the acceptor human framework has been shown to be necessary for retaining the full binding activity.

In practice, the number of framework changes required to design the CDR-grafted variable domain depends upon the degree of homology between the framework of the donor mouse antibody and the acceptor human body. In general two approaches have been described. In the first a generic human framework is chosen usually based on the availability of an X ray structure, *e.g.*, KOL for V_H and REI for V_L. This framework is then modified to accept the CDR loops of a specific antibody to be grafted. In the second approach, human frameworks are chosen from a database of known antibody sequences that show greatest homology to the frameworks of the donor mouse antibody. The V_L and V_H frameworks are not necessarily from the same antibody. Some fine tuning of the frameworks may still then be necessary. A further design consideration is the packing of the two domains. For the most part the contact residues at the V_H/V_L interface are conserved between mouse and human antibodies. However if the human frameworks chosen for grafting are not from the same antibody the interface residues should be checked to ensure compatibility（相容性，适应性）across the V_H V_L interface.

4.3.2 Construction of CDR-grafted variable domains（互补决定区移植可变区的构建）

The manipulation of antibody variable regions to produce grafted antibodies has been carried out in a number of ways. The first CDR-grafted variable domain genes were constructed by site-directed mutagenesis of a single-stranded DNA template. This method is time-consuming since three rounds of mutagenesis are required to incorporate each CDR sequence into each variable domain. In addition, the yield of each triple mutant variable domains is relatively low, around 5%. In an alternative approach, Queen *et al.* (1989) described the assembly of the entire CDR-grafted variable regions from 12×20 base pair oligonucleotides using DNA polymerase in combination with DNA ligase. This totally synthetic approach is expensive in terms of reagents and again gives relatively poor yields of the correct product. Improvements to both these methods have been described in which the polymerase chain reaction has been used to direct the synthesis of the complete variable domain. Lewis and Crowe (1991) have adapted the PCR strand overlap method of mutagenesis to replace the CDRs in a human variable domain sequence

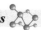

with those from a rodent antibody. Although several rounds of PCR amplification are required to build the CDR-grafted variable domain, correctly assembled sequences are obtained in high yield. As an alternative Daugherty *et al.* (1991) have used PCR to synthesize each CDR-grafted domain in one step using six overlapping 80 bp oligonucleotides (Fig. 4-3). This is theretofore the most rapid method for producing CDR-grafted genes but may suffer from a higher error rate. Consequently several PCR assembled variable region genes may have to be sequenced to obtain an error-free product.

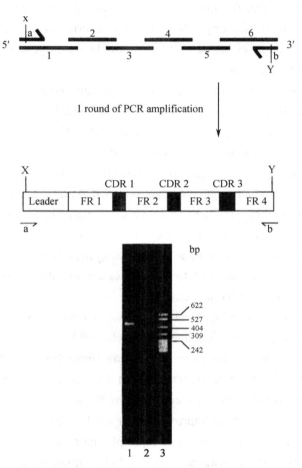

Fig. 4-3   Synthesis of CDR-grafted variable region genes by PCR amplification. The diagram shows the strategy for assembling variable region genes from overlapping oligonucleotides by the polymerase chain reaction. Six 80 bp oligonucleotides (Nos. 1-6, 1 pmol each) are mixed with two 20 bp flanking primers (a and b using the conditions: 94℃ 1 min; 55℃ 1 min; 72℃ 1 min for 30 cycles. The results of one round of PCR amplification are shown in track 2 of the photograph of an agarose gel. A further round of amplification using the product from the first round and primers a and b leads to an increased yield of the synthetic variable domain gene (track 1). DNA size marker are shown in track 3.

Construction of Fv and single-chain Fv fragments（Fv 与单链 Fv 片段的构建）

Immunoglobulins are multi-domain glycoproteins that may be dissected（切细，仔细分析）into individual domains using proteases. Typically, cleavage of an antibody hinge yields divalent $F(ab')_2$ or monovalent Fab fragments plus the Fc. Further careful proteolytic digestion may be used to generate the Fv fragment, which comprises the paired light and heavy chain variable domains only. Fragments of antibodies have proved valuable in the resolution of immunoglobulin structure by X ray crystallography and in the preparation of diagnostic reagents for use both *in vitro* and *in vivo*. The preparation of homogeneous antibody fragments by enzymatic digestion can be difficult and often conditions have to be optimized for each antibody. By contrast, recombinant DNA technology can be used to produce defined fragments of any immunoglobulin for study, *e.g.*, recombinant Fab fragments, recombinant Fc fragments and recombinant Fvs.

However, this technology is not limited to the production of conventional immunoglobulin fragments and has been extended to the generation of novel fragments, in particular those based on Fvs. Fvs may have an advantage over Fab fragments since they can be coupled to other effector molecules, *e.g.*, enzymes or drugs, without incurring a large penalty in terms of molecular size. Recombinant Fv fragments have been produced by either isolating the variable region gene segment or by inserting stop codons into heavy and light chain genes.

The resulting Fv fragments have been expressed in both mammalian and microbial cell systems and shown to retain the antigen-binding activity of the parent molecule. However, the variable domains of an Fv are only held together by relatively weak non-covalent interactions. It has been observed that at low concentration, certain Fvs dissociate whereas others appear to be more stable. One strategy that has been developed to improve the utility of Fv fragments has been to link the two domains together into a single polypeptide to produce the so-called single chain antibody (SCA) or single-chain Fv (sFv). A number of different linkers have been used to join the variable domains, including synthetic oligomers of (Gly4Ser) and natural sequences derived from proteins of known three dimensional structure. The length of the linker affects the folding of the sFv polypeptide and a joining peptide of 14 or 15 amino acids appears to be optimal. Although longer sequences of up to 25 residues are tolerated, linkers shorter than 14 residues result in a reduction in stability and binding activity.

sFv constructs have been made using a variety of monoclonal antibodies to both small molecular weight haptens, for example, phosphorylcholine fluorescein (磷酰胆碱荧光素) and 2-phenyloxazalone and complex polypeptide antigens, for example, human fibrin fragment D dimer and human IL-2 receptor. In most cases, the sFv has been shown to retain the antigen-binding affinity of the monovalent Fab′ fragment. Furthermore, for sFvs to tumor cell antigens, the relatively small size of the sFvs (25 kDa) compared to the Fab′ (50 kDa), results in improved tumor localization in mouse tumor xenograft models. This is presumably due to a combination of more rapid plasma clearance and greater tissue penetration. However, many antigen-antibody interactions involve both combining sites of the antibody either in binding to a molecule with more than one antigenic determinant or in bridging two separate cell surface molecules. Therefore, the monovalent binding of sFvs may limit their effective use. This is indicated by the following two studies. Milenic *et al.* (1991) observed that the sFv of the antibody CC49 that recognizes the multivalent tumor antigen, TAG72, had only one eighth the binding activity of the whole parent antibody. Condra *et al.* (1990) showed that sFv to ICAM (细胞间黏附分子), the cellular receptor for rhinovirus (鼻病毒), had a reduced potency in protecting cells from virus infection compared to intact antibody. This loss of activity was attributed to the inability of the sFv to cross-link cellular receptors. The potential benefits of an antibody fragment with high avidity (亲合力，抗体亲抗原性) may be obtained by joining two sFvs together. Two strategies have been reported to produce bi-sFv fragments. In the first a cysteine residue introduced at the C terminus of the sFv can be used to covalently link two sFvs via a disulfide bridge or heterobifunctional cross-linker. The second approach involves the addition of a short amphipathic helix to the C terminus of the sFv which results in the self-assembly of the sFv into non-covalently linked dimers.

Germline（种系，生殖细胞系）V region genes and the "Best Fit" strategy

A good candidate can be found in most cases by striking a balance between acceptor and donor V region homology, and acceptor V gene frequency in the population.

What may be crucial for efficacy in the therapeutic situation is how long, in how many repeated doses and at what frequency can an antibody be administered to a patient before an antiglobulin（抗球蛋白）response is likely to preclude further useful therapy. It seems likely that through the use of fully reshaped antibodies benefits will be obtained because of the longer periods over which the antibody can be administered before an antiglobulin response negates the effect.

The future approach to humanization will become more subtle than at present. It will no longer be sufficient to simply transplant the donor region CDRs into the framework of any acceptor human V region, greater consideration must be given to the amino acid sequence of the final product and how likely this is to be immunogenic in the human population. The acceptor V region will be carefully selected so as to be one which is well conserved within the population and well represented in the expressed repertoire, thus increasing the number of people to which it can be administered without it being seen as foreign. The use of well characterized human germline genes as acceptors will eliminate potential immunogenic sites caused by somatic mutation or by sequence errors. Ultimately, as knowledge of antibody structure improves, the sequence of the donor V region may simply be used to provide data enabling human germline CDR sequences to be modified to acquire the desired antigen binding properties. In other words, the aim is not to humanize the donor antibody, but to use data derived from it to predict the sequence of a true human antibody with the same antigen binding specificity.

In addition, it should not be forgotten that in the use of humanized antibodies the appropriate choice of both specificity and isotype is likely to be of great importance in deciding the clinical efficacy.

Antibodies from human patients or vaccine recipients

It is possible to exploit human immune reactions in the discovery of monoclonal antibodies. Simply put, the human immune response works in the same way as that in a mouse or other non-human mammal. Therefore, persons experiencing a challenge to their immune system, such as an infectious disease, cancer or vaccination are a potential source of monoclonal antibodies directed at that challenge. This approach seems especially apt（适宜的，恰当的）for the development of anti-viral therapies that exploit the principles of passive immunity. Variants of this approach have been demonstrated in principle and some are finding their way into commercial development.

Future Strategies for reshaping

To date, the major factor which has governed the choice of human acceptor V-regions used in humanization exercises has been the desire to retain antigen binding specificity and affinity in the final humanized antibody. However, of equal importance is the need to reduce the immunogenic potential of the antibody (in humans) to the minimum possible, after all, it is this which is the driving force behind the humanization process. By allowing our knowledge of immunoglobulin V region gene genetics, gene expression and affinity maturation to influence the final choice of human acceptor V-region, it should be possible to improve on past performance and reduce the immunogenic potential of humanized monoclonal antibodies still further.

4.4　Fully human antibodies（全人源抗体）

Some of the early attempts at generating fully human mAbs used human hybridomas. However, numerous difficulties, including the instability of the human hybridomas, a preponderance（优势，多数）of low affinity IgM mAbs, and the difficulty or ethical problems of finding humans immunized against the target antigen, resulted in this technology being used only rarely. Others have chimerized mAbs by linking the murine variable region to human constant regions. While requiring only relatively simple antibody engineering techniques, chimerized mAbs still may cause a human anti-chimeric antibody (HACA) response, an immune response in humans because of the fully murine framework and complementarity determining region (CDR) sequences of the antibody variable regions.

Antibodies for human therapy derived without using mice

There are technologies that completely avoid the use of mice or other non-human mammals in the process of discovering antibodies for human therapy. Examples of such systems include various "display" methods (primarily phage display) as well as methods that exploit the elevated B-cell levels that occur during a human immune response.

4.4.1　Phage display-derived human antibodies（噬菌体展示法制备全人源抗体）

Display methods

These employ the selective principles of specific antibody production but exploit microorganisms (as in phage display) or even cell free extracts (as in ribosome display). These systems rely on the creation of antibody gene "libraries" which can be wholly derived from human RNA isolated from peripheral blood. The immediate products of these systems are antibody fragments, normally Fab or scFv.

This means that, although antibody fragments created using display methods are of fully human sequence, they are not full antibodies. Therefore, processes in essence identical to humanization are used to incorporate and express the derived affinities within a full antibody.

Phage display technology has become one of the primary means for obtaining human antibodies, and some of them have been applied in clinical practice. Adalimumab（阿达木单抗）(Humira) is an example of an antibody approved for human therapy that was created through phage display.

Surface display of antibody fragments（抗体片段的表面展示）

Phage display of antibody libraries is an important *in vitro* technology for the discovery of monoclonal antibodies with therapeutic or diagnostic potential or value in basic research. The principle of phage display technology is to insert a foreign gene into one of the coat protein-encoding genes of the M13 phage to maintain the relative spatial structure and biological activity of the heterologous protein and present it on the surface of the phage.

Phage display technology was established by Smith (1985), who first described the use of filamentous phage (*e.g.*, M13 and Fd) for the expression of heterologous polypeptide sequences. A few copies of gene III protein cpIII (about four copies per virion) are normally expressed at the tip of the virion fd phage and are responsible for attachment to the F pilus of *E. coli* cells, and has been used to display peptide epitopes at the surface of the phage. By constructing a library of different peptides each fused to the cpIII of an individual virion, this expression method has been used to isolate specific peptide epitopes（表位，抗

原决定部位) by sequential panning (淘筛) and growth of the phage. Later this expression system has been applied to the surface display of antibody fragments, both sFvs and Fabs, and became one of the most successful methods in fully human antibody production.

Basic protocols for antibody library construction and selection of binder with the desired specificity

To carry out this procedure a few essential steps are required.

PCR cloning of variable region genes and the phage display system have been combined in the generation of libraries of V domain sequences. Antibody diversity is restricted to the variable regions (V_H and V_L). Functional antibody fragments can be displayed on the surface of phages by fusing the coding sequence of the antibody variable (V) regions to that of the phage minor coat protein pIII. These gene fragments are inserted into a specific vector in frame with the sequence encoding the phage protein pIII. Once assembled, the phage particle will expose the functional antibody fragment fused to the amino terminus of the minor coat protein III. Complete antibody V domains can be displayed on the surface of fd bacteriophage, that the phage binds specifically to antigen and that rare phage (one in a million) can be isolated after affinity chromatography.

In the creation of an antibody library several different choices can be made: a)which form of antibody fragment to use; b) the source of V regions repertoire. In general, successful approaches have employed either the single-chain fragment variables (scFv) format, consisting in a V_L and V_H regions linked by flexible linker, or the Fab (Fragment antigen-binding-) format, in which V_H-C_{H1} and V_L-C_L associate non-covalently. McCafferty *et al.* (1990) joined the heavy (V_H) and light (V_L) chain variable (V) domains by a flexible linker $(Gly_4-Ser)_3$, to allow expression of both on the same polypeptide, and the single-chain- Fv fragment (scFv) cloned into an fd phage vector (fdCAT1) at the N-terminal region of the gene III protein.

By creating large libraries, antibodies with affinities comparable to those obtained using traditional hybridoma technology can be isolated by a series of cycles of selection on the antigen of interest. A similar system based on fusion to the gene VIII coat protein permitting a multivalent display of antibody fragments has also been reported.

A particular application of this technology has been the isolation of novel human antibodies from both immune and non-immune B cells. Thus mRNA is isolated from B lymphocytes or spleen cells and all expressed heavy and light chain V region genes are cloned by PCR using framework 1 primers (see Fig. 4-3). Two libraries are constructed, one for the heavy chain variable domains and one for the light chain. These two libraries are genetically combined such that any V_H can pair with any V_L and be displayed on the surface of the phage as cpIII fusions. The expression library is then screened by panning to enrich for specificities to particular antigens. By increasing the stringency of antigen binding, high affinity fragments can be selected. In this way human Fab fragments to RSV (劳斯肉瘤病毒), tumor necrosis factor, HIV, and a number of other infectious agents have been isolated.

Natural V region repertoires can be recovered by RT-PCR amplification starting from lymphocytes which may or may not have undergone antigen stimulation. Such V genes are amplified using primers that recognize the 5′ end of the V genes and the 3′ end of the J genes. These naive (天然的) libraries turned out to be robust sources of antibodies potentially against any target, including those poorly antigenic in animals. As an alternative, synthetic antibody libraries have been created by introducing diversity artificially using oligonucleotides into frameworks with desirable properties. To generate diversity, completely degenerate oligonucleotides were used, although recently it has been found that diversity

Fundamentals, Approaches and Breakthroughs in R & D Genetically Engineered Biotherapeutics*

restricted to only few amino acids can provide antibodies with similar high affinities.

Before proceeding to the selection procedures the clonal diversity of the library, either naive or synthetic, needs to be assessed. Next generation sequencing is now routinely used to measure diversity and validate the design of displayed libraries.

Once a library is created, the enrichment of antigen-specific phage antibodies is carried out by "phage panning", using immobilized or labeled antigens.

In this process, the antigen of interest is directly immobilized on a solid support, such as microplate wells or is coupled to magnetic beads. The phage particles are then added to allow the binding of phages displaying appropriate antibody. After extensive washing to remove all nonspecifically bound material, phages displaying specific antibodies are retained while low affinity or unspecific phages are washed away. The selection procedure is repeated for two to five rounds usually decreasing antigen concentration and increasing stringency of washing steps, leading to the isolation of phages expressing the desired antibodies (*i.e.*, those that bind the antigen of interest). Bound phages are then eluted from the target antigen and used to infect bacteria for binding analysis. The expression of functional antibody fragments in the periplasmic space of *Escherichia coli* is the essential element for evolving the antibody phage display technique. The possibility of performing successive rounds of selection allows the isolation of binders present in very low numbers in a population of billions of different phages. A typical selection round is illustrated in Fig. 4-4.

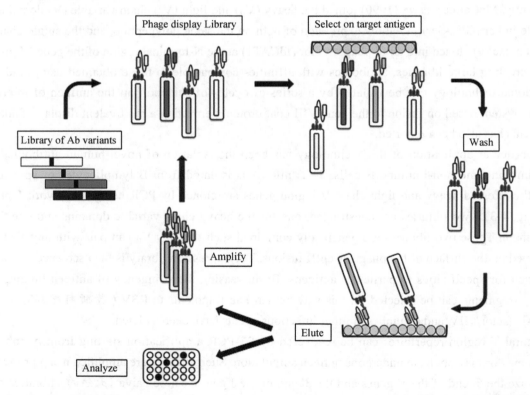

Fig. 4-4   Phage display selection cycle. Up to five rounds of selection over a specific target are performed; in each round, unreactive clones are removed, and reactive clones are amplified. Positive clones are successively isolated and identified by DNA sequencing.

At the end, specific antibodies for a given antigen are identified through an ELISA screening within

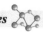

several random clones, and isolated genetic details are easily identified by DNA sequencing. At this point, the sequence can be subjected to downstream genetic engineering — antibody genes can be recovered simultaneously with selection and can be easily further engineered, for example by increasing their affinity to levels unobtainable in the immune system (through the generation of mutated antibodies secondary libraries), or by modulating their specificity and building full-length immunoglobulin with the desired effector functions (*e.g.*, by recloning into a full-length immunoglobulin scaffold).

Antibody libraries with varying size and sources are described, mainly comprising single-chain variable fragments (scFv) or Fab- based phage display libraries, which predominantly attempt to mirror the diversity of natural human antibody repertoires. However, for most therapeutic applications, the final antibody candidate favors a bivalent immunoglobulin G (IgG) format, due to its particular effector function, half-life, and avidity.

Selection of Phage Antibodies Using Biotinylated Antigen and Streptavidin-Paramagnetic Beads

An alternative to select antibodies bound to plastic plates is to select the antibodies in solution. This solves problems related to antigens that change conformation when directly coated onto solid surfaces. Furthermore, affinity selections are more straightforward with this method allowing a precise control of the interaction between the phage particle and the antigen that takes place in solution. The antigen is labeled by biotinylation (using kits that are sold by many companies) and incubated with the phage antibody library, after both have been appropriately blocked. Once interaction between the two has occurred the complex can be retrieved by using magnetic beads coated with streptavidin. Specificity is achieved by washing the beads several times. Phages are eluted from the beads with either acid or alkaline solution.

PCR Amplification and Fingerprinting of selected Clones

After positive clones have been identified, it is important to determine how many different antibodies have been selected.

A simple and fast method involves the use of PCR — heat to 95℃ for 10 min using the PCR-block, this is needed to break open the bacteria and release the template DNA — to amplify the scFv regions and then to digest the DNA samples with a frequently cutting restriction enzyme, such as *Bst*NI or *Hae*III. The digested DNA fragments are separated on an agarose gel and the various clones are characterized by their own DNA fragment patterns.

HuCAL®

The first version of the Human Combinatorial Antibody Library (HuCAL®) is a single-chain Fv-based phage display library (HuCAL®-scFv) with 2×10^9 members optimized for high-throughput generation and targeted engineering of human antibodies. 61% of the library genes code for functional scFv as judged by sequencing.

It is a fully synthetic antibody library, which is based on modular and expression-optimized consensus frameworks. Each of the V_H- and V_L-subfamilies frequently used in human immune responses is represented by a consensus framework resulting in a total of 49 different frameworks. These master genes were designed in such a way that unfavorable residues promoting protein aggregation were eliminated. Furthermore, unique restriction sites leading to modular composition of the genes were introduced. In HuCAL®-scFv, both the V_H- and V_L-CDR3 encoding regions of the 49 master genes were randomized by using trinucleotide mixtures. The modular design of HuCAL®, in contrast to PCR-derived recombinant antibody libraries, dramatically simplifies DNA rearrangements due to HuCAL®'s unique restriction sites not only flanking all important segments of the antibodies but also the various phage display and expression vector modules. This not only allows the rapid interconversion of HuCAL®-derived antibodies between different formats, such as scFv, Fab, multivalent miniantibodies and full-length immunoglobulins of different subclasses, but also simplifies any further improvement of HuCAL®-scFv and the addition of defined effector functions or tags to the antibodies for various purposes.

Construction of HuCAL®-immunoglobulin expression vectors

Heavy chain cloning. The multiple cloning site of pcDNA3.1+ (Invitrogen) was removed (*NheI/ApaI*), and a stuffer compatible with the restriction sites used for HuCAL®-design was inserted for the ligation of the leader sequences (*NheI/EcoRI*), V_H-domains (*EcoRI/BlpI*) and the immunoglobulin constant regions (*BlpI/ApaI*). The leader sequence was equipped with a Kozak sequence. The constant regions of human IgG_1, IgG_4 and serum IgA_1 were made synthetically by dissecting the sequences into overlapping oligonucleotides with lengths of about 70 bases. Silent mutations were introduced to remove restriction sites non-compatible with the HuCAL®-design. The oligonucleotides were spliced by overlap extension-PCR.

Light chain cloning. The multiple cloning site of pcDNA3.1/Zeo+ (Invitrogen) was replaced by two different stuffers. The K-stuffer provided restriction sites for the insertion of a K-leader (*NheI/EcoRV*), HuCAL®-scFv VK-domains (*EcoRV/BsiWI*) and the K-chain constant region (*BsiWI/ApaI*). The corresponding restriction sites in the λ-stuffer were *NheI/EcoRV* (λ-leader), *EcoRV/HpaI* (Vλ-domains) and *HpaI/ApaI* (λ-chain constant region). The K-leader as well as the λ-leader were both equipped with Kozak sequences. The constant regions of the human K- and λ-chain were assembled by overlap extension-PCR as described above.

Conversion of HuCAL®-scFv antibodies into other formats. Taking advantage of the modular design of HuCAL®, the antibody formats such as miniantibodies, human Fab, human IgG could generally be constructed within a few days, and specific, fully human antibodies for certain antigens were able to be isolated.

Since HuCAL®-scFv proved well suited for selecting antibodies, and since the antibodies are very efficiently expressed in *E. coli*, protocols for the high-throughput automated panning (AutoPan®) and screening (AutoScreen®) were developed. These protocols, optimized for 96- and 384-well compatible pipetting, dispensing and washing stations, allow rapid processing of packages of antigens in batches within a few weeks. In a first run, HuCAL®-scFv was successfully used to enrich and screen in parallel scFv antibodies against 30 antigens of different composition (haptens, peptides, proteins, glycoproteins).

The unique modular design of HuCAL® enables, if necessary, the directed affinity-maturation of HuCAL® antibodies by replacing the originally selected CDRs with different, high-quality and pre-prepared CDR cassette libraries. By this method, all framework residues of the antibody are preserved, which might be important for therapeutic applications due to immunogenicity concerns. The affinity maturation of a HuCAL® antibody fragment resulted in an about 100-fold improved monovalent K_D after optimization of two CDRs.

It is well known that the choice of antibody format strongly influences the outcome of pre-clinical and clinical assays. For instance, (i) the absence of the Fc-portion in scFv, Fab and di- or tetrameric miniantibodies lowers the background binding caused by Fc-receptor bearing cells; (ii) low molecular weight antibody fragments penetrate tissues more efficiently than the larger immunoglobulins; (iii) body clearance rates of unmodified scFv and Fab are much higher than for full-length immunoglobulins; (iv) scFv/Fab and miniantibodies or immunoglobulins display different valencies and, hence, different binding kinetics; and (v) each immunoglobulin subclass exerts a different biological response, for example, IgG_1 usually leads to a depletion of targeted cells, whereas IgG_4 mainly coats (and blocks) cells without depletion. The modular design of HuCAL® permits rapid and parallel access to and analysis of all antibody formats.

The immediate availability of these formats enables the early pre-selection of antibodies that are best suited for further evaluation. The modularity of the HuCAL®-genes also facilitates the construction of an infinite range of antibody fusion proteins such as tagging with immunotoxins, the green fluorescent protein or enzymes like alkaline phosphatase, which allows rapid and sensitive antibody validation.

In short, besides being a rich source of human therapeutic antibodies, the automated high-throughput antibody generation makes HuCAL®-scFv a valuable tool for functional genomics. The wealth of data collected about all antibody-antigen pairs in combination with the unique modular design of the HuCAL®-antibody genes enables the rapid and targeted engineering of further improved HuCAL®-versions. HuCAL®'s modularity allows the development of human antibodies by optimization procedures well known from classical low molecular weight drug development.

HuCAL®-EST

A generally applicable method, designated HuCAL®-EST had been developed for the high-throughput generation of antibodies to EST-encoded polypeptides.

This method had been developed for the high-level expression of expressed sequence tags (ESTs) as inclusion bodies in *Escherichia coli* by C-terminal fusion to the N1-domain of g3p of filamentous phage M13. The soluble fusion protein was obtained by an efficient refolding procedure. Frisch *et al*. (2003) had applied such protein preparations to the selection of human antibody fragments from specially detect, *e.g.*, in immunohistochemistry, the maternal full-length protein corresponding to the protein fragment. This expression technology, in combination with the automated HuCAL® antibody generation (AutoCAL™), had proven to be useful for the rapid, high-throughput generation of high-quality human antibodies against EST-encoded protein fragments for target research. Antibodies against dozens of EST-encoded polypeptides, derived mainly from target identification programs, had been generated at that time. Due to the fully human composition of these antibodies, they may immediately serve as lead candidates for drug development.

The main advantages of this approach comprise (i) high-throughput, (ii) delivery of antibodies recognizing the maternal protein, (iii) high numbers of IHC-grade antibodies and (iv) good overall success rates.

AmpIYFst

Screening for specific target binding ("hits") can be conveniently performed in high throughput by using soluble Fab molecules expressed in *E. coli*. However, for comprehensive functional testing and in-depth biophysical characterization of the antibody, especially when the desired final format is an IgG, reformatting of identified Fab hits into IgG, followed by IgG expression and purification, becomes indispensable.

Tiller *et al*. (2014) developed the fully synthetic human Fab phage display antibody library Ylanthia®, which covers a broad range of diverse CDR structures with biophysically optimal V_H/V_L pairings. Within iterative selection rounds (referred to "panning"), in which the Fab is displayed at the surface of the phage and presented to the antigen of interest ("target"), target-specific Fab-displaying phage are getting enriched.

Ylanthia comprises three major vector systems, each with different features. The display phagemid vector pYPdis10 enables the Fab to be presented at the surface of the phage covalently linked via a cysteine disulfide bridge to the phage coat protein pIII. The bacterial expression vector, pYBex10, is required for Fab expression and screening of crude *E. coli* lysates and is complemented by a mammalian expression vector, pYMex10, for full-length IgG production. While the subcloning of Ig heavy and light chain sequences from pYPdis10 into the bacterial expression vector pYBex10 system is a straightforward one-step cloning procedure (Fig. 4-5A), the transfer of the Fab antibody sequences into the mammalian pYMex10 vector requires in standard protocols two cloning steps. This is due to the essential exchange of the prokaryotic expression cassette (present in pYPdis10 and pYBex10) with a cassette containing a cytomegalovirus (CMV，巨细胞病毒) promotor and polyA sequence region suited for mammalian expression, in addition to the transfer of the antibody variable region segments from the bacterial to the mammalian vector system (Fig. 4-5B).

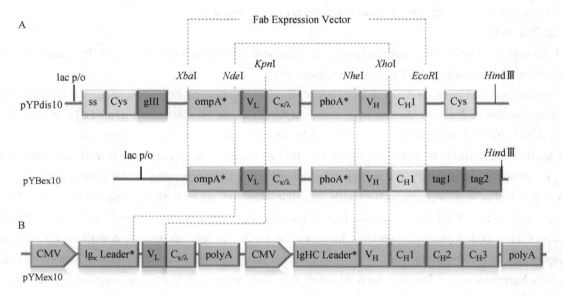

Fig. 4-5 A. Modular design and compatible restriction sites allow easy subcloning between pYPdis10 Fab display and pYBex10 Fab bacterial expression vectors via *Xba*I and *Eco*RI. B. Conversion between Fab and full-length IgG format is accomplished by transferring the antibody sequence via *Nde*I and *Xhd*I, followed by the introduction of a mammalian expression cassette with a polyA and a CMV-driven promotor sequence via *Kpn*I and *Nhe*I. *ompA**, *phoA** are modified leader sequences. V_L and V_H indicate the variable regions, Cκ/λ and C_H1, C_H2. C_H3 depict the constant region domains of the antibody's light and heavy chain, respectively. Cys: cysteine, *lac* p/o: lac promoter/operator sequence, gIII: gene III encoding for phage coat protein pIII. Schematic distances and sizes are not to scale.

The Ylanthia Vector System

Phage Fab Display Vector pYPdis10. In the tri-cistronic phagemid Fab display vector pYPdis10 the variable region (V) light and heavy chain sequences of the Fab are preceded by modified prokaryotic *ompA** and *phoA** leader sequences, respectively. Upstream of the V region sequence is the gIII sequence encoding for the phage coat protein pIII. N-terminally (for pIII) and C-terminally (for Fd chain)

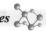

introduced cysteine residues are the basis for the formation of disulfide-linked Fd-pIII complexes during phage assembly and the subsequent incorporation of the complete Fab-pIII complex into the phage particle.

Bacterial Fab Expression Vector pYBex10. In the bacterial Fab expression vector pYBex10, the variable light and heavy chain sequences of the Fab are preceded by modified prokaryotic *ompA** and *phoA** leader sequences, respectively. Upstream of the V region is an isopropyl β-D-thiogalactopyranoside (IPTG) and lactose inducible promotor. The sequence section between the *Kpn*I and *Nhe*I restriction sites consists of the light chain constant region sequence, and the modified *phoA** leader sequence that precedes the V region of the heavy chain (Fig. 4-6).

Mammalian IgG Expression Vector: pYMex10. In the mammalian IgG expression vector pYMex10, the V region light and heavy chain sequences of the IgG are encoded on one plasmid (Fig. 4-7). They are preceded by the natural V_{kappa} leader and a consensus V_H leader sequence, respectively. Each chain is translated together with its N-terminal leader sequence from a separate transcript. Transcription is driven by two cytomegalovirus (CMV) promotor sites. The acceptor vector backbone contains the constant region of the heavy chain, the polyA sequence of human growth hormone (hGH), the Amp^r resistance gene, and a CMV promotor site (Fig. 4-8A). The eukaryotic expression cassette between *Kpn*I and *Nhe*I is comprised of the constant light chain region, a Simian-Virus (SV40) (for pYMin_Ig$_{kappa}$) (pYMin, pYMin mammalian expression cassettes) or an hGH (for pYMin_Ig$_{lambda}$) polyA region, one CMV promotor site, and the leader sequence for the heavy chain (Fig. 4-8B).

Sterner *et al*. (2017) present an optimized subcloning method, termed **AmpIYFast**, for the fast and convenient conversion of phage-displayed monovalent Fab fragments into full-length IgG or immunoglobulins of any other isotype.

Classical cloning methods to switch antibody formats from Fab to IgG utilize established standard technologies based on size-dependent electrophoretic separation methods. These usually require high amounts of both, donor and acceptor vector DNA for restriction digest and subsequent DNA purification

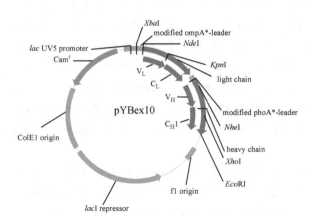

Fig. 4-6   Schematic map of the pYBex10 bacterial Fab expression vector. The pYBex10 plasmid carries a chloramphenicol resistance gene (cam^r) and an origin for double-stranded (ColE1 *ori*) DNA replication. *Xba*I, *Nde*I, *Kpn*I, *Nhe*I, *Xho*I, and *Eco*RI indicate conserved restriction sites for cloning or exchange of domains. *ompA** and *phoA** are modified leader sequences.

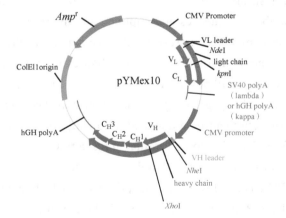

Fig. 4-7   Schematic map of the pYMex10 mammalian IgG expression vector. The pYMex10 plasmid carries an ampicillin resistance gene (amp^r) and an origin for double-stranded (ColE1 *ori*) DNA replication. *Nde*I, *Kpn*I, *Nhe*I, and *Xho*I indicate conserved restriction sites for cloning or exchange of domains.

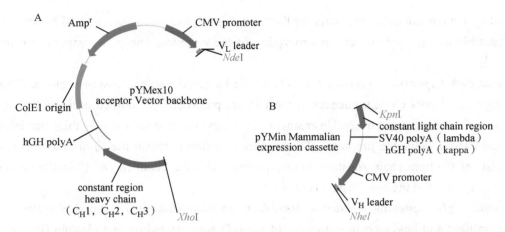

Fig. 4-8   A. The pYMex10 acceptor vector backbone and; B. pYMin mammalian expression cassette insert.

steps via laborious preparative agarose gel electrophoresis and gel extraction. Especially, the preparative gel electrophoresis procedure is very inconvenient and time consuming when dealing with high numbers of samples. Furthermore, purification of DNA from agarose gels is very often accompanied by significant loss of DNA yields, making an upscaling of the input DNA material absolutely inevitable.

By using biotinylated primers, unique mammalian expression vectors, and multi-well plates, AmpIYFst circumvents these downsides. AmpIYFast combines the rapid amplification, degestion, and ligation of recombinant Ig heavy and light chain sequences in an easy-to-operate high-throughput manner, and represents a rapid method for convenient and efficient parallel cloning of many antibody V region encoding donor DNA inserts (*e.g.*, derived from pYP-dis10, pYBex10) into an acceptor vector backbone (*e.g.*, from the pYMex10 vector series). The protocol described above concerning the Ylanthia® vector system can easily be adapted, if modified accordingly by appropriate primer design, to any other vector system. The AmpIYFast procedure is subdivided into two parts. Each part comprises a PCR applying one biotinylated and one unmodified primer, a purification step with streptavidin-coupled beads, a restriction digest, and a ligation step. In the first part of AmpIYFast, the "Fab vector backbone" and variable antibody sequences are amplified and the bacterial expression cassette is replaced by a cassette suitable for mammalian expression. The second part of the method includes the transfer of the antibody sequence in conjunction with the mammalian expression cassette to the acceptor vector backbone which defines the final antibody format. By the use of biotinylated primers and streptavidin-coupled megnetic beads, the need for agarose gel purification steps becomes obsolete. Furthermore, most steps of the AmpIYFast procedure can be automated, allowing a fast reformatting of hundreds of different antibody sequences from the Fab into IgG format in just a few days.

In the first part of AmpIYFast. "Fab vector" backbone and antibody sequences are amplified by PCR (PCR-I) employing specific primers, of which one is biotinylated. The resulting biotinylated PCR product (PCR-Product-I) is subsequently bound to magnetic streptavidin beads facilitating its purification after amplification and the isolation of the desired DNA fragment after subsequent sequential restriction digests without the need of conventional gel electrophoresis and gel extraction. Thereafter, a pre-prepared "ready to use" DNA fragment (pYMin Mammalian Expression Cassette) suitable for mammalian expression is inserted by ligation via the respective restriction sites (Fig. 4-9).

The second part of AmpIYFast includes the transfer of DNA fragment comprising the antibody

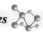
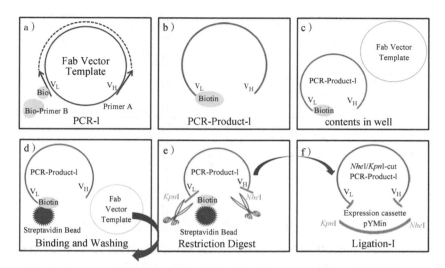

Fig. 4-9 Schematic outline of AmplYFast PART 1. (a) The antibody and "Fab vector" backbone sequences are getting amplified by PCR employing specific primers, of which one is biotinylated. The resulting biotinylated PCR product (PCR-Product-I) (b, c) is subsequently bound to magnetic streptavidin beads (d) facilitating its purification after amplification and restriction digest (e) without the need of conventional gel electrophoresis. Thereafter, the "ready to use" (pYMin) cassette suitable for mammalian expression is inserted by ligation via the respective restriction sites (Ligation-Product-I) (f).

sequence in connection with the mammalian expression cassette ("insert") (PCR-Product-II) to the acceptor vector backbone that defines the final antibody format. Therefore, the respective DNA fragment is amplified in a second PCR reaction, using the ligation product (Ligation-Product-I) as template DNA (PCR-II). The resulting biotinylated PCR product (PCR-Product-II) is subsequently bound to magnetic streptavidin coupled beads facilitating its purification and the isolation of the desired DNA fragment after subsequent sequential restriction digests without the need of conventional gel electrophoresis and gel extraction. Subsequently, the relevant digested DNA fragment is ligated into a "ready to use" mammalian acceptor vector backbone to obtain the final vector construct (IgG vector construct) (Fig. 4-10).

Thus, AmplYFast improves quality and efficiency in DNA cloning and significantly minimizes timelines for antibody lead identification.

pDong3

The previously reported phage display systems mainly display scFv and Fab. ScFv is easy to synthesize in bacteria and has good tolerance to bacteria, but its stability is poor and easy to aggregate. Compared to scFv, Fab is more stable and has more expression products in bacteria, but its structure is different from that of natural antibodies, and monovalent binding lowers its affinity relative to that of full-length antibodies.

Full-length antibodies are a natural form in organisms. Compared to scFv and Fab that are monovalent, the full-length antibody with two antigen-binding sites has high stability and a higher affinity hence activity. For the development of antibody pharmaceuticals, scFv or Fab needs to be transferred to IgG for further evaluation in some cases. A full-length antibody display system that can express IgG will help save developing time and down the cost. Rhiel *et al.* (2014) developed a full-length display system with yeast cells through an Fc-binding domain and could isolate one clone from 10^6 yeast cells.

Zhang *et al.* (2021) constructed a new phage display system that can display full-length IgG antibodies on M13 phage. They constructed a vector that can be directly used for both full-length antibody phage

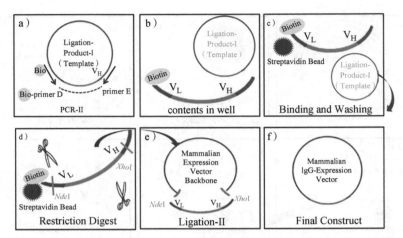

Fig. 4-10　Schematic outline of AmpIYFast PART 2. The second part of AmpIYFast includes the transfer of the antibody sequence in connection with the mammalian expression cassette ("insert") to the acceptor vector backbone which defines the final antibody format. First, the insert is amplified by PCR utilizing one biotinylated and one unmodified primer (a) and the Ligation-Product-I as templated DNA (PCR-Product-II). The biotinylated PCR-Product-II, comprising the variable antibody sequences of the individual starting clones and the constant sequences originating from the "ready to use" pYMin expression cassette (b), is captured on magnetic streptavidin beads (c) for convenient purification after digest (d) with the respective restriction enzymes. (e) Subsequently, the digested PCR-Product-II is ligated into the "ready to use" acceptor vector backbone to obtain the final vector construct(f).

display and antibody expression, which will provide an efficient tool for antibody pharmaceutical research and development.

Design and construction of vector pDong3

In Zhang's study, a phage display system pDong3 was constructed to successfully display the full-length antibody on the surface of the M13 phage, and the binding activity of the full-length antibody to the antigen was confirmed by ELISA. They displayed the full-length antibody on protein III of the M13 phage (Fig. 4-11B).

Genes encoding the heavy chain and light chain of nivolumab (Niv) were designed for *E. coli* expression and synthesized. Polymerase chain reaction (PCR) was carried out to amplify the genes for the heavy chain and for the light chain. After purification, the heavy chain gene was digested with *Nco*I and *Eag*I. It was recovered after separation on a 1% agarose gel. The Recovered DNA was ligated with *Nco*I/*Eag*I-digested pDong1/Fab. The ligation mixture was used to transform XL10-Gold competent cells and cultivated overnight. Colony PCR was carried out to screen a colony harboring a plasmid containing the Niv heavy chain gene. The plasmid containing the heavy chain gene was digested with *Sal*I/*Asc*I, ligated with the *Sal*I/*Asc*I-digested light chain gene, and screened with colony PCR. Plasmids containing the heavy and light chain genes of Niv were designated as pDong3-Niv. The schemes for vector construction are shown in Fig. 4-11A.

Considering the potential use of the system for screening human antibodies, the human C_H1-C_H2-C_H3 and kappa chain were employed. The vector contains open reading frames (ORFs) encoding the heavy and light chains of the antibody. *Nco*I/*Xho*I restriction enzyme sites were used to clone the variable region of the antibody heavy chain into the heavy chain ORF, and *Sal*I/*Not*I sites were used to clone the light chain variable region. *Sna*BI and *Sbf*I restriction enzyme sites were designed between the cloning sites of heavy and light chains, respectively, to increase the cloning efficiency. Two transglutaminase terminators

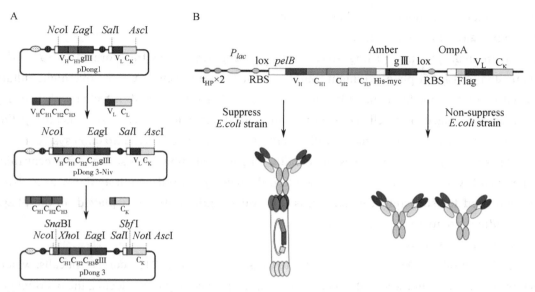

Fig. 4-11 (A) The construction and (B) the functions of the pDong3 vector. V_H: variable region of the antibody heavy chain; C_H1, 2, and 3: constant regions 1, 2, and 3 of the antibody heavy chain; V_L: variable region of the antibody light chain; Cκ: kappa chain of the antibody; t_{HP}: transglutaminase terminators; P_{lac}: lac promoter; RBS: ribosome binding site.

were set upstream of the *lac* promoter gene to prevent undesirable transcription leakage under non-induced conditions. His-myc and FLAG tags were fused to the heavy and light chains, respectively, for the detection and purification of the expressed antibody.

To construct a general vector for full-length antibody phage display, a DNA cassette containing a DNA spacer and C_H1-C_H2-C_H3 gene was amplified with corresponding primers and digested with *Nco*I and *Eag*I. Another DNA cassette containing a spacer and kappa chain was amplified by PCR using the corresponding primers and cloned into pDong3-IgG with enzymes *Sal*I and *Asc*I. The resulting plasmid was designated as pDong3.

There are two recombinant enzyme recognition sites, loxp2272 and loxp511, in the upstream and downstream regions of V_H-C_H1-C_H2-C_H3-gⅢ. The diversity of the phage library can be increased by using the system to construct a phage library with *E. coli* expressing Cre recombinant enzyme. An amber codon is set between the V_H-C_H1-C_H2-C_H3 and pⅢ genes to control the fusion state of the heavy chain and pⅢ by changing the host phenotype. Suppressive *E. coli* strains, such as TG-1, will display full-length antibodies on phages, whereas non-suppression strains, such as HB2151, secrete full-length antibodies into the culture medium, which makes the system convenient for obtaining soluble full-length antibodies.

Application scenarios of pDong3

Genes coding for the V_H and V_L of other monoclonal antibodies of interest were amplified. The PCR products were recovered after electrophoresis separation. Restriction endonucleases *Nco*I/*Xho*I/*Sna*BI and *Sal*I/*Not*I/*Sbf*I were used to treat the target fragments and pDong3, which were ligated with Ligation high Ver.2 (Toyobo Biological). The ligation mixture was used to transform *E. coli* XL10-Gold competent cells, which were evenly cultivated on LBAG plates overnight. PCR was carried out to screen positive clones which were further cultivated for plasmid extraction. Plasmids with accurate sequences — pDong3-mAbs, and/or the plasmid-containing bacteria, were properly kept, waiting for downstream process operation for monoclonal antibody production.

Full-length antibody phage display

The recombinant plasmid, pDong3-Niv or other pDong3-mAb was transformed into *E. coli* TG-1 and cultivated on LBAG plate overnight. Single colonies were selected, and the overnight culture was inoculated in a liquid medium and cultivated until A_{600} of 0.4 was reached. Infected with helper phage KM13, then centrifuged. The cell sediment was suspended and cultured again. After centrifugation, the supernatant was recovered and extracted with PEG/NaCl aqueous two-phase extraction system (20% PEG 6000/2.5M NaCl). The precipitate was dissolved with phosphated-buffered saline. After centrifugation, the supernatant was collected as a phage solution displaying the full-length antibody (*e.g.*, Niv-IgG-phage) and used for subsequent experiments. The full-length antibody displayed on the phage had obvious binding activity to its corresponding antigen.

Full-length IgG expression

pDong3-Niv or other pDong3-mAb was used to transform *E. coli* HB2151 competent cells, which are a non-suppression strain, and were cultivated overnight. A single colony was selected, the overnight culture was inoculated and cultivated in LBA liquid medium (1% V/V) and induced with IPTG when A_{600} of 0.5 was reached. The bacterial suspension was harvested the next day. The supernatant was collected, and the soluble full-length antibody was purified using a Protein A MagBeads according to the manufacturer's protocol (GenScript Biotechnology Co., Ltd.). The system can be used to produce functional full-length antibodies — the secreted IgGs have antigen-specificity and binding activity similar to those of the positive controls.

The pDong3 system uses two pⅢ protein molecules for antibody display, which makes phage displaying more efficient. Meanwhile it uses only one promoter, which is a single mRNA with the heavy chain placed in front of the light chain — this design balances the ratio of heavy and light chains, thereby ensuring a greater antibody expression yield. It can be used for antibody library panning.

Limitation

There are no carbohydrate chains attached to the antibodies expressed in *E. coli*, which are different from the antibodies produced in eukaryotes, though Zhang's results did not show any impact on the antigen-binding characteristics. The pDong3 system may be further engineered using those *E. coli* strains to prepare full-length antibodies with glycosylation to reacquire their original properties.

The pDong3 system is the first phage display system to display full-length antibodies and will provide theoretical and technical guidance for the future development of antibody pharmaceuticals.

Prospect

Antibody phage display technology plays an important role in the development of monoclonal antibodies, humanization, and affinity evolution of antibodies. Adalimumab, the first fully human antibody approved by the U.S. Food and Drug Administration for the treatment of rheumatoid arthritis and ankylosing spondylitis, was prepared by phage display technology. Since then, many specific neutralizing antibodies have been prepared using phage display technology, such as those against the influenza virus, snake venom, and Ebola virus. The phage display technique would still be one of the most attractive options for the production of fully human antibody in the near future.

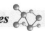

4.4.2   Transgenic and trans-chromosomic mouse-derived human antibodies（转基因、转染色体小鼠法制备全人源抗体）

More sophisticated technologies such as humanization and phage display use tools of molecular biology and prokaryotic genetics to re-engineer antibodies to resemble their human counterparts. Humanization technology starts with a murine antibody with the desired characteristics and then changes, from a mouse-like to human-like usage, those amino acids thought to be non-critical to antigen recognition. Typically, this technology requires individual tailoring for each antibody, including extensive molecular modeling and manipulation of the DNA encoding the mAb. Even then, amino acid changes that would be predicted to have little effect on the antibody could unexpectedly abrogate（废除）antibody function. Finally, humanization leaves murine amino acids in the antibody, allowing the possibility of a HAMA response. In phage display technology, combinatorial libraries of human naive variable regions displayed on the surface of bacteriophage are used to develop antigen-specific antibodies. However, this technology typically requires successive rounds of *in vitro* mutagenesis, V gene shuffling and/or panning to produce antibodies with sub-nanomolar affinity. The synthesis of a complete mAb from phage display technology requires that the DNA encoding the *in vitro* affinity-matured V regions be further manipulated by functionally linking them to DNA encoding constant regions in a suitable expression vector, expressing the construct in a tissue culture system, and finally confirming that the synthetic human mAb does indeed have the desired function.

An alternative strategy for producing human mAbs is to alter the mouse humoral（体液的）immune system so that it will produce fully human antibodies, obviating the need for re-engineering of the actual antibodies themselves and leaving intact the powerful natural mechanisms for class switching and affinity maturation. This strategy would require considerable effort up front（预先）to genetically engineer the mouse, but the resulting technology would be user friendly, enabling the end-user to produce high-affinity human antibodies against human antigens using only standard hybridoma procedures. The **Humab-Mouse** and **XenoMouse** technologies represent the success of this vision（憧憬）.

HumAb-Mouse™

During 1991-1997, a transgenic mouse platform called HumAb-Mouse had been set up and developed. Double- transgenic/double-deletion mice are constructed. Such mice are homozygous for each of two different targeted deletions: a deletion of the endogenous heavy-chain J gene segments (J_HD mutation), that prevents VDJ rearrangement and expression of mouse IgM, and a deletion of the endogenous κ-light-chain J and C gene segments (JCκD mutation), that prevents VJ rearrangement and expression of mouse Igκ. In addition, the mice are either hemizygous（半合子的）or homozygous for the presence of each of two different types of transgene: a germline configuration, human, heavy-chain, minilocus transgene, and a germline configuration, human, κ-light-chain transgene.

The heavy-chain minilocus in each of the mice is the HC2 transgene. HC2 includes 4 V_H gene segments, 16 D segments, all 6 J_H segments, Cμ, and Cγ1 (human γ1 constant regions is expressed via intratransgene class switching).

The light chain transgene is derived in part from a yeast artificial chromosome clone that includes nearly half of the germline human Vκ region. Mice with two different light-chain miniloci were used. The KCo4 light-chain transgene includes 4 Vκ gene segments, all 5 Jκ segments, and Cκ. The second light-chain transgene, KCo5 includes the entire KCo4 minilocus, together with a 450 kb YAC (y17) that includes sequences spanning most, if not all, of the distal portion of the human Vκ region.

10 distinct Vκ genes have been identified within YAC y17. These 10 Vκ genes span a 365-kb region of the human κ locus, which encompasses most of the 390-kb distal Vκ cluster. The distal cluster potentially encodes 23 functional Vκ segments and, because it represents an inverted repeat of a large fraction of the proximal Vκ cluster, encodes gene segments that are substantially homologous to many of the gene segments encoded by the rest of the Vκ locus. Therefore, this single YAC clone is likely to include a significant fraction of the primary V gene diversity encoded by the human κ locus.

Expression of at least four YAC-derived and two plasmid-clone-derived Vκ segments had been detected. The four YAC-derived expressed segments span approximately 200 kb of genomic DNA, from VκA10 to VκL24, thus demonstrating that a significant fraction of the introduced YAC has been incorporated into the genome and is expressed.

Multiple high-avidity human sequence lgGκ Mabs directed against a human antigen have been generated using this novel strain of human immunoglobulin transgenic mice, *e.g.*, human IgGκ Mabs that are specific for the human T-cell marker CD4 have been isolated, with high binding avidities, and immunosuppressive *in vitro*.

The human Mab-secreting hybridomas display properties similar to those of wild-type mice including stability, growth, and secretion levels. Since Mabs with four distinct specificities were derived from a single transgenic mouse, an extensive diversity in the primary repertoire encoded by the transgenes was demonstrated. Hence these human immunoglobulin transgenic mice provide a method of obtaining human monoclonal antibodies (Mabs) using conventional hybridoma technology.

XenoMouse

XenoMouse construction for the facile generation of therapeutic human monoclonal antibodies

XenoMouse strains are genetically engineered mice in which the murine IgH and Igκ loci have been functionally replaced by their human Ig counterparts on yeast artificial chromosome (YAC) transgenes. These human Ig transgenes carry the majority of the human variable repertoire and can undergo class switching from IgM to IgG isotypes. The large and complex human V repertoires on the YAC transgenes support development of a large B cell population and the formation of a broad and diverse primary immune repertoire. The human genes are compatible with mouse enzymes mediating class switching from IgM to IgG as well as somatic hypermutation and affinity maturation. The immune system of the XenoMouse strains recognizes administered human antigens as foreign, with a concomitant strong human humoral immune response. The use of XenoMouse mice in conjunction with well established hybridoma procedures reproducibly（可再生产地）results in IgG mAbs with sub-nanomolar affinities for human antigens and with suitability for repeated administration to humans.

Engineering of mice to produce fully human IgM and IgG

Recapitulation（重演，再现）of a robust human humoral immune response in mice required two types of major genetic modifications of the mouse genome (Fig. 4-12). Mouse embryonic stem cells（ES cells，胚胎干细胞）were used as the vehicle for altering the mouse genome because of their proven utility for introducing precise mutations, followed by efficient transmission into the germline. The first modification, ablation of the ability of the mouse to produce murine Ig, was achieved through inactivation of the endogenous murine IgH and Igκ loci using well-defined techniques of homologous recombination. Deletion of the murine J_H region inactivated the IgH locus, and deletion of the mouse Cκ region inactivated the mouse Igκ locus. Successive crosses of $mJ_H^{-/+}$ mice to $mCκ^{-/+}$ mice H and their resulting progeny yielded double inactivated $mJ_H^{-/-}$; $mCκ^{-/-}$ (DI) strains, a genetic background with all of the *trans*-acting factors regulating rearrangement and expression of Ig genes intact and suitable for introduction of the human Ig transgenes.

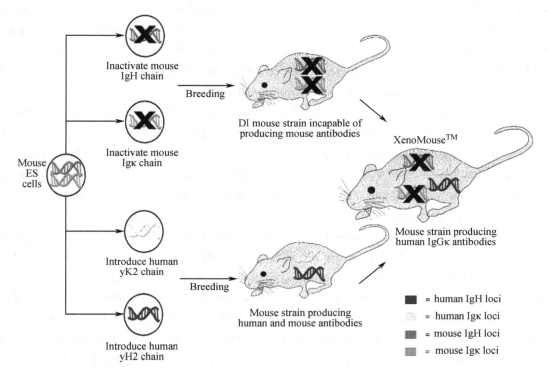

Fig. 4-12   Schematic for the genetic engineering of XenoMouse mice to produce fully human antibodies in the absence of mouse antibodies. The endogenous murine IgH and Ig κ genes were inactivated separately using homologous recombination in mouse embryonic stem cells. Germline transmission of the mutated loci and subsequent interbreeding（异种交配，使杂交）and backcrossing（回交）produced the DI mouse strain, which is homozygous（纯合子的）for the inactivated IgH and Ig κ loci and is incapable of generating murine antibodies (top path). The human IgH and Ig κ loci contained on the yH2 and yK2 YACs were integrated intact into the ES cell genome, and used to generate transgenic mice. The progeny of the subsequent interbreeding of the yH2 and yK2 transgenic mice produced human and mouse antibodies (bottom path). The yH2; yK2 mice were bred to the DI mice and subsequently backcrossed to produce XenoMouse strains, mouse strains with four genetic alterations, integration of intact yH2 and yK2 into the genome, and homozygous for the inactivated alleles of the murine IgH and Ig κ loci. XenoMouse animals, with functional human IgH and Ig κ loci but non-functional mouse IgH and Ig κ loci, produce fully human IgH κ antibodies without contaminating murine IgH κ antibodies.

The second genetic modification made to the mouse genome was the insertion of the human Ig loci cloned on YACS. Unrearranged human immunoglobulin loci are very large (IgH, 1.5 Mb; Igk, 2 Mb; Igl, 1 Mb) and possess around a hundred gene segments including the V, (D), J and constant regions, as well as interspersed *cis*-regulatory elements that act in a concert to encode and control the expression of the huge diversity of the humoral immune response. The transfer of the bulk of this rich potential of the human antibody response to mice required an ability to clone and introduce very large portions of the human Ig loci in their germline configuration（布局，排列，配置）.

Two technological advances potentiated（使成为可能）the introduction of the majority of the human IgH and Igκ loci into mice. First, YAC technology allowed the cloning and facile（易做到的）manipulation of megabase-size, germline-configured fragments of DNA in yeast. Second, development of yeast spheroplast-ES cell fusion technology enabled the efficient introduction and integration of intact and unrearranged mega-based sized YACs into the mouse genome and germline.

Reconstruction of human heavy and κ light chain loci on YACs

YACs which span large portions of megabase-sized loci containing the desired elements of human heavy and κ light chain immunoglobulin genes were combined into single YACs containing large contiguous fragments of the human heavy and kappa (κ) light chain immunoglobulin loci in nearly germline configuration. This stepwise YAC recombination scheme utilized the high frequency of meiotic-induced homologous recombination in yeast and the ability to select the desired recombinants by the yeast markers present on the vector arms of the recombined TACs.

Four YACs, 1H (240 kb), 17H (280 kb), 3H (290 kb) and 4H (345 kb), which span 860 out of the 1 000 kb of the human heavy chain variable region on chromosome 14q were used to reconstruct the locus (Fig. 4-13A). 1H, the YAC introduced into first generation xenomouse, is comprised of the human C_δ, C_μ, J_H, and D_H regions and the first five V_H genes in germline configuration. The other three YACs cover the V_H region from $V_H 2\sim5$ to $V_H 3\sim65$, thus contributing approximately 61 additional V_H genes. Each of the four YACs contained overlapping portions of the human IgH locus, and were thus used to recombine with each other in yeast by a stepwise recombination strategy to generate 970-kb recombinant YAC (Fig. 4-13A). Then the YAC acentric (无着丝粒的) arm was targeted with a vector bearing the complete human γ2 constant region, mouse 3′ enhancer and the neomycin gene, to yield the final 1,020-kb heavy chain YAC, yH2. As part of the recombination scheme, a hypoxanthine phosphoribosyltransferase (HPRT) selectable marker was retrofitted (改进, 改装) into this YAC at the 5′-end of the yH2 core. This YAC contained 80% of the human variable region with approximately 66 V_H genes, all 23 unique D_H regions, all six J_H regions, and two constant regions C_μ and C_δ, all in germline configuration. Finally, a DNA cassette containing a human constant region Cγ gene with the control elements for Ig class switching and the murine 3′ enhancer was appended downstream of the Cδ gene using gene targeting in yeast. Three different versions of this cassette generated three different YACs, differing in that they contain either Cγ1, Cγ2, or Cγ4 constant regions.

A similar stepwise recombination strategy was applied for reconstruction of the human κ chain locus from the three YACs designated 1K, 2K and 3K. 1K, a 180-kb YAC introduced into the first generation xenomouse, contained the κ deleting element, (Kde), the κ 3′ and intronic enhancers, C_K, J_K, and the three Vκ genes on the B cluster. 2K (480 kb), and 3K (380 kb) together encompass most of the κ chain proximal variable region (the κ distal region largely duplicates the proximal region and the proximal Vκ genes are the ones most commonly used in humans) on chromosome 2p, with an approximate 100-kb deletion spanning the L5~L13 region (Fig. 4-13B). Through the homologous recombination of all three YACs, an 800-kb recombinant YAC, yK, was generated, with 32 Vκ genes in germline configuration except for the described deletion in the Lp region (Fig. 4-13B). yK2 centric and acentric arms contained the HPRT selectable marker (on the 5′ YAC arm) and neomycin selectable markers, respectively. Thus, the Vκ genes represented on yK2 capture 80% of the Vκ repertoire commonly used in humans. In addition to its Vκ gene segments, yK2 contains the entire Jκ region, Cκ, the Kde, and the Igκ intronic and 3′ enhancers, all in germline configuration, plus an inserted HPRT selectable marker on the 5′ YAC arm.

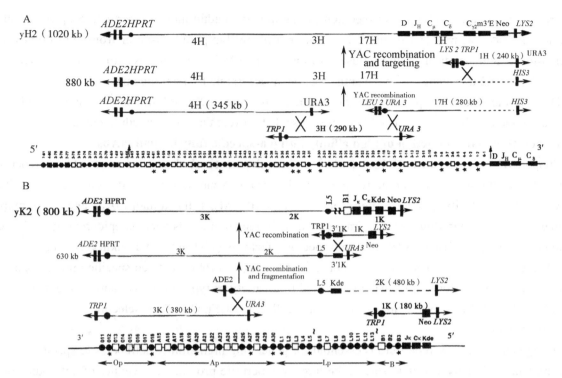

Fig. 4-13　Schematic representation of reconstructed, human heavy chain (A) and κ chain (B) loci YACs introduced into xenomouse II strains. YACs spanning the human heavy chain (1H, 17H, 3H, and 4H) and the human κ chain proximal (1K, 2K and 3K) loci were cloned from human-YAC libraries. The locations of the different YACs with respect to the human Ig loci, their sizes, and non-Ig sequences are indicated (not shown to scale). The YACs were recombined in yeast in a two-step procedure to reconstruct the human heavy and κ light chain YACs, yH2 (further retrofitted with human γ2 sequences) and yK2, respectively. The YAC vector elements: telomere (▶), centromere (●), mammalian (*HPRT*, neo) and yeast (*TRP*1, *ADE*2, *LYS*2, *LEU*2, *URA*3, *HIS*3) selectable markers on the YAC vector arms are indicated. VH segments are classified as genes with open reading frames (●), pseudogenes (□), and non-rearranged genes with the open reading frames that can be also classified as pseudogenes(gray circle). Vκ segments are classified as genes with the open reading frames (●) and pseudogenes (□). The V genes to be utilized by xenomouse II are marked (*). The VH gene region contained on yH2 is marked by arrows.

　　Fusion of yeast spheroplasts containing yH2 or yK2 with the ES cells lacking mouse HPRT function, E14.TG3B1 followed by selection of HPRT$^+$ cell clones, resulted in integration of yH2 and yK2 into the ES cell genome. Chimeric mice produced by microinjection of ES clones into blastocysts（囊胚）subsequently transmitted yH2 and yK2 into the mouse germline, without apparent rearrangements or deletions. Successive rounds of breeding of the yH2 and yK2 transgenics with the DI mice produced XenoMouse — yH2; yK2; DI, mice genetically engineered to produce fully human IgMκ and IgGκ in the absence of mouse heavy and κ light chain antibodies.

The large and complex V repertoire of XenoMouse mice is essential for efficient restoration of B cell development and a human-like humoral immune response

　　Production of high levels of human μ, γ, and κ demonstrated successful class switching from human IgM to human IgG and secretion of Ig in XenoMouse mice. After immunization of XenoMouse animals, the human γ chain levels increase to 2.5~4.0 mg/ml, indicative of a robust（富有活力的，强有力的）class switching after antigen stimulation.

　　The developing B cells in XenoMouse mice use the endowment（才能，天资）of a large V repertoire to create a broad array of antibody specificities that mirror an adult human repertoire. Sequencing of in-frame（框内的，符合读框的）transcripts from peripheral lymphoid tissue or from hybridomas from XenoMouse animals revealed diverse usage of the different V, D, and J genes across the entire length of the yH2 and yK2 transgenes, with the entire loci being accessible for rearrangement.

Data for the antibody repertoire and the antibody structure in XenoMouse strains show that yH2 and yK2 drive the development of an antibody response that mirrors that found in adult humans.

Generation and production of high affinity antigen-specific fully human mAbs

Supported by reconstituted（重建，重组）B cell development and a broadly diverse antibody repertoire, XenoMouse strains allowed the derivation of high affinity (XenoMouse animals consistently produced mAbs of high affinity, generally between 10^{-11} and 10^{-9} M), fully human mAbs against numerous human antigens. XenoMouse strains immunized with human antigens such as epidermal growth factor receptor (EGFr), interleukin-8 (IL-8), tumor necrosis factor α (TNF-α), interleukin-6 (IL-6), L-selectin, GROα, and CD147, amongst others, mounted（组织，发动）a robust antigen-specific immune response. Moreover, the XenoMouse mice have responded to a variety of types of human antigens, either soluble, *e.g.*, IL-8, IL-6, TNF-α, or membrane-bound on a cell, *e.g.*, EGFr, CD147, L-selectin.

Advantages

A large and diverse V repertoire is essential for generating high affinity antibodies to specific epitopes on antigens. Critically（极为重要地），the large V repertoire provided a diversity of antibodies in the primary immune and subsequent secondary immune response, including a subset with infrequently used V genes, thereby increasing the chances of finding antibodies with the desired epitope specificity.

The large number of different human V regions supports the development of a broad primary repertoire in XenoMouse strains, one comparable in diversity and functionality to that found in adult humans. While the broad primary immune repertoire of XenoMouse strains, in turn, allows the recognition of diverse epitopes on an antigen.

In XenoMouse strains, the *in vivo* secondary immune response, including efficient class switching and affinity maturation, exploits the broad primary immune response, to produce a diversity of high affinity IgG antibodies. The design of the different yH2 transgenes in the XenoMouse strains, all with the same core V_H, D_H, J_H, Cμ and Cδ regions, and differing only at the single Cγ gene, either Cγ1, Cγ2, or Cγ4, permits the production of only a single IgG isotype from each strain. This built-in strategy for the XenoMouse strains ensures that the desired antigen-specific mAb will also be the desired isotype.

By relying on the finely-tuned *in vivo* immune response of the mouse and well-established procedures for generation of hybridomas, the identification of hybridomas secreting antigen-specific fully human mAbs, from immunization to ELISA screening, reproducibly takes about 3 months when using XenoMouse animals. The ability to use hybridomas directly to produce mAbs can significantly shorten the time of pre-clinical development and initiation of pre-clinical trials. Other technologies, such as humanization or combinatorial libraries, can suffer from the need for extensive and sophisticated *in vitro* manipulation to re-engineer or enhance the characteristics of the antibody, followed by subsequent engineering of an expression system, and finally demonstration of the functionality of the engineered antibody. In contrast, the speed and reliability of the XenoMouse technology can reduce the time to initiation of product development to 6~18 months.

The XenoMouse technology also offers manufacturing flexibility, allowing production of mAbs either

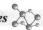

directly from hybridomas or from recombinant cell lines, transgenic animals or plants. Hybridomas derived from XenoMouse strains are stable and are amenable (可用某种方式处理的) to adaptation to serum-free medium and subsequent process development.

The first transgenic mouse-derived fully human mAb to be administered to a human, ABX-IL8, was generated from a XenoMouse animal and produced from a hybridoma. The antibody had a $t_{1/2}$ of 21 days, without any detectable human anti-human antibody responses. Thus, a human mAb from XenoMouse animals, when administered to humans, appears to be safe and well-tolerated and appears to possess the kinetics of normal serum Ig, further validating the use of XenoMouse mice for generation and production of therapeutic fully human mAbs against human antigens.

The germline-configured yH2 and yK2 human IgH and Igκ transgenes on a genetic background of inactivated murine IgH and Igk loci form **the core of the XenoMouse technology**. The *trans*-acting factors of the mouse humoral immune system activate and regulate these YAC transgenes. This enables yH2 and yK2, with their large and complex V repertoires and with their *cis*-acting regulatory elements intact, to fuel the development of a mature B cell population, and to restore the bone marrow and the peripheral lymphoid compartments, with $\geqq 95\%$ of the B cells expressing fully human IgHκ antibodies.

TC Mouse

The size of the human Ig loci, which stretch over 1~2 megabases (Mb), has provided quite a challenge to the transgenic approach for the successful introduction of entire human Ig loci into mice because of some technical difficulties in manipulating YACs. For instance, the requirement of complicated processes to reconstruct large contiguous loci from small YACs by homologous recombination in the yeast cell, or the difficulty of cloning YAC clones containing all of the human Ig C regions. In addition, the constant region of the human *IgH* locus is known to contain sequences difficult to be cloned.

Furthermore, these mice produce only human IgM and a single subclass of IgGs (IgG2), and for therapeutic purposes, recombinant DNA techniques may be required to change the isotype.

Consequently, it was very difficult, even using a YAC vector, to clone such over megabase-sized DNA fragments encompassing whole human *Ig* loci and to introduce them into mice. It occurred to researchers that it might be possible to use a human chromosome itself as a vector for transgenesis. Hence **trans-chromosomic (TC) technology has been applied to the construction of the TC Mouse™, which incorporates entire human immunoglobulin (hIg) loci.**

Ishida's group has developed a novel procedure that allows the introduction of very large pieces (> 1 MB) of foreign genetic material into mice by using a Chromosome itself as a "vector", thus producing chimeric mice bearing and functionally expressing a single human chromosome or its fragment.

The first examples of "trans-chromosomic (TC) mice" or "TransChromo (TC) Mouse™" containing a heritable foreign chromosome were demonstrated in *1997*. Then the method was applied to the creation of TC mice containing fragments of human chromosomes (hChrs) 14 and 2 bearing the immunoglobulin heavy (Ig-H) and (Ig-κ) loci respectively and for expressing fully human antibodies.

Human chromosome (hChr.) 14, 22, or a hChr. 2-derived fragment, which contains an Ig heavy, λ, or κ locus was demonstrated to be transferrable into mouse ES cells by **microcell-mediated chromosome transfer (MMCT)** strategy. In the chimeric mice produced from the resultant microcell-hybrid ES (MH (ES)) cells, the transferred chromosomes were retained, and the transcripts of several human genes including Igs were expressed in a proper tissue-specific manner.

Production of chimeric mice retaining hChrs

The approach for introducing a hChr into mice is outlined in Fig. 4-14. As shown, pSTneoB, which bears a G418-resistant gene (G418^r) whose promoter is active in ES cells, was transfected into human fibroblast cells and underwent random integration into human chromosomes. A pool of G418^r human fibroblast cells were fused with A9 mouse cells to prepare microcells, which were then fused with A9 cells to affect chromosome transfer and selected with G418 in order to obtain a library of A9 clones containing various pSTneoB-tagged human chromosomes or chromosome fragments. This library, including about 700 independent clones, was screened with PCR primer pairs specific to a human chromosome to identify A9 clones containing the hChr fragment of interest. Microcells prepared from these A9 clones were transferred to mouse ES cells (TT2: 40, XY or TT2F: 39, XO). The generation of microcells from these human cells and their subsequent fusion with mouse ES cells (TT2: 40, XY; or TT2F; 39, XO) allowed the transfer of human chromosomes into these cells. Following G418 selection, it was possible to isolate ES cells that bore a pSTneoB-tagged human chromosome or chromosome fragment. The resultant microcell hybrid ES [MH (ES)] cells were injected into 8-cell stage embryos of albino MCH (ICR) mice, and the injected embryos were then transferred into the uteri or oviducts of pseudopregnant mice. Chimeric mice could be identified by their patches of agouti（刺鼠，深浅环纹毛皮）coat color, and the percentage of agouti color provided an indicator of the MH (ES) cell contribution to the chimera.

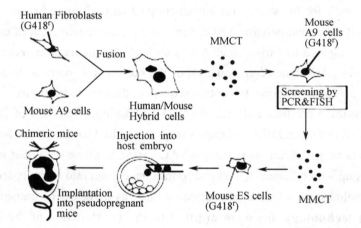

Fig. 4-14 A schematic diagram showing the construction of MH(ES) cells to express human genes on the transferred chromosomes. G418^r: G418-resistant gene.

In the B cell lineage of these chimeras, human antibody genes on the transferred hChr fragments undergo rearrangement and are transcribed properly to express functional human antibodies. In addition, examination of the expression of other human genes on the hChr fragments showed that they too were expressed only in appropriate tissues and therefore were under proper tissue-specific transcriptional regulation in the chimeras.

Further investigation has shown that, while various hChr fragments could be introduced into mice via ES cells, the hChr 14 fragment employed displayed superior of retention to that of chromosome fragments derived from hChr 2 and hChr 22.

Improvement of instability of the hChr

A general approach has been developed to solve the issue of introducing and stably maintaining hChrs

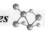

containing defined regions in mice. A chromosome-cloning system has been developed that employs a combination of *Cre/loxP-mediated* chromosome translocation with telomere-directed chromosome truncation in homologous recombination-proficient chicken DT40 cells. Using this approach, it is possible to introduce very large (> 1 Mb) and well-defined hChr regions into a stably maintained hChr 14 fragment-based mini-chromosome vector. Fig. 4-15 presents a schematic summary of this unique cloning system.

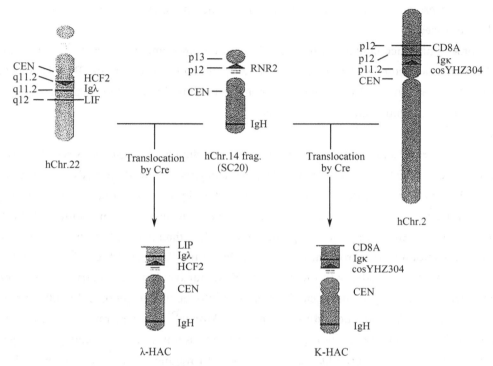

Fig. 4-15   The whole scheme of the System. DT40 cells containing the IgH locus-bearing hChr 14 fragment, a potential human mini-chromosome vector, were transfected with the targetted *lox*P insertional vector to integrate a *lox*P sequence to *RNR2* locus at 14p12 to make a cloning site for chromosome inserts. The chromosome insert containing Ig-light chain λ locus derived from hChr 22 was prepared by truncation of hChr 22 at *LIF locus* and insertion of a *lox*P sequence at *HCF2* locus in DT40 cells. The region between *HCF2* and *LIF* loci containing Igλ locus on hChr 22 is cloned into the *RNR* locus on the short arm of the hChr 14 mini-chromosome vector by Cre-recombinase mediated translocation in DT40 cells. Similarly, hChr 2 was truncated at *CD8A* locus and a *lox*P sequence was inserted into *WHZ30-4* locus.

Cre/*lox*P-mediated chromosome translocation is one of the simplest site-specific recombination systems, which is derived from the lysogenic bacteriophage Pl, which encodes a 38-kilodalton (kDa) protein, Cre, that recombines DNA between specific 34-basepair (bp) sequences, *lox*P sites. The recombination is initiated by Cre proteins binding to 13-bp inverted repeat regions in the *lox*P sites and promoting synapsis (联会) (or joining) of a pair of sites. Cre proteins then catalyze strand exchange between the pair of sites within an asymmetric 8-bp central spacer sequence by concerted cleavage and rejoining reactions, which involve a transient DNA-protein covalent linkage.

The chicken pre-B cell line DT40 is known to be homologous recombination-proficient and enables the efficient modification of human chromosomes by gene targeting. The human chromosome 22 was transferred into DT40 cells from mouse A9 cells by MMCT method, **where human telomeric repeat (TTAGGG)$_n$ was integrated** into the *LIF* locus at 22q12 **on the chromosome** just distal to the *Ig*λ.

In the chromosome-cloning system, a defined human chromosomal region was cloned into a stable human minichromosome vector by a combination of Cre/*lox*P-mediated chromosome translocation and telomere-directed chromosome truncation in homologous recombination-proficient chicken DT40 cells. By cloning into the minichromosome vector, a 10 Mb human chromosome region defined by a *lox*P-integration site and telomere-truncation site containing the immunoglobulin λ-light chain (Igλ) locus on the mitotically unstable hChr22 fragment was stabilized in mouse embryonic stem (ES) cells. Chimeric mice were produced stably maintaining this human artificial chromosome (HAC) carrying the hChr22-derived insert, and showed that the human Igλ gene on the chromosomal insert in the HAC was functionally expressed.

Trans-chromosomic mice contains a heritable foreign chromosome and reveals that the chromosome itself can be used as a vector for transgenesis, thereby extending the size limit of DNA fragment currently used to create transgenic mice. This technology opened an alternative way to produce a variety of human antibodies in mice containing entire human Ig loci.

KM Mouse™

TC Mouse™ expresses a fully diverse repertoire of hIgs, including all the subclasses of IgGs (IgG1~G4). Immunization of the TC Mouse™ with various human antigens produced antibody responses comprised of human antibodies. Furthermore, it was possible to obtain hybridoma clones expressing fully human antibodies specific for the target human antigen. However, because of the instability of the Igκ locus bearing HCF2, the efficiency of hybridoma production was less than one-tenth of that observed in normal mice. An instant solution to this problem was to cross-breed the Kirin TC Mouse™ carrying the HCF14, which was stable in mouse cells, with the Medarex YAC-transgenic mouse carrying about 50% of the hIgVκ gene segments as a region that is stably integrated into the mouse genome. In **2002**, a novel mouse line for fully human mAb production, **dubbed the KM Mouse™** was generated by the combination of knockout and transgenic mouse technologies. **The resulting mouse,** lacks the endogenous genes for Ig H and L chains and instead carries a human chromosome 14 fragment containing the entire human Ig H chain loci and the human L chain segments, **performed as well as normal mice with regard to immune responsiveness and efficiency of hybridoma production.** Consequently, it has become easy and convenient to produce fully human mAbs against all kinds of antigens by using splenocytes derived from the KM mouse for use in mouse/mouse hybridoma techniques.

The HumAb strains, XenoMouse strains, TC mouse strains, and KM mouse strains are powerful tools for the generation of high affinity fully human mAbs suitable for use in humans as therapeutic agents. By using those animals, extensive and successive rounds of antibody engineering by the user are unnecessary because the required engineering, genetic engineering of large portions of the native human Ig loci into the mouse germline, was performed at a much earlier stage. Thus, with the human Ig transgenes/ trans-chromosomes functionally replacing their murine counterparts, the progressively and innovatively improved technology platforms Humab, XenoMouse, TC mouse and KM mouse utilize the natural ability of the murine immune system to create high affinity human antibodies. Those strategies have been repeatedly validated, with a 100% success rate in the generation of high affinity antigen-specific human mAbs to many different antigens.

Technologies for the facile generation of high affinity, antigen-specific fully human monoclonal against human antigens have revolutionized the use of therapeutic mAbs in the clinic. Fully human antibodies are likely to allow repeated dosing without the risk of immunogenic or allergic responses, and increase their safety for use in chronic disease in individuals with functioning immune systems. Those platforms provide proven, user-friendly techniques for the rapid generation of fully human mAbs and should help support and accelerate the development of therapeutic mAbs.

Analysis of thousands of VDJ rearrangements in this study now clearly demonstrates that enormous variability of the Ig gene loci could exist within the human population. This study has shown that the functional IGH haplotypes that encode the IgH chain are incredibly diverse, and that this diversity includes a surprisingly high frequency of deletion and duplication polymorphisms. Where genes are present, dramatic variations are also seen in rearrangement frequencies, particularly with the genes of the IGHD locus. Together, this variation suggests that the repertoire of VDJ rearrangements may vary substantially between individuals. It may well be that individual variation in the genes of the Ig loci, and resulting repertoire variation, emerge as important contributors to individual variation in immunocompetency and individual susceptibility to Ab-mediated immunopathology. Similarly, when a donor's genome was adopted to construct a genomic library for selecting gene fragments or chromosome fragments pertinent to fully human antibody production, what the vector carries (restricted by the current databases) may only represent a portion of the allelic diversity present within the human species, rather than all.

4.5 Expression of engineered antibodies in mammalian cells（工程抗体在哺乳动物细胞中的表达）

The requirements for expression of engineered antibodies will range from the rapid preparation of small amounts of material for research purposes through to（直到）the production of large quantities of antibody for clinical trials. Antibodies are authentically glycosylated and secreted at high levels from mammalian cells (see Table 4-1).

Table. 4-1 Expression of recombinant B72.3 antibodies

	Promoter	Host cell	Selectable marker	Yield	Reference
Chimeric IgG1	Ig	Sp2/0	gpt/neo	50-60	Gillies *et al.*, 1989
	Ig	Sp2/0	DHFR (amplified)	120-150	Gillies *et al.*, 1989
Chimeric IgG4	hCMV	CHO	gpt/neo	35-100	King *et al.*, 1992
	hCMV	NSO	GS (amplified)	560	Bebbington *et al.*, 1992
Chimeric Fab'	hCMV	CHO	gpt/neo	20-120	King *et al.*, 1992
	TAC	*E. coli*	Kan	50-100	N. Weir and A. Mountain, unpublished data
Fv	hCMV	CHO	GS (amplified)	4	King *et al.*, 1993
	TAC	*E. coli*	Kan	450 mg/L	King *et al.*, 1993

Low copy vectors（低拷贝载体）

The earliest examples of the expression of immunoglobulins in mammalian cells involved the re-introduction of antibody genes into lymphoid cells. Gene expression was directed by either viral (*e.g.*, Simian virus 40) or immunoglobulin promoters/enhancers. However antibody production from recombinant myelomas（骨髓瘤）(10~100 mg/L) rarely approaches（接近）that obtained from the original hybridoma from which the heavy and light chain genes were cloned.

As an alternative, immunoglobulin genes have been expressed in a number of different nonlymphoid cell types. Although the expression levels reported in these early studies were relatively low (< 1 mg/L) they indicated that more efficient expression systems developed for non-myeloid cells（非骨髓细胞）may be applicable to antibodies. Chinese hamster ovary cells (CHO) in particular have been used for the production of a number of recombinant proteins. It has been found that one of the most efficient promoter systems for use in CHO cells is the major intermediate early gene promoter element from human cytomegalovirus（巨细胞病毒）. An expression vector incorporating this promoter has been developed and used to direct the expression of immunoglobulin genes in CHO cells. Stable cell lines expressing a chimeric version of the tumor-specific antibody, B72.3, were constructed by first transfecting the cells with a vector containing the light chain gene. The highest producing cell line was then re-transfected with the heavy chain vector and again the best producer selected. In this way CHO cell lines producing up to 50 mg/L B72.3 antibody were obtained. While the alternative of introducing both heavy and light chain genes into cells at the same time does not give high yielding cell lines with these low copy number vectors.

Later a variant CHO cell line has been developed at Celltech that constitutively expresses a modified version of the E1a transcriptional activator from human adenovirus. This protein increases transcription from a number of viral promoters, including the hCMV promoter, leading to increased expression of recombinant proteins from vectors containing such promotors. A particular use of this cell line is the rapid production of relatively small quantities of proteins such as antibodies. Thus cells co-transfected with heavy and light chain genes yield up to 1~2 μg antibody/ml of culture media in only 4~5 days.

Vector amplification（载体扩增）

Significant improvements in expression levels in CHO cells can be achieved by vector amplification. An amplifiable marker gene usually encodes an enzyme that is both essential for cell survival and one for which an inhibitor with high affinity binding is available. By applying increasing amounts of the inhibitor to the cells expressing the desired product, variant clones that are resistant to higher levels of inhibitor are selected. Resistance is usually the result of an increase in the number of copies of the marker gene, *i.e.*, amplification, integrated into the genome of the cells. The region that is amplified is usually larger than that occupied by the marker gene, hence associated sequences including the gene encoding the product also become amplified. This results in higher expression levels of the product. The most commonly used system of vector amplification is based on the enzyme dihydrofolate reductase (DHFR) which is inhibited by methotrexate (MTX). Expression vectors for this system carry the DHFR gene and are transfected into a dhfr-CHO cell line. Copy numbers in excess of 2000 copies/cell have been achieved after repeated rounds of MTX selection. However the fact that multiple rounds of selection are required in order to obtain maximal levels of expression is a major disadvantage of this approach since it is very time consuming.

A number of other amplifiable markers are available. The use of one in particular appears to overcome the limitations of DHFR. This is the enzyme, **glutamine synthetase (GS)** which catalyzes the formation of glutamine from glutamate and ammonia and is inhibited by L-methionine sulfoximine (MSX, L-蛋氨酸亚砜亚胺). GS can be used as a dominant selectable marker in a variety of different cell types and is maximally amplified in a single round by increasing the concentration of MSX applied to the transfected cells.

In order to adapt a vector amplification system for the production of antibodies both heavy and light chain genes are required to be integrated in close proximity to the amplifiable marker. One approach is to use separate amplifiable markers on separate vectors for each chain, *e.g.*, DHFR for the light chain and adenosine deaminase for the heavy chain. A simpler approach would be to co-amplify the heavy and light chains expressed on the same vector. In this situation the order of the genes appears to be important, since there is the possibility of the occlusion (闭塞) of a downstream promoter by transcription read-through from an upstream promoter. By placing the light chain before the heavy chain any transcriptional interference is likely to lead to an excess of the light chain. This may be preferable to excess free heavy chain since it has been reported that excess heavy chain can be toxic to cells. Using the GS amplifiable marker and such a configuration of immunoglobulin genes, yields of up to 200 mg/L of antibody has been obtained in CHO cells. Similar expression levels have been reported for an antibody produced using DHFR in CHO cells. However in this case cells transfected with a double gene construct proved to be unstable and a re-transfection strategy had to be used. The GS system has recently applied to the expression of antibodies in myeloma cells. In these cells even higher yields of antibody have been reported, up to 560 mg/L. A plasmid vector for expressing antibody genes using the GS selectable marker is shown in Fig. 4-16A.

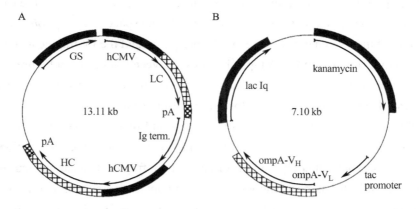

Fig. 4-16   Plasmid vectors for expressing recombinant antibodies. A: represents a plasmid vector for the co-expression of immunoglobulin heavy and light chain in mammalian cells. Abbreviations: GS = glutamine synthetase selectable marker gene; hCMV = human cytomegalovirus promoter; LC = light chain gene; HC = heavy chain gene; pA = polyadenylation signal; Ig term = immunoglobulin transcriptional terminator. B: represents a plasmid vector for the co-expression of Fv fragments in *Escherichia coli*. ompA-V$_H$-heavy chain variable region gene fused to the gene segment encoding the leader sequence; ompA-V$_L$ = the equivalent construct for light chain variable region gene.

Expression of engineered antibodies in microbial cells（工程抗体在微生物细胞中的表达）

Although whole immunoglobulins have been expressed in microbial cells both *E. coli* and yeast, the yields of active antibody were poor. By contrast microbial systems have emerged as the method of choice for the production of antibody fragments, in particular Fabs, Fvs and sFvs (see Table 4-1). Most work has been carried out on the development of expression vectors for *E. coli* cells which appear to have significant advantages over the major alternative, yeast cells, in terms of speed and yield. Two alternative routes are possible for *E. coli* expression systems, namely, intracellular synthesis or secretion.

A variation of the secretion route is also possible involving the display of the antibody fragments on the surface of bacterial phage particles. This has opened up the possibility of screening a large number of antibody variants to isolate novel or improved binding activities.

Intracellular vs. secretion（细胞内表达与分泌表达）

Fabs, Fvs and sFvs have all been produced by intracellular expression in *E. coli*. One of the earliest reports was that of the Fab fragments of an anti- (carcinoembryonic antigen; CEA) antibody（抗癌胚抗原抗体）. The expression of the genes encoding the Fd′ fragment of the heavy chain and light chain was driven by the *trp* promoter in separate cells. Both polypeptides accumulated as insoluble inclusion bodies in the *E. coli* cells. However, anti-CEA activity was obtained by reconstituting the Fd′ and light chain polypeptides *in vitro*. Similarly a functional Fv fragment of the anti- (lysozyme) antibody, GLOOP2, was produced following co-expression of the V_H and V_L genes in the same *E. coli* cells. It was found that the variable domain polypeptides accumulated up to 7% of total bacterial cell protein providing a protease deficient strain of *E.coli* (lon⁻, htpr⁻) was used as the host cell.

The production of antibody fragments as secreted products greatly simplifies the purification of the fragment in an active form. Experiments by Skerra and Plückthun (1988) and Better *et al*. (1988) showed that assembled antibody fragments could be formed by secretion of the component polypeptide chains into the periplasmic space of *E.coli*. Skerra and Plückthun (1988) used an expression vector containing the V_H and V_L genes for the anti-(phosphorylcholine) antibody（抗磷酸胆碱抗体）, McPC603, controlled by the inducible *lac* promoter. A different prokaryotic leader sequence was fused to each of these genes capable of directing the expressed polypeptide to the periplasmic space of the *E. coli* cells (ompA V_H and phoA V_L). Assembly of the two chains occurred in the periplasm and the Fv fragment could be purified in a single step by affinity chromatography. A typical expression vector is shown in Figure 4-16B.

In the Better *et al*. (1988) experiments, a chimeric mouse-human Fab′ fragment was produced. This group used the same leader sequence, *pelB*, for directing the secretion of both heavy and light chain polypeptides. Both genes were again located on the vector and their expression controlled by the *araB* promoter of *S. typhimurium*（鼠伤寒沙门菌）. It was found that although the polypeptides were directed to the periplasmic space, approximately 2 mg/L of active Fab′ fragments accumulated in the cell media supernatant. More recently it has been shown that Fv fragments also accumulate in the culture media following expression from a secretion vector with yields of up to 40 mg/L obtained in shaking culture. The smaller Fv and sFv fragments of antibodies are obtained in higher yields than Fab′ fragments in the cell media following expression in *E. coli*. Large quantities of active Fab′ can however be recovered from the periplasm of the cells.

4.6   Summary and prospect（总结及展望）

A number of recent technological developments have greatly facilitated the genetic engineering of immunoglobulins. The use of PCR has permitted the variable regions to be rapidly cloned either from a specific hybridoma source or as a gene library from non-immunized cells. The conversion of the rodent antibody into a humanized version, even a human version is now well established. To develop these antibodies for clinical use has required the development of high level expression systems. For the expression of large multimeric glycoproteins, mammalian cell systems generally provide the highest levels of secreted product and therefore are the methods of choice for producing whole recombinant antibodies. Novel antigen-binding units have been developed by joining the two variable domains of an antibody into single-chain polypeptides. Such fragments can be produced in high yield by secretion from *E. coli* raising the prospect（前途，预期）of bulk preparation of these antibody fragments for the development of low-cost immunopurification and assay reagents.

The ability to screen for antigen binding by displaying immunoglobulin variable regions on the surface of filamentous bacteriophages has opened up the possibility of bypassing the immune system to generate novel antibody specificities *in vitro*. Meanwhile, transgenic and trans-chromosomic technologies have been continuing to invigorate and promote the research and development of antibody therapeutics. As the demand for monoclonal antibodies in research and clinical applications continues to increase, the necessity to develop even more efficient molecules is crucial. Antibody engineering has become a key discipline for generation of innovative antibodies-based molecules used in research, diagnostics, and therapy.

References

［1］ 李元.基因工程药物.2版.北京：化学工业出版社，2007.

［2］ 夏焕章，熊宗贵.生物技术制药.2版.北京：高等教育出版社，2006.

［3］ Stanley T C, Branda F B, Rosanne M C, et al.Antisense technology: an overview and prospectus. Nature Reviews/Drug Discovery，2021, 20：427-453.

［4］ William R S. Compilation and analysis of DNA sequences associated with apparent streptomycete promoters. Nucleic Acids Research, 1992, 20(5): 961-974.

［5］ Jozef A, Bárbara M, Jan V I, et al. Recombinant protein production and streptomycetes. Journal of Biotechnology, 2012, 158: 159-167.

［6］ Maria V, Puri F. Simian Virus-40 as a Gene Therapy Vector. DNA and Cell Biology, 2004, 23(5): 271-281.

［7］ David S S. Gene Therapy Using SV40-Derived Vectors: What Does the Future Hold? Journal of cellular physiology, 1999, 181:375-384 .

［8］ Louis B,Pierre C. Potential of Recombinant SV40-Based Vectors for Gene Therapy. Recent Patents on DNA & Gene Sequences,2007, 1: 93-99.

［9］ Smith B J. Quantification of Proteins on polyacrylamide gels. The Protein Protocols Handbook.3rd ed, 2009,1:479-486.

［10］ Wayne R S. Quantification of Radiolabeled Proteins in Polyacrylamide Gels. The Protein Protocols Handbook.3rd ed, 2009, 1:443-448.

［11］ Raymond J O, Robert J Y. The genetic engineering of monoclonal antibodies. Journal of Immunological Methods, 1994, 168: 149-165.

［12］ Michael J M, Larry L G, Jose R F, et al.Functional transplant of megabase human immunoglobulin loci recapitulates human antibody response in mice. Nature genetics, 1997, 15: 146-156.

［13］ Larry L G. Antibody engineering via genetic engineering of the mouse: XenoMouse strains are a vehicle for the facile generation of therapeutic human monoclonal antibodies. Journal of Immunological Methods, 1999, 231: 11-23.

［14］ Isao I, Hitoshi Y, Kazuma T. Production of a Diverse Repertoire of Human Antibodies in Genetically Engineered Mice. Microbiol Immunol, 1998, 42(3): 143-150.

［15］ Isao I, Kazuma T, Hitoshi Y. Trans Chromo Mouse ™, Biotechnology and Genetic Engineering Reviews, 2002, 19:1, 73-83.

［16］ Heiner N, Alexander K, Angelika S. Production of Biopharmaceuticals in Transgenic Animals. Pharmaceutical Biotechnology: Drug Discovery and Clinical Applications. 2nd ed. 2012,1:71-111.

［17］ Zhang L, Cong Y, Li H，et al. Construction of a full-length antibody phage display vector. Journal of Immunological Methods, 2021, 494: 113052.

［18］ Andrea S,Carolin Z. High-Throughput IgG Conversion of Phage Displayed Fab Antibody Fragments by AmpIYFast. Thomas Tiller (ed.), Synthetic Antibodies: Methods and Protocols, Methods in Molecular Biology, 2017, 1575: 121-143.